Nutrients in Infancy

Special Issue Editors

Colin Binns

Mi Kyung Lee

Masaharu Kagawa

MDPI • Basel • Beijing • Wuhan • Barcelona • Belgrade

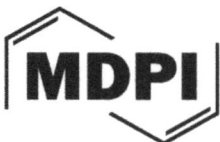

MDPI

Special Issue Editors

Colin Binns
Curtin University
Australia

Mi Kyung Lee
Murdoch University
Australia

Masaharu Kagawa
Kagawa Nutrition University
Japan

Editorial Office
MDPI AG
St. Alban-Anlage 66
Basel, Switzerland

This edition is a reprint of the Special Issue published online in the open access journal *Nutrients* (ISSN 2072-6643) from 2016–2017/ (available at: http://www.mdpi.com/journal/nutrients/special_issues/nutrients_infancy).

For citation purposes, cite each article independently as indicated on the article page online and as indicated below:

Author 1; Author 2. Article title. *Journal Name* **Year**, *Article number*, page range.

First Edition 2017

ISBN 978-3-03842-560-1 (Pbk)
ISBN 978-3-03842-561-8 (PDF)

Table of Contents

About the Special Issue Editors

Colin Binns MBBS MPH PhD (Hon Inje) FRACGP FAFOEM FAFOHM, John Curtin Distinguished Professor, Curtin University. Graduated in medicine from the University of Western Australia and worked in hospitals in Perth and in Papua New Guinea. In PNG he became interested in nutrition and received a scholarship to complete a MPH degree at Harvard. He was appointed foundation Head of the School of Public Health Curtin University a position held for 21 years and continues as Professor of Public Health. He was Vice-President of the Asia Pacific Academic Consortium for Public Health for five years; foundation head of the National Drug Research Institute (Curtin University); held visiting professorial positions at Kagawa Nutrition University Tokyo, University of Ryukus Okinawa, Tonji Medical College Wuhan and Inje University, Republic of Korea. He has served on 21 committees of the NHMRC and including Australian Dietary Guidelines and Infant Feeding Guidelines Committee He is a member of numerous government advisory and research groups. Awards include of Senior Western Australian of the Year (WA), Lifetime Achievement Award for medical research by Research Australia and Fellow of the Nutrition Society of Australia, Asia Pacific Clinical Nutrition Society and the Dieticians Association of Australia. Current research interests include breastfeeding, international health and public health nutrition. He has 550+ publications in nutrition and public health.

Mi Kyung Lee, GradDipHSc MA PhD, is a senior lecturer in School of Health Professions, Murdoch University, Australia. As a health professional Dr. Lee feels passionate about raising awareness of healthy living and improving the long term health of the disadvantaged in our society and in our region. Dr. Lee's research projects revolve around her interests in public health nutrition and multicultural issues in education. Current projects include: (1) Joint research on 'Dietary Guidelines in the Asia-Pacific region' (Australia, China, Japan, Korea, Malaysia, Singapore, Papua New Guniea) and reviewing 'Dietary Supplements within the Asia-Pacific region; (2) Continued collaboration in research in infant nutrition in our region. She serves as a committee member of the Nutrition Society of Australia (NSA) Perth Regional Group; an executive council member of the Korean Academy of Scientists and Engineers Australasia (KASEA) and chairperson of the KASEA WA. She is an external expert for the Tertiary Education Quality and Standards Agency (TEQSA).

Masaharu Kagawa, BSc(Hons), PhD, is an Associate Professor and the Deputy Director of the Institute of Nutrition Sciences, Kagawa Nutrition University. He has been also appointed as Adjunct Professor of the Faculty of Public Health, Mahidol University in Thailand, a Visiting Associate Professor of the School of Public Health at Curtin University in Australia, and an Adjunct Associate Professor of the School of Exercise and Nutrition Sciences as well as a member of the Institute of Health and Biomedical Innovation (IHBI) at Queensland University of Technology (QUT) in Australia. Dr. Kagawa's research interests include all topics associated with anthropometry and body composition assessments in the fields of Public Health and Nutrition, particularly in relation to obesity and health screening, body image, maternal and child health, and sports science. Dr. Kagawa's recent works include identification of influencing factors on body image of young Japanese females, investigation of anthropometric indices to monitor sports performance of athletes, and the development of 3D imaging to reflect anthropometric and body composition values of individuals that can be utilized for health promotion of the general public as well as health education for athletes. Dr. Kagawa is a Registered Public Health Nutritionist with the Nutrition Society of Australia (NSA) and also the first Japanese Level 3 Anthropometrist as well as one of the eight Photoscopic Somatotype Raters in the world, both accredited by the International Society for the Advancement of Kinanthropometry (ISAK). Dr. Kagawa also serves as a member of editorial board for journals Body Image, Obesity Science and Practice, and Perceptual and Motor Skills.

Preface to "Nutrients in Infancy"

This monograph based on a special issue of Nutrients contains 31 papers: 5 reviews and 26 original publications that reflect the wide spectrum of current research on nutrients and infancy. The papers include populations from many countries including Australia, Canada, China, Ireland, Italy, Malaysia, Mexico, Netherlands, Norway, Singapore, Spain, Sweden, Thailand, United Kingdom and USA. The largest group of papers are on the nutrient composition of breastmilk and the timing and factors that influence the nutrient content of breastfeeding. The age range of the subjects studied was from preterm VLBW babies to older infants.

There are two key objectives for infant nutrition: survival and to lay the foundations for growth and development that will optimise health throughout a long lifespan. Besides the ethical problems associated with infant research there is the obvious difficulty of conducting lifespan research in humans[1]. Continued infant nutrition research will rely on retrospective epidemiological studies and increasing knowledge of health and lifespan biomarkers.

In compiling this special issue there were two issues that the editors found to be important. Definitions have always been central to successful research and the definition used determines the results presented in relation to breastfeeding and complementary feeds. Much has been written about definitions of breastfeeding, but there is still little standardisation in publications[2–4]. At the very least authors should adhere to the standard WHO definitions of exclusive breastfeeding, but then describe what they have actually done to allow others to accurately interpret their results.

The ethics of research are always important in all publications, but particularly so in the area of infant nutrition. The editors of this monograph summarised the ethical principles involved in infant nutrition research[5]. In recent years the influence of early nutrition on later health and longevity has been increasingly studied. This means that extra care must be taken with any early life intervention studies.

One third of the articles are on breastmilk composition from countries around the globe and several more on factors associated with breastfeeding duration. This reflects the centrality of breastmilk to the supply of nutrients in infancy, its importance for lifelong health and development and that we still have to learn. The results of several studies have implications for public health nutrition programs. It is estimated that 1.9 billion people live in areas of the world subject to subclinical iodine deficiency which is important for cognitive development in infancy?[6]. The study by Jorgenson and her colleagues demonstrate that in Australia with a food fortification program and the recommendation of pregnant women to take 150mcg iodine supplements daily the iodine content of breastmilk is generally adequate[7].

In the NHANES study from the USA an analysis of NHANES data on iron, calcium, and zinc among children in the second year of life using two days of dietary intake data found that one in four children and one in ten children had usual intakes below the RDA for iron and calcium, respectively[8].

The relationship between nutrients and growth will be a continued area of interest. The prevalence of stunting is still relatively high in some world regions and is a priority of the UN Sustainable Development Goals (SDGs)[9]. At the other end of the continuum of development child obesity is now a major problem and is also an important target[9]. Micro nutrient deficiency may influence stunting and undernutrition but more research is still required to complete our understanding. The review on iron and zinc supplementation found that low dose of daily iron and zinc use during 6–23 months of age had a positive effect on child's iron and zinc status[10]. However, this did not translate into a reduction in the proportion of children with stunting. Further research is required into stunting to achieve the UNSDGs. The role of protein in over nutrition and the development of obesity has been a fertile area of research[11]. The lower protein level of breastmilk compared to the higher protein levels of many infant formulae provides a biological basis for understanding the protective effects of breastmilk against obesity[12].

An area of continued interest is the relationship between the human microbiomes and nutrition. In 2007 the National Institutes of Health launched the Human Microbiome Project to promote research into the ways in which health outcomes are linked to changes in the microbiome[13,14]. The human microbiome is exceedingly complex, both in its composition and in its interrelation with nutrients. Nutrients can change the nature of the microbiome and in turn the microbiome has effects on metabolism[15]. It is now well understood that infant feeding method, mechanism of delivery and the use of perinatal antibiotics can influence the composition of the microbiome[16]. One of the mechanisms responsible for protection against obesity provided by breastfeeding may be by through the development of a healthy microbiome[17]. There is increasing evidence of links between early development (particularly in the perinatal period) and later mental illness[18,19]. Again this linkage may be through changes to the human microbiome[20–22]. The use of pre-lacteal feeds and complementary feeds (i.e., not exclusively breastfeeding), C-section delivery and use of antibiotics (particularly in the perinatal period) changes the composition of the microbiome[23,24]. From a public health perspective the increasing rates of operative delivery, widespread antibiotic use and low rates of exclusive breastfeeding may be associated with increased rates of obesity, diabetes and other metabolic disorders and mental illness. Exclusive breastfeeding remains as important as ever as the basis of infant and maternal health[25]. As long term changes to the microbiome may be one mechanism by which early life dietary intake can modify health in later life, research into nutrients and microbiome health will be important.

We believe this collection is a useful summary of progress in many areas of infant nutrition. It also points to many research needs to better understand infant nutrient requirements, growth and healthy development. With the present rate of progress it may only be few years before another volume is required.

Colin Binns, Mi Kyung Lee and Masaharu Kagawa
Special Issue Editors

References

1. Binns, C.; Lee, M.K.; Kagawa, M. Ethical challenges in infant feeding research. *Nutrients* **2017**, 9.
2. Khanal, V.; Lee, A.H.; Scott, J.A.; Karkee, R.; Binns, C.W. Implications of methodological differences in measuring the rates of exclusive breastfeeding in nepal: Findings from literature review and cohort study. *BMC Pregnancy Childbirth* **2016**, 16, 389.
3. Inoue, M.; Binns, C.W.; Otsuka, K.; Jimba, M.; Matsubara, M. Infant feeding practices and breastfeeding duration in japan: A review. *Int. Breastfeed. J.* **2012**, 7, 15.
4. Binns, C.W.; Fraser, M.L.; Lee, A.H.; Scott, J. Defining exclusive breastfeeding in australia. *J. Paediatr. Child health* **2009**, 45, 174–180.
5. Binns, C.W.; Lee, M.K.; Tang, L.; Yu, C.; Hokama, T.; Lee, A. Ethical issues in infant feeding after disasters. *Asia-Pac. J. Public Health/Asia-Pac. Acad. Consort. Public Health* **2012**, 24, 672–680.
6. Zimmermann, M.B.; Andersson, M. Update on iodine status worldwide. *Curr. Opin. Endocrinol. Diabetes Obes.* **2012**, 19, 382–387.
7. Jorgensen, A.; O'Leary, P.; James, I.; Skeaff, S.; Sherriff, J. Assessment of breast milk iodine concentrations in lactating women in western australia. *Nutrients* **2016**, 8.
8. Hamner, H.C.; Perrine, C.G.; Scanlon, K.S. Usual intake of key minerals among children in the second year of life, nhanes 2003-2012. Nutrients 2016, 8.
9. United Nations. Transforming Our World Sdg Goals and Targets. Available online: https://sustainabledevelopment.Un.Org/content/documents/21252030%20agenda%20for%20sustain able%20development%20web.Pdf (accessed on 4 september 2017).
10. Petry, N.; Olofin, I.; Boy, E.; Donahue Angel, M.; Rohner, F. The effect of low dose iron and zinc intake on child micronutrient status and development during the first 1000 days of life: A systematic review and meta-analysis. *Nutrients* **2016**, 8.
11. Koletzko, B.; Brands, B.; Grote, V.; Kirchberg, F.F.; Prell, C.; Rzehak, P.; Uhl, O.; Weber, M.; Early Nutrition Programming, P. Long-term health impact of early nutrition: The power of programming. *Ann. Nutr. Metab.* **2017**, 70, 161–169.
12. Bischoff, S.C.; Boirie, Y.; Cederholm, T.; Chourdakis, M.; Cuerda, C.; Delzenne, N.M.; Deutz, N.E.; Fouque, D.; Genton, L.; Gil, C., et al. Towards a multidisciplinary approach to understand and manage obesity and related diseases. *Clin. Nutr.* **2017**, 36, 917–938.

13.   Young, V.B. The role of the microbiome in human health and disease: An introduction for clinicians. *BMJ-Br. Med.J.* **2017**, *356*.

14.   Proctor, L.M. The human microbiome project in 2011 and beyond. *Cell Host Microbe* **2011**, *10*, 287–291.

15.   Xu, Z.J.; Knight, R. Dietary effects on human gut microbiome diversity. *Br. J. Nutr.* **2015**, *113*, S1–S5.

16.   Azad, M.B.; Konya, T.; Persaud, R.R.; Guttman, D.S.; Chari, R.S.; Field, C.J.; Sears, M.R.; Mandhane, P.J.; Turvey, S.E.; Subbarao, P., et al. Impact of maternal intrapartum antibiotics, method of birth and breastfeeding on gut microbiota during the first year of life: A prospective cohort study. *BJOG* **2016**, *123*, 983–993.

17.   Houghteling, P.D.; Walker, W.A. Why is initial bacterial colonization of the intestine important to infants' and children's health? *J. Pediatr. Gastroenterol. Nutr.* **2015**, *60*, 294–307.

18.   Guintivano, J.; Kaminsky, Z.A. Role of epigenetic factors in the development of mental illness throughout life. *Neurosci.Res.* **2016**, *102*, 56–66.

19.   Maccari, S.; Polese, D.; Reynaert, M.L.; Amici, T.; Morley-Fletcher, S.; Fagioli, F. Early-life experiences and the development of adult diseases with a focus on mental illness: The human birth theory. *Neuroscience* **2017**, *342*, 232–251.

20.   Deans, E. Microbiome and mental health in the modern environment. *J. Physiol. Anthropol.* **2016**, *36*.

21.   Dinan, T. How the gut influences the brain: The intestinal microbiome as a new dimension for understanding mental health. *Eur. Neuropsychopharmacol.* **2016**, *26*, S23–S24.

22.   Logan, A.C.; Jacka, F.N.; Craig, J.M.; Prescott, S.L. The microbiome and mental health: Looking back, moving forward with lessons from allergic diseases. *Clin. Psychopharmacol. Neurosci.* **2016**, *14*, 131–147.

23.   Leclercq, S.; Mian, F.M.; Stanisz, A.M.; Bindels, L.B.; Cambier, E.; Ben-Amram, H.; Koren, O.; Forsythe, P.; Bienenstock, J. Low-dose penicillin in early life induces long-term changes in murine gut microbiota, brain cytokines and behavior. *Nat. Commun.* **2017**, *8*, 15062.

24.   Moya-Perez, A.; Luczynski, P.; Renes, I.B.; Wang, S.; Borre, Y.; Anthony Ryan, C.; Knol, J.; Stanton, C.; Dinan, T.G.; Cryan, J.F. Intervention strategies for cesarean section-induced alterations in the microbiota-gut-brain axis. *Nutr. Rev.* **2017**.

25.   Binns, C.W.; Lee, M.K.; Kagawa, M.; Low, W.Y.; Liqian, Q.; Guldan, G.S.; Hokama, T.; Nanishi, K.; Oy, S.; Tang, L., et al. Dietary guidelines for the Asia Pacific region. *Asia-Pac. J. Public Health* **2017**, *29*, 98–101.

![nutrients logo] **nutrients**

![MDPI logo]

Review

Probiotics and Time to Achieve Full Enteral Feeding in Human Milk-Fed and Formula-Fed Preterm Infants: Systematic Review and Meta-Analysis

Arianna Aceti [1,2], **Davide Gori** [2,3], **Giovanni Barone** [2,4], **Maria Luisa Callegari** [2,5], **Maria Pia Fantini** [2,3], **Flavia Indrio** [2,6,7], **Luca Maggio** [2,4,7], **Fabio Meneghin** [2,8], **Lorenzo Morelli** [2,5], **Gianvincenzo Zuccotti** [2,9] and **Luigi Corvaglia** [1,2,7,*]

[1]   Neonatology and Neonatal Intensive Care Unit, Department of Medical and Surgical Sciences (DIMEC), University of Bologna, S.Orsola-Malpighi Hospital, Bologna 40138, Italy; arianna.aceti2@unibo.it

[2]   Task Force on Probiotics of the Italian Society of Neonatology, Milan 20126, Italy; dedegori27@gmail.com (D.G.); gbarone85@yahoo.it (G.B.); marialuisa.callegari@unicatt.it (M.L.C.); mariapia.fantini@unibo.it (M.P.F.); f.indrio@alice.it (F.I.); luca.maggio@fastwebnet.it (L.Ma.); fabio.meneghin@asst-fbf-sacco.it (F.M.); lorenzo.morelli@unicatt.it (L.Mo.); gianvincenzo.zuccotti@unimi.it (G.Z.)

[3]   Department of Biomedical and Neuromotor Sciences (DIBINEM), University of Bologna, Bologna 40138, Italy

[4]   Neonatal Unit, Catholic University, Rome 00168, Italy

[5]   Institute of Microbiology, UCSC, Piacenza 29122, Italy

[6]   Department of Pediatrics, Aldo Moro University, Bari 70124, Italy

[7]   Study Group of Neonatal Gastroenterology and Nutrition of the Italian Society of Neonatology, Milan 20126, Italy

[8]   Division of Neonatology, Children Hospital V. Buzzi, ICP, Milan 20154, Italy

[9]   Department of Pediatrics, Children Hospital V. Buzzi, University of Milan, Milan 20154, Italy

*   Correspondence: luigi.corvaglia@unibo.it; Tel./Fax: +39-051-342-754

Received: 13 June 2016; Accepted: 26 July 2016; Published: 30 July 2016

Abstract: Probiotics have been linked to a reduction in the incidence of necrotizing enterocolitis and late-onset sepsis in preterm infants. Recently, probiotics have also proved to reduce time to achieve full enteral feeding (FEF). However, the relationship between FEF achievement and type of feeding in infants treated with probiotics has not been explored yet. The aim of this systematic review and meta-analysis was to evaluate the effect of probiotics in reducing time to achieve FEF in preterm infants, according to type of feeding (exclusive human milk (HM) vs. formula). Randomized-controlled trials involving preterm infants receiving probiotics, and reporting on time to reach FEF were included in the systematic review. Trials reporting on outcome according to type of feeding (exclusive HM vs. formula) were included in the meta-analysis. Fixed-effect or random-effects models were used as appropriate. Results were expressed as mean difference (MD) with 95% confidence interval (CI). Twenty-five studies were included in the systematic review. In the five studies recruiting exclusively HM-fed preterm infants, those treated with probiotics reached FEF approximately 3 days before controls (MD -3.15 days (95% CI $-5.25/-1.05$), $p = 0.003$). None of the two studies reporting on exclusively formula-fed infants showed any difference between infants receiving probiotics and controls in terms of FEF achievement. The limited number of included studies did not allow testing for other subgroup differences between HM and formula-fed infants. However, if confirmed in further studies, the 3-days reduction in time to achieve FEF in exclusively HM-fed preterm infants might have significant implications for their clinical management.

Keywords: probiotics; preterm infants; human milk; full enteral feeding; systematic review

1. Introduction

Nutrition during critical time windows in early life can affect long-term health [1]. Early provision of optimal enteral nutrition to preterm infants might improve neurodevelopmental outcome by decreasing the rate of several complications of prematurity, such as extrauterine growth restriction, necrotizing enterocolitis (NEC), sepsis, bronchopulmonary dysplasia, and retinopathy of prematurity [2].

Late introduction and slow advancement of enteral feeding may alter gastrointestinal motility and disrupt microbial colonization [3], leading to a delay in establishing full enteral feeding (FEF). The consequent prolonged need for parenteral nutrition can have serious infectious and metabolic complications, which might prolong hospital stay, increase morbidity and mortality, and affect growth and development [4].

Several clinical variables and interventions have been proposed as predictors of the time to FEF achievement in preterm and very-low-birth-weight (VLBW) infants. Among these variables, the influence of type of feeding was also documented, as FEF achievement was delayed in formula-fed infants compared to human milk (HM)-fed infants [5].

Recently, probiotic use has been associated with a reduced time to achieve FEF and better feeding tolerance [6], as well as a reduction of NEC [7,8] and late-onset sepsis [9]. Probiotics are live microorganisms which, when ingested in adequate amounts, confer a health benefit to the host, by modifying the composition and function of gut microbiota and the immunological responses in the host [10]. The role of probiotics in attaining a more rapid achievement of FEF could be related to their favorable effect on the physiological intestinal dysbiosis of preterm infants [11], which is the result of the exposure to a unique environment and to several iatrogenic manipulations, such as broad spectrum antibiotics [12]. It is well known that gut microbiota in HM-fed infants is different compared to formula-fed infants [13]; data from an observational study also suggest a feeding-dependent effect of probiotics, as in that study NEC incidence was reduced in infants treated with probiotics and receiving HM, but not in those exclusively formula-fed [14]. However, the relationship between probiotics and type of feeding in attaining a more rapid achievement of FEF has not been explored yet, even in the most recent meta-analysis on this topic [6].

Thus, the aim of the present paper was to evaluate the effect of probiotics on time to FEF achievement according to type of feeding (exclusive HM vs. formula), by performing a systematic review and meta-analysis of currently available literature on this topic.

2. Materials and Methods

2.1. Literature Search

The study protocol was designed by the members of the Task Force on Probiotics of the Italian Society of Neonatology. PRISMA guidelines [15] were followed in order to perform a systematic review of published studies reporting the relationship between probiotic use and time to FEF achievement in preterm infants according to type of feeding.

In order to be included in the meta-analysis, studies had to meet the following inclusion criteria: randomized or quasi-randomized clinical trials involving preterm infants (gestational age (GA) <37 weeks) who received, within one month of age, any probiotic compared to placebo or no treatment, and reporting on type of feeding. The outcome of interest was time for FEF achievement (any definition). Only English-written studies and studies involving humans were included in the meta-analysis.

A search was conducted for studies published before 2 March 2016 in PubMed [16], the Cochrane Library [17], and Embase [18]. The following search string was used for the PubMed search: ((preterm infant OR pre-term infant) OR (preterm infants OR pre-term infants) OR (preterm neonate OR pre-term neonate) OR (preterm neonates OR pre-term neonates) OR (preterm newborn OR pre-term newborn) OR (preterm newborns OR pre-term newborns) OR (premature infant OR premature infants) OR (premature neonate OR premature neonates) OR (premature newborn OR premature newborns)

OR infant, extremely premature (MeSH Heading (MH)) OR premature birth (MH) OR infant, low birth weight (MH) OR infant, very low birth weight (MH)) AND (full enteral* OR feed*) AND (probiotic OR probiotics OR pro-biotic OR pro-biotics OR probio*)) NOT (animals (MH) NOT humans (MH).

The string was built up by combining all the terms related to probiotics and FEF achievement: PubMed MeSH terms, free-text words, and their combinations obtained through the most proper Boolean operators were used. The same criteria were used for searching the Cochrane Library and Embase.

Arianna Aceti and Luigi Corvaglia performed the literature search: relevant studies were identified from the abstract; full-texts of relevant studies were examined, as well as their reference lists in order to identify additional studies.

2.2. Data Extraction and Meta-Analysis

Study details (population, characteristics of probiotic and placebo, type of feeding, and outcome assessment) were evaluated independently by Arianna Aceti and Luigi Corvaglia, and checked by Davide Gori. Study quality was evaluated independently by Arianna Aceti and Davide Gori using the risk of bias tool as proposed by the Cochrane collaboration (Chapter 8 of the Cochrane Handbook of Systematic Reviews) [19].

The corresponding authors of the studies in which days to FEF achievement were not reported as mean ± standard deviation (SD) were contacted by email. When data were not provided, the study was not included in the meta-analysis.

The association between probiotic use and FEF achievement according to type of feeding was evaluated by a meta-analysis conducted by AA and DG using the RevMan software (Cochrane Informatics and Knowledge Management Department, version 5.3.5) downloaded from the Cochrane website [20]. Mean difference (MD) in days to achieve FEF between infants receiving probiotics and those receiving placebo or no treatment was calculated using the inverse variance method, and reported with 95% confidence interval (CI).

For the analysis, we planned to use at first a fixed effect model. Heterogeneity was measured using the I^2 test: if significant heterogeneity was present ($p < 0.05$ from the χ^2 test) and/or the number of studies was $\leqslant 5$, a random-effects model was used instead.

3. Results

Literature Search

Overall, 372 papers were identified through the literature search, 155 in PubMed [16], 73 in the Cochrane Library [17], and 144 in Embase [18].

As shown in Figure 1, 35 studies met the inclusion criteria [21–55]. Fourteen additional papers were identified from the reference lists of included studies or by "snowballing" techniques [52,56–68].

Twenty-four studies were excluded after examining the full-texts [28,29,31–33,35,42–47,51,53–55,57–59, 62,63,65,69]. Twenty-five studies were then suitable for inclusion in the systematic review (Table 1) [21–27, 30,34,36–41,48–50,56,60,61,64,66,68,70].

Among them, only eight studies reported FEF achievement according to type of feeding: infants were fed exclusively HM, either own mother's (OMM) or donor human milk (DHM), in six studies [22,38,50,56,60,70], while two studies reported FEF in exclusively formula-fed infants [41,61].

The corresponding authors of four of these papers were contacted by email, as data for FEF achievement were not suitable for inclusion in the meta-analysis: mean ± SD of days for FEF achievement were provided for one study [22], while data were unavailable for three studies [41,61,70]; these three studies were thus excluded from the meta-analysis.

Overall, five studies were included in the meta-analysis: in all these studies, infants were fed exclusively HM, either OMM or DHM (Figure 1) [22,38,50,56,60].

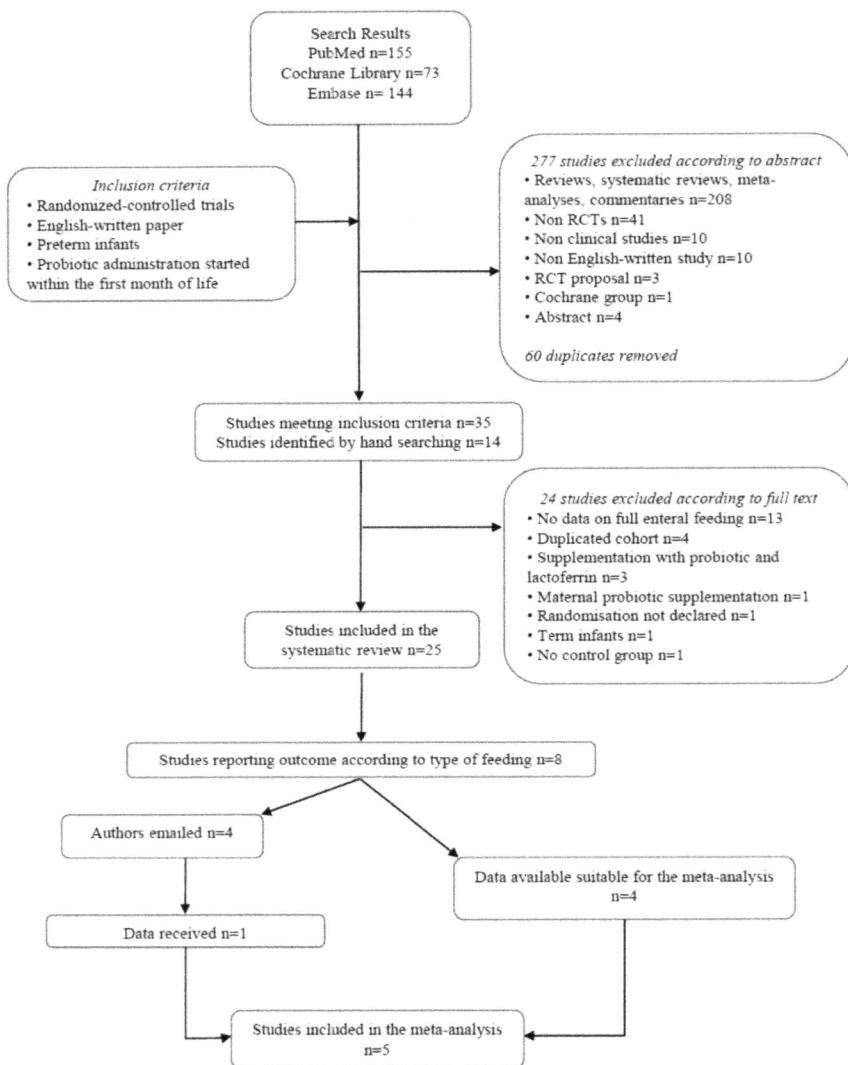

Figure 1. Flow chart of the search strategy used for the systematic review. The relevant number of papers at each point is given.

Table 1. Studies included in the systematic review.

Author, Year	Study Details	Study Population	Intervention Specie — Dose (D) / Start of Treatment (S) / End of Treatment (E)	Milk	Placebo	FEF Definition
Bin-Nun, 2005 [40]	P, B, R, C	Preterm infants with BW <1500 g, who began enteral feeding on a weekday	*B. infantis, Str. thermophilus, B. bifidus*; D: 0.35 × 10⁹ CFU each, OD; S: start of enteral feeding; E: 36 w postconceptual age	OMM, PFM	HM or FM	100 mL/kg/day
Braga, 2011 [60]	P, DB, R, C	Inborn infants with BW 750–1499 g	*L. casei, B. Breve*; D: 3.5 × 10⁷ CFU to 3.5 × 10⁹ CFU OD; S: day 2; E: day 30, NEC diagnosis, discharge, death, whichever occurred first	HM (± PFM from w3)	Extra HM	150 mL/kg/day
Costalos, 2003 [41]	P, R, C	GA 28–32 w; No major GI problem; Not receiving antibiotics; Not receiving breast milk	*Saccharomyces boulardii*; D: 1 × 10⁹ CFU BD; S: non-specified; Median duration of probiotic supplementation: 30 days	PFM	MDX	Not defined
Costeloe, 2015 [64]	P, DB, R, C, Multic.	Preterm infants with GA 23–30 + 6 weeks, without any lethal malformation or any malformation of the GI tract	*Bifidobacterium breve BBG-001*; D: 8 · 3–8 · 8 log₁₀ CFU/day; S: as soon as possible after randomisation; E: 36 w PMA or discharge if sooner	OMM, DHM, FM	Corn starch powder	150 mL/kg/day
Demirel, 2013 [27]	P, B, R, C	Preterm infants with GA ⩽ 32 weeks and BW ⩽ 1500 g, who survived to feed enterally	*S. boulardii*; D: 5 × 10⁹ CFU OD; S: first feed; E: discharge	HM, FM	None	Not defined
Dilli, 2015 [49]	P, DB, R, C, Multic.	Preterm infants with GA < 32 weeks and BW < 1500 g, born at or transferred to the NICU within the first week of life and fed enterally before inclusion	*B. lactis*; D: 5 × 10⁹ CFU; S: beyond d7 after birth; E: death or discharge (max 8 weeks)	HM, FM	MDX powder	100 mL/kg/day (FEF for hydration); 150 mL/kg/day (FEF for growth)

Table 1. *Cont.*

Author, Year	Study Details	Study Population	Intervention Specie — Dose (D), Start of Treatment (S), End of Treatment (E)	Milk	Placebo	FEF Definition
Fernández-Carrocera, 2013 [30]	P	Preterm infants with	*L. acidophilus* 1×10^9 CFU/g, *L. rhamnosus* 4.4×10^8 CFU/g, *L. casei* 1×10^9 CFU/g, *L. plantarum* 1.76×10^8 CFU/g, *B. infantis* 2.76×10^7 CFU/g, *Str. thermophilus* 6.6×10^5 CFU/g	OMM, PFM	None	Not defined
	DB	BW <1500 g	Total D: 1 g powder OD			
	R	Infants with NEC stage 1A and stage 1B were excluded	S: start of enteral feeding			
	C		E: non specified			
Hays, 2014 [66]	P	Preterm infants with GA 25–31 weeks, BW 700–1600 g, AGA, enteral feeding initiated before day 5	Probiotic group composed of 3 subgroups:	OMM, DM or PFM	MDX	Not defined
	DB		P1 *B. lactis*			
	R	Infants with NEC stage ≥ 1B, malformations or severe medical or surgical conditions were excluded	P2 *B. longum*			
	C		P3 *B. lactis + longum*			
	Multic.		D: 1×10^9 CFU each probiotic daily			
			Duration: 4 weeks for infants ≥29 w/6 weeks for infants ≤28 w GA			
Hikaru, 2010 [68]	P	Extremely low birth weight and very low birth weight infants	*B. breve*	OMM, PFM	None	Not defined
	R		D: 0.5×10^9 CFU BD			
	C		S: birth			
			E: discharge from NICU			
Jacobs, 2013 [25]	P	Preterm infants with GA <32 weeks and BW <1500 g	*B. infantis* BB-02 300 CFU $\times 10^6$, *Str. thermophilus* Th-4 350 CFU $\times 10^6$, *B. lactis* BB-12 350 CFU $\times 10^6$	HM, FM	MDX powder	Enteral feeds of 120 mL/kg for ≥3 days
	DB		Total D: 1×10^9 CFU + 1.5 g MDX powder OD			
	R		S: enteral feed ≥ 1 mL every 4 h			
	C		E: discharge or term corrected age			
	Multic.					

Table 1. *Cont.*

Author, Year	Study Details		Study Population	Intervention Specie Dose (D) Start of Treatment (S) End of Treatment (E)	Milk	Placebo	FEF Definition
Lin, 2008 [39]	P		Preterm infants with GA < 34 weeks and BW ≤ 1500 g, who survived to feed enterally	*L. acidophilus NCDO 1746, B. bifidum NCDO 1453* 10⁹ CFU	HM, FM	None	Oral intake of 100 mL/kg/day
	B			D: 1 × 10⁹ CFU each probiotic (= 125 mg/kg) BD			
	R			S: day 2 of age			
	C			Duration: 6 weeks			
	Multic.						
Manzoni, 2006 [56]	P		Infants with BW < 1500 g, ≥3 day of life, who started enteral feeding with HM	*L. casei subspecies rhamnosus LGG*	OMM, DM	None	Not defined
	DB			D: 6 × 10⁹ CFU/day			
	R			S: day 3 of life			
	C			E: end of the 6th week or discharge			
Mihatsch, 2010 [36]	P		Preterm infants with GA < 30 weeks and BW ≤ 1500 g	*B. lactis BB12*	OMM, PFM	Indistinguishable powder	150 mL/kg/day
	R			D: 2 × 10⁹ CFU/kg 6 times a day			
	C			S: start of enteral feeding			
				E: non specified			
Oncel, 2014 [24]	P		Preterm infants with GA ≤ 32 weeks and BW ≤ 1500 g, who survived to feed enterally	*L. reuteri DSM 17938*	HM, FM	Oil base	Not defined
	DB			D: 1 × 10⁸ CFU OD			
	R			S: first feed			
	C			E: death or discharge			
Patole, 2014 [23]	P		Preterm infants with GA < 33 weeks and BW < 1500 g	*B. breve*	HM, FM	Dextrin	150 mL/kg/day enteral feeding
	DB			D: 3 × 10⁹ CFU OD (1.5 × 10⁹ CFU OD for newborn ≤ 27 w until they reached 50 mL/kg/day enteral feeds)			
	R			S: start of enteral feed			
	C			E: corrected age of 37 w			
Rougé, 2009 [37]	P		Preterm infants with GA < 32 weeks and BW < 1500 g, ≤2 weeks of age, without any disease other than those linked to prematurity, who started enteral feeding before inclusion	*B. longum* BB536, *L. rhamnosus* GG BB536-LGG	OMM, DM or PFM	MDX	Not defined
	DB			Total D: 1 × 108 CFU/day			
	R			S: start of enteral feeding			
	C			E: discharge			
	Bic.						

Table 1. *Cont.*

Author, Year	Study Details	Study Population	Intervention Specie / Dose (D) / Start of Treatment (S) / End of Treatment (E)	Milk	Placebo	FEF Definition
Roy, 2014 [50]	P	Preterm infants (GA < 37 weeks) and BW < 2500 g, with stable enteral feeding within 72 h of birth	*L. acidophilus* 1.25×10^9 CFU × 1 g, *B. longum* 0.125×10^9 CFU × 1 g, *B. bifidum* 0.125×10^9 CFU × 1 g, *B. lactis* 1×10^9 CFU × 1 g	HM	Sterile water	120 mL/kg/day for ≥3 d
	DB		D: half a 1 g sachet			
	R		S: from 72 h of life			
	C		E: after 6 w or at discharge			
Saengtawesin, 2014 [48]	P	Preterm infants with GA ≤ 34 weeks and BW ≤ 1500 g	*L. acidophilus* 1×10^9 CFU, *B. bifidum* 1×10^9 CFU	HM, PFM	None	150 mL/kg/day
	R		D: 125 mg/kg BD			
	C		S: start of feeding			
			E: 6 w of age or discharge.			
Samanta, 2008 [38]	P	Preterm infants with GA < 32 weeks and BW < 1500 g, who started enteral feeding and survived beyond 48 h of age	*B. infantis, B. bifidum, B. longum, L. acidophilus*	HM	None	Not defined
	DB		D: 2.5×10^9 CFU each probiotic, BD			
	R		S: start of enteral feeding			
	C		E: discharge			
Sari, 2011 [34]	P	Preterm infants with GA < 32 weeks or BW < 1500 g, who survived to feed enterally	*L. sporogenes*	HM, FM	None	Not defined
	B		D: 0.35×10^9 CFU OD			
	R		S: first feed			
	C		E: discharge			
Serce, 2013 [26]	P	Preterm infants with GA ≤ 32 weeks and BW ≤ 1500 g, who survived to feed enterally	*S. boulardii*	HM, FM	Distilled water	100 mL/kg/day enteral feeding
	M		D: 0.5×10^9 CFU/kg BD			
	R		S: non specified			
	C		E: non specified			
Stratiki, 2007 [61]	P	Preterm infants with GA 27–32 weeks, formula-fed, without major congenital anomalies	*Bifidobacterium lactis*	FM	None	150 mL/kg/day
	B		D: 2×10^7 CFU/g of milk powder			
	R		S: start of enteral feeding			
	C		E: not specified			

8

Table 1. *Cont.*

Author, Year	Study Details	Study Population	Intervention Specie — Dose (D) / Start of Treatment (S) / End of Treatment (E)	Milk	Placebo	FEF Definition
Tewari, 2015 [70]	P	Preterm infants with GA < 34 weeks	*Bacillus clausii*	OMM, DHM	Sterile water	180 mL/kg/day
	DB	Excluded if: NEC, congenital anomaly, outborn and >10 days of with sepsis	D: 2.4×10^9 CFU/day			
	R	Stratified as extreme preterm (GA 27–30 + 6) and very preterm (GA 31–33 + 6)	S: by day 5 in asymptomatic and by day 10 in symptomatic infants			
	C		E: 6 weeks of age, discharge or death (whichever occurred first)			
Totsu, 2014 [21]	P		*B. bifidum*	HM, FM	Dextrin	Postnatal day at which the amount of enteral feeding exceeded 100 mL/kg/day
	DB		D: 2.5×10^9 CFU, divided in two doses			
	CLR	Infants with BW < 1500 g	S: within 48 h after birth			
	C		E: body weight 2000 g			
	Multic.					
Van Niekerk, 2014 [22]	P	Preterm infants with GA < 34 weeks and BW < 1250 g, exposed and non-exposed to HIV (only infants unexposed to HIV are included in the meta-analysis)	*L. rhamnosus*, *B. infantis*	HM	MCT oil	"when infants no longer required the use of IV fluids"
	DB		D: 0.35×10^9 CFU each probiotic			
	R		S: start of enteral feeding			
	C		E: day 28 postconceptual age			

P: prospective; B: blinded; R: randomized; C: controlled; DB: double-blinded; Multic: multicentric; M: masked; CLR: cluster-randomized; BW: birth weight; GA: gestational age; HM: human milk; L.: Lactobacillus; B.: Bifidobacterium; Str.: Streptococcus; S.: Saccharomyces; CFU: colony forming unit; OD: once daily; NEC: necrotizing enterocolitis; BD: twice daily; OMM: own mother's milk; PFM: preterm formula; FM: formula; MDX: maltodextrin; PMA: postmenstrual age; AGA: appropriate for gestational age.

Data from 359 infants in the probiotic group and 360 infants in the control group were evaluated: probiotic use was associated with a reduction in the time for FEF achievement (MD -3.15 days (95% CI $-5.25/-1.05$), $p = 0.003$; Figure 2a). The funnel plot did not show any clear asymmetry (Figure 2b).

2a

Study or Subgroup	Probiotic Mean	SD	Total	Control Mean	SD	Total	Weight	Mean Difference IV, Random, 95% CI
Braga, 2011	15.2	5.2	119	17.4	5.7	112	21.9%	-2.20 [-3.61, -0.79]
Manzoni, 2006	15	8	39	17	9	41	13.8%	-2.00 [-5.73, 1.73]
Roy, 2014	11.22	5.04	56	15.41	8.07	56	18.1%	-4.19 [-6.68, -1.70]
Samanta, 2009	13.76	2.28	91	19.2	2.02	95	23.8%	-5.44 [-6.06, -4.82]
Van Niekerk, 2014	9.63	2.42	54	11.14	4.15	56	22.4%	-1.51 [-2.77, -0.25]
Total (95% CI)			359			360	100.0%	-3.15 [-5.25, -1.05]

Heterogeneity: Tau² = 4.71; Chi² = 41.69, df = 4 (P < 0.00001), I² = 90%
Test for overall effect: Z = 2.94 (P = 0.003)

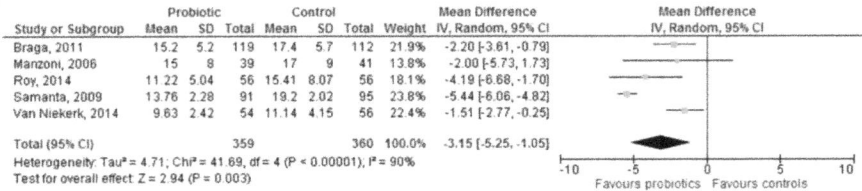

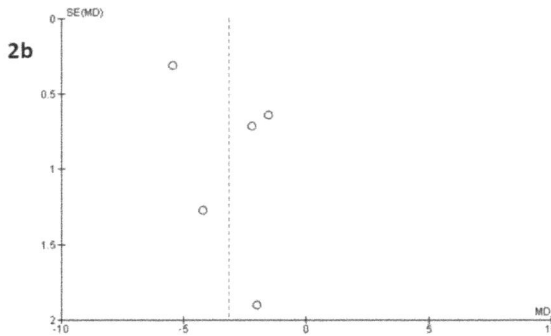

Figure 2. Forest plot (**2a**) and funnel plot (**2b**) showing the association between the use of probiotics and achievement of full enteral feeding in exclusively human milk-fed preterm infants. IV: inverse variance method.

Three studies were not included in the meta-analysis because data on FEF were not available as mean ± SD [41,61,70]. One study reported the use of *Bacillus clausii* in preterm infants with GA < 34 weeks, fed expressed breast milk or DHM [70] and stratified as extreme preterm (GA 27–30 + 6 weeks) and very preterm (GA 31–33 + 6 weeks). In both groups, probiotic use was associated with a reduced time to achieve FEF (risk ratio 0.82 (95% CI 0.74–0.88) and 0.67 (95% CI 0.32–0.77), respectively).

The other two studies reported probiotic use in exclusively formula-fed infants: in the study by Costalos et al., infants born at 28–32 weeks gestation and fed exclusively preterm formula received *Saccharomyces boulardii* or placebo for approximately 30 days [41]. In the study by Stratiki et al., formula-fed infants with a similar gestational age (27–32 weeks) received *Bifidobacterium lactis* vs. no treatment [61]. Neither of these two studies reported any significant difference between groups in terms of time to FEF achievement.

All the studies included in the meta-analysis, except one [50], recruited exclusively infants with birth weight <1500 g. The study by Roy et al. [50] reported specific data for extremely low birth weight (ELBW) infants: time to reach FEF in ELBW infants treated with probiotics was significantly lower than in controls (mean ± SD 13.22 ± 5.04 vs. 17.41 ± 8.07, respectively, $p = 0.014$). None of the studies included in the meta-analysis reported separate data on intrauterine growth restricted (IUGR) infants.

In all the studies, except one [56], a probiotic mix was used: the meta-analysis performed after the exclusion of the study by Manzoni et al., where a single-strain product containing Lactobacillus GG was used, confirmed the results of the overall analysis (MD -3.33 days (95% CI $-5.63/-1.04$), $p \leqslant 0.004$).

4. Methodological Study Quality

Evaluation of the quality of the studies included in the meta-analysis according to the risk of bias tool as proposed by the Cochrane Collaboration [19] is shown in Table 2.

Table 2. Evaluation of the quality of the studies included in the meta-analysis according to the risk of bias tool as proposed by the Cochrane collaboration.

Study	Random Sequence Generation	Allocation Concealment	Blinding	Incomplete Outcome Data	Selective Outcome Reporting	Other Sources of Bias
Braga, 2011 [60]	Low	Low	Low	Low	Unclear	Low
Manzoni, 2006 [56]	Low	Low	Low	Unclear	Unclear	Low
Roy, 2014 [50]	Low	Unclear	Low	Low	Unclear	Unclear
Samanta, 2008 [38]	Low	Low	Low	Unclear	Unclear	Unclear
Van Niekerk, 2014 [22]	Low	Unclear	Low	Unclear	Unclear	Unclear

5. Discussion

The present meta-analysis shows that the use of probiotics in preterm, VLBW infants fed exclusively HM is associated with 3-days reduction in the time to FEF achievement. The only two studies included in the present systematic review in which infants were exclusively formula-fed did not report any difference between the probiotic and the control group.

The single previous meta-analysis investigating FEF as primary outcome showed an overall smaller reduction in the time to FEF achievement, but did not report separate data for HM-fed and formula-fed infants [6]. The studies included in the meta-analysis by Athalye-Jape et al. are almost the same as those included in our systematic review; quite surprisingly, in the majority of the studies included in these two reviews, both HM and formula-fed infants were recruited, but no detailed information on the relationship between type of feeding and outcome was provided.

Type of feeding might modulate the relationship between probiotics and neonatal clinical outcome [14]. It has been previously shown that HM feeding is associated with shorter time to achieve FEF compared to formula feeding [5]. Our meta-analysis, which included only studies where infants were exclusively HM-fed, showed a significant reduction in the time to achieve FEF attributable to probiotics. Despite the limitation given by the small number of studies, a probiotic-related 3-days reduction in time to achieve FEF in preterm infants fed exclusively HM has strong clinical implications and deserves further consideration. When OMM is not available or contraindicated, the use of pasteurized DHM is recommended for preterm infants: pasteurization inactivates most viral and bacterial agents, but at the same time affects some nutritional and immunological properties of HM, including endogenous probiotics [71]. It can be speculated that the beneficial effect of probiotics documented in exclusively HM-fed infants could be attributed to a synergic action exerted by the prebiotic components of HM and the exogenous probiotic, which partially restores the symbiotic properties of naïve HM [72]. In the present meta-analysis, no separate data for OMM-fed and DHM-fed infants were available; for this reason, it is not possible to clarify whether the beneficial effect of HM on FEF achievement applies both to OMM and to DHM.

Heterogeneity among included studies was high; however, given the small number of papers, our ability to explore sources of heterogeneity was limited. In the five included studies, different probiotic strains were used. We aimed to perform strain-specific sub-meta-analyses, in order to clarify whether there was any probiotic product showing a significant benefit in terms of reduction in the time to achieve FEF. However, such analyses were not feasible, as none of the studies used the same probiotic strain or mix. Similarly, it was not possible to explore additional sources of heterogeneity, such as the characteristics of probiotic administration (dose, duration, infant age at probiotic initiation, etc.). In addition, we were unable to test for subgroup differences between HM-fed and formula-fed infants, which might have partially explained the different results in terms of FEF achievement.

Apparently, studies were homogeneous in terms of included populations, as almost all of them recruited only VLBW infants. However, few data on "high-risk" infants, such as ELBW and IUGR infants, could be extrapolated from the main results of the included studies.

The use of probiotics should be weighed against their potential side effects. There are some reports about the occurrence of sepsis in preterm newborns, potentially linked to probiotic administration [73].

However, none of the studies included in the systematic review reported any side effect related to the use of probiotics.

6. Conclusions

According to the results of the present meta-analysis, the use of probiotics is linked to 3-days reduction in time to achieve FEF in preterm VLBW infants fed exclusively HM. If confirmed in further studies, this reduction might have strong clinical implications for this high-risk population.

Acknowledgments: No funding was received to produce the present paper.

Author Contributions: Each author listed on the manuscript has seen and approved the submission of this version of the manuscript and takes full responsibility for the manuscript. Specifically, all the authors, as part of the Task Force on Probiotics of the Italian Society of Neonatology, conceived and designed the study protocol. A.A. and L.C. performed the literature search and assessed study details, which were checked by D.G. A.A. and D.G. evaluated study quality and performed the meta-analyses. A.A. and L.C. wrote the first draft of the paper, which was critically revised by all the other authors.

Conflicts of Interest: The authors declare no conflict of interest.

References

1. Faldella, G.; Aceti, A.; Corvaglia, L. Formula milk and neurodevelopmental and cognitive outcomes: Where are we now? *Early Hum. Dev.* **2011**, *87S*, S5–S8. [CrossRef] [PubMed]
2. Hsiao, C.-C.; Tsai, M.-L.; Chen, C.-C.; Lin, H.-C. Early optimal nutrition improves neurodevelopmental outcomes for very preterm infants. *Nutr. Rev.* **2014**, *72*, 532–540. [CrossRef] [PubMed]
3. Berrington, J.E.; Stewart, C.J.; Embleton, N.D.; Cummings, S.P. Gut microbiota in preterm infants: Assessment and relevance to health and disease. *Arch. Dis. Child. Fetal Neonatal Ed.* **2013**, *98*, F286–F290. [CrossRef] [PubMed]
4. The SIFT Investigators Group. Early enteral feeding strategies for very preterm infants: Current evidence from Cochrane reviews. *Arch. Dis. Child. Fetal Neonatal Ed.* **2013**, *98*, F470–F472.
5. Corvaglia, L.; Fantini, M.P.; Aceti, A.; Gibertoni, D.; Rucci, P.; Baronciani, D.; Faldella, G. Predictors of full enteral feeding achievement in very low birth weight infants. *PLoS ONE* **2014**, *9*. [CrossRef] [PubMed]
6. Athalye-Jape, G.; Deshpande, G.; Rao, S.; Patole, S. Benefits of probiotics on enteral nutrition in preterm neonates: a systematic review. *Am. J. Clin. Nutr.* **2014**, *100*, 1508–1519. [CrossRef] [PubMed]
7. Aceti, A.; Gori, D.; Barone, G.; Callegari, M.L.; Di Mauro, A.; Fantini, M.P.; Indrio, F.; Maggio, L.; Meneghin, F.; Morelli, L.; et al. Probiotics for prevention of necrotizing enterocolitis in preterm infants: Systematic review and meta-analysis. *Ital. J. Pediatr.* **2015**, *41*, 89. [CrossRef] [PubMed]
8. Alfaleh, K.; Anabrees, J.; Bassler, D. Probiotics for prevention of necrotizing enterocolitis in preterm infants. *Cochrane Database Syst. Rev.* **2014**, CD005496. [CrossRef] [PubMed]
9. Rao, S.C.; Athalye-jape, G.K.; Deshpande, G.C.; Simmer, K.N.; Patole, S.K. Probiotic supplementation and late-onset sepsis in preterm infants: A meta-analysis. *Pediatrics* **2016**, *137*, e20153684. [CrossRef] [PubMed]
10. Sanders, M.E.; Guarner, F.; Guerrant, R.; Holt, P.R.; Quigley, E.M.M.; Sartor, R.B.; Sherman, P.M.; Mayer, E.A. An update on the use and investigation of probiotics in health and disease. *Gut* **2013**, *62*, 787–796. [CrossRef] [PubMed]
11. Murguía-Peniche, T.; Mihatsch, W.A.; Zegarra, J.; Supapannachart, S.; Ding, Z.-Y.; Neu, J. Intestinal mucosal defense system, Part 2. Probiotics and prebiotics. *J. Pediatr.* **2013**, *162*, S64–S71. [CrossRef] [PubMed]
12. Martin, C.R.; Walker, W.A. Probiotics: Role in pathophysiology and prevention in necrotizing enterocolitis. *Semin. Perinatol.* **2008**, *32*, 127–137. [CrossRef] [PubMed]
13. Carlisle, E.M.; Morowitz, M.J. The intestinal microbiome and necrotizing enterocolitis. *Curr. Opin. Pediatr.* **2013**, *25*, 382–387. [CrossRef] [PubMed]

14. Repa, A.; Thanhaeuser, M.; Endress, D.; Weber, M.; Kreissl, A.; Binder, C.; Berger, A.; Haiden, N. Probiotics (*Lactobacillus acidophilus and Bifidobacterium bifidum*) prevent NEC in VLBW infants fed breast milk but not formula. *Pediatr. Res.* **2015**, *77*, 381–388. [CrossRef] [PubMed]

15. Moher, D.; Liberati, A.; Tetzlaff, J.; Altman, D.G. Preferred reporting items for systematic reviews and meta-analyses: The PRISMA statement. *PLoS Med.* **2009**, *6*, e1000097. [CrossRef] [PubMed]

16. PubMed. Available online: http://www.ncbi.nlm.nih.gov/pubmed (accessed on 28 July 2016).

17. Cochrane Library. Available online: http://www.cochranelibrary.com/ (accessed on 28 July 2016).

18. Embase. Available online: http://store.elsevier.com/en_US/info/30800006 (accessed on 28 July 2016).

19. Higgins, J.P.; Green, S. *Cochrane Handbook for Systematic Reviews of Interventions*; The Cochrane Collaboration: London, UK, 2011.

20. RevMan Software. Available online: http://tech.cochrane.org/revman/download (accessed on 28 July 2016).

21. Totsu, S.; Yamasaki, C.; Terahara, M.; Uchiyama, A.; Kusuda, S. Bifidobacterium and enteral feeding in preterm infants: Cluster-randomized trial. *Pediatr. Int.* **2014**, *56*, 714–719. [CrossRef] [PubMed]

22. Van Niekerk, E.; Kirsten, G.F.; Nel, D.G.; Blaauw, R. Probiotics, feeding tolerance, and growth: A comparison between HIV-exposed and unexposed very low birth weight infants. *Nutrition* **2014**, *30*, 645–653. [CrossRef] [PubMed]

23. Patole, S.; Keil, A.D.; Chang, A.; Nathan, E.; Doherty, D.; Simmer, K.; Esvaran, M.; Conway, P. Effect of Bifidobacterium breve M-16V supplementation on fecal bifidobacteria in preterm neonates—A randomised double blind placebo controlled trial. *PLoS ONE* **2014**, *9*, e89511. [CrossRef] [PubMed]

24. Oncel, M.Y.; Sari, F.N.; Arayici, S.; Guzoglu, N.; Erdeve, O.; Uras, N.; Oguz, S.S.; Dilmen, U. Lactobacillus Reuteri for the prevention of necrotising enterocolitis in very low birthweight infants: A randomised controlled trial. *Arch. Dis. Child. Fetal Neonatal Ed.* **2014**, *99*, F110–F115. [CrossRef] [PubMed]

25. Jacobs, S.E.; Tobin, J.M.; Opie, G.F.; Donath, S.; Tabrizi, S.N.; Pirotta, M.; Morley, C.J.; Garland, S.M. Probiotic effects on late-onset sepsis in very preterm infants: A randomized controlled trial. *Pediatrics* **2013**, *132*, 1055–1062. [CrossRef] [PubMed]

26. Serce, O.; Benzer, D.; Gursoy, T.; Karatekin, G.; Ovali, F. Efficacy of saccharomyces boulardii on necrotizing enterocolitis or sepsis in very low birth weight infants: A randomised controlled trial. *Early Hum. Dev.* **2013**, *89*, 1033–1036. [CrossRef] [PubMed]

27. Demirel, G.; Erdeve, O.; Celik, I.H.; Dilmen, U. Saccharomyces boulardii for prevention of necrotizing enterocolitis in preterm infants: A randomized, controlled study. *Acta Paediatr.* **2013**, *102*, 560–565. [CrossRef] [PubMed]

28. Rojas, M.A.; Lozano, J.M.; Rojas, M.X.; Rodriguez, V.A.; Rondon, M.A.; Bastidas, J.A.; Perez, L.A.; Rojas, C.; Ovalle, O.; Garcia-Harker, J.E.; et al. Prophylactic probiotics to prevent death and nosocomial infection in preterm infants. *Pediatrics* **2012**, *130*, e1113–e1120. [CrossRef] [PubMed]

29. Sari, F.N.; Eras, Z.; Dizdar, E.A.; Erdeve, O.; Oguz, S.S.; Uras, N.; Dilmen, U. Do oral probiotics affect growth and neurodevelopmental outcomes in very low-birth-weight preterm infants? *Am. J. Perinatol.* **2012**, *29*, 579–586. [CrossRef] [PubMed]

30. Fernández-Carrocera, L.A.; Solis-Herrera, A.; Cabanillas-Ayón, M.; Gallardo-Sarmiento, R.B.; García-Pérez, C.S.; Montaño-Rodríguez, R.; Echániz-Aviles, M.O.L. Double-blind, randomised clinical assay to evaluate the efficacy of probiotics in preterm newborns weighing less than 1500 g in the prevention of necrotising enterocolitis. *Arch. Dis. Child. Fetal Neonatal Ed.* **2013**, *98*, F5–F9. [CrossRef] [PubMed]

31. Havranek, T.; Al-Hosni, M.; Armbrecht, E. Probiotics supplementation increases intestinal blood flow velocity in extremely low birth weight preterm infants. *J. Perinatol.* **2013**, *33*, 40–44. [CrossRef] [PubMed]

32. Chrzanowska-Liszewska, D.; Seliga-Siwecka, J.; Kornacka, M.K. The effect of Lactobacillus rhamnosus GG supplemented enteral feeding on the microbiotic flora of preterm infants-double blinded randomized control trial. *Early Hum. Dev.* **2012**, *88*, 57–60. [CrossRef] [PubMed]

33. Campeotto, F.; Suau, A.; Kapel, N.; Magne, F.; Viallon, V.; Ferraris, L.; Waligora-Dupriet, A.-J.; Soulaines, P.; Leroux, B.; Kalach, N.; Dupont, C.; Butel, M.-J. A fermented formula in pre-term infants: Clinical tolerance, gut microbiota, down-regulation of faecal calprotectin and up-regulation of faecal secretory IgA. *Br. J. Nutr.* **2011**, *105*, 1843–1851. [CrossRef] [PubMed]

34. Sari, F.N.; Dizdar, E.A.; Oguz, S.; Erdeve, O.; Uras, N.; Dilmen, U. Oral probiotics: Lactobacillus sporogenes for prevention of necrotizing enterocolitis in very low-birth weight infants: A randomized, controlled trial. *Eur. J. Clin. Nutr.* **2011**, *65*, 434–439. [CrossRef] [PubMed]
35. Indrio, F.; Riezzo, G.; Raimondi, F.; Bisceglia, M.; Cavallo, L.; Francavilla, R. Effects of probiotic and prebiotic on gastrointestinal motility in newborns. *J. Physiol. Pharmacol.* **2009**, *60*, 27–31. [PubMed]
36. Mihatsch, W.A.; Vossbeck, S.; Eikmanns, B.; Hoegel, J.; Pohlandt, F. Effect of Bifidobacterium lactis on the incidence of nosocomial infections in very-low-birth-weight infants: A randomized controlled trial. *Neonatology* **2010**, *98*, 156–163. [CrossRef] [PubMed]
37. Rougé, C.; Piloquet, H.; Butel, M.-J.; Berger, B.; Rochat, F.; Ferraris, L.; Des Robert, C.; Legrand, A.; de la Cochetiere, M.-F.; N'Guyen, J.-M.; et al. Oral supplementation with probiotics in very-low-birth-weight preterm infants: A randomized, double-blind, placebo-controlled trial. *Am. J. Clin. Nutr.* **2009**, *89*, 1828–1835. [CrossRef] [PubMed]
38. Samanta, M.; Sarkar, M.; Ghosh, P.; Ghosh, J.K.; Sinha, M.K.; Chatterjee, S. Prophylactic probiotics for prevention of necrotizing enetrocolitis in very low birth weight newborns. *J. Trop. Pediatr.* **2008**, *55*, 128–131. [CrossRef] [PubMed]
39. Lin, H.-C.; Hsu, C.-H.; Chen, H.-L.; Chung, M.-Y.; Hsu, J.-F.; Lien, R.; Tsao, L.-Y.; Chen, C.-H.; Su, B.-H. Oral probiotics prevent necrotizing enterocolitis in very low birth weight preterm infants: A multicenter, randomized, controlled trial. *Pediatrics* **2008**, *122*, 693–700. [CrossRef] [PubMed]
40. Bin-Nun, A.; Bromiker, R.; Wilschanski, M.; Kaplan, M.; Rudensky, B.; Caplan, M.; Hammerman, C. Oral probiotics prevent necrotizing enterocolitis in very low birth weight neonates. *J. Pediatr.* **2005**, *147*, 192–196. [CrossRef] [PubMed]
41. Costalos, C.; Skouteri, V.; Gounaris, A.; Sevastiadou, S.; Triandafilidou, A.; Ekonomidou, C.; Kontaxaki, F.; Petrochilou, V. Enteral feeding of premature infants with *Saccharomyces boulardii*. *Early Hum. Dev.* **2003**, *74*, 89–96. [CrossRef]
42. Dani, C.; Biadaioli, R.; Bertini, G.; Martelli, E.; Rubaltelli, F.F. Probiotics feeding in prevention of urinary tract infection, bacterial sepsis and necrotizing enterocolitis in preterm infants. *Biol. Neonate* **2002**, *82*, 103–108. [CrossRef] [PubMed]
43. Stansbridge, E.M.; Walker, V.; Hall, M.A.; Smith, S.L.; Millar, M.R.; Bacon, C.; Chen, S. Effects of feeding premature infants with Lactobacillus GG on gut fermentation. *Arch. Dis. Child.* **1993**, *69*, 488–492. [CrossRef] [PubMed]
44. Millar, M.R.; Bacon, C.; Smith, S.L.; Walker, V.; Hall, M.A. Enteral feeding of premature infants with Lactobacillus GG. *Arch. Dis. Child.* **1993**, *69*, 483–487. [CrossRef] [PubMed]
45. Indrio, F.; Riezzo, G.; Raimondi, F.; Bisceglia, M.; Cavallo, L.; Francavilla, R. The effects of probiotics on feeding tolerance, bowel habits, and gastrointestinal motility in preterm newborns. *J. Pediatr.* **2008**, *152*, 801–806. [CrossRef] [PubMed]
46. Al-Hosni, M.; Duenas, M.; Hawk, M.; Stewart, L.A.; Borghese, R.A.; Cahoon, M.; Atwood, L.; Howard, D.; Ferrelli, K.; Soll, R. Probiotics-supplemented feeding in extremely low-birth-weight infants. *J. Perinatol.* **2012**, *32*, 253–259. [CrossRef] [PubMed]
47. Savino, F.; Ceratto, S.; Poggi, E.; Cartosio, M.E.; Cordero di Montezemolo, L.; Giannattasio, A. Preventive effects of oral probiotic on infantile colic: A prospective, randomised, blinded, controlled trial using Lactobacillus reuteri DSM 17938. *Benef. Microbes* **2014**. [CrossRef]
48. Saengtawesin, V.; Tangpolkaiwalsak, R.; Kanjanapattankul, W. Effect of oral probiotics supplementation in the prevention of necrotizing enterocolitis among very low birth weight preterm infants. *J. Med. Assoc. Thail.* **2014**, *97*, S20–S25.
49. Dilli, D.; Aydin, B.; Fettah, N.; Özyazıcı, E.; Beken, S.; Zenciroğlu, A.; Okumuş, N.; Özyurt, B.; İpek, M.; Akdağ, A.; et al. The propre-save study: Effects of probiotics and prebiotics alone or combined on necrotizing enterocolitis in very low birth weight infants. *J. Pediatr.* **2015**, *28*, 1537–1541. [CrossRef] [PubMed]
50. Roy, A.; Chaudhuri, J.; Sarkar, D.; Ghosh, P.; Chakraborty, S. Role of enteric supplementation of Probiotics on late-onset sepsis by Candida species in preterm low birth weight neonates: A randomized, double blind, placebo-controlled trial. *N. Am. J. Med. Sci.* **2014**, *6*, 50–57. [PubMed]
51. Oncel, M.Y.; Arayici, S.; Sari, F.N.; Simsek, G.K.; Yurttutan, S.; Erdeve, O.; Saygan, S.; Uras, N.; Oguz, S.S.; Dilmen, U. Comparison of Lactobacillus reuteri and nystatin prophylaxis on Candida colonization and infection in very low birth weight infants. *J. Matern. Neonatal Med.* **2014**, 1–5. [CrossRef]

52. Millar, M.; Wilks, M.; Fleming, P.; Costeloe, K. Should the use of probiotics in the preterm be routine? *Arch. Dis. Child. Fetal Neonatal Ed.* **2012**, *97*, F70–F74. [CrossRef] [PubMed]

53. Rinaldi, M.; Manzoni, P.; Meyer, M.; Casa, E.D.; Pugni, L.; Mosca, F.; Stolfi, I.; Messner, H.; Memo, L.; Laforgia, N.; et al. Bovine lactoferrin supplementation for prevention of necrotising enterocolitis in preterm very-low-birth-weight neonates: A randomised trial. *Early Hum. Dev.* **2012**, *88*, S102. [CrossRef]

54. Manzoni, P.; Meyer, M.; Stolfi, I.; Rinaldi, M.; Cattani, S.; Pugni, L.; Romeo, M.G.; Messner, H.; Decembrino, L.; Laforgia, N.; et al. Bovine lactoferrin supplementation for prevention of necrotizing enterocolitis in very-low-birth-weight neonates: A randomized clinical trial. *Early Hum. Dev.* **2014**, *90*, S60–S65. [CrossRef]

55. Benor, S.; Marom, R.; Tov, A.B.; Domany, K.A.; Zaidenberg-Israeli, G.; Dollberg, S. Probiotic supplementation in mothers of very low birth weight infants. *Am. J. Perinatol.* **2014**, *31*, 497–504. [PubMed]

56. Manzoni, P.; Mostert, M.; Leonessa, M.L.; Priolo, C.; Farina, D.; Monetti, C.; Latino, M.A.; Gomirato, G. Oral supplementation with Lactobacillus casei subspecies rhamnosus prevents enteric colonization by Candida species in preterm neonates: A randomized study. *Clin. Infect. Dis.* **2006**, *42*, 1735–1742. [CrossRef] [PubMed]

57. Kitajima, H.; Sumida, Y.; Tanaka, R.; Yuki, N.; Takayama, H.; Fujimura, M. Early administration of Bifidobacterium breve to preterm infants: Randomised controlled trial. *Arch. Dis. Child. Fetal Neonatal Ed.* **1997**, *76*, F101–F107. [CrossRef] [PubMed]

58. Mohan, R.; Koebnick, C.; Schildt, J.; Schmidt, S.; Mueller, M.; Possner, M.; Radke, M.; Blaut, M. Effects of Bifidobacterium lactis Bb12 supplementation on intestinal microbiota of preterm infants: A double-blind, placebo-controlled, randomized study. *J. Clin. Microbiol.* **2006**, *44*, 4025–4031. [CrossRef] [PubMed]

59. Lin, H.-C.; Su, B.-H.; Chen, A.-C.; Lin, T.-W.; Tsai, C.-H.; Yeh, T.-F.; Oh, W. Oral probiotics reduce the incidence and severity of necrotizing enterocolitis in very low birth weight infants. *Pediatrics* **2005**, *115*, 1–4. [PubMed]

60. Braga, T.D.; da Silva, G.A.P.; de Lira, P.I.; de Carvalho Lima, M. Efficacy of Bifidobacterium breve and Lactobacillus casei oral supplementation on necrotizing enterocolitis in very-low-birth-weight preterm infants: A double-blind, randomized, controlled trial. *Am. J. Clin. Nutr.* **2011**, *93*, 81–86. [CrossRef] [PubMed]

61. Stratiki, Z.; Costalos, C.; Sevastiadou, S.; Kastanidou, O.; Skouroliakou, M.; Giakoumatou, A.; Petrohilou, V. The effect of a bifidobacter supplemented bovine milk on intestinal permeability of preterm infants. *Early Hum. Dev.* **2007**, *83*, 575–579. [CrossRef] [PubMed]

62. Manzoni, P.; Rinaldi, M.; Cattani, S.; Pugni, L.; Romeo, M.G.; Messner, H. Bovine lactoferrin supplementation for prevention of late-onset sepsis in very-low-birth-weight neonates. *JAMA* **2009**, *302*, 1421–1428. [CrossRef] [PubMed]

63. Li, Y.; Shimizu, T.; Hosaka, A.; Kaneko, N.; Ohtsuka, Y.; Yamashiro, Y. Effects of bifidobacterium breve supplementation on intestinal flora of low birth weight infants. *Pediatr. Int.* **2004**, *46*, 509–515. [CrossRef] [PubMed]

64. Costeloe, K.; Hardy, P.; Juszczak, E.; Wilks, M.; Millar, M.R. Bifidobacterium breve BBG-001 in very preterm infants: A randomised controlled phase 3 trial. *Lancet* **2015**, *387*, 649–660. [CrossRef]

65. Dutta, S.; Ray, P.; Narang, A. Comparison of stool colonization in premature infants by three dose regimes of a probiotic combination: A randomized controlled trial. *Am. J. Perinatol.* **2015**, *32*, 733–740. [PubMed]

66. Hays, S.; Jacquot, A.; Gauthier, H.; Kempf, C.; Beissel, A.; Pidoux, O.; Jumas-Bilak, E.; Decullier, E.; Lachambre, E.; Beck, L.; et al. Probiotics and growth in preterm infants: A randomized controlled trial, PREMAPRO study. *Clin. Nutr.* **2014**. [CrossRef] [PubMed]

67. Romeo, M.G.; Romeo, D.M.; Trovato, L.; Oliveri, S.; Palermo, F.; Cota, F.; Betta, P. Role of probiotics in the prevention of the enteric colonization by Candida in preterm newborns: Incidence of late-onset sepsis and neurological outcome. *J. Perinatol.* **2011**, *31*, 63–69. [CrossRef] [PubMed]

68. Hikaru, U.; Koichi, S.; Yayoi, S.; Hiromici, S.; Hiroaki, S.; Yoshkazu, O.; Seigo, A.; Satoru, N.; Toshiaki, S.; Yuichiro, Y. Bifidobacteria prevents preterm infants from developing infection and sepsis. *Int. J. Probiotics Prebiotics* **2010**, *5*, 33–36.

69. Patole, S.K.; Keil, A.D.; Nathan, E.; Doherty, D.; Esvaran, M.; Simmer, K.N.; Conway, P. Effect of *Bifidobacterium breve* M-16V supplementation on fecal bifidobacteria in growth restricted very preterm infants -analysis from a randomised trial. *J. Matern. Fetal Neonatal Med.* **2016**. [CrossRef] [PubMed]

70. Tewari, V.V.; Dubey, S.K.; Gupta, G. Bacillus clausii for prevention of late-onset sepsis in preterm infants: A randomized controlled trial. *J. Trop. Pediatr.* **2015**, *61*, 377–385. [CrossRef] [PubMed]
71. Bertino, E.; Giuliani, F.; Baricco, M.; Di Nicola, P.; Peila, C.; Vassia, C.; Chiale, F.; Pirra, A.; Cresi, F.; Martano, C.; Coscia, A. Benefits of donor milk in the feeding of preterm infants. *Early Hum. Dev.* **2013**, *89*, S3–S6. [CrossRef] [PubMed]
72. Zivkovic, A.M.; German, J.B.; Lebrilla, C.B.; Mills, D.A. Human milk glycobiome and its impact on the infant gastrointestinal microbiota. *Proc. Natl. Acad. Sci. USA* **2011**, *108*, 4653–4658. [CrossRef] [PubMed]
73. Bertelli, C.; Pillonel, T.; Torregrossa, A.; Prod'hom, G.; Fischer, C.J.; Greub, G.; Giannoni, E. Bifidobacterium longum bacteremia in preterm infants receiving probiotics. *Clin. Infect. Dis.* **2015**, *60*, 924–927. [CrossRef] [PubMed]

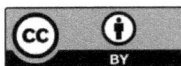

nutrients

MDPI

Review

Ethical Challenges in Infant Feeding Research

Colin Binns [1,*], Mi Kyung Lee [2] and Masaharu Kagawa [3]

[1] John Curtin Distinguished Emeritus Professor of Public Health, Curtin University, Perth 6845, Australia
[2] Department, School of Health Professions, Murdoch University, Perth 6150, Australia;
     m.k.lee@murdoch.edu.au
[3] Institute of Nutrition Sciences, Kagawa Nutrition University, Saitama 350-0214, Japan; mskagawa@eiyo.ac.jp
*   Correspondence: c.binns@curtin.edu.au; Tel.: +61-8-9266-2952

Received: 17 November 2016; Accepted: 9 January 2017; Published: 11 January 2017

Abstract: Infants have a complex set of nutrient requirements to meet the demands of their high metabolic rate, growth, and immunological and cognitive development. Infant nutrition lays the foundation for health throughout life. While infant feeding research is essential, it must be conducted to the highest ethical standards. The objective of this paper is to discuss the implications of developments in infant nutrition for the ethics of infant feeding research and the implications for obtaining informed consent. A search was undertaken of the papers in the medical literature using the PubMed, Science Direct, Web of Knowledge, Proquest, and CINAHL databases. From a total of 9303 papers identified, the full text of 87 articles that contained discussion of issues in consent in infant feeding trials were obtained and read and after further screening 42 papers were included in the results and discussion. Recent developments in infant nutrition of significance to ethics assessment include the improved survival of low birth weight infants, increasing evidence of the value of breastfeeding and evidence of the lifelong importance of infant feeding and development in the first 1000 days of life in chronic disease epidemiology. Informed consent is a difficult issue, but should always include information on the value of preserving breastfeeding options. Project monitoring should be cognisant of the long term implications of growth rates and early life nutrition.

Keywords: Infant feeding; research; ethics; consent; breastfeeding; trials

1. Introduction

Infants are not just small adults. They have a complex set of nutrient requirements and interactions to account for the high metabolic rate, growth, immunological and cognitive development, etc. Infant nutrition lays the foundation for a healthy life. Centuries of observation and research have described the relationship between appropriate nutrition and child growth and survival. In the past century major advances have been made in understanding basic nutrient needs and applying this data to the benefit of humanity and particularly to infants and children. It is appropriate that the collection of original research papers and reviews on infant nutrition is being published in this volume of "Nutrients" at the beginning of the United Nations Decade of Action on Nutrition 2016–2025 [1]. The goals of the decade include increasing rates of exclusive breastfeeding to six months, reducing wasting and stunting and reducing the rates of low birthweight. However the progress in infant nutrition has only served to make the ethical issues around research in this age group even more complex. In this review and discussion paper we will outline progress in infant nutrition and the ethical issues facing infant nutrition researchers and the wider scientific community, particularly the difficulties in defining an adequate consent process.

Progress in Infant Nutrition

This year our world will welcome 131 million new infants, but around 5.5 million will die before reaching the age of five years. While this number is still unacceptably high it is only one fifth of the number dying 50 years ago [2]. The global under-5 years mortality rate has fallen by 53% since 1990 to 42.5 per 1000 live births in 2015, still a heavy burden for families to bear. The difference between regions is great with an under-5 years death rate of 98.7 in West Africa compared to 17.1 in Europe. In some individual countries, such as China, Korea, and Vietnam, the rate of decline has been more rapid than the average improvement for the developing world. In the Republic of Korea the under-5 mortality dropped from 330 per 1000 live births to 3.8 between 1950 and 2014, an unrivalled rate of progress. While the improvement has been rapid, the present rates are still far too high and should be seen as a call to further action to improve infant nutrition and health.

One of the most important factors in declining child mortality has been in the improvements made to the food supply and the scientific understanding of the global food supply and nutrient requirements [3,4]. The history of nutrition is a fascinating journey that encompasses a wide spectrum of scientific disciplines from epidemiology and public health to biochemistry and genomics [5]. Many of the advances in nutrition have been driven by clinical necessity as exploring the causation of deficiency syndromes has led to understanding the roles of specific nutrients. Good examples are vitamin C, vitamin A, and thiamin where clinical syndromes led eventually to the understanding of biochemical pathways [6–9]. During the 19th and 20th centuries the role of nutrients in producing structural, biochemical and behavioural deficiencies was unravelled [10,11]. The bone deformities of children with vitamin D deficiencies have almost gone from the industrialised world and knowledge of iodine and folate has meant that supplementation can reduce the neurological deficiencies they cause [12–16]. In the last half of the 20th century the work of Scrimshaw, the Jelliffes, and Widdowson improved the understanding of the relationships between poor nutrition, growth and infectious diseases, a major factor in the decline of child deaths [17–21].

The simple models of a linear relationship between nutrient intake and function has been replaced with the knowledge that it is often a U-shaped curve that may be made more complex by genomics or interactions with other nutrients [22]. There are many nutrients where a deficiency or an excess of a nutrient, such as vitamin A, can have pathological effects, while amounts consistent with the nutrient reference values (or dietary reference values) result in optimal health outcomes [23,24]. For many infants in vitamin A-deficient regions supplementation has been of considerable benefit. However while vitamin A supplementation in mothers and infants has been widely practised its benefits on a broad scale are still being evaluated [25–28]. Vitamin D supplementation reduces bone pathology in deficient infants and is recommended in breastfed infants in some countries but, again, the longer-term outcomes of country programs are uncertain [29].

As food supplies have improved and utilisation efficiency has increased with the control of infections, excess of energy intake over expenditure has resulted in our current epidemics of obesity. The double burden of nutrition has made nutrition education so much more complex as we grapple with the difficulty of discussing deficient and excess energy intakes within the same country or even within the same family [30].

While probiotics have been in use for many years the complexity of the human microbiome and the relationships of any changes to nutritional status has been the subject of much recent research. In 2007 the National Institutes of Health launched the Human Microbiome Project to stimulate research in an area with potential for human health benefits and much progress has been made in our understanding of this area [31]. Disruption of the human microbiome is now recognised as a potentially important mechanism in the development of obesity in in infants and children [32,33]. The behavioural sciences have always been important in nutrition. New generations are forgetting what "normal" infants and children look like and the image of overweight or obesity has become the new idealised normal [34]. Parents and health professionals have to be re-educated about the importance of growth management as a component of paediatric nutrition.

One of the most far reaching developments has been our understanding of the relationships between early growth and development and later disease, the Developmental Origins of Health and Disease (DOHAD) hypothesis [35–39]. The structure of health care has been segmented by ages and paediatricians never get to see the cardiac problems of middle age. But this can no longer be the case. The way infants and children are managed has implications for lifelong health, leading to the emphasis on the first 1000 days from conception [40]. If antibiotics are used at birth (and in parts of Asia 100% of mothers receive antibiotics during childbirth) or infant formula is given as the first feed it may disrupt the microbiome with potential lifelong implications for conditions such as obesity or diabetes [41–43]. Long term changes to the microbiome may be one mechanism by which early life dietary intake can modify health in later life [44,45].

The development of the knowledge-base of infant nutrition has made many advances in the last decade confirming the supremacy of breastmilk over other sources of infant nutrition. Information is now available on the short- and long-term results of infant feeding decisions making research into infant nutrition very complex as any intervention that diminishes the likelihood of exclusive breastfeeding to six months is likely to be unethical. Once breastfeeding has stopped or been compromised by partial supplementation, it is very difficult, if not impossible, to resume full breastfeeding. The task of those involved in infant nutrition research is to ensure that the highest ethical standards are followed so that breastfeeding is not compromised.

The ethical issues of infant nutrition research extend into the way that human milk substitutes are sometimes marketed [46–49]. Infant nutrition is being subjected to an unprecedented amount of advertising to parents and promotion to health professionals and formula sales are increasing [49–51]. Parents in the newly-rich countries seek to give their children the best possible start in life. Advertisers often distort advances in science. For example if a nutrient is present in breastmilk the formula companies assume that it will be equally beneficial if added as a pure chemical to a manufactured milk mixture. This ignores the complexity of breastmilk which contains thousands of complex chemicals, living cells, and probiotics [52]. The international news media are quick to draw attention to the existence of any contaminants in breastmilk, ignoring the fact that it is still safer and more beneficial than artificial formula. Professionals involved in human lactation and infant formula research should ensure that their work is not misused in marketing in contravention of the WHO Code [53,54].

Several centuries of infant nutrition research can be summarised in two phrases: "Breast is best" and "Babies were born to breastfeed" [55–57]. All international and national infant feeding guidelines reiterate the premier role of breastfeeding, including the benefits of promoting breastmilk for low birth-weight and preterm infants in neonatal intensive care units [58]. The objective of this paper is to discuss the implications of developments in infant nutrition for the ethics of infant feeding research and the implications for obtaining informed consent.

2. Materials and Methods

To compile this narrative review a search of databases for papers relevant to infant feeding research ethics was undertaken for publications in the past 25 years. The databases searched were PubMed, Science Direct, Web of Knowledge, Proquest, and CINAHL using combinations of the keywords "Infant Feeding", "Ethics", "Trial(s)", "Research", "Guidelines", and "Consent". Additional searches were made in several relevant journals including the Journal of Human Lactation, Breastfeeding Medicine, Breastfeeding Review, Public Health Ethics, Hastings Review, New England Medical Journal, JAMA, and Pediatrics. The policy documents from selected regulators in the USA, European Union, Canada, and Australia were reviewed. An additional database of infant feeding studies (5846 entries) continuously compiled by the authors was also used. From the potential 9303 papers identified the full text of 87 articles that contained discussion of issues of consent in infant feeding trials were obtained and read. The papers were further assessed and when issues related to the principles of ethical decisions in infant feeding studies were discussed they have been included in this review. Papers were excluded if they were related to adults, children (not infants), or were not directly related to consent in infant feeding trials. A further 45 papers were excluded in this way, leaving 42 papers that were included in the narrative review.

3. Results and Discussion

3.1. The Ethics of Infant Nutrition Research

In order for infants to benefit from an improved understanding of nutrition and possible improvements in clinical outcomes research must ultimately be conducted on human subjects, and this means research using infants. The ethics of infant nutritional research are becoming more complex. Ethical approval prior to research commencement is a universal requirement for publication and all of the papers describing trials that were read for this review had received ethical approval. The major principles of medical research have evolved over many centuries and include the minimisation of risk to participants, informed consent, confidentiality, and the right to withdrawal without prejudice. The National Health and Medical Research Council (Australia) states that the values in human research include "respect for human beings, research merit and integrity, justice, and beneficence" and these help to shape the research relationship "as one of trust, mutual responsibility and ethical equality" [59]. The practical implementation of these principles has in the past lagged behind the theory and in the 1950s and 1960s, Pappworth (in the UK and Europe), and Beecher on the opposite side of the Atlantic, drew attention to the violations of ethical research practices occurring on a daily basis [60–64]. In the 19th and early 20th centuries, for example, it was convenient to use children in institutions, invariably from lower socio-economic backgrounds for trials, including smallpox and pertussis vaccination and the transmission of hepatitis and HIV [65,66]. There were many further examples found of research that were clearly unethical on which discussions could be based [67]. The widespread discussion of ethical issues in human research that resulted led to a tightening of research ethics requirements for all research involving humans and the publication of the Helsinki Declaration [68]. Human research ethics committees became mandatory and no journal editor today would knowingly publish a study where there was doubt about the ethics of the study. The International Committee of Medical Journal Editors has built on the Helsinki declaration and has standards for the publication of journal articles that include reference to the ethics of research [69,70]. However, these do not have any special reference to research on infants, other than inclusion as one of the especially dependent groups.

More recently attention has been given to research ethics guidelines that specifically include infants [71]. The Early Nutrition Academy (ENA) and the European Society for Pediatric Gastroenterology, Hepatology, and Nutrition (ESPGHAN) have developed a position statement on infant feeding research [72]. The statement recognises the need for special considerations for infants and breastfeeding mothers. They include an important statement on breastfeeding:

"Breast-feeding is recognised as the optimal feeding choice for healthy infants and should be actively protected and promoted. Conditions of studies performed in breastfeeding women and infants, in particular the strategies for subject recruitment and the interaction with parents and health care professionals, should ensure that there is no interference with breastfeeding [72]". The statement reiterates in a useful way, the many established principles of human subject research. However there are several issues of infant feeding research ethics that are not mentioned in detail. These include who can give consent, what does informed consent mean in the context of breastfeeding, and how are potential life-long effects of not-breastfeeding to be accounted for. In a review of the standards for intervention trials on feeding of infants, Woodside et al. recommend that "trial duration must be long enough to show changes in the primary outcome measure" [73]. No papers were found which mentioned monitoring to minimise possible long term adverse outcomes such as early signs of obesity.

3.2. Breastfeeding and Randomised Controlled Trials

In most clinical research randomised controlled trials are ranked higher than cohort studies and other observational research, but the random allocation of a control group to "non-breastfeeding" is not ethical and usually other study designs must be used. Perhaps the best known study of health outcomes of breastfeeding is the PROBIT trial conducted in Belarus which overcame the ethical issues in a unique way [74]. This was a cluster randomised controlled trial of a breastfeeding promotion intervention, which resulted in higher rates of exclusive breastfeeding in the trial hospitals. As well as analysing the results by hospital (intention to treat analysis), analyses were done where the infants who were exclusively breastfed were compared to those who were breastfed, but not exclusively. Individual breastfeeding status was measured at one month and this could have resulted in misclassification if prelacteal, or other early complementary feeds, had been given. The potential misallocation is important as it is now known that the microbiome can be modified by even short-term formula use. This study design overcame the important ethical issues that would have been involved if infants had been directly allocated to breastfeeding and non-breastfeeding groups, but eliminated a true control group of non-breastfed infants. There are also issues of consent to be considered as some individual choice is lost in cluster randomisation [75]. In the case of PROBIT, the trial is really of a breastfeeding education intervention, but it may be the most practical design for an ethical breastfeeding randomized controlled trial (RCT). However the PROBIT data is also analysed as a comparison of longer and more exclusive breastfeeding versus shorter and less exclusive breastfeeding. In this case the allocation to groups at one month may be a critical distinction since even a short duration of breastfeeding could be protective against certain diseases or adverse outcomes, if compared with no breastfeeding at all, as in the Pima studies [76,77].

3.3. Consent in Infant Feeding Trials

Consent in infant feeding studies is a basic ethics consideration. Noel-Weiss discusses studies of lactation and describes how the USA distinguishes between studies that would benefit only the neonate or both the infant and mother (infant mother breastfeeding dyad) [78]. In the former case both parents are required to give consent while the involvement of the mother-infant dyad requires only the consent of the mother [79]. In Canada there are similar requirements and Menon and colleagues have documented the consent process in studies of children in critical care studies [80,81]. One of their concerns was how a lower rate of consent may bias results of the study. The situations they studied raise similar issues to infant feeding studies in neonatal intensive care units and demonstrate the potential conflict between the desire to obtain informed consent and the needs of the research project to obtain a high consent rate to minimise bias.

In Europe the study must comply with usual ethical principles with an emphasis on potential benefit to the participants and community [82,83]. In Australia the National Health and Medical Research Council oversees the implementation of the National Ethical statement which requires the consent on one parent [59]. There is no reference to the situation where parents have separated and a family court (or equivalent judicial body) mandated joint custody agreement is in place.

Consent implies that it is informed and parents must be given adequate and accurate information. There is no dispute; breastfeeding is best for infants. However, is there an inherent right of an infant to be breastfed? There are some medical contraindications to breastfeeding [84]. There are also the rights of the mother to make an informed decision about breastfeeding. In all cases of infant feeding trials the benefit to an infant to be breastfed should not be interfered with. In preterm infants there is benefit to infants who are breastfed, although some may require additional special feeding regimes. Mothers should be encouraged to continue to express breastmilk to maintain their supply, so that breastfeeding can ultimately be commenced (and continued?).

Screening for metabolic disorders and nutritional deficiencies is now routine in neonatal paediatrics. When a new disease or deficiency is added to a routine screening program, commonly referred to as a pilot study this should be considered to be research and ethics approval and informed consent are required [85].

3.4. Beneficence

Beneficence literally means "doing good to others" and in the context of research ethics also includes "non-maleficence", avoiding doing harm [59]. The National Health and Medical Research Council then concludes this section (4.2.5) "the circumstances in which the research is conducted should provide for the child's safety, emotional and psychological security, and wellbeing" and (Section 4.2.13) "Before including a child in research, researchers must establish that there is no reason to believe that such participation is contrary to that child's best interest [59]".

In light of the research into the disadvantages of not breastfeeding and the advantages of breastfeeding the principle of beneficence means that, wherever possible, an infant should receive breastmilk. Ideally the recommendations of the WHO should be followed: "exclusive breastfeeding for six months followed by continued breastfeeding while complementary foods are also given" [56]. Where this is not possible any breastfeeding is better than none [56]. In any infant nutrition research it is important that there be no interference with the mother's intention to breastfeed [86].

3.5. Monitoring of Infant Feeding Trials

The principle of beneficence extends to longer term risk. Fewtrell describes the change in infant nutrition research from just eliminating nutritional deficiencies to promoting optimal health which then requires a longer term perspective. "This approach necessitates identifying appropriate outcome measures for both safety and efficacy, and also introduces the additional challenges of longer-term follow-up of study participants [87]. There is increasing evidence for early life influences, including nutrition, on later health, the developmental origins of health and disease (DOHAD) [35–39]. The rate of infant growth, too slow or too rapid may be related to later health.

Research that involves the use of human milk substitutes in both preterm and term infants has used growth and survival as primary objectives for evaluation. To these should also be added longer term objectives including potential for excessive growth (obesity), alterations to and disruptions of the microbiome and longer term chronic disease outcomes (DOHAD). Infant feeding researchers need to be cognisant of possible life-long implications of their research. For example the development of protocols to promote rapid catch up growth in low birth weight infants may possibly be related to increased adult morbidity [88,89].

Further research into relevant clinical markers of long term outcomes is required, but those known to be significant are growth, growth velocity and, perhaps, microbiome alterations. The role of an independent monitoring committee should include checking the rate of individual growth to ensure that it is not too rapid and would increase risk of obesity or later chronic morbidity. "Catch-up growth" of very low birth weight (VLBW) infants is important to ensure survival, but until more is known about long-term risk. A prudent policy is to aim for growth in the middle centile. It is obviously impractical to monitor infant feeding trials for a lifetime for adverse effects, but monitoring of growth rates and signs of early obesity is important. The role and challenges of monitoring committees in clinical trials has been described by De Mets and colleagues [90]. Monitoring of the impact of nutrition interventions on the microbiome may also become advisable as the available technology improves. The principles of ethics applicable to infant feeding studies will need to be kept under review as nutrition science makes further progress.

4. Conclusions

A balanced approach to infant nutrition is required. Some infants will require an infant formula and some mothers will choose not to breastfeed. There is no doubt that advances in infant nutrition applied to infant formula have substantially improved infant and child health outcomes. It is essential that this research continues within the constraints of research ethics and the public health imperative of continuing to promote breastfeeding. For infant feeding research involving breastmilk substitutes, the strict implementation of research guidelines is required. As knowledge of the benefits of breastfeeding and the importance of early nutrition, growth, and development on later health, this has increased the responsibility of researchers to strictly apply the ethical principles of beneficence by improving the quality of the information given when obtaining informed consent. This particularly includes the provision of information for informed consent that includes the benefits of breastfeeding and the importance of maintaining lactation. The principle of beneficence would seem to require long-term monitoring of growth and metabolic parameters to minimise any risk to long-term health. In the future, the requirements for ethics approval and longer term monitoring of research outcomes are likely to be strengthened as further advances in research occur.

Acknowledgments: No funding was received for this project.

Author Contributions: CWB conceived the project. All authors contributed equally to researching, writing and editing the paper.

Conflicts of Interest: The authors declare no conflict of interest.

References

1. World Health Organization (WHO). United Nations Decade of Action on Nutrition 2016–25. Available online: http://www.Who.Int/nutrition/en/ (accessed on 5 November 2016).
2. United Nations Children's Fund. The State of the World's Children 2016. Available online: https://www.Unicef.Org/sowc2016/ (accessed on 5 November 2016).
3. McKeown, T. Medical issues in historical demography. *Int. J. Epidemiol.* **2005**, *34*, 515–520. [CrossRef] [PubMed]
4. McKeown, T.; Brown, R.G.; Record, R.G. An interpretation of the modern rise of population in Europe. *Popul. Stud. (Camb.)* **1972**, *26*, 345–382. [CrossRef] [PubMed]
5. Carpenter, K.J. A short history of nutritional science: Part 1 (1785–1885). *J. Nutr.* **2003**, *133*, 638–645. [PubMed]
6. Schreier, P.; Binns, C.W.; Högger, P.; Wu, D. It began with citrus. *Nutr. Med.* **2013**, *1*, 5.
7. Khounnorath, S.; Chamberlain, K.; Taylor, A.M.; Soukaloun, D.; Mayxay, M.; Lee, S.J.; Phengdy, B.; Luangxay, K.; Sisouk, K.; Soumphonphakdy, B.; et al. Clinically unapparent infantile thiamin deficiency in Vientiane, Laos. *PLoS Negl. Trop. Dis.* **2011**, *5*, e969. [CrossRef] [PubMed]
8. Barennes, H.; Sengkhamyong, K.; Rene, J.P.; Phimmasane, M. Beriberi (thiamine deficiency) and high infant mortality in northern Laos. *PLoS Negl. Trop. Dis.* **2015**, *9*, e0003581. [CrossRef] [PubMed]
9. Sommer, A. Preventing blindness and saving lives: The centenary of vitamin A. *JAMA Ophthalmol.* **2014**, *132*, 115–117. [CrossRef] [PubMed]
10. Spector, A.A.; Kim, H.Y. Discovery of essential fatty acids. *J. Lipid Res.* **2015**, *56*, 11–21. [CrossRef] [PubMed]
11. Semba, R.D. The discovery of the vitamins. *Int. J. Vitam. Nutr. Res.* **2012**, *82*, 310–315. [CrossRef] [PubMed]
12. National Health and Medical Researh Council. *Iodine Supplementation during Pregnancy and Lactation: Literature Review*; NHMRC: Canberra, Australia, 2009.
13. Brough, L.; Jin, Y.; Shukri, N.H.; Wharemate, Z.R.; Weber, J.L.; Coad, J. Iodine intake and status during pregnancy and lactation before and after government initiatives to improve iodine status, in Palmerston North, New Zealand: A pilot study. *Mater. Child Nutr.* **2015**, *11*, 646–655. [CrossRef] [PubMed]
14. World Health Organisation. *Guideline: Optimal Serum and Red Blood Cell Folate Concentrations in Women of Reproductive Age for Prevention of Neural Tube Defects*; WHO: Geneva, Switzerland, 2015.
15. Angermayr, L.; Clar, C. Iodine supplementation for preventing iodine deficiency disorders in children. *Cochrane Database Syst. Rev.* **2004**. [CrossRef]
16. Wu, T.; Liu, G.J.; Li, P.; Clar, C. Iodised salt for preventing iodine deficiency disorders. *Cochrane Database Syst. Rev.* **2002**. [CrossRef]
17. Scrimshaw, N.S. Historical concepts of interactions, synergism and antagonism between nutrition and infection. *J. Nutr.* **2003**, *133*, 316S–321S. [PubMed]
18. Scrimshaw, N.S.; Taylor, C.E.; Gordon, J.E. Interactions of nutrition and infection. *Monogr. Ser. World Health Organ.* **1968**, *57*, 3–329. [PubMed]
19. Jelliffe, D.B. World trends in infant feeding. *Am. J. Clin. Nutr.* **1976**, *29*, 1227–1237. [PubMed]
20. Jelliffe, D.B.; Jelliffe, E.F. The uniqueness of human milk. An overview. *Am. J. Clin. Nutr.* **1971**, *24*, 1013–1024. [PubMed]

21. Widdowson, E.M. Adventures in nutrition over half a century. *Proc. Nutr. Soc.* **1980**, *39*, 293–306. [CrossRef] [PubMed]
22. Binns, C.; Low, W.Y. Nutrition in the 21st century: Riding the U-shaped wave. *Asia-Pac. J. Public Health/Asia-Pac. Acad. Consort. Public Health* **2014**, *26*, 444–446. [CrossRef] [PubMed]
23. Food and Nutrition Board Institute of Medicine. *Nutrient Recommendations: Dietary Reference Intakes (DRI)*; National Institutes of Health Office of Dietary Supplements: Washington, DC, USA, 2016.
24. National Health and Medical Research Council. *Nutrient Reference Values for Australia and New Zealand Including Recommended Dietary Intakes*; National Health and Medical Research Council (NHMRC): Canberra, Australia, 2006.
25. Darlow, B.A.; Graham, P.J.; Rojas-Reyes, M.X. Vitamin A supplementation to prevent mortality and short- and long-term morbidity in very low birth weight infants. *Cochrane Database Syst. Rev.* **2016**. [CrossRef]
26. Imdad, A.; Ahmed, Z.; Bhutta, Z.A. Vitamin A supplementation for the prevention of morbidity and mortality in infants one to six months of age. *Cochrane Database Syst. Rev.* **2016**, *9*. [CrossRef]
27. Benn, C.S.; Aaby, P.; Arts, R.J.; Jensen, K.J.; Netea, M.G.; Fisker, A.B. An enigma: Why vitamin A supplementation does not always reduce mortality even though vitamin a deficiency is associated with increased mortality. *Int. J. Epidemiol.* **2015**, *44*, 906–918. [CrossRef] [PubMed]
28. Mason, J.; Greiner, T.; Shrimpton, R.; Sanders, D.; Yukich, J. Vitamin A policies need rethinking. *Int. J. Epidemiol.* **2015**, *44*, 283–292. [CrossRef]
29. Kumar, G.T.; Sachdev, H.S.; Chellani, H.; Rehman, A.M.; Singh, V.; Arora, H.; Filteau, S. Effect of weekly vitamin D supplements on mortality, morbidity, and growth of low birthweight term infants in India up to age 6 months: Randomised controlled trial. *BMJ* **2011**, *342*, d2975. [CrossRef] [PubMed]
30. Richter, L.M.; Daelmans, B.; Lombardi, J.; Heymann, J.; Boo, F.L.; Behrman, J.R.; Lu, C.; Lucas, J.E.; Perez-Escamilla, R.; Dua, T.; et al. Investing in the foundation of sustainable development: Pathways to scale up for early childhood development. *Lancet* **2016**, *389*, 103–118. [CrossRef]
31. Proctor, L.M. The human microbiome project in 2011 and beyond. *Cell Host Microbe* **2011**, *10*, 287–291. [CrossRef] [PubMed]
32. Aceti, A.; Gori, D.; Barone, G.; Callegari, M.L.; Fantini, M.P.; Indrio, F.; Maggio, L.; Meneghin, F.; Morelli, L.; Zuccotti, G.; et al. Probiotics and time to achieve full enteral feeding in human milk-fed and formula-fed preterm infants: Systematic review and meta-analysis. *Nutrients* **2016**, 471. [CrossRef] [PubMed]
33. Yoo, J.Y.; Kim, S.S. Probiotics and prebiotics: Present status and future perspectives on metabolic disorders. *Nutrients* **2016**, *8*, 173. [CrossRef] [PubMed]
34. Chen, S.; Binns, C.W.; Maycock, B.; Zhao, Y.; Liu, Y. Chinese mothers' perceptions of their child's weight and obesity status. *Asia Pac. J. Clin. Nutr.* **2014**, *23*, 452–458. [PubMed]
35. Barker, D.; Barker, M.; Fleming, T.; Lampl, M. Developmental biology: Support mothers to secure future public health. *Nature* **2013**, *504*, 209–211. [CrossRef] [PubMed]
36. Barker, D.J. The fetal and infant origins of adult disease. *BMJ* **1990**, *301*, 1111. [CrossRef] [PubMed]
37. Barker, D.J. The origins of the developmental origins theory. *J. Intern. Med.* **2007**, *261*, 412–417. [CrossRef] [PubMed]
38. Eriksson, J.G. Developmental origins of health and disease-from a small body size at birth to epigenetics. *Ann. Med.* **2016**, *48*, 456–467. [CrossRef] [PubMed]
39. Chu, D.M.; Meyer, K.M.; Prince, A.L.; Aagaard, K.M. Impact of maternal nutrition in pregnancy and lactation on offspring gut microbial composition and function. *Gut Microbes* **2016**, *7*, 459–470. [CrossRef] [PubMed]
40. World Health Organization. *Essential Nutrition Actions: Improving Maternal, Newborn, Infant and Young Child Health and Nutrition*; WHO: Geneva, Switzerland, 2016.
41. Cho, I.; Yamanishi, S.; Cox, L.; Methe, B.A.; Zavadil, J.; Li, K.; Gao, Z.; Mahana, D.; Raju, K.; Teitler, I.; et al. Antibiotics in early life alter the murine colonic microbiome and adiposity. *Nature* **2012**, *488*, 621–626. [CrossRef] [PubMed]
42. Azad, M.B.; Konya, T.; Persaud, R.R.; Guttman, D.S.; Chari, R.S.; Field, C.J.; Sears, M.R.; Mandhane, P.J.; Turvey, S.E.; Subbarao, P.; et al. Impact of maternal intrapartum antibiotics, method of birth and breastfeeding on gut microbiota during the first year of life: A prospective cohort study. *BJOG* **2016**, *123*, 983–993. [CrossRef] [PubMed]
43. Bailey, L.C.; Forrest, C.B.; Zhang, P.; Richards, T.M.; Livshits, A.; DeRusso, P.A. Association of antibiotics in infancy with early childhood obesity. *JAMA Pediatr.* **2014**, *168*, 1063–1069. [CrossRef] [PubMed]

44. Beaumont, M.; Goodrich, J.K.; Jackson, M.A.; Yet, I.; Davenport, E.R.; Vieira-Silva, S.; Debelius, J.; Pallister, T.; Mangino, M.; Raes, J.; et al. Heritable components of the human fecal microbiome are associated with visceral fat. *Genome Boil.* **2016**, *17*, 189. [CrossRef] [PubMed]

45. Soderborg, T.K.; Borengasser, S.J.; Barbour, L.A.; Friedman, J.E. Microbial transmission from mothers with obesity or diabetes to infants: An innovative opportunity to interrupt a vicious cycle. *Diabetologia* **2016**, *59*, 895–906. [CrossRef] [PubMed]

46. Binns, C.W.; Lee, M.K.; Tang, L.; Yu, C.; Hokama, T.; Lee, A. Ethical issues in infant feeding after disasters. *Asia-Pac. J. Public Health* **2012**, *24*, 672–680. [CrossRef] [PubMed]

47. Brady, J.P. Marketing breast milk substitutes: Problems and perils throughout the world. *Arch. Dis. Child.* **2012**, *97*, 529–532. [CrossRef] [PubMed]

48. Cattaneo, A.; Pani, P.; Carletti, C.; Guidetti, M.; Mutti, V.; Guidetti, C.; Knowles, A. Advertisements of follow-on formula and their perception by pregnant women and mothers in Italy. *Arch. Dis. Child.* **2015**, *100*, 323–328. [CrossRef] [PubMed]

49. Singh, J.A.; Daar, A.S.; Singer, P.A. Shared principles of ethics for infant and young child nutrition in the developing world. *BMC Public Health* **2010**, *10*, 321. [CrossRef] [PubMed]

50. Rios, R.; Riquelme, H.; Beshlawy, S.E. Prescribing under the influence: The business of breastmilk substitutes. *Soc. Sci.* **2016**, *5*, 53. [CrossRef]

51. Baker, P.; Smith, J.; Salmon, L.; Friel, S.; Kent, G.; Iellamo, A.; Dadhich, J.P.; Renfrew, M.J. Global trends and patterns of commercial milk-based formula sales: Is an unprecedented infant and young child feeding transition underway? *Public Health Nutr.* **2016**, *19*, 2540–2550. [CrossRef] [PubMed]

52. Hassiotou, F.; Beltran, A.; Chetwynd, E.; Stuebe, A.M.; Twigger, A.J.; Metzger, P.; Trengove, N.; Lai, C.T.; Filgueira, L.; Blancafort, P.; et al. Breastmilk is a novel source of stem cells with multilineage differentiation potential. *Stem Cells* **2012**, *30*, 2164–2174. [CrossRef] [PubMed]

53. McInnes, R.J.; Wright, C.; Haq, S.; McGranachan, M. Who's keeping the code? Compliance with the international code for the marketing of breast-milk substitutes in greater Glasgow. *Public Health Nutr.* **2007**, *10*, 719–725. [CrossRef] [PubMed]

54. World Health Organization. *International Code of Marketing of Breast-Milk Substitutes*; WHO: Geneva, Switzerland, 1981.

55. U.S. Department of Health and Human Services. *The Surgeon General's Call to Action to Support Breastfeeding*; Department of Health and Human Services Office of the Surgeon General: Washington, DC, USA, 2011.

56. World Health Organization. *The World Health Organization's Infant Feeding Recommendation*; WHO: Geneva, Switzerland, 2016.

57. Lessen, R.; Kavanagh, K. Position of the academy of nutrition and dietetics: Promoting and supporting breastfeeding. *J. Acad. Nutr. Diet.* **2015**, *115*, 444–449. [CrossRef] [PubMed]

58. Froh, E.B.; Spatz, D.L. An ethical case for the provision of human milk in the NICU. *Adv. Neonatal Care* **2014**, *14*, 269–273. [CrossRef] [PubMed]

59. National Health and Medical Research Council; Australian Research Council; Australian Vice -Chancellors' Committee. *National Statement on Ethical Conduct in Human Research 2007*; NHMRC: Canberra, Australia, 2015.

60. Pappworth, M.H. "Human guinea pigs"—A history. *BMJ* **1990**, *301*, 1456–1460. [CrossRef] [PubMed]

61. Pappworth, M.H. Setting the limits. *World Health* **1976**, *19*, 14–17.

62. Harkness, J.; Lederer, S.E.; Wikler, D. Laying ethical foundations for clinical research. *Bull. World Health Organ.* **2001**, *79*, 365–366. [PubMed]

63. Beecher, H.K. Ethics and clinical research. *N. Engl. J. Med.* **1966**, *274*, 1354–1360. [CrossRef] [PubMed]

64. Jones, D.S.; Grady, C.; Lederer, S.E. "Ethics and clinical research"—The 50th anniversary of beecher's bombshell. *N. Engl. J. Med.* **2016**, *374*, 2393–2398. [CrossRef] [PubMed]

65. Burns, J.P. Research in children. *Crit. Care Med.* **2003**, *31*, S131–136. [CrossRef] [PubMed]

66. Chin, R. Chapter 15-ethics and institutional review board capacity building. In *Global Clinical Trials Playbook*; Academic Press: San Diego, CA, USA, 2012; pp. 175–196.

67. Chadwick, G.L. Historical perspective: Nuremberg, Tuskegee, and the radiation experiments. *J. Int. Assoc. Physicians AIDS Care* **1997**, *3*, 27–28. [PubMed]

68. World Medical Association. Declaration of Helsinki. Recommendations guiding physicians in biomedical research involving human subjects. *JAMA* **1997**, *277*, 925–926.

69. International Committee of Medical Journal Editors. Uniform Requirements for Manuscripts Submitted to Biomedical Journals: Writing and Editing for Biomedical Publication. 2008. Available online: http://www.Icmje.Org/icmje-recommendations.Pdf (accessed on 5 November 2016).

70. International Committee of Medical Journal Editors. Recommendations for the Conduct, Reporting, Editing, and Publication of Scholarly Work in Medical Journals. 2016. Available online: http://www.Icmje.Org/icmje-recommendations.Pdf (accessed on 5 November 2016).

71. McIntosh, N.; Bates, P.; Brykczynska, G.; Dunstan, G.; Goldman, A.; Harvey, D.; Larcher, V.; McCrae, D.; McKinnon, A.; Patton, M.; et al. Guidelines for the ethical conduct of medical research involving children. Royal college of paediatrics, child health: Ethics advisory committee. *Arch. Dis. Child.* **2000**, *82*, 177–182. [PubMed]

72. Koletzko, B.; Benninga, M.A.; Godfrey, K.M.; Hornnes, P.J.; Kolacek, S.; Koletzko, S.; Lentze, M.J.; Mader, S.; McAuliffe, F.M.; Oepkes, D.; et al. Public-private collaboration in clinical research during pregnancy, lactation, and childhood: Joint position statement of the early nutrition academy and the european society for pediatric gastroenterology, hepatology, and nutrition. *J. Pediatr. Gastroenterol. Nutr.* **2014**, *58*, 525–530. [CrossRef] [PubMed]

73. Woodside, J.V.; Koletzko, B.V.; Patterson, C.C.; Welch, R.W. Scientific standards for human intervention trials evaluating health benefits of foods, and their application to infants, children and adolescents. *World Rev. Nutr. Dietet.* **2013**, *108*, 18–31.

74. Kramer, M.S.; Chalmers, B.; Hodnett, E.D.; Sevkovskaya, Z.; Dzikovich, I.; Shapiro, S.; Collet, J.P.; Vanilovich, I.; Mezen, I.; Ducruet, T.; et al. Promotion of breastfeeding intervention trial (PROBIT): A randomized trial in the republic of belarus. *JAMA* **2001**, *285*, 413–420. [CrossRef] [PubMed]

75. McRae, A.D.; Bennett, C.; Brown, J.B.; Weijer, C.; Boruch, R.; Brehaut, J.; Chaudhry, S.; Donner, A.; Eccles, M.; Grimshaw, J.; et al. Researchers' perceptions of ethical challenges in cluster randomized trials: A qualitative analysis. *Trials* **2013**, *14*, 1. [CrossRef] [PubMed]

76. Pettitt, D.J.; Forman, M.R.; Hanson, R.L.; Knowler, W.C.; Bennett, P.H. Breastfeeding and incidence of non-insulin-dependent diabetes mellitus in Pima Indians. *Lancet* **1997**, *350*, 166–168. [CrossRef]

77. Martens, P.J. What do Kramer's baby-friendly hospital initiative probit studies tell us? A review of a decade of research. *J. Hum. Lact.* **2012**, *28*, 335–342. [CrossRef] [PubMed]

78. Noel-Weiss, J.; Woodend, A.K.; Kujawa-Myles, S. Lactation and breastfeeding research studies: Who should provide consent for the neonate? *J. Hum. Lact.* **2010**, *26*, 180–182. [CrossRef] [PubMed]

79. U.S. Department of Health and Human Resources. *Code of Federal Regulations: Title 45-Public Welfare, part 46-Protection of Human Subjects*; U.S. Department of Health and Human Resources: Washington, DC, USA, 2005.

80. Menon, K.; Ward, R.; Canadian Critical Care Trials Group. A study of consent for participation in a non-therapeutic study in the pediatric intensive care population. *J. Med. Ethics* **2014**, *40*, 123–126. [CrossRef] [PubMed]

81. Menon, K.; Ward, R.E.; Gaboury, I.; Thomas, M.; Joffe, A.; Burns, K.; Cook, D. Factors affecting consent in pediatric critical care research. *Intensive Care Med.* **2012**, *38*, 153–159. [CrossRef] [PubMed]

82. Gill, D.; Ethics Working Group of the Confederation of European Specialists in Paediatrics. Ethical principles and operational guidelines for good clinical practice in paediatric research. Recommendations of the ethics working group of the confederation of European specialists in paediatrics (CESP). *Eur. J. Pediatr.* **2004**, *163*, 53–57. [CrossRef] [PubMed]

83. Dalla-Vorgia, P.; Mason, S.; Megone, C.; Allmark, P.; Bratlid, D.; Gill, A.B.; Morrogh, P.; Plomer, A.; Reiter-Theil, S. Overview of European legislation on informed consent for neonatal research. *Arch. Dis. Child. Fetal Neonatal Ed.* **2001**, *84*, F70–73. [CrossRef] [PubMed]

84. World Health Organization. *Acceptable Medical Reasons for Use of Breastmilk Substitutes*; WHO: Geneva, Switzerland, 2009.

85. Botkin, J.R.; Lewis, M.H.; Watson, M.S.; Swoboda, K.J.; Anderson, R.; Berry, S.A.; Bonhomme, N.; Brosco, J.P.; Comeau, A.M.; Goldenberg, A.; et al. Parental permission for pilot newborn screening research: Guidelines from the NBSTRN. *Pediatrics* **2014**, *133*, e410–e417. [CrossRef] [PubMed]

86. Franck, L.S. Research with newborn participants: Doing the right research and doing it right. *J. Perinat. Neonatal Nurs.* **2005**, *19*, 177–186. [CrossRef] [PubMed]

87. Fewtrell, M.S. Clinical safety assessment of infant nutrition. *Ann. Nutr. Metab.* **2012**, *60*, 200–203. [CrossRef] [PubMed]
88. Gat-Yablonski, G.; Phillip, M. Nutritionally-induced catch-up growth. *Nutrients* **2015**, *7*, 517–551. [CrossRef] [PubMed]
89. Brennan, A.M.; Murphy, B.P.; Kiely, M.E. Optimising preterm nutrition: Present and future. *Proc. Nutr. Soc.* **2016**, *75*, 154–161. [CrossRef] [PubMed]
90. DeMets, D.L.; Ellenberg, S.S. Data monitoring committees-expect the unexpected. *N. Engl. J. Med.* **2016**, *375*, 1365–1371. [CrossRef] [PubMed]

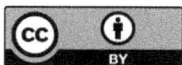

nutrients

MDPI

Review

Early Taste Experiences and Later Food Choices

Valentina De Cosmi [1], Silvia Scaglioni [2] and Carlo Agostoni [3,*

[1]   Valentina De Cosmi Pediatric Intensive Care Unit, Fondazione IRCCS Cà Granda Ospedale Maggiore
     Policlinico, Branch of Medical Statistics, Biometry, and Epidemiology "G. A. Maccacaro",
     Department of Clinical Sciences and Community Health, University of Milan, 20122 Milan, Italy;
     valentina.decosmi@gmail.com
[2]   Silvia Scaglioni Fondazione De Marchi Department of Pediatrics, Fondazione IRCCS Cà Granda Ospedale
     Maggiore Policlinico, 20122 Milan, Italy; silviascaglioni50@gmail.com
[3]   Carlo Agostoni Pediatric Intermediate Care Unit, Fondazione IRCCS Cà Granda Ospedale Maggiore
     Policlinico, Department of Clinical Sciences and Community Health, University of Milan, 20122 Milan, Italy
*   Correspondence: carlo.agostoni@unimi.it; Tel.: +39-025-503-2497

Received: 4 November 2016; Accepted: 24 January 2017; Published: 4 February 2017

Abstract: Background. Nutrition in early life is increasingly considered to be an important factor influencing later health. Food preferences are formed in infancy, are tracked into childhood and beyond, and complementary feeding practices are crucial to prevent obesity later in life. Methods. Through a literature search strategy, we have investigated the role of breastfeeding, of complementary feeding, and the parental and sociocultural factors which contribute to set food preferences early in life. Results. Children are predisposed to prefer high-energy, -sugar, and -salt foods, and in pre-school age to reject new foods (food neophobia). While genetically determined individual differences exist, repeated offering of foods can modify innate preferences. Conclusions. Starting in the prenatal period, a varied exposure through amniotic fluid and repeated experiences with novel flavors during breastfeeding and complementary feeding increase children's willingness to try new foods within a positive social environment.

Keywords: early taste; food preferences; breastfeeding; complementary feeding; feeding strategy; children obesity; food choices

---

1. Introduction

Childhood is a period of very rapid growth and development. In this critical phase, food preferences are formed, are tracked into childhood and beyond, and foundations are laid for a healthy adult life [1]. The characterization of feeding practices is important for the determination of which factors of the early environment can be modified and thus are amenable to intervention. Since early life exposures may contribute to the risk of obesity [2], the topic is highly recognized to be of social and public health interest [3,4].

Infants' and children's eating and activity behaviors are influenced by both intrinsic (genetics, age, gender) and environmental (family, peers, community, and society) factors [5]. These factors are fully displayed in Figure 1.

Firstly, prenatal exposure, and then breastfeeding, have been associated with flavor stimulation and moderately lower childhood obesity risk in many studies [2,6,7]. Later on, the period of complementary feeding is also crucial, both for obesity prevention and for setting taste preferences and infant attitude towards food. Parents act by teaching children in different ways how, what, when, and how much to eat and by transmitting cultural and familial beliefs and practices surrounding food and eating [8]. Parents' influence is significant: it is reflected both by what is on the plate and the context in which it is offered [9].

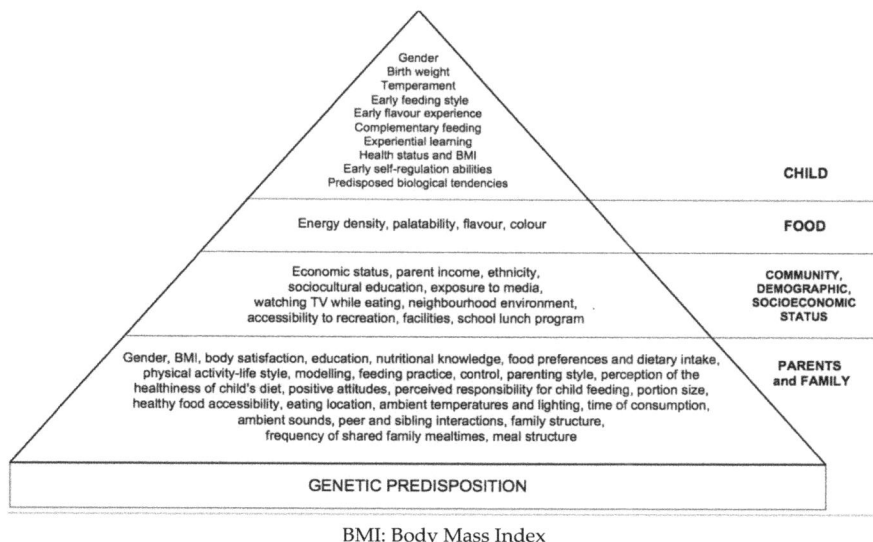

Figure 1. Environmental factors that influence child eating behavior.

Obesity is a burden social disease, linked to lifestyle and food choices changes, characterized by low level of physical activity, high energy density, and free sugar-rich food. As nutritional habits are tracked from infancy to adulthood, we investigated factors inside the child milieu, possibly connected to flavor learning and feeding practices. In particular, we focused on strictly child-related factors. Parental influence is only described in terms of food offering feeding style, while parental modeling is not a topic of our review. We reviewed (1) the biological and social early-life exposures; (2) the prenatal influence of the amniotic fluid; (3) how breast milk and formula may influence taste development; (4) the role of complementary feeding; (5) the parental and sociocultural factors associated with trajectories of health in adulthood.

2. Methods—Literature Search Strategy

Electronic databases (Pubmed, Medline, Embase, Google Scholar) were searched to locate and appraise relevant studies. We carried out the search to identify articles published in English on the relation between children's early taste experiences and their food choices during childhood. Relevant articles published after 2005 and up to August 2016 were identified using the following search words in various combinations. The literature search was not aimed to conduct a systematic review or meta-analysis of all of the available literature on this topic, but to explore the pertinent observations in a period of 10 years. Our work is a narrative review, and search terms were inserted individually and using the booleans AND and OR. The following terms were included in the search strategy: ("early taste experiences" OR "early food preferences") & ("food choices in childhood") OR ("parental feeding practices" OR "parent's feeding strategies" OR "parental modeling") & ("family environmental factors" OR "family eating environments") & ("early exposure" AND "obesity risk" AND "childhood obesity risk factors") & ("amniotic fluid" OR "breast milk" AND "taste AND flavor development") & ("early diet experiences" OR "development of eating habits") & ("Food choices"). More than 5000 references matched the terms of the search, and around 1500 had been published in the past 10 years. The authors selected the articles and assessed the potentially relevant ones.

2.1. Effects of Early Taste Experiences

According to a working hypothesis, the first thousand days of life represent a sensitive period for the development of healthy eating habits, and for this reason, interventions are likely to have a strong impact on health outcomes later during childhood and adulthood. This critical period starts with feeding through the cord during gestation, passes toward oral feeding with milk, and then the complementary feeding begins and the infant discovers a variety of foods and flavors. Humans generally have inborn positive responses to sugar and salt, and negative responses to bitter taste [10]. Genetically determined individual differences also exist, and interact with experience to ensure that children are not genetically restricted to a narrow range of foodstuffs [11]. Children are also predisposed to prefer high-energy foods, to reject new foods, and to learn associations between food flavors and the post-ingestive consequences of eating [12]. This genetic predisposition appears to have evolved over thousands of years when foods—especially those high in energy density—were scarce. Few children—PROP (6-*n*-propylthiouracil) tasters—are sensitive to bitter taste and have higher liking and consumption of bitter foods, such as cruciferous vegetables. Additionally, those children who are unable to taste PROP (nontasters) like and consume more dietary fat and are prone to obesity; thus, genetic variation in the ability to taste bitter compounds may have important implications as a marker for dietary patterns and chronic health in children. The available literature suggests that some children may require additional strategies to accept and consume bitter-tasting fruits and vegetables and that genetic predisposition may be modified by repeated exposures [13,14].

2.2. Amniotic Fluid and Breast Milk

The ability to recognize a variety of flavors involves multiple chemosensory sensations, primarily the sense of taste and smell. Food experiences begin prenatally, since chemosensory systems have an adaptive and evolutionary role and are functional before birth [10]. The exposure to an in utero environment may cause permanent effects on the developing tissue. These effects are referred to as "programming", and are important risk factors for chronic diseases in later adulthood [15].

Children usually prefer foods that are high in sugar and salt over those which are sour and bitter tasting, such as some vegetables. Preferences for salt and the refusal of bitter can be modified early through repeated exposure to flavors in amniotic fluid, mother's milk, and solid foods during complementary feeding. Flavor senses are well developed at birth, and continue to change throughout childhood and adolescence, serving as gatekeepers throughout the life span, controlling whether to accept or reject a foreign substance. Since amniotic fluid and breast milk both reflect to a variable degree the food composition of the maternal diet, a repeated exposure to their flavors increases infants' acceptance of foods [16]. While the knowledge of the influence of the maternal diet on breast milk is mostly indirect [17], the sensory experiences with food flavors in mothers who ate a varied diet may explain why their breastfed children tend to be less picky [18] and more willing to try new foods during childhood [11,19,20]. A cohort study [21] on 1160 mother–infant pairs showed that preponderance of breastfeeding in the first 6 months of life and breastfeeding duration were associated with less maternal restrictive behavior and less pressure to eat. Accordingly, compared with bottle-feeding, breastfeeding may promote maternal feeding styles that are less controlling and more responsive to infant cues of hunger and satiety, thereby allowing infants to develop a greater self-regulation of energy intake [21].

2.3. Formula-Fed Infants

The early flavor experience of formula-fed infants is markedly different from that of breast-fed infants. Exclusively formula-fed children do not benefit from the ever-changing flavor profile of breast milk. Their flavor experience is more monotone and lacks the flavors of the foods of the mother's diet. There are striking differences in flavors among the different types of formulas and brands of formulas, and formula-fed infants learn to prefer the flavors of the formula they are fed and foods containing these flavors [11]. There is a plethora of infant formulas on the market that differ in macronutrient composition. When evaluating the effect of diet composition on growth and health outcomes, it may no longer be appropriate to consider all formula-fed infants as a homogeneous group, because infant formulas may also differ in both fat and carbohydrate composition/structure as well as protein composition, and these differences may in turn affect growth and flavor development [22]. Consequently, it is important to understand the composition of the diet to which breastfeeding is being compared before drawing conclusions. European and US populations reveal an association between breastfeeding and a reduced prevalence of obesity in a meta-analysis; however, in a large randomized controlled trial, there was no effect of breastfeeding on body mass index in later childhood [23]. When infants are fed with a formula that is more similar in protein content to breast milk (lower vs. higher protein), their weight-for-length at 24 months of age does not differ from breastfed infants [24]. Another difference is found in infants consuming protein hydrolysate formula when compared with cow's milk formula: they are satiated sooner and have a less excessive rates of weight gain [25]. The mechanism of this effect is currently unknown, but is hypothesized to be related to differences in free glutamate (which is abundant in human breast milk) [26,27].

2.4. Complementary Feeding and Future Consumption of Fruits and Vegetables during Childhood

Early learning about flavours continues during the complementary feeding period, through the introduction of solids and changing exposures to a variety of new foods. In this peculiar time of the child's life, there is the transition from breast/formula feeding to a complementary solid diet, and infants discover the sensory (texture, taste, and flavour) and nutritional properties (energy density) of the foods that will ultimately compose their adult diet [28]. Being exposed to a variety of foods during the complementary feeding period helps modulate the acceptance of new foods in the first year, whereas exposure in the second year may have a more limited impact [29].

Young children (especially 2–5 years old) exhibit heightened levels of food neophobia during this time. This means that they are unwilling to eat novel foods; it is interpreted as an adaptive behaviour, ensuring children consume foods that are familiar and safe [30].

Distaste—dislike of the sensory characteristics of a food—appears to be the strongest driver of neophobia in young children [31]. Indeed, the two strongest predictors of young children's food preferences are familiarity and sweetness, reflecting unlearned preferences. However, these innate tendencies are paired with a predisposition to learn from early experiences through associative learning and repeated exposure, allowing the child to learn how to accept and prefer the foods that are available within his particular environment [30]. Repeated exposures to a food increase their familiarity, and it is one of the primary determinants of its acceptance. Several studies have shown that a food is consumed more and is judged as more liked by the infant after several offers. For instance, an increase in acceptance of a new green vegetable was observed after at least eight exposures to this food [31]. The effect of repeated exposure is potent enough to increase the acceptance of foods which had been previously identified by the mother as being refused by her infant during the beginning of the complementary feeding, which were most often green vegetables, but also pumpkin [32]. However, despite the efficacy of this mechanism, foods are most often only presented a limited number of times (often less than five times) before the parents decide that the infant dislikes this food [33–35].

Reactions towards new foods differ according to food groups [28]. Lange et al. (2013) asked mothers to report their infant's reactions to new foods at the beginning of complementary feeding, and they found that fruits and vegetables, which are firstly offered to infants, are less accepted than other food groups [36].

A study of de Launzon et al. investigated the long-term effects of early parental feeding practices on fruit and vegetable intake. The study used data from four European cohorts, in which data on fruits and vegetables consumption were assessed with a questionnaire. These cohorts reported different findings. Fruit and vegetable intake in early childhood varied with an average intake of <1 vegetable/day in the Greek EuroPrevall study and >3 vegetables/day in the Generation XXI Birth Cohort. Moreover, longer breastfeeding duration was found in Generation XXI than in the others.

The timing of complementary feeding varied too: complementary foods were introduced mainly between 3 and 4 months of age in ALSPAC (British Avon Longitudinal Study of Parents and Children), at ≈4 months in Generation XXI, and at ≈5 months in Greek Euro-Prevall. In EDEN (French Etude des De'terminants pre et postnatals de la sante' et du de'veloppement de l'Enfant), there was no peak age for introduction to complementary foods.

A concordant positive association between breastfeeding duration and fruit and vegetable intake was found in different cultural contexts, with a longer breastfeeding duration consistently related to higher fruit and vegetable intake in young children, whereas the associations with age of introduction to fruit and vegetable intake were weaker and less consistent [37].

Similarly, 2- to 8-year old children who were breastfed for three or more months were more likely to eat vegetables, as compared to children who were breastfed for a shorter time [28,38]. Taste may impact the acceptance of new foods, since vegetables added with salt or a salty ingredient are more easily accepted [39]. However, this observation should not encourage parents to use salt or salty ingredients, because sodium is not recommended for infants [2,35]. Furthermore, acceptance of green beans appears more difficult than that of carrot, in part due to the difference in the tastes of the two vegetables, since carrots are sweeter than beans [35].

Therefore, the attraction towards new foods in the absence of imprinting and/or learning seems to depend on their tastes and on the sensory properties of foods. At the same time, some individuals may be more sensitive to taste features. In particular, for the sour, sweet, and umami tastes, the individual sensitivity to taste in water solutions at the age of 6 months was predictive of the positive reaction towards foods bearing these tastes [39].

Nicklaus and coworkers in 2014 studied the effect of repeated exposure and of flavor-flavor learning on toddlers' (2–4 years) acceptance of a non-familiar vegetable, and concluded that repeated exposure is the simplest choice to increase vegetable intake in the short and long term [29,35]. The NOURISH is a randomized controlled trial which evaluated an intervention commencing in infancy to provide anticipatory guidance to first-time mothers on a "protective" pattern of complementary feeding practices that were hypothesized to reduce childhood obesity risk. In agreement with the results, investing in early advice on training mothers about responsive complementary feeding can improve maternal feeding practices, and suggests that complementary feeding practices promoting the self-regulation of intake and preference for healthy foods may have positive effects on obesity risk up to 5 years of age [15,40].

Early experiences with nutritious foods and flavour variety may maximize the likelihood that children will choose a healthier diet as they grow, because they like the tastes and the variety of the foods it contains. A recent investigation demonstrated that early exposure to a rotation of vegetable flavours first added to milk and then to cereals increased the intake and liking of these vegetables. Infants assigned to the intervention ate more of the target vegetables in the laboratory and at home than those assigned to the control group [12].

During childhood, the strongest predictors of what foods young children eat are (1) whether they like how the foods taste; (2) how long they were breastfed and whether their mothers ate these foods; and (3) whether they had been eating these foods from an early age [20,41]. During early childhood, infants are more likely to accept new foods, and parents should promote a varied diet and the child's curiosity towards food to reduce neophobia in toddlers [41,42]. After the age of 3–4 years, reported dietary patterns/food habits remained quite stable, further highlighting the importance of getting children on the right track from the initial stages of learning to eat [43].

2.5. Sociocultural and Family Environment

Social support plays a key role starting from birth. Accordingly, the initiation and continuation of breastfeeding and cultural beliefs—shared through kin, friend, and neighbors networks—may serve to promote or limit breastfeeding [2]. Parents create food environments for children's early experiences with food and eating, and also influence their children's eating by modeling their own eating behaviors, taste preferences, and food choices. As children grow and become more independent, familial influences on eating behavior may diminish, and other factors such as those of peers may become more influential [44]. Parents and caregivers play a role in structuring early feeding, which in turn is embedded in the larger micro- and macro-environments that shape parental beliefs, decisions, and practices [45]. It has been shown that forcing a child to eat a particular food will decrease the liking for that food, and that restricting access to particular foods increases rather than decreases preferences [14].

Social influences become increasingly important for the development of food preferences throughout infancy, and may either support or contrast the preferences learned during the prenatal and early postnatal periods [30]. Beauchamp and Moran [46] examined the preference for sweet solutions versus water in approximately 200 infants. At birth, all of the infants preferred sweet solutions to water, but by 6 months of age, the preference for sweetened water was linked to the infants' dietary experience. Infants who were routinely fed sweetened water by their mothers showed a greater preference for it than did infants who were not. Therefore, offering complementary foods without added sugars and salt may be advisable not only for short-term health but also to set the infant's threshold for sweet and salty tastes at lower levels later in life [14]. Neophobic tendencies can be reduced and preferences can be increased by exposing infants and young children repeatedly to novel foods. Children need to be exposed to a novel food between 6 and 15 times before increases in intake and preferences are seen. A recent study found that repeatedly exposing children to a novel food within a positive social environment was especially effective in increasing children's willingness to try it. These findings suggest the importance of both the act of repeatedly exposing children to new foods and the context within which this exposure occurs [30].

3. Discussion

The prevalence of childhood obesity is rising, and multiple studies indicate that most of the risk factors develop during the early phases of life. These factors may range from the prenatal to postnatal period.

Within this context, strategies to successfully promote better acceptance of vegetables should be identified. In spite of a huge body of literature, practical aspects and the results of their application are still poorly understood. This is due to the high complexity related to physiological mechanisms underlying early sensory experiences and the development of sensory preferences.

Breast-fed infants more easily accept a new vegetable, and have higher acceptance of new foods as they are introduced into the infant's diet. There are many factors which influence infants' feeding behaviours; they interact and contribute to the creation of future eating habits. Mothers who consume an array of healthy foods themselves throughout pregnancy and lactation—and subsequently feed their children these foods at the complementary feeding period—can promote healthful eating habits in their children and families. Although a large part of food-preference development occurs during early childhood, food preferences continue to change during adolescence up to adulthood, and the factors that influence these changes become more complex through the years [30]. While it is emphasized that an excessive intake of foods high in salt and refined sugars early in life may be associated with later non-communicable disorders, the individual genetic background and sensitivity to specific nutrients makes it difficult to substantiate a precise cause and effect dose-dependent relationship.

On the other side, food likes and dislikes are learned, and the learning process begins early and depends on biological and sociocultural attitudes.

4. Conclusions

Attention should be paid to the different socio-cultural contexts of eating in future studies, and cohort studies are needed to quantify the effect of early stimulation of taste and preferences. Randomized controlled trials on early diet, focusing on both caregivers and children's behaviours and adjusted for food-related genotype are also essential for understanding how preferences can be modified to promote healthful diets across the life course [30].

Acknowledgments: The authors thank all the members of the Pediatric Unit for their kindly support.

Author Contributions: Valentina De Cosmi, Silvia Scaglioni, Carlo Agostoni contributed equally in the writing and revising of the manuscript.

Conflicts of Interest: The authors declare no conflict of interest.

References

1. Alles, M.S.; Eussen, S.R.; Van Der Beek, E.M. Nutritional challenges and opportunities during the weaning period and in young childhood. *Ann. Nutr. Metab.* **2014**, *64*, 284–293. [CrossRef] [PubMed]
2. Amanda, L.T.; Margaret, E. The critical period of infant feeding for the development of early disparities in obesity. *Soc. Sci. Med.* **2013**. [CrossRef]
3. Benyshek, D.C. The developmental origins of obesity and related health disorders–prenatal and perinatal factors. *Coll. Antropol.* **2007**, *31*, 11–17. [PubMed]
4. Gillman, M.W. Developmental origins of health and disease. *N. Engl. J. Med.* **2005**, *353*, 1848–1850. [CrossRef] [PubMed]
5. Bellows, L.L.; Johnson, S.L.; Davies, P.L.; Anderson, J.; Gavin, W.J.; Boles, R.E. The Colorado LEAP study: Rationale and design of a study to assess the short term longitudinal effectiveness of a preschool nutrition and physical activity program. *BMC Public Health* **2013**. [CrossRef] [PubMed]
6. Arenz, S.; Rückerl, R.; Koletzko, B.; von Kries, R. Breast-feeding and childhood obesity—A systematic review. *Int. J. Obes.* **2004**, *28*, 1247–1256. [CrossRef] [PubMed]
7. Owen, C.G.; Martin, R.M.; Whincup, P.H.; Smith, G.D.; Cook, D.G. Effect of infant feeding on the risk of obesity across the life course: A quantitative review of published evidence. *Pediatrics* **2005**, *115*, 1367–1377. [CrossRef] [PubMed]
8. Birch, L.L.; Fisher, J.O. Development of eating behaviours among children and adolescents. *Pediatrics* **1998**, *101*, 539–549. [PubMed]
9. Mitchell, G.L.; Farrow, C.; Haycraft, E.; Meyer, C. Parental influences on children's eating behaviour and characteristics of successful parent-focussed interventions. *Appetite* **2013**, *60*, 85–94. [CrossRef] [PubMed]
10. Robinson, S.; Fall, C. Infant nutrition and later health: A review of current evidence. *Nutrients* **2012**, *4*, 859–874. [CrossRef] [PubMed]
11. Mennella, J.A. Ontogeny of taste preferences: Basic biology and implications for health. *Am. J. Clin. Nutr.* **2014**, *99*, 704S–711S. [CrossRef] [PubMed]
12. Hetherington, M.M.; Schwartz, C.; Madrelle, J.; Croden, F.; Nekitsing, C.; Vereijken, C.M.J.L.; Weenen, H. A step-by-step introduction to vegetables at the beginning of complementary feeding. The effects of early and repeated exposure. *Appetite* **2015**, *84*, 280–290. [CrossRef] [PubMed]
13. Keller, K.L.; Adise, S. Variation in the Ability to Taste Bitter Thiourea Compounds: Implications for Food Acceptance, Dietary Intake, and Obesity Risk in Children. *Annu. Rev. Nutr.* **2016**, *36*, 157–182. [CrossRef] [PubMed]
14. Agostoni, C.; Decsi, T.; Fewtrell, M.; Goulet, O.; Kolacek, S.; Koletzko, B.; Shamir, R. Complementary feeding: A commentary by the ESPGHAN Committee on Nutrition. *J. Pediatr. Gastroenterol. Nutr.* **2008**, *46*, 99–110. [CrossRef] [PubMed]
15. Muniandy, N.D.; Allotey, P.A.; Soyiri, I.N.; Reidpath, D.D. Complementary feeding and the early origins of obesity risk: A study protocol. *BMJ Open* **2016**. [CrossRef] [PubMed]
16. Forestell, C.A. The Development of Flavor Perception and Acceptance: The Roles of Nature and Nurture. *Nestle Nutr. Inst. Workshop Ser.* **2016**, *85*, 135–143. [PubMed]
17. Bravi, F.; Wiens, F.; Decarli, A.; Dal Pont, A.; Agostoni, C.; Ferraroni, M. Impact of maternal nutrition on breast-milk composition: A systematic review. *Am. J. Clin. Nutr.* **2016**, *104*, 646–662. [CrossRef] [PubMed]
18. Galloway, A.T.; Lee, Y.; Birch, L.L. Predictors and consequences of food neophobia and pickiness in young girls. *J. Am. Diet. Assoc.* **2003**, *103*, 692–698. [CrossRef] [PubMed]
19. Skinner, J.D.; Carruth, B.R.; Bounds, W.; Ziegler, P.; Reidy, K. Do food-related experiences in the first 2 years of life predict dietary variety in school-aged children? *J. Nutr. Educ. Behav.* **2002**, *34*, 310–315. [CrossRef]

20. Cooke, L.J.; Wardle, J.; Gibson, E.L.; Sapochnik, M.; Sheiham, A.; Lawson, M. Demographic, familial and trait predictors of fruit and vegetable consumption by pre-school children. *Public Health Nutr.* **2004**, *7*, 295–302. [CrossRef] [PubMed]

21. Taveras, E.M.; Scanlon, K.S.; Birch, L.; Rifas-Shiman, S.L.; Rich-Edwards, J.W.; Gillman, M.W. Association of breastfeeding with maternal control of infant feeding at age 1 year. *Pediatrics* **2004**, *114*, e577–e583. [CrossRef] [PubMed]

22. Trabulsi, J.C.; Mennella, J.A. Diet, sensitive periods in flavour learning, and growth. *Int. Rev. Psychiatry* **2012**, *24*, 219–230. [CrossRef] [PubMed]

23. Martin, R.M.; Patel, R.; Kramer, M.S.; Guthrie, L.; Vilchuck, K.; Bogdanovich, N.; Rifas-Shiman, S.L. Effects of promoting longer-term and exclusive breastfeeding on adiposity and insulin-like growth factor-I at age 11.5 years: A randomized trial. *JAMA* **2013**, *309*, 1005–1013. [CrossRef] [PubMed]

24. Koletzko, B.; von Kries, R.; Closa, R.; Escribano, J.; Scaglioni, S.; Giovannini, M.; Sengier, A. Lower protein in infant formula is associated with lower weight up to age 2 y: A randomized clinical trial. *Am. J. Clin. Nutr.* **2009**, *89*, 1836–1845. [CrossRef] [PubMed]

25. Mennella, J.A.; Ventura, A.K.; Beauchamp, G.K. Differential growth patterns among healthy infants fed protein hydrolysate or cow-milk formulas. *Pediatrics* **2011**, *127*, 110–118. [CrossRef] [PubMed]

26. Ventura, A.K.; Beauchamp, G.K.; Mennella, J.A. Infant regulation of intake: The effect of free glutamate content in infant formulas. *Am. J. Clin. Nutr.* **2012**, *95*, 875–881. [CrossRef] [PubMed]

27. Larnkjær, A.; Bruun, S.; Pedersen, D.; Zachariassen, G.; Barkholt, V.; Agostoni, C.; Michaelsen, K.F. Free Amino Acids in Human Milk and Associations with Maternal Anthropometry and Infant Growth. *J. Pediatr. Gastroenterol. Nutr.* **2016**, *63*, 374–378. [CrossRef] [PubMed]

28. Nicklaus, S. The role of food experiences during early childhood in food pleasure learning. *Appetite* **2016**, *104*, 3–9. [CrossRef] [PubMed]

29. Bouhlal, S.; Issanchou, S.; Chabanet, C.; Nicklaus, S. 'Just a pinch of salt'. An experimental comparison of the effect of repeated exposure and flavor-flavor learning with salt or spice on vegetable acceptance in toddlers. *Appetite* **2014**, *83*, 209–217. [CrossRef] [PubMed]

30. Ventura, A.K.; Worobey, J. Early influences on the development of food preferences. *Curr. Biol.* **2013**, *23*, R401–R408. [CrossRef] [PubMed]

31. Sullivan, S.A.; Birch, L.L. Infant dietary experience and acceptance of solid foods. *Pediatrics* **1994**, *93*, 271–277. [PubMed]

32. Maier, A.; Chabanet, C.; Schaal, B.; Issanchou, S.; Leathwood, P. Effects of repeated exposure on acceptance of initially disliked vegetables in 7-month old infants. *Food Qual. Preference* **2007**, *18*, 1023–1032. [CrossRef]

33. Carruth, B.R.; Ziegler, P.J.; Gordon, A.; Barr, S.I. Prevalence of picky eaters among infants and toddlers and their caregivers' decisions about offering a new food. *J. Am. Diet. Assoc.* **2004**, *104*, S57–S64. [CrossRef] [PubMed]

34. Maier, A.; Chabanet, C.; Schaal, B.; Leathwood, P.; Issanchou, S. Food-related sensory experience from birth through weaning: Contrasted patterns in two nearby European regions. *Appetite* **2007**, *49*, 429–444. [CrossRef] [PubMed]

35. Nicklaus, S. Complementary Feeding Strategies to Facilitate Acceptance of Fruits and Vegetables: A Narrative Review of the Literature. *Int. J. Environ. Res. Public Health* **2016**. [CrossRef] [PubMed]

36. Lange, C.; Visalli, M.; Jacob, S.; Chabanet, C.; Schlich, P.; Nicklaus, S. Maternal feeding practices during the first year and their impact on infants' acceptance of complementary food. *Food Qual. Preference* **2013**, *29*, 89–98. [CrossRef]

37. De Lauzon-Guillain, B.; Jones, L.; Oliveira, A.; Moschonis, G.; Betoko, A.; Lopes, C.; Charles, M.A. The influence of early feeding practices on fruit and vegetable intake among preschool children in 4 European birth cohorts. *Am. J. Clin. Nutr.* **2013**, *98*, 804–812. [CrossRef] [PubMed]

38. Wadhera, D.; Phillips, E.D.C.; Wilkie, L.M. Teaching children to like and eat vegetables. *Appetite* **2015**, *93*, 75–84. [CrossRef] [PubMed]

39. Schwartz, C.; Chabanet, C.; Lange, C.; Issanchou, S.; Nicklaus, S. The role of taste in food acceptance at the beginning of complementary feeding. *Physiol. Behav.* **2011**, *104*, 646–652. [CrossRef] [PubMed]

40. Daniels, L.A.; Mallan, K.M.; Nicholson, J.M.; Thorpe, K.; Nambiar, S.; Mauch, C.E.; Magarey, A. An early feeding practices intervention for obesity prevention. *Pediatrics* **2015**, *136*, e40–e49. [CrossRef] [PubMed]

41. Northstone, K.; Emmett, P.M. Are dietary patterns stable throughout early and mid-childhood? A birth cohort study. *Br. J. Nutr.* **2008**, *100*, 1069–1076. [CrossRef] [PubMed]
42. Skinner, J.D.; Carruth, B.R.; Bounds, W.; Ziegler, P.J. Children's food preferences: A longitudinal analysis. *J. Am. Diet. Assoc.* **2002**, *102*, 1638–1647. [CrossRef]
43. Singer, M.R.; Moore, L.L.; Garrahie, E.J.; Ellison, R.C. The tracking of nutrient intake in young children: The Framingham Children's Study. *Am. J. Public Health* **1995**, *85*, 1673–1677. [CrossRef] [PubMed]
44. Kral, T.V.; Rauh, E.M. Eating behaviors of children in the context of their family environment. *Physiol. Behav.* **2010**, *100*, 567–573. [CrossRef] [PubMed]
45. Savage, J.S.; Fisher, J.O.; Birch, L.L. Parental influence on eating behavior: Conception to adolescence. *J. Law Med. Ethics* **2007**, *35*, 22–34. [CrossRef] [PubMed]
46. Mennella, J.A.; Kennedy, J.M.; Beauchamp, G.K. Vegetable acceptance by infants: Effects of formula flavors. *Early Hum. Dev.* **2006**, *82*, 463–468. [CrossRef] [PubMed]

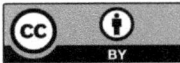

nutrients

MDPI

Review

The Essentiality of Arachidonic Acid in Infant Development

Kevin B. Hadley [1], Alan S. Ryan [2,*], Stewart Forsyth [3], Sheila Gautier [1] and Norman Salem Jr. [1]

[1] DSM Nutritional Products, 6480 Dobbin Road, Columbia, MD 21045, USA; kevin.hadley@dsm.com (K.B.H.); sheila.gautier@dsm.com (S.G.); norman.salem@dsm.com (N.S.Jr.)

[2] Clinical Research Consulting, 9809 Halston Manor, Boynton Beach, FL 33473, USA

[3] School of Medicine, Dentistry & Nursing, University of Dundee, Ninewells Hospital and Medical School, Dundee, UK; stewartforsyth@btinternet.com

* Correspondence: alan_s_ryan@yahoo.com; Tel.: +1-857-488-0512

Received: 17 February 2016; Accepted: 5 April 2016; Published: 12 April 2016

Abstract: Arachidonic acid (ARA, 20:4n-6) is an n-6 polyunsaturated 20-carbon fatty acid formed by the biosynthesis from linoleic acid (LA, 18:2n-6). This review considers the essential role that ARA plays in infant development. ARA is always present in human milk at a relatively fixed level and is accumulated in tissues throughout the body where it serves several important functions. Without the provision of preformed ARA in human milk or infant formula the growing infant cannot maintain ARA levels from synthetic pathways alone that are sufficient to meet metabolic demand. During late infancy and early childhood the amount of dietary ARA provided by solid foods is low. ARA serves as a precursor to leukotrienes, prostaglandins, and thromboxanes, collectively known as eicosanoids which are important for immunity and immune response. There is strong evidence based on animal and human studies that ARA is critical for infant growth, brain development, and health. These studies also demonstrate the importance of balancing the amounts of ARA and DHA as too much DHA may suppress the benefits provided by ARA. Both ARA and DHA have been added to infant formulas and follow-on formulas for more than two decades. The amounts and ratios of ARA and DHA needed in infant formula are discussed based on an in depth review of the available scientific evidence.

Keywords: arachidonic acid; docosahexaenoic acid; infant formula; growth; human milk; long-chain polyunsaturated fatty acids

1. Introduction

During the first year of life, infants have special nutritional requirements to maintain a healthy body and support rapid growth and development. Human milk is typically the sole source of nutrition that must supply the infant with appropriate amounts of energy and nutrients. The long-chain polyunsaturated fatty acids (LCPUFA), docosahexaenoic acid (DHA, 22:6n-3) and arachidonic acid (ARA, 20:4n-6) are always present in human milk. These fatty acids play key roles in the structure and function of human tissues, immune function, and brain and retinal development during gestation and infancy [1,2]. Although breastfeeding is considered the ideal way to nourish infants, recent nutrition surveys report that the majority of infants in developed countries receive at least some infant formula during the first year of life [3,4].

Both ARA and DHA have been added to infant formulas in the United States since 2001, although supplementation began in Europe much earlier. Most infant formulas contain 0.2% to 0.4% of total fatty acids as DHA and between 0.35% and 0.7% of total fatty acids as ARA based on worldwide averages of DHA and ARA content in human milk [5] and the recommendations from a number of international expert groups [6–9]. Thus, all commercially available infant formulas contain preformed

ARA at levels equal to or higher than the DHA content in order to maintain adequate DHA and ARA status in non-breastfed infants.

Both α-linolenic acid (ALA, 18:3*n*-3) and linoleic acid (LA, 18:2*n*-6) are regarded as nutritionally essential fatty acids [10]. However, as Lauritzen *et al.* [10] point out, all classic signs of essential fatty acid (EFA) deficiency can be completely reversed by the administration of *n*-6 fatty acids alone, particularly ARA. With respect to infants, the presence of a relatively fixed level of preformed ARA in human milk and the active accumulation of ARA by tissues throughout the body support the concept of the essentiality of ARA. Previously, a description of the essentiality of ARA during infancy has not been considered in detail, although a brief outline of the essentiality of *n*-6 and *n*-3 polyunsaturated fatty acids was presented by Lauritzen *et al.* [10] in 2001.

The purpose of this paper is to review the essentiality of ARA for infant growth and development. We consider both animal models and human studies of ARA. We describe: (1) ARA accumulation and function in brain and tissues; (2) ARA content in human milk and in various tissues, including rates of accretion during gestation and early infancy; (3) the structure and biosynthesis of ARA from LA and its role as a precursor to leukotrienes, prostaglandins, and thromboxanes, collectively known as eicosanoids; (4) dietary intakes of ARA during late infancy and early childhood when non-breast milk food items are introduced into the diet; (5) immune system development and the dual role of PGE_2 and its receptors in modulating the inflammatory response during infancy; (6) bone metabolism and growth; (7) regulation of cardiac function; (8) consequences of ARA deficiency; (9) the importance of ARA for optimal brain and central nervous system development; (10) the history, reasons for, and nutritional effects of adding both DHA and ARA to infant formulas, with an emphasis on the effects of ARA; (11) the importance of ARA in infant health; and (12) the regulatory requirements for ARA and DHA in infant formulas. Based on a detailed review of the scientific literature presented herein, recommendations for dietary intakes ARA during infancy are provided.

2. ARA Accumulation and Function in Brain and Tissue

Over the last decade, there has been increased understanding of the molecular roles that the *n*-3 and *n*-6 PUFA play in brain and cellular function. The variety of functions shown to be related to ARA indicates its importance and essentiality in the metabolic chain of events leading to brain structural lipid development, signaling, and many basic cellular functions.

ARA is indispensable for brain growth where it plays an important role in cell division and signaling [11]. The brain in mammals consists of 60% fat, which requires DHA and ARA for its growth and function [12]. Across different species of mammals there is little variation in DHA and ARA composition of the brain. ARA is one of the most abundant fatty acids in the brain, and compared with DHA, ARA is present in similar quantities [13,14]. The two fatty acids account for approximately ~25% of its total fatty acid content predominately in the form of phospholipids and thus are major structural components of neural cellular membranes.

ARA rapidly accumulates in the brain during development [1,14,15] which takes place from the beginning of the third trimester of gestation up to about 2 years of age [16] (Figure 1). As shown in brain kinetics in fetal baboons, [17] in addition to maternal preformed ARA, LA may be transported across the blood-brain barrier despite its very low content within brain lipids. The brain has an active desaturation/elongation system that converts LA to ARA [17]. ARA activity is higher in brain than in other organs such as the liver. However, the conversion of LA to ARA is low (see below).

The maximum rate of brain growth is primarily associated with myelination [14]. In animal models, approximately 50% of the adult amounts of ARA and DHA accumulate in rat brain during the period before myelination and at 15 days after birth when myelination has just started [14]. Diets low in LCPUFA adversely affect the development of the myelin lipids needed early in brain development [14].

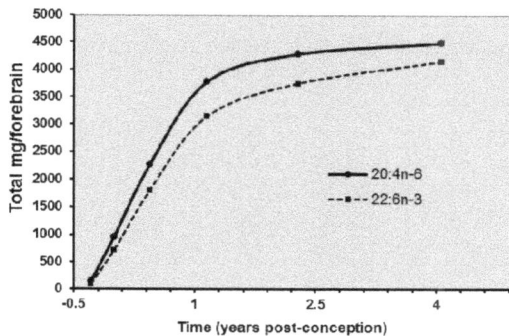

Figure 1. Long-chain polyunsaturated fatty acids (LCPUFA) accretion in the human brain during perinatal development (Data from Martinez [15]).

ARA has several functions in the brain. ARA mediates neuronal firing [18], signaling [19], and long-term potentiation [20]. ARA also helps maintain membrane order and hippocampal plasticity [21], defends the brain against oxidative stress in the hippocampus by activating the peroxisome proliferator-activated receptor gamma (PPARγ), and aids in the synthesis of new protein in tissue [22].

A potentially important aspect of ARA metabolism *in vivo* is its function as an immediate precursor for adrenic acid (22:4n-6) [23]. Adrenic acid is the third most abundant PUFA in the brain that is found in large quantities in myelin lipids, particularly in phosphatidylethanolamine (PE) [1]. Rapid accumulation of adrenic acid, like ARA, occurs during the early post-natal period of the brain growth spurt in infants. The conversion of ARA to adrenic acid may represent an important pathway for ARA utilization in infants in order to meet the rapid increase of adrenic acid needed for neural tissue development.

Using a single dose of U-^{13}C-labeled ARA to investigate preformed ARA utilization in baboon neonates, Wijendran *et al.* [23] reported that a major portion of ARA consumed (79%–93%) was accumulated as ARA in tissue lipids, consistent with its primary function as a principal constituent of membrane lipids. Approximately 5% to 16% of ARA was converted to adrenic acid. Based on tracer data, net accretion of ARA and adrenic acid during the first 4 weeks of age in the neonate baboon brain was 17% and 8%, respectively, corresponding to efficiencies (*i.e.*, percentage of dose recovered in brain) of 0.48% and 0.54% of dietary levels, respectively.

To determine the effects that differing DHA to ARA ratios have on tissue fatty acids, twelve-week-old full term baboons were randomized to one of three diets: control (no DHA or ARA), moderate (0.33% DHA, 0.67% ARA) and high LCPUFA (1.00% DHA, 0.67% ARA) [24]. In all groups, DHA levels increased significantly in liver, heart, plasma and in the central nervous system (CNS) regions (precentral gyrus, frontal cortex, inferior and superior colliculi, globus pallidus, and caudate). The formula with the highest level of DHA significantly reduced ARA levels in two areas of the brain (superior colliculus and globus pallidus), indicating its competition with ARA and the importance of a proper balance of DHA to ARA.

Phosphatidylcholine (PC) is a lipid class that is a major component of most intracellular membranes [25]. Some intracellular lipid bilayers include PC containing ARA (ARA-PC). ARA-PC functions as a retrograde messenger in long-term potentiation of synapses in the hippocampus CA1 region [26] and is involved in migration of neurons in the cerebral cortex [27].

Using imaging mass spectrometry, Yang *et al.* [25] characterized the distribution of ARA-PC within cultured neurons of the superior cervical ganglia and found an increasing gradient of ARA-PC along the proximodistal axonal axis that may provide a source for free ARA release [25]. Released free ARA is known to activate protein kinases and ion channels, inhibit neurotransmitter uptake, and enhance synaptic transmission [11]. Free ARA therefore modulates neuronal excitability. As ARA mediates intracellular signaling the concentration of free ARA must be maintained at precise levels within the cells. A higher concentration of ARA-PC near the axon terminal might provide a timely source of ARA when needed during the activated period [25].

ARA also is responsible for the activation of syntaxin-3 (STX-3), a plasma membrane protein involved in the growth and repair of neurites [28]. Growth of neurite processes from the cell body is a critical step in neuronal development. STX-3 serves as a single effector molecule and direct target for ARA [28]. Neurite growth closely correlates with the ability of ARA to activate STX-3 in membrane expansion at growth cones [28].

ARA also enhances the engagement of STX-3 with the fusogenic soluble N-ethylmaleimide-sensitive factor attachment protein receptors (SNARE complex), proteins that form a ternary complex that drives exocytosis [29]. In the brain, at the neuromuscular junction, and in endocrine organs, a set of three SNARE proteins has a primary role in producing fusion of vesicular and plasma membranes. The formation of this SNARE complex drives membrane fusion which leads to the release of vesicular cargo into the extracellular spaces [29]. Darios and colleagues [29] report that α-synuclein, a synaptic modulatory protein implicated in the development of Parkinson disease, can sequester ARA and thereby block the activation of the SNARE complex. This finding underlines the importance of ARA for the regulation of synaptic transmission and transport.

Detergent resistant microdomains, also referred to as lipid rafts, are specialized regions within plasma membranes [30]. These microdomains serve as platforms for biomechanical interactions between the lipid and protein components of signal transduction pathways [30–32]. The outer leaflet of lipid rafts is highly enriched with glycol-sphingolipids and cholesterol [32]. The inner, or cytosol facing leaflet is enriched with alkenyl forms of PE which have been termed plasmenylethanolamine. Electrospray ionization/mass spectrometric analysis has shown that the ARA-containing plasmenylethanolamine represents as much as 50% of the phospholipids of the cytosolic leaflet [31]. This is consistent with a role of PE as an important source of ARA within the cell.

Stearoyl-2-arachidonoyl is a highly abundant species of phosphatidylinositol (PI) found in the phosphorylated forms of PI, the phosphoinositides [33–38]. In addition to serving as a substrate for phospholipase C to produce inositol-triphosphate and diacylglycerol, phosphoinositides serve important biochemical functions including lipid signaling, cell signaling and membrane trafficking. Phosphoinositides perform these roles in part by serving as adaptors for protein-protein and protein-membrane interactions in order to facilitate and/or regulate G-receptor protein activity and signal transduction, and trafficking of various metabolites such as cholesterol or calcium, or other ions, between cellular compartments [39–43]. These biochemical functions of ARA demonstrate its importance for cell signaling, trafficking and regulation of spatial-temporal interactions between cellular structures.

3. Levels of ARA in Human Milk, Brain, and Tissues

Fat is a critical component of human milk that provides energy and nutrients needed for the development of the CNS [10]. DHA and ARA are the principal LCPUFA found in human milk. The synthesis of DHA and ARA is limited in infants [5] and both DHA and ARA must be obtained from dietary sources. Amounts of DHA and ARA in human milk tend to vary by diet, nutritional status, and other factors [5]. Based on data from 65 studies of human milk from 2474 women, the mean concentration of ARA (by weight) was 0.47% ± 0.13% (range 0.24% to 1.0%) whereas the mean concentration of DHA was 0.32% ± 0.22% (range 0.06% to 1.4%) [5]. The DHA concentration in human milk is lower and more variable than ARA. The level of ARA in human milk is much more stable. The relatively stable content of ARA in human milk is biologically important because it provides preformed ARA consistently at a time when brain growth and development is most critical. The majority of ARA in human milk does not derive from dietary LA but rather from maternal stores of ARA [44]. The correlation between DHA and ARA is low, which may reflect a higher degree of variability in the ratio of DHA to ARA in individual human milk samples [5].

The composition of the brain is dominated by ARA and DHA [45]. During pregnancy, both ARA and DHA are preferentially transferred across the placenta [46] and sequestered in the developing brain from the earliest phases of its growth. After birth, human milk provides both DHA and ARA to the breastfed infant [47] with a rapid rise towards adult levels of DHA and ARA in the brain within the first two years of life [48]. ARA is found at a level comparable to that of DHA in neural membranes, particularly those of the brain [49].

Based on estimated total body content of ARA from fetal organ weights during the last trimester of pregnancy and early infancy the relative amount of brain ARA decreases, but because of brain growth the absolute amount of ARA increases [50]. In fact, the absolute amount of ARA increases in all organs with increasing gestational age while the relative contribution (g per 100 g fatty acids; g %) decreases [50]. At 25 weeks gestation, the whole fetal body contains about 1.1 g ARA which increases to 4.2 g ARA at 35 weeks gestation. A full-term infant (3500 g) has about 7.6 g of ARA. The accretion rate of ARA is estimated to be 6.1 mg/day during the first 25 weeks and increases to 95.2 mg/day by 35–40 weeks gestation. The fetal accretion rate for ARA is 2-fold that of DHA [50]. Most of the bodily ARA at 25 and 40 weeks is located in skeletal muscle, adipose tissue and the brain, in that order [50].

In human infant central nervous tissue (cerebral cortex and retina) ARA comprises approximately 10%–12% of total fatty acids [49]. The amount of ARA in central nervous tissue appears to be influenced to a greater extent by postnatal age than by dietary ARA supply [49]. Samples of frontal cerebral cortex obtained from 58 human autopsies (mean age 40 ± 29 years) indicated that the relative levels of PUFA expressed as a percentage of total fatty acids generally decrease with age with the exception of DHA [51].

The distribution of *n*-6 and *n*-3 PUFA was determined in various viscera and tissues within the whole body of rats fed a diet containing 10 wt % fat (15% linoleate and 3% α-linolenate) until 7 weeks of age when they were sacrificed [52] (Figure 2).

The rat whole body was comprised of primarily saturated fatty acids (48.4% of total fatty acids) while the monounsaturated fatty acids were present in the second greatest amount (34.8%). The total amount of *n*-6 PUFA was 12.0% and was more than 5-fold greater than the total *n*-3 PUFA. The *n*-6 PUFA with the highest content was LA (10.1%) followed by ARA (1.4%). ARA was the major PUFA in nearly every tissue and was the major PUFA in most internal organs. The tissues with the highest content of ARA were plasma (25.3%) followed by kidney, red blood cells (RBC), and spleen, ranging from 18.7% to 23.5%. Brown adipose, white adipose and the eye contained very low amounts of ARA (<1.0%). For each compartment in the rat body, the total ARA/organ was highest for muscle, then liver, adipose, and carcass. In terms of fatty acid composition expressed as a percentage, ARA was highest in the circulation, kidney, and the spleen.

As shown in rat pups, when tissues are deprived of *n*-3 PUFA, the accretion of ARA from LA is increased and ARA is further metabolized to produce docosapentaenoic acid (22:5*n*-6, DPA) which accumulates in tissues [53], particularly in the nervous system. The accumulated DPA in turn reciprocally replaces lost DHA in tissue [53].

Pigs fed varying amounts of ARA and DHA levels after birth and then sacrificed at day 28 showed that dietary ARA had little effect on tissue DHA accretion [54], but heart tissue was particularly sensitive to ARA intake. These observations are particularly notable because the pigs were fed ARA at a level of 0.53% of total fatty acids. This level is slightly above the worldwide ARA mean in human milk and 0.67% of total fatty acids is the level currently added to many infant formulas and is near the high end of human milk ARA levels [5]. Neonatal pigs serve as a practical biomedical model of human infant development due to their similar metabolic responses, genetics of the fatty acid desaturases, and rates of perinatal brain growth [5]. The importance of ARA for the heart is discussed in greater detail in Section 8.

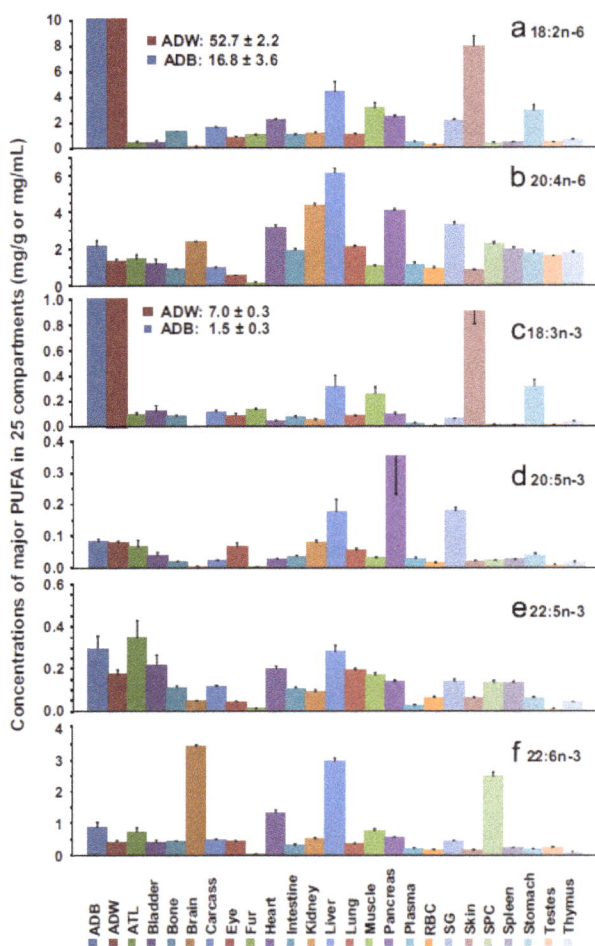

Figure 2. Distribution of fatty acids in 25 different tissue compartments in young male rats. Abbreviations: ATL, adrenal gland, thyroid gland, mandibular gland, and lymph nodes; RBC, red blood cell; SG, salivary gland; ADB, brown adipose tissue; ADW, white adipose tissue (from Salem *et al.* [52]).

4. ARA Biosynthesis and Metabolism

ARA is an *n*-6 polyunsaturated 20-carbon essential fatty acid formed by biosynthesis from LA [10]. ARA is a precursor to leukotrienes, prostaglandins, and thromboxanes, collectively known as eicosanoids [55,56]. ARA is found in membrane phospholipids throughout the body and is particularly abundant in the brain, muscles and liver. The metabolic pathways of the *n*-6 series and *n*-3 series are shown in Figure 3.

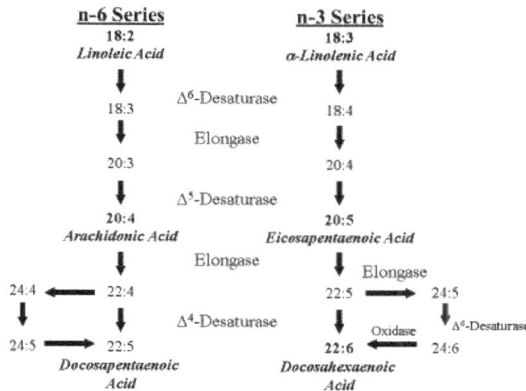

Figure 3. Metabolic pathways of linoleic and α-linolenic acid (Adapted from Lauritzen *et al.* [10]).

The use of stable isotope labelled fatty acids to investigate essential fatty acid metabolism was pioneered in the 1930s with the first identifiable study done by Schoenheimer and Rittenberg [57]. Several decades later, Nichaman *et al.* [58] gave four adult subjects ^{14}C-labeled LA and found a very small but significant incorporation into plasma phospholipid ARA acid based on responses in gas-radiochromatography. Similarly, ^{14}C-labeled LA was shown to be converted to ^{14}C-ARA in human fetal liver microsomes, *in vitro* [59]. El Boustani *et al.* [60] studied the conversion of deuterated dihommo-gamma linoleic acid (20:3*n*-6, DGLA) into ARA in plasma phospholipid and triglyceride fractions *in vivo* in diabetic patients. After a 2 g isotope ingestion, a maximum of 5 mg of labelled ARA/L was observed in plasma. The authors stated that "this was consistent with the very low Δ5 desaturase activity observed *in vitro* in the human liver".

In the 1980s, Emken and colleagues [61] developed stable isotope technology in adult humans. In an early study of deuterated-LA metabolism *in vivo*, when a large dose of over 14 g of isotope was given, the authors concluded that "interconversion products such as deuterium-labeled ... 20:3 and 20:4 were not detected in any of the lipid classes" [62]. They calculated that a conversion of as little as 0.00012% would have been detectable. The absence of any LA metabolism to ARA was confirmed in a subsequent study even where labelled-ALA was clearly incorporated into EPA and DHA [61].

In 1995, Demmelmair *et al.* [63] used natural abundance ^{13}C measurements in corn oil fed infants to demonstrate LA conversion to ARA. They observed conversion but concluded that "the activity of the enzyme system seems to be limited". Shortly afterwards, the conversion of LA to ARA was conclusively and directly demonstrated in newborn infants using stable isotope technology by Salem *et al.* [64]. The D5-LA was used together with a highly sensitive NCI GC/MS method after PFB derivatization [65]. With this new methodology, the deuterated fatty acid could be chromatographically separated from its corresponding endogenous analogue and so the signal of the stable isotope labeled metabolite would not be obscured by the much larger signal from the endogenous fatty acid. A crude estimate was made of the net accretion of ARA over the six day period of the study which was 53 mg, or about 9 mg ARA/day. Such estimates of "net synthesis" treated the organism as if the synthesis was occurring within the bloodstream and this is clearly not the case. In addition, what was being measured is the synthesis, minus the catabolism, plus the transport/release into a compartment such as the bloodstream where it can be sampled. Carnielli *et al.* [66] used a similar methodology to confirm the conversion of LA to ARA in very low birth-weight infants using ^{13}C-labeled LA.

Pawlosky *et al.* [67] studied stable isotope labeled LA and DGLA metabolism to ARA in 10 newborn human infants within the first week of life *in vivo* and performed compartmental modeling to provide an estimate of the synthetic rates. Formula and breast milk intakes were considered so that ARA and other PUFA intake could be estimated; LA and ARA intake was estimated at 3 g/kg/day and

2.8 mg/kg/day, respectively. They concluded that "the mean daily rate of synthesis and turnover of 20:4*n*-6 in plasma of infants were estimated to be from 0.06 to 2.1 mg/day ... and from 0 to 51 mg/day (mean 10.2)" [67]. They went on to say that "such rates of synthesis are incapable of sustaining plasma 20:4*n*-6 concentrations in nearly all of these subjects necessitating an intake of ~4 mg/kg/day from either human milk or a supplement". The fractional rate of conversion (FRC) observed in this study was 2.7% which is even more than that observed by Sauerwald *et al.* [68] who calculated an FSR of 0.4% to 1.1% depending upon the ALA content of the formula.

Carnielli and colleagues in 2007 [69] studied LA conversion to ARA using natural abundance ^{13}C measurements in preterm infants *in vivo* in those fed LCPUFA or no LCPUFA-containing formulas at 1, 3 and 7 months of age. These authors show that ARA synthesis is decreasing with age as it fell from 26.7 mg/kg/day to 14.4 mg/kg/day and then to 11.6 mg/kg/day from 1 to 3 to 7 months of age, respectively. It seems that the endogenous synthesis rate in these infants was inadequate as the ARA plasma phospholipid level fell from 5.6 mol% in the ARA fed group to 1.9 mol% in the no ARA group, a 66% drop. This underlines the inadequacy of LA alone as a source of ARA and the requirement for preformed ARA in the infant diet if blood levels of ARA are to be maintained similar to those in breastfed infants.

5. Global Intake of ARA in Early Life

In contrast to *n*-3 LCPUFA, there are few data relating to dietary intakes of *n*-6 LCPUFA in early life. In relation to dietary ARA, many regulatory agencies have tended to assume that beyond the age of 6 months, the endogenous synthesis of ARA will meet the needs of infants and young children during this period of rapid growth and development [70,71]. However, studies have shown that the endogenous synthesis of both DHA and ARA may be insufficient with evidence of blood and tissue concentrations decreasing after birth if there is not an exogenous supply [49,72].

The World Health Organization (WHO) [73,74] and the American Academy of Pediatrics [75] recommend that infants should be exclusively breastfed for the first six months of life to achieve optimal growth, development and health. Thereafter, to meet their dietary requirements during growth, infants should receive nutritionally adequate and safe complementary foods while breastfeeding continues for up to two years of age or beyond [73,74]. However, there is widespread variation in compliance with this recommendation in both developed and developing countries. In an evaluation of 33 developing countries, where the health benefits of this policy could have the greatest impact, exclusive breastfeeding occurred in 46% of countries, the median duration of breastfeeding was 18.6 months and over 30% received complementary foods before 6 months of age [76]. The extent to which variation in feeding practices may influence global intakes of ARA and infant growth and development in early life needs to be further evaluated.

5.1. ARA Intake from Human Milk

In exclusively breastfed infants, the mean human milk intake at 6 months has been measured to be 854 g/day [73,74]. Based on those data and an estimation that 4.2% of human milk is composed of fatty acids [77] the average ARA and DHA intakes in exclusively breastfed infants at 6 months of age are about 169 mg/day and 115 mg/day, respectively. Moreover, many infants continue to receive human milk throughout the first year of life and longer. It is estimated that at 12 months of age the intake of human milk is in the range of 600–900 g/day [73,74]. This amount provides infants with an ARA intake from human milk in the range of 118–178 mg/day. The mean estimated ARA intake is approximately 12–18 mg/kg/day when adjusted for body weight using weight-for-age percentiles [78].

5.2. ARA Intake from Infant Formula

Infant formulas typically contain levels of ARA and DHA at 140 mg/day and 100 mg/day, respectfully, based on worldwide averages of ARA and DHA content in human milk [5]. Therefore, intakes of ARA and DHA from infant formula are similar to those provided from human milk.

5.3. ARA Intake from Weaning Foods

In both developed and developing countries weaning foods contain low amounts of fat, which results in a sharp transition from adequate fat intake during breastfeeding to significantly lower fat intake when children are weaned from the breast [79,80]. The main food sources of ARA are beef, poultry, eggs and seafood. Complementary foods in low-income countries are typically cereal-based and therefore LCPUFA dietary intake from these weaning foods may be minimal [79]. Countries with the lowest gross national product (GNP) (e.g., Malawi, Ethiopia, Bangladesh, Burkina Faso, Ghana and India) had a mean percentage of total PUFA from animal source foods of 4.9% *vs.* countries with a higher GNP (Vietnam, Bolivia, Indonesia, Guatemala, China, South Africa, Mexico) where the mean percentage of total PUFA from animal food sources was 18.1% [79].

Intakes of ARA (mean mg/day and estimated mean mg/kg/day) from several developing and developed countries are presented in Table 1. In the village of Keneba, Gambia, estimated mean intake of ARA during the period of 0–6 months when infants are predominantly breastfed was 90 mg/day and as complementary foods were introduced the ARA intake fell steadily to 10 mg/day at 24 months [81]. In Heqing County, Yunnan Province China, the mean intake of ARA was 55 mg/day at 1 to 3 years of age and 50 mg/day at 4 to 5 years of age [82].

Vulnerable infants and young children need energy- and nutrient-dense foods to grow and develop both physically and mentally [83]. For these reasons, dietary diversity is now included as a specific recommendation in the guidance for complementary feeding of the breastfed child aged 6 to 23 months [83]. Many factors contribute to limited dietary diversity including economic limitations, religious beliefs, and a concern that infants under 1 year of age cannot digest animal sourced foods [84,85]. There is also a widely held perception by parents that fish may be associated with allergic reactions [85,86].

Even in developed countries where dietary diversity is higher and meat and eggs contribute more to the complementary diet, the detrimental impact of the introduction of complementary feeding with low amounts of ARA and DHA content is evident. For example, mean ARA intake in German infants/toddlers decreased from 72 mg/day at 6 months of age to 24 mg/day at 9 months of age [87] (Table 1). In a separate study, these authors reported that predominately breastfed German infants had an ARA intake of 103 mg/day at 3 months of age and this amount declined to 24 mg/day at 9 months when human milk represented only 20% of the diet [88].

One hundred-seventy-four Italian breastfed children were followed from birth to 12 months of age [89]. Human milk samples were analyzed. The mean ARA intake from human milk was 95.6 mg/day at 1 month, 109.6 mg/day at 2 months, and 101.1 mg/day at 3 months. However, at 6 months of age, ARA intake sharply declined to 58.7 mg/day.

In Belgium, mean intakes of ARA were very low at 2.5 to 3 years of age and at 4 to 6.5 years of age (17 and 18 mg/day, respectively) [90] (Table 1). In Australia, national intake data indicated that 2 to 3 year-old and 4 to 7 year-old children consumed 16 mg/day and 22 mg/day of ARA, respectively [91]. Much higher mean ARA intakes were reported for Canadian children living in Vancouver where intakes ranged from 133 to 260 mg/day among children 1.5 to 5 years of age [92]. However, in children aged 4 to 7 years of age from Ontario, Canada, mean intake of ARA was lower (57 mg/day) [93].

Based on food records from the National Health and Nutrition Examination Survey (NHANES 2003–2008), the mean intake of ARA in American children at 1 to 4 years of age was 60 mg/day [94]. Most of the ARA was obtained from poultry (32.5%), eggs (27.5%), and meat dishes (20.9%). The latest NHANES data from 2015 indicate that the mean ARA intake of American children at 2 to 5 years of age increased to 80 mg/day [95].

Table 1. ARA intakes in developed and developing countries during the first 2 years of life.

Country	Age	Method	Mean ARA Intake (mg/Day) (mg/kg/Day) [1]
Australia [91]	2–3 years	1-day weighed food record	16 (1.3)
		1-day weighed food record	22 (1.8)
Belgium [90]	2–5 years	3 days food record	17 (1.4)
	4–6.5 years	3 days food record	18 (1.0)
Canada [92,93]	1.5–2 years	1 day food frequency	133 (11.0)
	2.1–3 years	I day food frequency	260 (22.0)
	3.1–5 years	1 day food frequency	226 (15.0)
	4–7 years	3-days food records	57 (2.9)
China [82]	1–3 years	3 days 24 h recall	55 (4.6)
	4–5 years	3 days 24 h recall	50 (2.5)
Gambia [82]	0–6 months	1 day weighed food monthly	90 (15.0)
	7–12 months	1 day weighed food monthly	70 (7.8)
	13–17 months	1 day weighed food monthly	60 (6.7)
	24 months	1 day weighed food monthly	10 (0.8)
Germany [87,88]	6 months	3 days weighed food record	72 (12.0)
	9 months	3 days weighed food record	24 (2.7)
Italy [89]	1 month	Human milk composition	95.6 (29.0)
	2 months	Human milk composition	109.6 (33.0)
	3 months	Human milk composition	101.1 (16.9)
	6 months	Human milk composition	58.7 (9.8)
U.S. 2003–2008 [94]	1–4 years	1 day weighed food record	60 (5.0)
U.S. 2015 [95]	2–5 years	1 day weighed food record	80 (6.7)

Notes: [1] Estimated mean intake for ARA (9 mg/kg/day) for ages 0 month to 3 years was calculated using median weight-for-age percentiles for boys, birth to 36 months, and from median body mass index for ages 4 through 19 years; from the Centers for Disease Control and Prevention-Growth Charts (CDC, [78]).

Based on these dietary intakes from local and national surveys, it is clear that the diets of young children contain low levels of ARA. Reported mean intakes of ARA at 10 to 18 mg/day in developing and developed countries are only about 10% of the amount of ARA available to infants fed human milk or infant formulas containing DHA and ARA.

Birch *et al.* [96] reported that despite the introduction of a variety of solid foods at 17 weeks of age, infants who did not receive an infant formula supplemented with ARA and DHA throughout the first year of life had significantly lower levels of both of these fatty acids in plasma. The clinical consequences of low intake of ARA have not been adequately investigated.

6. ARA and Its Role in Immune System Development and Function

There is growing evidence from preclinical and clinical studies that ARA plays an important role in maintaining infant health through its effects on the immune system and through the modulation of the inflammatory response [97]. The eicosanoids that ARA produces serve as both mediators and regulators of inflammation [98] (Table 2). These immunomodulatory effects have generated much interest in the potential roles that LCPUFA in general and ARA in particular have in common inflammatory conditions in childhood such as asthma, eczema, atopic dermatitis, and food allergies [97].

In cell membranes, ARA contributes to membrane order, has roles in signal transduction, and gene expression, and provides substrate for production of important chemical mediators [99]. Although ARA has been widely viewed as a pro-inflammatory agent, the eicosanoids that ARA produces serve as both mediators and regulators of inflammation [98]. ARA-derived eicosanoids, and other oxidized derivatives [98] are generated by the metabolic processes as shown in Figure 4.

Table 2. Pro- and anti-inflammatory effects of prostaglandin E_2 (PGE$_2$) and leukotriene B_4 (LTB$_4$) [1].

Eicosanoid	Effects
PGE$_2$	**Proinflammatory**
	Induces fever
	Increases vascular permeability
	Increases vasodilatation
	Causes pain
	Enhances pain caused by other agents
	Anti-inflammatory
	Inhibits production of TNF and IL-1
	Inhibits 5-LOX (decreases 4-series LT production)
	Induces 15-LOX (increases lipoxin production)
LTB$_4$	**Proinflammatory**
	Increases vascular permeability
	Enhances local blood flow
	Chemotactic agent for leukocytes
	Induces release of lysomal enzymes
	Induces release of oxygen species by granulocytes
	Increases production of TNF, IL-8, and IL-6

Notes: [1] IL, interleukin; LOX, lipoxygenase; TNF, tumor necrosis factor. From Calder [98].

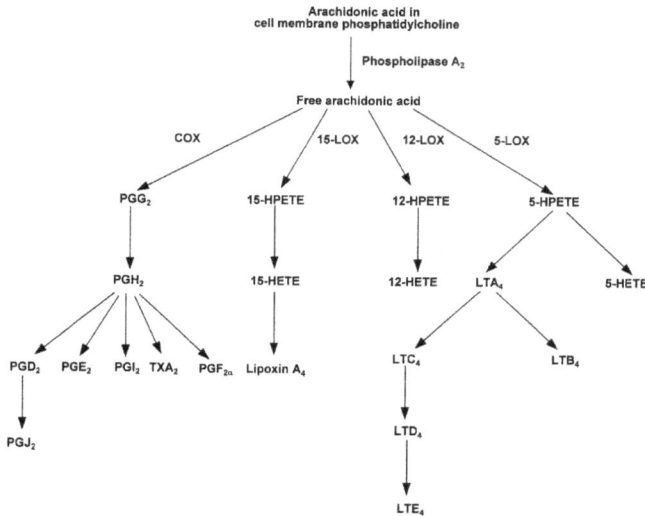

Figure 4. Generalized pathway for the conversion of ARA to eicosanoids. COX, cyclooxygenase; HETE, hydroxyeicosatetraenoic acid; HPETE, hydroperoxyeicosatetraenoic acid; LOX, lipoxygenase; LT, leukotriene; PG, prostaglandin; TX, thromboxane (from Calder [98]).

Another example of the dual role of PGE$_2$ and its receptors in modulating the inflammatory response has been described by Riccioti and FitzGerald [100]. During neuro-inflammation, the LPS-induced PGE$_2$ synthesis causes adverse effects in neurons resulting in lesions and enhanced pain [101]. However, PGE$_2$ also mediates bradykinin-induced neuroprotection by blocking LPS and ATP-induced cytokine synthesis in microglia and in neuron-glia co-cultures [102]. The anti-inflammatory and neuro-protective effects of PGE$_2$ are mediated by microglial EP2- and EP4-receptors [100].

ARA is the substrate for the biosynthesis of prostaglandins. Prostaglandins and thromboxane A_2 are collectively called prostanoids. Prostanoids are formed when ARA is released from the plasma membrane by phospholipase and metabolized by the sequential actions of prostaglandin G/H synthase, or cyclooxygenase (COX), and by respective synthesis [100]. Prostanoids serve a variety of functions. The adhesion-type prostaglandins as well as prostacyclin are important in vasodilation and in anti-thrombus formation [103]. The E series prostaglandins act to dilate arterioles and capillaries to bring about a drop in blood pressure, relax vascular smooth muscle, open the bronchi of the lungs, and enhance blood flow through the kidney [104]. Prostaglandins are also involved in sleep regulation [105], febrile response [106], and in pain perception [107].

As discussed by Calder [98], the overall physiologic (or pathophysiologic) outcome associated with the production of eicosanoids depends on the cells present, the nature of the stimulus, the timing of eicosanoid production, and the sensitivity of the target cells and tissues to the type of eicosanoids that are produced [98,108]. For example, studies have shown that prostaglandin PGE_2, acting as a pro-inflammatory agent, induces cyclooxygenase 2 (COX-2) in fibroblast cells and by doing so up-regulates its own production [109] which in turn stimulates the production of IL-6 by macrophages (see Astudillo *et al.* [108] for a review of ARA metabolism by inflammatory cells). As an anti-inflammatory agent, PGE_2 inhibits 5-lipoxygenase (5-LOX) thereby decreasing production of the 4-series leukotrienes [110].These 4-series leukotrienes induce 15-LOX which in turn promotes the formation of lipoxins that aid the resolution phase of inflammation [110]. Thus, the ARA-derived PGE_2 has both pro- and anti-inflammatory effects (Table 2).

Leukotrienes, eoxins, lipoxins, and hydroperoxyeicosatetranoic acids (HPETEs) are synthesized from ARA by lipoxgenase enzymes and metabolized to LTA_4 [108]. LTA_4 is unstable and can be rapidly converted into LTB_4 or LTC_4. These three leukotrienes constitute the slow-reacting substances involved in anaphylaxis that act in allergic response [111]. They contract smooth muscle and affect vascular permeability. Eoxins are generally proinflammatory and are produced in the same manner as leukotrienes, but by the action of 15-lipoxgenase [108]. Lipoxins are produced by transcellular biosynthesis and have anti-inflammatory properties and are involved in the resolution of inflammation [112].

In vitro and animal studies suggest that ARA has a critical role in immune cell growth in the thymus, and in differentiation, migration, and proliferation of immune cells [98]. During early growth, there is substantial accretion of ARA in the mouse thymus which corresponds to the enrichment of the placental ARA for the fetus [98].

The immune system is composed of an integrated network of organs, tissues, cells and molecules that work together to resist infection, but maintain tolerance to harmless factors such as "self", antigens, and allergens [113]. When a challenge is detected (e.g., an allergen or pathogen), cell signaling between immune cells produces a coordinated immune response involving the release of cytokines and eicosanoids, which under normal circumstances allows cells to communicate with each other to neutralize and eliminate the challenge [114,115].

ARA is highly abundant in platelet membranes and is closely linked to many platelet functions [116]. Due to their high numbers (*i.e.*, normal platelet count of $1.50\text{--}4.00 \times 10^{11}$ platelets per liter of blood [117] and their ability to release inflammatory mediators, platelets perform several sentinel tasks and can quickly communicate with the cells of the immune system [118]. For example, in inflammatory skin disorders, platelets recognize bacterial pathogens through interactions with Toll-like receptors leading to the elimination of bacteria by release of antimicrobial peptides or by aggregation of platelets around the bacteria [119]. An array of receptors present on platelet membranes facilitate transduction of signals and coordinate release of chemokines, cytokines, and other inflammatory mediators to regulate inflammation and respond to invading pathogens [118,119].

Inflammation is the immune's systems response to infection and injury [98]. Inflammation disorders are observed in infants, particularly those born prematurely [120]. Inflammation is characterized by the production of inflammatory cytokines, inflammatory agents such as reactive oxygen species, adhesion molecules, and the ARA-derived eicosanoids, and other oxidized derivatives [98]. *N*-3 LCPUFA decrease the production of the inflammatory mediators (eicosanoids, cytokines, and reactive oxygen species) and expression of adhesion molecules [98] by replacing ARA as an eicosanoid substrate and inhibiting ARA metabolism [98,121]. Aspirin and nonsteroidal anti-inflammatory drugs (NSAIDs) also inhibit the cyclooxygenase-catalyzed conversion of ARA to prostaglandins [122].

Although inflammation is perceived to be a serious health problem, the inflammation process is in fact an intrinsically beneficial event. Offending factors are removed or destroyed and as a result the affected tissues and physiological functions are restored. During the acute phase of inflammation, there is a rapid influx of blood granulocytes, typically neutrophils, followed by monocytes that mature into inflammatory macrophages [100]. The macrophages proliferate and affect the functions of resident tissue macrophages. This initial acute phase causes the usual signs of inflammation: redness, heat, swelling, and pain [100]. Once the initial adverse stimulus is removed via phagocytosis, the inflammation reaction typically decreases and ultimately resolves. During the resolution phase of inflammation, granulocytes are eliminated and macrophages and lymphocytes return to their normal pre-inflammatory levels [100]. The usual outcome of the acute inflammatory process is successful resolution and repair of tissue damage.

Eicosanoids and Their Effects on Hormones and Bone Formation

The typical definition of a hormone is a chemical substance produced in the body that controls and regulates the activity of certain cells or organs [123]. Many hormones are secreted by special glands, such as thyroid hormone produced by the thyroid gland. Eicosanoids are recognized as different from hormones because they are not synthesized or stored in select tissues or endocrine organs. Eicosanoids are synthesized in almost all tissues and exert their biological effect near the site of their synthesis rather at a distance such as other hormones [124]. Despite these differences, eicosanoids are generally classified as hormones [125]. Eicosanoids directly affect other hormones including glycoprotein hormones. The glycoprotein hormones include luteinizing hormone, somatostatin, and glucagon. Somatostatin is an important growth hormone that controls and regulates growth and cell division [126]. It is the main hormone that stimulates cell proliferation and growth, and this hormone must be regulated so that growth is controlled [126]. Insulin and glucagon release are also affected by the eicosanoid derivatives, epoxy-eicosatrienoic acids [124].

ARA also plays an important role in the hormonal regulation of normal bone formation and whole body mineral metabolism during infant and childhood growth (Table 3). During skeletal development, the eicosanoids relay cellular, organ, and systemic signals to balance the calcium and phosphate needs for bone formation and other metabolic activities [127,128]. During long bone growth, when bone tissue is created, [127–130] ARA mediates vitamin D_3-regulated chondrocyte maturation [131] and proliferation [127,132–134] for the mineralization of skeletal growth plates (Figure 5).

A product of ARA, prostaglandin PGE_2 is a potent regulator of cartilage formation or chondrogenesis and resorption [135–139]. At low levels, PGE_2 stimulates bone formation by increasing the production of insulin-like growth factor, a powerful growth stimulator for bone, cartilage, and muscle [140]. At high levels, PGE_2 has the opposite effect: bone formation is reduced and resorption is increased [140].

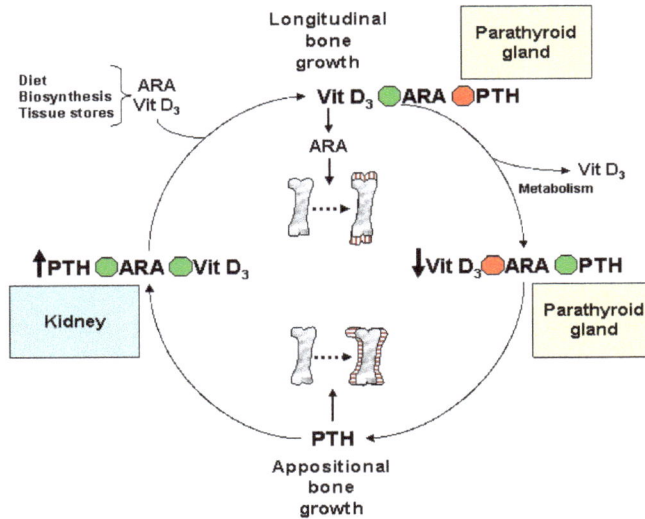

Figure 5. The role of ARA in bone development and homeostatic regulation of vitamin D_3 and parathyroid hormone (PTH) levels along the parathyroid gland-kidney axis during growth. ARA and vitamin D_3 are acquired from the diet and/or from endogenous sources. ARA mediates vitamin D_3 regulation of chondrocyte proliferation and growth plate mineralization during bone elongation. As vitamin D_3 is metabolized and levels subside, ARA-dependent PTH suppression is diminished and PTH production by the parathyroid gland is upregulated. This results in increased periosteal bone mineral content (appositional bone growth). In kidney, PTH induces the ARA-mediated increase in vitamin D_3 activation and secretion, elevating the amount of vitamin D_3 in circulation. The cycle continues as the restoration of vitamin D_3 results in the ARA-dependent suppression of PTH and stimulates longitudinal bone growth.

These differential effects of osteoclast formation and resorption are mediated through multiple subtypes of G-protein coupled PGE_2 cell surface receptors (EP1, EP2, and EP4) [141]. Activation of the EP2 and EP4 receptor subtypes are linked to an elevated level of cyclic adenosine monophosphate (cAMP) and bone formation. EP2 also acts as a selective agonist which has the ability to heal long bone fractures as demonstrated in animal models [141,142].

PGE_2 is also critically important for bone strength [141]. When different doses (3 or 6 mg PGE2/kg/day) of prostaglandin PGE_2 were given to Sprague-Dawley rats for 3 weeks an increase in bone and hard tissue mass, calcified cartilage cores, and a decrease in osteoclasts were observed [143]. PGE_2 increased metaphyseal calcified tissue mass by depressing hard tissue resorption and stimulating the replication and differentiation of osteoblast precursors to form new bone [143].

Other prostaglandins play multiple roles for bone metabolism and remodeling by regulating various signaling pathways [144]. For example, PGF2α, through the activation of protein kinase C (PKC), stimulates the Na-dependent inorganic phosphate transport in osteoblasts [144]. PGF2α also up-regulates interleukin (IL-6) to stimulate osteoclast formation and increases vascular endothelial growth factor (VEGF) associated with the growth of blood vessels from pre-existing vasculature [144]. PKCα, in particular, appears to play a critical role in the regulation of osteoblastic function under load-bearing conditions [145]. During exposure to mechanical strain, PKCα is activated in osteoblast-like cells [146] while PKC signaling has been implicated in the regulation of various mechanically response genes including the osteoblast differentiation marker osteocalcin [147,148].

Table 3. Roles of ARA in bone formation, metabolism, and mineral balance.

Metabolic Effector	Physiological Roles of ARA
ARA [149]	Maintain normal balance between bone mineral accrual and bone resorption during infant development
ARA, growth hormones [150,151]	Increase insulin-like growth factor gene expression and induction of osteoblast-dependent bone formation
Vitamin D_3 [128,133]	Mediate vitamin D_3 coordination of chondrocyte proliferation in the epiphyseal growth plates of long bones. Parathyroid hormone secretion
Calcium and phosphorous [152]	Regulation of parathyroid hormone secretion in response to blood mineral concentrations
Parathyroid hormone [149,150]	ARA mediated/activated pathway involved in the activation and secretion of vitamin D_3 by kidneys
Physical activity [153]	ARA mediates bone adaptation to changes in physical stress through mechanisms which mediate resorption and remodeling

In studies of piglets fed formulas with differing levels of ARA (0.30%, 0.45%, 0.60% or 0.75% of fat) plus the same level of DHA (0.1% of fat), proportions of ARA in plasma, liver and adipose were dose dependent but bone modeling was not [150]. Whole-body bone mineral content was elevated in the piglets fed the highest levels of ARA (0.60% and 0.75%) and was best predicted by dietary ARA [150,154]. In addition, the 0.60% and 0.75% ARA groups had bone mineral content values closest to that of a reference group of suckled piglets [150,155].

Overall, dietary provision of ARA serves a number of important roles in skeletal metabolism. ARA functions as an important modulator of vitamin D regulation of chondrocyte proliferation and growth plate mineralization. ARA derived metabolites are important inducers of osteoclast [156,157] and osteoblast differentiation [158,159], and in modulating resorption of bone [139,149] by increasing IGF-1 gene expression [104,151] and circulating levels of IGF-1 [150]. ARA also responds to changes in stress and mechanical loading [153,160], and accelerates bone repair and healing [142,161]. Additionally, in term infants, cord blood ARA levels correlate positively with bone mineral density [155]. Thus, ARA represents an important nutrient for infant and childhood bone development and metabolism.

7. ARA in Skeletal and Cardiac Muscle

Several animal studies have shown that the concentration of ARA in the heart is highly sensitive to levels and ratios of ARA and DHA of the diet [24,54,162–164]. The amount of ARA in cardiac tissue muscle is at concentrations 2 to 3 times greater than observed in skeletal muscle [52]. Analysis of the phospholipid composition of skeletal muscle biopsies collected from 56 children <2 years of age indicated that ARA represented 16.5% of the total percentage of LCPUFA in muscle phospholipids [165].

Repetitive force loading and unloading during ATP-dependent contraction of actin filaments are major mechanical functions of heart muscle, and to a lesser extent, skeletal muscle [166]. ARA is critical for muscle contraction [166–168]. In skeletal muscle, excitation–contraction coupling is the process by which muscles contract [166] when a muscle action potential in the muscle fiber causes the myofibrils to contract [169]. Excitation–contraction coupling relies on a direct coupling between key proteins, the sarcoplasmic reticulum calcium release channel (the release of Ca^{2+} ions), and the voltage-gated L-type calcium channels [170]. The release of Ca^{2+} ions from the sarcoplasmic reticulum causes binding between actin and myosin to induce muscle contraction. This cycle is reset as calcium declines back to resting levels [166]. Cardiac and skeletal muscle require tight regulation of voltage-gated calcium channels and calcium homeostasis to coordinate the excitation-contraction coupling process [170].

Phosphatidylinositol (4,5) bisphosphate (PIP_2), a phospholipid component of cell membranes, serves as an important regulator for Ca^{2+} release from the sarcoplasmic reticulum and assists in the maintenance of normal calcium signaling to control contractile forces [167,168,171]. The fatty acids of PIP_2 are variable in different species and tissues, but studies show the most common fatty acids are stearic in position 1 and ARA in position 2 [37].

Calcium homeostasis, regulation and maintenance are critical elements for normal muscle function. Wolf *et al.* [34] have shown that the endoplasmic reticulum is directly responsible for the regulation of intracellular Ca^{2+} concentrations. ARA plays an important cooperative role with myo-inositol 1,4,5-triphosphate (IP_3) in glucose-induced calcium mobilization and insulin secretion by pancreatic islets.

PIP_2 and phosphatidylinositol 3,4,5-triphosphate (PIP_3) are also critical for cardiac function [172]. In the heart, PIP_2, as a key second messenger, controls the activity of ion channels involved with the modulation of heart rhythm. PIP_3, on the other hand, is primarily involved in the control of cardiomyocyte apoptosis, hypertrophy, and contractility [172]. In adults, deregulation of the phosphoinositide metabolism is associated with the onset and progression of several cardiovascular pathologies including atherosclerosis and heart failure [172].

Muscle growth and atrophy depend on the balance between the rates of protein synthesis and degradation [173]. *In vitro* experiments with animal and human skeletal and cardiac muscle tissue indicate that prostaglandins are involved in the regulation of protein synthesis and degradation in various types of striated muscle [173,174]. While PGE_2 increases degradation of muscle in young rats and causes net protein balance to become more negative, $PGF_{2\alpha}$ causes a large stimulation of protein synthesis in muscle tissue [173]. These findings are consistent with the many important roles played by prostaglandins PGE_2 and $PGF_{2\alpha}$ in muscle protein balance and indicate that overall, ARA serves multiple functions in cardiac and skeletal muscle function and physiology.

8. Biomagnification and Accretion of ARA in Infants

Biomagnification is when infants have higher levels of LCPUFA in plasma lipid fractions and erythrocytes as compared with their mothers [45]. Biomagnification can be especially marked for ARA with levels more than 2-fold of that from the maternal side and independent from the amount of its precursor LA available maternally. The stability of LA content implies that any conversion to ARA is not keeping up with the fetal demand for ARA [45]. Biomagnification by the placenta serves to preferentially obtain preformed ARA and DHA from the mother in order to deliver it to and nourish the fetus [45].

As shown by Kuipers *et al.* [175], biomagnification is independent of maternal ARA status at both delivery and at 3 months of age and is found to be similar across different populations with differing diets. These findings indicate that biomagnification as a biological process seeks to achieve a uniform ARA status in infants at the expense of their mothers. The process of biomagnification suggests that a certain level of infant prenatal ARA status must be maintained for optimal infant growth.

Infants with the lowest birthweights have the lowest levels of ARA, and those born earliest have the lowest levels of DHA [45]. The process of biomagnification initially protects vascular growth which is a requirement for brain growth. Vascular growth must precede brain growth to meet the brain's demand for energy, which can be as high as 70% of the total fetal demand for energy in the last trimester of pregnancy [45].

At delivery, as shown by Luxwolda *et al.* [176], the maternal RBC-ARA content is consistently higher than that at 3 months postpartum. At delivery, infant RBC-ARA content is similar or higher than their mother's RBC-ARA contents. From delivery to 3 months postpartum, maternal RBC-ARA increases while infant RBC-ARA decreases. The decrease in RBC-ARA content may be due to a lower conversion of LA to ARA since the infant's capacity to synthesize LCPUFA decreases dramatically after delivery [69] and has been shown to decrease with gestational age at birth [64].

There appears to be a tightly regulated synergism between DHA and ARA at low DHA status and an antagonism at high DHA status [50]. Intrauterine DHA biomagnification in mothers with low fish intakes aims at a synergistic increase of fetal DHA to maintain a balance with ARA. Bioattenuation at higher DHA status may in turn prevent abundant passage of DHA across the placenta that leads to antagonism with ARA. Since ARA is important for fetal growth [177] and is rapidly accreted in the fetal brain [178,179] any competition from gestational DHA must be tightly regulated and balanced for optimal neurodevelopment after birth [50]. Dietary depletion of ARA in early infancy may have adverse consequences for brain development [178,179].

9. Consequences of ARA Deficiency

Essential fatty acid (EFA) deficiency impairs lipid and energy metabolism, cell membrane structures, lipid signaling pathways, and ultimately leads to death [180,181]. Mammals are dependent on a dietary supply of LA and ALA which are converted into *n*-6 and *n*-3 PUFA, respectively. Δ6-fatty acid desaturase (FADS2) converts LA to γ-linolenic acid (C18:3*n*-6) and Δ5-fatty acid desaturase (FADS1) converts dihommo-γ-linolenic acid (C20:3*n*-6) to ARA [182].

Early studies of EFA deficiency considered the effect that various dose levels of intake of LA, ARA and ALA esters (0% to 10% of total calories for 100 days) had on the fatty acid composition in the liver of rats [183]. Fat deficiency symptoms (necrotic tail and scaly feet) appeared in all animals fed LA at less than 0.6% of calories and ARA at less than 0.25% of calories. ARA was 3-fold more effective than LA in liver incorporation and mitigating deficiency. Fat deficiency symptoms affecting the skin were not surprising. In the skin, as in all organs, EFA are principally found in glycolipids and phospholipids. Most of the epidermal fatty acid PUFA is ARA [184]. EFA deficiency causes skin flaking in humans, dogs, and mice, symptoms that can be restored with LA dietary therapy [184].

Since LA deficiency results in disruption of the skin's water barrier function [185] and heat loss from skin [186] the side effects make it difficult to distinguish the specific effects of ARA deficiency independent from those related to LA deficiency. The fads2$^{-/-}$ mouse allows for the specific investigation of ARA deficiency without the underlying complications of LA deficiency [181]. The mutation eliminates Δ-6 desaturase activity leading to a dramatic decrease in the accumulation of ARA in tissues and subsequently, ARA conversion to PGE, TXB, prostacyclin and leukotrienes. Platelet aggregation and thrombosis are therefore also limited.

When fads2$^{-/-}$ mice were followed for several weeks and fed a diet lacking Δ6-fatty acid desaturase products but containing ample amounts of LA, the lack of PUFA and eicosanoids did not impair lifespan but all the mice were sterile, developed ulcerative dermatitis, splenomegaly, and ulceration in the duodenum and ileocecal junction [182]. Liver levels of ARA and DHA declined by 95% and somewhat smaller decreases were observed in the brain and testes (~50%). The absence of γ-linolenic conversion in the fads2$^{-/-}$ mouse deprived the cyclooxygenase and lipoxygenase pathways of their substrates, including the elimination of PGE synthesis, the failure of synthesis of TXBs by thrombocytes, and the failure to produce leukotrienes [181]. PUFA supplementation completely restored the adverse symptoms observed in fads2$^{-/-}$ mice. The mechanism by which ARA prevented dermatitis may be due, at least in part, to lower levels of prostaglandin D$_2$ (PGD$_2$) when skin ARA is decreased [182].

The ulceration of the small intestine in the fads2$^{-/-}$ mouse may have been associated with the decline of prostaglandin synthesis, similar to the effect often seen with the long-term use of NSAIDs [187]. NSAIDs block prostaglandin synthesis by inhibiting cyclooxygenases, leading to an erosion and then ulceration of the mucosal layer of the stomach and small intestine. However, loss of organized stratification of proliferating cells into defined zones is a common feature of EFA deficiency [188].

The Δ6-fatty acid desaturase gene FADS2 was cloned in 1999 [189]. An adult human case of Δ6-fatty acid desaturase deficiency was identified and described in the literature [190]. The patient exhibited growth retardation accompanied by skin abnormalities, corneal ulceration, and feeding intolerance. Treatment with dietary DHA and ARA restored normal growth and eliminated most of the symptoms [190].

A novel genetic model, the FADS1 ($\Delta 5$ desaturase) knockout mouse was used to determine the role that the ARA-derived 2-series eicosanoids had in mucosal physiology and inflammation [191]. Fads1$^{-/-}$ mice have very low levels of ARA in tissues (colon mucosa, liver, spleen, serum and fatty acid profiles). The deficiency in ARA resulted in a massive enhancement of dihomo-y-linolenic acid, the 1-series prostaglandin substrate in tissues and a decrease in 2-series-derived prostaglandins or PGE$_2$. Fads1$^{-/-}$ mice failed to thrive, gradually dying at 5 to 6 weeks of age with no survivors past 12 weeks of age [191]. The lack of PGE$_2$ was associated with disturbed intestinal crypt proliferation, altered immune cell homeostasis, and a heightened sensitivity to acute inflammatory challenge [191]. Dietary supplementation with ARA extended the longevity of fads1$^{-/-}$ mice to levels comparable with normal wild-type mice (Figure 6).

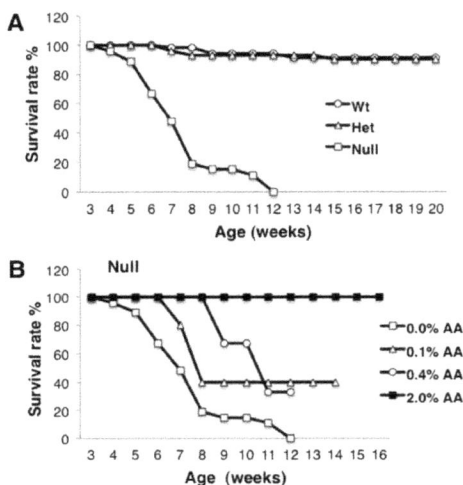

Figure 6. Kaplan-Meier survival curves of *Fads1* mice, AA = ARA. (**A**) *Fads1* null mice exhibited low viability when fed a standard AA-free diet; $n = 37$ for wild-type, $n = 44$ for heterozygous, $n = 11$ for Null; (**B**) Dietary supplementation with AA (0.1% and 0.4%, w/w) partially reversed the *Fads1* null mouse phenotype; $n = 5$ for Null + 0.1% AA, $n = 3$ for Null + 0.4% AA. Supplementation with 2.0% AA completely reverse the Null phenotype; $n = 4$ for Null $\pm$ 2% AA (from Fan *et al.* [191]).

Although fads1$^{-/-}$ and fad2$^{-/-}$ mice are useful to examine the function of ARA *in vivo* PUFA are transferred through the placenta from the heterozygous mother into the homozygous fetus. Additionally, the amount of DHA and ARA in the brain tends to remain tightly controlled even under conditions of PUFA deprivation, but at the expense of other tissues to protect the brain [182]. Lpiat1$^{-/-}$ mice have a mutation that affects the synthesis of ARA-containing PI. PI is unique in its fatty acid composition, *i.e.*, most of the fatty acid that is attached to the sn-2 position of PI is ARA [33]. Other membrane phospholipids such as PC and PE contain other PUFA including DHA.

Lee *et al.* [33] showed that Lpiat1$^{-/-}$ mice had a reduced content of ARA in PI and had deficits in cortical lamination during brain development, delayed neuronal processes in the cortex, and reduced neurite outgrowth *in vitro*. Lpiat1$^{-/-}$ mice died within a month and showed atrophy of the cerebral cortex and hippocampus. These results demonstrate the importance of ARA-containing PI in normal cortical development in mice. By eliminating LPIAT1 in Lpiat1$^{-/-}$ mice, the enzyme responsible for the incorporation of ARA into PI, it was shown that the ARA-containing PI is essential for brain development in mammals [33].

Newborn pups of Δ6-fatty acid desaturase knockout mice were administered artificial milks that contained 3.7% ALA and 16% LA with or without 1.2% ARA and/or 1.2% DHA for 18 days immediately after birth [192]. Compared with wild-type mice, the body weight of the mice fed the control diet was significantly lower, particularly after 6 weeks of age. However, body weights of knockout mice fed milks with DHA and ARA+DHA were similar to that of the wild-type mice. Motor activities of the knockout mice fed ARA were elevated compared with the wild-type mice and those fed the control diet. Better motor performance was also observed in knockout mice fed the ARA + DHA diet. The authors concluded that ARA corrected the decrease in body weight and the combination of ARA and DHA improved the motor dysfunction caused by the deficit of Δ6-fatty acid desaturase.

Taken together, results from these investigations indicate the importance of ARA and its derivatives for the coordination of cellular differentiation, organogenesis, and function during early growth and development.

10. Animal Studies of ARA Supplementation

10.1. Immunomodulatory Effects of ARA and DHA Supplementation

The activation of peroxisomal proliferator-activated receptors (PPARs) has been shown to be protective in brain ischemic and oxidative injury and in many neurological diseases that may affect infants [193] (Figure 7). In addition, transcription of the gene for the Major Facilitator Superfamily of the domain-containing protein 2a (MFSD2A) has been identified as being an important transporter for the uptake of DHA across the blood brain barrier [194] and is under the control of PPAR [195]. Studies indicate that LCPUFA and their metabolites are ligands to PPARs. Diets containing an *n*-6:*n*-3 ratio of about 1-2:1 supplied during pregnancy and lactation appear to be optimal for the expression of neuron-specific enolase, glial fibrillary acidic protein and myelin basic protein, markers related to the growth and maturation of neurons, astrocytes and myelin [193].

To investigate the immunomodulatory effects of different PUFA, weanling rats were fed a high-fat diet (178 g/kg) that contained 4.4 g of ALA, γ-linolenic, ARA, EPA, or DHA/100 g total diet [196] for 6 weeks. The proportion of total PUFA content (~35 wt %) was held constant and the *n*-6 to *n*-3 ratio was maintained at 5.8 to 7.0. PGE_2 production was enhanced in leukocytes from rats fed the ARA-rich diet and was decreased from leukocytes in rats fed the EPA or DHA diets. ARA did not affect lymphocyte proliferation, NK cell activity, or the cell-mediated immune response. Lack of an effect on T-lymphocyte proliferation and Con A in splenocyte cultures was also observed in mice fed a safflower oil ethyl ester diet +1% ARA for 10 days [197]. The lack of an immunological effect of ARA agrees with findings from a human study that considered 1.5 g of ARA/day for 50 days on the proliferation response of peripheral blood mononuclear cells to Con A, phytohemagglutinin, or poke-weed mitogen [198]. Human peripheral blood NK activity was also unaffected by the consumption of ARA.

Prostaglandins which are involved in inflammatory processes also play a major role in the recovery of intestinal barrier function in ischemia-injured porcine ileum by converting ARA to PGH_2 [199]. The importance of ARA and ARA-derived eicosanoids in the intestinal epithelium was reviewed by Ferrer and Moreno [200]. In a study that considered the effect of supplemental ARA on intestinal barrier repair in ischemia-injured porcine ileum pigs were fed a formula containing no LCPUFA (0% ARA), 0.5% ARA, 5% ARA, or 5% EPA for 10 days. Piglets that were fed 5% ARA exhibited enhanced recovery compared with piglets fed 0% ARA or 0.5% ARA [201]. The EPA-fed piglets had enhanced recovery comparable with piglets fed 0% ARA. The enhanced recovery response observed with 5% ARA was supported by reduction in the mucosal-to-serosal flux of ^{3}H-mannitol and ^{14}C-inulin compared with the other dietary groups. Jacobi *et al.* [201] concluded that piglets fed a high-ARA diet are less susceptible to ischemia-induced epithelial cell sloughing and that feeding elevated levels of LCPUFA, including ARA, enhances acute recovery of ischemia-injured porcine ileum. For infants affected by necrotizing enterocolitis (NEC) where physiological repair of the intestines is necessary elevated LCPUFA intake including ARA enhances recovery of damaged tissues [201].

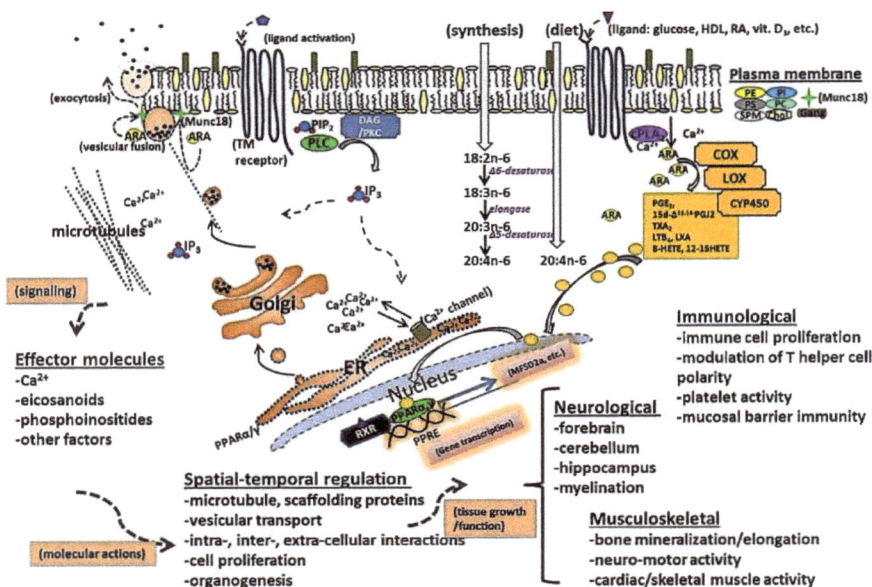

Figure 7. Schematic summary of molecular events and functional outcomes involved in metabolism of ARA. ARA is derived from endogenous synthesis or directly from the diet and is incorporated into cellular membrane complex lipids. Within the lipid bilayer, ARA is enriched in PE and PI in the inner membrane. Coordination of spatial-temporal interactions between molecular and cellular components and activities are mediated by metabolites of, or molecules associated with metabolism of ARA. Metabolism of ARA is triggered by activation of transmembrane receptors as a result of binding a ligand. A few examples of receptor-mediated activation of ARA metabolism include glucose, vitamin D_3, Ca^{2+}, or antigen presentation or detection by immune cells. ARA released from the membrane by the actions of PLA_2 or metabolized by enzymes such as COX, CYP450, and/or LOX can act directly or serve as a substrate for various enzymes to produce second-messengers. ARA-derived eicosanoids, including prostaglandins, leukotrienes, lipoxins, and HETEs regulate numerous activities including passage of ions between subcellular compartments, interactions between various structures or cells, and nuclear regulation of gene transcription by PPARs activators. Within the inner leaflet of cell membranes, ARA is enriched in micro-domains and is involved in regulation of receptor mediated activities. In addition, micro-domains serve as foundations for biophysical interactions between subcellular structures such as microtubules and other cytoskeletal activities including vesicular transport. The consequences of temporal-spatial regulation include coordinated release of hormones, expression of various cell functions, and/or alterations in phenotypes, and cellular motility. Examples of PPAR-regulated gene products involved tissue uptake of LCPUFA and oxidation of stored lipids: MFSD2A, major facilitator of superfamily domain-containing protein 2A. Membrane components: Chol, cholesterol; Gang, gangliosides; PC, phosphatidylcholine; PE, phosphatidylethanolamine; PI, phosphatidylinositol; PS, phosphatidylserine; SPM, Sphingomyelin. Nuclear transcription factors: PPAR, peroxisome-proliferator activator receptors; RXR, retinoid X receptors. TM, transmembrane receptors. Enzymes: COX, cyclooxygenase; CYP450, cytochrome P450; LOX, lipoxygenase; PLA_2, Phospholipase A2; PLC, Phospholipase C. Signaling molecules: PG, prostaglandin (Adapted from Pike [32]).

EFA deficiency also leads to hepatic steatosis. When rats were administered varying amounts of DHA and ARA to determine whether exclusive supplementation with DHA or ARA could prevent

EFA deficiency and inhibit the development of hepatic steatosis mice fed at least 2% of their calories from DHA and 1% of the calories from ARA did not develop clinical or biochemical evidence of EFA deficiency disease or hepatic steatosis [202]. Although hepatic steatosis is an adult disease, the fact that mice fed at least 2% of their calories from DHA and 1% of the calories from ARA prevent the development of EFA deficiency suggests the importance of ARA throughout the lifespan.

To investigate the ability of ARA- and ARA + DHA-enriched formula to modulate immune response in neonatal piglets to an inactivated influenza virus vaccine Bassaganya-Riera *et al.* [203] considered a diet with ARA + DHA in sow milk fed at birth. The diet modulated antigen-specific T-cell responses to an inactivated influenza virus and up-regulated IL-10 expression [203]. Although ARA and DHA have been suggested to elicit opposing immunomodulatory actions, the immunologic outcome in the study was beneficial [203]. The authors concluded that ARA + DHA enriched formulas, with the approximate 2:1 ratio fed during the neonatal period, may prevent or manage autoimmune and allergic reactions in infants by down-modulating T-cell reactions.

10.2. Retinal and Neurodevelopmental Effects of ARA and DHA Supplementation

The retinal DHA content in guinea pigs was considered in relation to diets containing different *n*-6:*n*-3 ratios (from 72.0 to 2.5) [204]. Not surprisingly, diets with the highest *n*-6:*n*-3 PUFA ratios had the highest *n*-6 retinal fatty acid profiles. Weisinger *et al.* [204] reported that retinal function was altered by tissue DHA levels and responded according to an inverted "U-shaped" function. As DHA levels increased past an optimal amount found to be 19%, the result was poorer electroretinographic scores. However, there was no mention that as DHA increased there was a corresponding decrease in ARA levels due to ARA antagonism. The marked decrease in ARA levels may have been the variable of interest that was not fully considered and responsible for the electroretinographic changes at high DHA intakes.

Champoux *et al.* [205] used a neurodevelopmental battery to test the neurological behavior in rhesus macaques neonates fed a control formula without LCPUFA or a LCPUFA-supplemented formula with 1 wt % each of DHA and ARA. Macaque neonates fed the supplemented formula obtained higher scores on motor maturity and orientation than those fed a control formula. Champoux *et al.* [205] concluded that the results supported the view that preformed DHA and ARA in infant formulas are required for optimal neurological development.

Learning behavior in rats fed a diet supplemented with 3% safflower oil (Safflower, *n*-3 fatty acid deficient, high LA acid) was compared to those fed 3% perilla oil (Perilla, high ALA) [206]. Through two generations, the *n*-3 fatty acid deficient group exhibited decreased correct response ratios in a brightness-discrimination behavior test. The altered learning ability in the brightness-discrimination test was restored with supplementation of DHA after weaning, only after levels of ARA in the brain lipids were normalized. The authors concluded that *n*-3 fatty acid is essential for the maintenance of learning performance and that *n*-3 deficiency in the presence of *n*-6 fatty acid during gestation did not lead to irreversible damage to the brain [206]. Thus, both DHA and ARA affected learning performance and a balance of ARA and DHA levels must be maintained.

To investigate the effects that varying dietary levels of LCPUFA have on growth, brain fatty acid composition and behavior in mice, 5 groups of pregnant and lactating mice were fed diets with either very high *n*-6 to *n*-3 ratio of 49 (*n*-3 deficient), a more usual ratio of 4.0, or a low ratio of 0.32 for 15 weeks [207]. There was no effect of diet on birth weights of pups, but on days 15 and 22 the pups in the low *n*-6 to *n*-3 groups weighed less than those in the other treatment groups. Increasing levels of DHA in the diet increased brain DHA and decreased brain ARA. The differing ratios of *n*-6 to *n*-3 had no effect on the ability of mice to learn the place test or perform in the Morris water maze. However, the mice fed the low *n*-6 to *n*-3 ratio swam more slowly, unless ARA was substituted for LA as the source of the *n*-6. The lower body weight in the high *n*-6 to *n*-3 fed mice was not attributed to simply *n*-6 deficiency. The high *n*-3 to *n*-6 ratio led to the inhibition of Δ6-desaturase [207]. Thus, the conversion of LA to ARA was impeded and ARA became unavailable for growth. Mice fed high levels of DHA also had high levels of EPA showing a considerable amount of retroconversion. The findings showed the importance of balancing the amounts of ARA to DHA and that some deficits can be overcome if LA is replaced by ARA as the source of *n-6* fatty acid [207]. Wainright *et al.* [208] also reported that ARA supplementation increased ARA levels and decreased DHA levels in forebrain membrane phospholipids in Long-Evans rats, whereas DHA supplementation increased DHA levels and decreased ARA levels. Correlational analyses did not show a relationship between DHA and ARA levels in the forebrain and working memory performance [208,209].

Newborn infants of diabetic mothers have lower ARA and DHA levels in cord blood than newborns of normal mothers [210]. The lower levels of the LCPUFA in the newborns of diabetic mothers were associated with impaired and altered sensory-cognitive and psychomotor functions at birth and reduced visual and memory performance at 8 and 12 months [211,212]. Compared with normal controls, most rat models of diabetes are characterized by a lower level of brain ARA only and not a lower level of DHA [213]. Even though both ARA and DHA are important for neurodevelopment, brain accretion of ARA exceeds that of DHA during gestation [214], especially in the first two trimesters during the period of rapid proliferation of neuronal and glial elements [179,215]. When Sprague-Dawley diabetic, pregnant rats were fed either a control diet or an ARA (0.5%) supplemented diet throughout reproduction, the weaned offspring in the ARA group performed significantly better in the water maze and rotarod tests and showed greater exploratory behavior than control-diet offspring [216]. The results indicated that maternal hyperglycemia has long-term consequences during the initial stages of learning and that maternal supplementation with ARA positively influences learning outcomes.

Amusquivar *et al.* [217] reported that rat pups of dams fed diets with *n-3* fatty acids from fish oil compared with those fed *n-6* fatty acids from olive oil during pregnancy and lactation had smaller increases in postnatal body weight and length, and delayed body and psychomotor maturation indices. Slower growth and brain development occurred when both dams and fetuses were fed a moderate amount of fish oil (10%) as the only fat source [217]. In the study, the ARA level was lower than the DHA level in brain tissue of the offspring of dams fed high *n-3* fatty acid diets. The differences in postnatal development disappeared when the fish oil was supplemented with γ-linolenic acid, a precursor of ARA. The growth deficits were also eliminated by the inclusion of ARA in the diet [207]. The studies demonstrate the importance of maintaining adequate levels of ARA during development, and suggest that diets too high in *n-3* fatty acids during development may have negative effects on development by reducing tissue levels of ARA [218].

To investigate the effects that a DHA-rich maternal diet compared with an ARA-only diet have on brain fatty acid composition of Sprague-Dawley rats, Elsherbiny *et al.* [219] considered a control diet containing ARA (0.4 g/100 g of total fatty acid) *vs.* a DHA + ARA diet (0.9 g/100 of DHA and 0.4 g/100 g of ARA of total fatty acid). The results indicated that at three weeks postnatally the DHA-rich diet increased levels of DHA in the brain and decreased ARA by 12.8%. The brain of a three-week-old rat is at a comparable stage as that of a human toddler at 2–3 years of age [219]. At six weeks (comparable to a 12–18 years old human), the DHA-induced decreases in ARA were reversed and disappeared when DHA was continued (*i.e.*, DHA/control group). Thus, elevated dietary levels of DHA decrease the amount of ARA in brain without an adequate supply of dietary ARA.

Prepulse inhibition (PPI) is a normal suppression of a startle response when a low intensity stimulus that elicits little or no behavioral response immediately precedes an unexpected stronger startling response [220]. Deficits in PPI have been reported in individuals that have mental disorders including schizophrenia [220]. Various brain regions including the hippocampus have been associated with PPI problems. To determine whether dietary administration of LCPUFA enhances neurogenesis in the rat hippocampus and improves PPI response in wild-type mice and Pax6[+/−] mice (that exhibit PPI deficits) a control diet or diets supplemented with ARA (4%), DHA (4%) or ARA (4%) + DHA (4%) were administered [220]. Compared with the other diets, the administration of the ARA diet successfully increased neurogenesis not only in the Pax6[+/−] mice but also in the wild-type mice. Treating the

Pax6$^{+/-}$ mice with ARA also resulted in alleviating their PPI deficits. The authors suggested that the ARA diet as compared with the DHA or ARA + DHA diets positively affected postnatal neurogenesis in several regions of the brain including the hippocampus by influencing the fluidity of neuronal membranes and by regulating neuronal transmission [220].

11. Introduction of DHA and ARA in Infant Formulas

Both DHA and ARA have been added to infant formulas in the United States since 2001. In Europe, the addition of DHA and ARA in infant formulas began much earlier in 1994. Most infant formulas contain 0.2% to 0.4% total fatty acids of DHA and between 0.35% and 0.7% total fatty acids of ARA based on worldwide averages of DHA and ARA content in human milk [5]. Several international expert groups [6–9] support the addition of these levels of DHA and ARA in infant formulas to ensure optimal infant growth and development. Thus, all commercially available infant formulas contain preformed ARA at levels equal to or higher than the DHA content in formulas where these LCPUFA are added.

To determine the necessity of adding LCPUFA to infant formula, several studies were performed in the 1990s with preterm and term infants fed formulas containing DHA or EPA with and without ARA (see Fleith and Clandinin [221] for a review). No studies have examined supplementation of infant formula with ARA alone. In most studies, a control group without LCPUFA and/or a breastfed group were included. Studies also investigated the effect of adding ALA to ensure a sufficient endogenous synthesis of DHA [222,223], but not surprisingly, due to the limited conversion of ALA to DHA, the added ALA was not effective in raising DHA plasma status to the same level as that observed in breastfed infants ([223]. Some studies also considered experimental formulas containing added γ-linolenic acid from black current-seed oil, borage oil, or evening primrose oil, DHA and EPA from marine oil, and ARA from egg phospholipids [223–229]. The effects of feeding formula supplemented with soy oil and marine oils containing DHA/EPA showed no abnormalities on growth, tolerance, clotting function, erythrocyte membrane fluidity and vitamin A or E levels in low-birth-weight-term infants [230].

Infant formulas containing DHA and ARA from single cell oils (DHASCO® and ARASCO®, DSM, Columbia, MD, USA), respectively, were evaluated and found to maintain both DHA and ARA status in infants [178,231–233]. After 2001, DHASCO and ARASCO (DSM, Columbia, MD, USA) became predominant as the sources of DHA and ARA added to infant formulas in the United States. Both DHASCO and ARASCO are general recognized as safe (GRAS) for use in infant formulas in the United States and approved as novel foods in Canada [234,235]. DHASCO and ARASCO have an established history of use in Europe, Australia and New Zealand and are not considered novel foods and can be added to infant formulas (see Ryan *et al.* [236] for a review of the safety of single-cell oils).

The clinical studies used to evaluate the effects of DHA and ARA added to infant formulas measured infant growth, body and fatty acid composition, behavioral and sensory functions (retinal function, visual acuity and auditory function). Many of the early studies focused on preterm infants because they provided an opportunity to evaluate the effects of DHA- and ARA-enriched formulas in infants who may be deficient in these LCPUFA. Transfer across the placenta and accretion of ARA and DHA in the developing human brain and retina occurs mainly during the last trimester of pregnancy [179,215] when the rate of brain growth is most rapid [237]. Infants born prematurely thus may have an increased need for dietary ARA due to the interrupted supply during the last trimester [220,238,239].

Four studies with preterm infants considered formulas without added preformed ARA [240–243]. Each was influential in recognizing the importance of ARA for optimal growth. Two of the studies reported an increase in visual acuity at 2 or 4 months postmenstrual age (PMA) in preterm infants fed formulas supplemented with DHA and EPA from fish oil with a low or high ratio of DHA to EPA (2:1, 5:1, respectively) and no ARA [241,244–246].

In one study [240], infants fed formula with a low ratio of DHA to EPA until 79 weeks PMA, compared with controls, had significantly lower z-score values for weight, length and head circumference beginning at 40 weeks PMA. Poorer growth was also associated with lower scores of psychomotor development [244]. The supplemented group also had lower blood levels of ARA [177] suggesting that the effects of growth may have been related to the reduced availability of ARA as a result of the competitive inhibition by the high levels of EPA in marine oil. This finding was supported in a second study [241] in which preterm infants were fed formula with a high DHA to EPA ratio until 48 weeks PMA. Compared with controls, preterm infants fed a high ratio of DHA to EPA and with no ARA consistently had lower mean weight-for-length values at 2, 6, 9, and 12 months PMA, weighed less at 6 and 9 months PMA, and had smaller head circumferences at 9 months PMA [246].

In a third study, three premature infant formulas were compared in a double-blind parallel-group study of the growth of healthy, very-low-birth-weight infants (846–1560 g at birth) [242]. The DHA formula contained 0.34% of fat as DHA and the DHA +ARA formula contained 0.33% as DHA and 0.60% as ARA. The control formula contained no DHA or ARA. A reference group consisted of term infants who were predominately breastfed. Results indicated that infants fed formula with DHA + ARA gained significantly more weight than infants fed formula without DHA+ARA. At 48 and 57 weeks, weight of infants in the DHA + ARA group did not differ from the reference group of term infants. Length of infants in the DHA + ARA group was significantly greater than that of infants fed DHA alone at 40 and 48 weeks, but not at 57 weeks. The authors concluded that supplementation with ARA in addition to DHA supported growth of preterm infants [242].

In a fourth study [243], male but not female preterm infants fed formula with DHA and EPA from fish oil (0.2 wt %, 5:1 ratio) and no ARA, or a control formula to 59 weeks PMA, had significantly smaller gains in weight, length, and head circumference and lower fat-free mass as determined from total body electrical conductivity (TOBEC).

In the Carlson *et al.* [177,240] studies that reported slower growth in preterm infants a positive association between plasma ARA concentration and measures of growth (weight, length, z-score, weight-to-length, and head circumference) was observed. In the 1990s, when the studies were conducted, it was unknown whether the negative effects of DHA and/or EPA supplementation on growth could be overcome by adding ARA to infant formulas [177]. However, it was known that the bioactive metabolites of ARA mediate the secretion of several hormones associated with growth and basic metabolic functions [247]. These include luteinizing hormone, prolactin, adrenocorticotropic hormone (ATCH), and corticotropin-releasing hormone (CRH) [241] which could influence growth. ARA and its second messengers also appear to be involved in bone formation and resorption [248].

To maintain ARA status in preterm infants, additional studies were performed with infant formulas containing both ARA and DHA [221]. The addition of ARA at levels found in breast milk produced growth comparable to that observed in breastfed infants [221]. Adding both ARA and DHA to preterm infant formulas also resulted in beneficial effects on visual acuity as compared with infants fed a control formula [221].

Concern with a high level of DHA without a concomitant increase of ARA was raised in a randomized, controlled clinical trial of term infants administered formula with no LCPUFA, or differing levels of DHA intakes of 0.32%, 0.64% and 0.96% at the same ARA level of 0.64% [249,250]. There were no formula effects on tests of behavioral and psychophysiological indices of attention at 4, 6, and 9 months of age. However, infants supplemented at the two lower doses of DHA spent proportionally more time engaged in active stimulating processes (increased attention) than infants in the unsupplemented group [249]. Positive results were also observed on vocabulary (Peabody Picture Vocabulary), a card-shorting task, and an intelligence test (Wechler Primary Preschool Scales of Intelligence) at 3 to 6 years of age in the two lower doses of DHA (0.32% and 0.64%) [250]. However, performance of infants and children who were administered the highest dose of DHA (0.96%) but with a reduced ratio of ARA to DHA was attenuated [250]. The results demonstrated that a proper balance of DHA and ARA is needed for optimal cognitive performance as too much DHA may suppress the benefits provided by ARA.

The effects that different ratios of *n*-6 to *n*-3 had on preterm infant neurodevelopment were recently considered by Alshweki *et al.* [251]. Preterm infants (<1500 g and/or <32 weeks gestational age) were given infant formula with an *n*-6 to *n*-3 ratio of 2:1 or 1:1. The infants were followed for up to 2 years. Preterm infants fed formula with a 2:1 ratio of ARA to DHA had higher ARA blood levels during the first year of life and better psychomotor development compared with those fed a 1:1 ratio of ARA to DHA. However, despite the fact that one group received twice the amount of ARA than DHA (66% *vs.* 33%), there was almost no difference between the two groups in plasma *n*-6 to *n*-3 ratio. The balance between *n*-6 and *n*-3 is very complex, but appears to be maintained at a steady level when adequate supplementation of ARA and DHA are available [251].

To date, several systematic reviews of the literature and meta-analyses have been published to evaluate the effects of LCPUFA in preterm and term infants [221,229,252] on various outcomes including growth, cognition and vision. The reviews considered both the earlier and more recent studies on LCPUFA. Fleith and Clandinin [221], in one of the earliest reviews, reported that collectively the body of literature supported the view that LCPUFA are important for growth and development of preterm and term infants. Formula levels of ARA and DHA should be in the same range as those found in human milk and with the same ratio [221]. There needs to be a dietary supply of ARA and DHA to achieve similar accretion levels in plasma and in RBC as compared with breastfed infants [221,253,254].

A Cochrane review of LCPUFA supplementation in term infants reported that there was little evidence that supplementation conferred a benefit on visual or cognitive development [229]. In a recent meta-analysis of four clinical trials including data for preterm and term infants, LCPUFA supplementation was also shown to have no effect on Bailey Developmental scores at 18 months of age [252]. However, as pointed out by Colombo *et al.* [250], the lack of an observed effect at 18 months of age is consistent with the view that the Bailey Scales of Infant Development are not very sensitive to the effects of LCPUFA supplementation. The Bailey Scales of Infant Development yield a composite score obtained from the infant's attainment of normal developmental milestones and may not be able to provide detailed assays of specific cognitive mechanisms that are measured using more sophisticated laboratory tasks [250]. This raises the question of whether the Bailey Scales are appropriate for measuring the effects of LCPUFA on cognitive development in older infants/toddlers.

A systematic review of 20 randomized, controlled trials of term infants who received DHA and ARA supplemented formula or a control formula indicated that infants given formulas containing DHA levels close to the worldwide human milk mean of 0.32% of total fatty acids were more likely to yield positive results on cognitive and visual tests [255]. There was also clinical evidence to suggest than an ARA:DHA ratio greater than 1:1 was associated with improved cognitive outcomes [255].

Since the publication of the Hoffman *et al.* [255] review, several epidemiological and interventional studies of LCPUFA supplementation during infancy have appeared in the literature. These recent publications have been reviewed by Ryan *et al.* [256]. The most recent data indicate that maternal supplementation during pregnancy and/or lactation support the role for LCPUFA in the neurodevelopment of infants [256]. Supplementation with LCPUFA-containing infant formula for more than 6 months increased the likelihood of observing improved cognitive function during infancy [256,257].

The reasons that some studies failed to show a statistically significant association between LCPUFA intake and better neurological performance may have been related to limitations of study design and the use of varying amounts and sources of LCPUFA. For example, in the United States, most of the recent studies that have considered both neurocognitive function and growth have used infant formulas for preterm and term infants that contain DHA and ARA from single cell oils (DHASCO® and ARASCO®). Outside the United States, DHA may be obtained from fish oil [258,259] and ARA may be obtained from eggs [260,261]. As mentioned above, the early studies of the 1990s used a variety of experimental formulas with different sources and amounts of LCPUFA (many of these studies are cited by EFSA in their review, [71]). This is noteworthy because only DHA and ARA from single cell oils have been recently shown to enhance neurodevelopment in both preterm [262–264] and term infants [257,265]. The source of the oil is important because it significantly affects growth. Clandinin *et al.* [264] have shown that body weight at 118 days and length at 79 and 92 weeks of age in preterm infants fed formula containing ARA and DHA from single-cell oils were greater than in those than those fed a formula containing DHA from tuna oil. Additionally, for both weight and length, there were no differences between breastfed infants and those fed ARA and DHA from single-cell oils [264]. The possibility that ARA and DHA derived from single-cell oils or fish oil have differing effects on growth and neurodevelopment may also be due to the EPA at too high a level in fish oil and its propensity to antagonize ARA [257]. An ARA:DHA ratio greater than 1:1 with up to 0.65% of ARA of total fatty acids is associated with improved cognitive performance [255] and balances the potential competition caused by high levels of DHA.

12. The Benefits of ARA for Infant Health

LCPUFA are not only important for growth and neurodevelopment, but recent studies have shown that LCPUFA are also critical for infant health. In an early study, infants fed formula with ARA and DHA developed significantly less stage II and III NEC than those fed a control formula but had similar rates of bronchopulmonary dysplasia, septicemia and retinopathy of prematurity (ROP) [266]. In a recent retrospective cohort study of premature infants (<30 weeks gestation), the relationship between fatty acid profiles during the first postnatal month and infant morbidity due to chronic lung disease, ROP, and late-onset sepsis was analyzed [120]. Results indicated that fatty acid levels of DHA and ARA declined rapidly with a concomitant increase in LA. While the decreased DHA level was associated with increased risk of chronic lung disease, decreased ARA was associated with increased risk of late-onset sepsis. The authors noted that in premature infants, low levels of DHA and ARA contribute to dysregulation of immune and inflammatory responses, predisposing these infants to chronic lung disease and late-onset sepsis [120]. The DHA-derived resolvins decrease neutrophil infiltration and enhance macrophage phagocytosis [267]. DHA also downregulates nuclear factor kB activity in cells either directly or by stimulating the activation of peroxisome proliferator-activated receptors thereby limiting the pro-inflammatory signaling mediated by ARA [267]. Thus, a low level of DHA would predispose these infants to an increased inflammatory response as seen in chronic lung disease. In late-onset sepsis, a decreased ARA level increases the risk of inhibiting the innate immune response through decreased production of eicosanoids, particularly leukotrienes, which enhance chemotaxis of leukocytes, neutrophil activation, and activity of natural killer cells [97,120]. As a consequence, in premature infants, a balance of DHA and ARA levels must be maintained to help reduce the development of morbidity due to prematurity.

Studies have demonstrated that LCPUFA in human milk can modulate immunological responses and affect the T-helper cell (Th) type-1 (Th1)/Th2 balance [268,269]. Th1 cell effectors produce interferon-γ (IFN-γ) and TNF-α which regulate cellular immunity against infection whereas Th2 cells produce interleukin (IL)-4, IL-5, and IL-13 which help mediate immunity against parasitic infections [270,271]. For example, Barakat *et al.* [272] reported that supplementation for 14 days with 10 mg/kg of ARA in *Schistosoma mansoni*-infected schoolchildren induced moderate cure rates (50%) in children with light infection and modest cure rates (21%) in those with high infection. The cure rates associated with ARA were comparable to those produced by 40 mg/kg of praziquantel. The combination of ARA and praziquantel elicited 83% and 78% cure rates in children with light and heavy infections, respectively [272].

The relationship between maternal fatty acid desaturase (FADS) genotype and LCPUFA levels in human milk on infant blood T-cell profiles and cytokine production in 6-month old infants was recently considered [271]. LCPUFA levels in human milk were measured at 4 weeks of age and the FADS genotype was determined in both mothers and infants. Results indicated that ARA levels in human milk were inversely correlated with the production of the cytokines IL-10, IL-17, IL-5 and IL-13 and EPA levels were positively associated with counts of regulatory T-cells and cytotoxic T-cells and decreased T-helper cell counts. The minor FADS alleles were associated with lower ARA and EPA levels in human milk and a higher production of IL-10, Il-17, and IL-5. The major FADS alleles were associated with an increase in the level of ARA in human milk (19%–22%) compared with the minor alleles. There were no association between T-cell distribution and maternal or infant gene variants. Also, there was no relationship between cytokine levels in plasma and levels of LA, EPA, or DHA in human milk.

It has been shown that the FADs gene polymorphism may influence the risk of developing allergies in children [273]. In the study by Muc *et al.* [271] the strongest association between LCPUFA levels and cytokines was observed among those related to the activity of type-2 and type-17 *vs.* those from type-1 responses. The expression of type-2 and type-17 cells have been linked to increased airway inflammation in severe asthma [274]. By reducing type-2 and type-17 activity, LCPUFA including ARA found in human milk may help reduce the risk of childhood asthma and allergies [271].

Notably, Th17 cytokines were initially identified as key factors in the induction of inflammation and tissue destruction associated with a variety of autoimmune response such as multiple sclerosis, arthritis, colitis, celiac disease, and gluten sensitivity [275,276]. However, it is becoming apparent that T17 cells also provide protective immunity against various pathogens at different mucosal sites [270]. Thus, there is a fine balance between protection and pathological manifestation of Th17 responses. As a consequence, a balance of LCPUFA levels similar to that found in human milk is needed to help reduce the risk of developing autoimmune diseases in childhood.

Two studies have compared the frequency of common illnesses in infants fed formula with and without DHA and ARA [277,278]. Both studies used the same LCPUFA-supplemented formula that contained 0.32% DHA and 0.64% ARA of total fatty acids (17 mg of DHA/100 kcal and 34 mg of ARA/100 kcal). In the first study, infants fed the LCPUFA-supplemented formula experienced a lower incidence of bronchiolitis/bronchitis compared with infants fed formula without DHA and ARA [277]. The results from the second study were similar to those of the first. Infants who consumed formula with DHA and ARA had a lower incidence of bronchiolitis/bronchitis, nasal congestion, cough and diarrhea requiring medical attention than infants fed formula without DHA and ARA. The authors indicated that DHA and ARA at present levels in infant formula and follow-on formulas may have a positive effect on moderate to severe common infant illnesses, including diarrhea [277,278].

Two cohorts of children who had previously completed randomized, double-blind trials (one published [72], one unpublished) in which they received a LCPUFA-supplemented formula that contained 0.32%–0.36% DHA and 0.64%–0.72% ARA of total fatty acids or an unsupplemented formula (control) fed during the first year of life were followed up to 3 years of age to determine the incidence of allergies and common respiratory illnesses [279]. The LCPUFA-supplemented group had a significantly lower risk for developing upper respiratory infections, wheezing/asthma, atopic dermatitis, any allergy, and a longer time to first diagnosis than those given an unsupplemented formula.

A subset of children from the Kansas City cohort of the DIAMOND (DHA Intake and Measurement of Neural Development) study [96] were followed to 4 years of age to determine the incidence of childhood allergies [280]. As infants, they were fed either a control unsupplemented formula or one of three formulas with either 0.32%, 0.64% or 0.96% of total fatty acids as DHA with the same amount of ARA (0.64% of total fatty acids). All the different DHA dose and ARA supplemented subjects were pooled into a single supplemented cohort. Results indicated that the incidence of allergic illnesses in the first year of life was lower in the combined LCPUFA group compared with the control. By 4 years of age, LCPUFA supplementation significantly delayed time to first allergic illness and skin allergic illness. LCPUFA supplementation also reduced the risk of any allergic diseases and skin allergic diseases. If the mother had allergies, LCPUFA supplementation reduced the incidence of wheezing/asthma in her offspring. The results of these allergy studies add to the evidence that supplementation of infant formula with both ARA and DHA in the first year of life delays the onset of allergy and may have a protective effect against allergy in early childhood.

Crawford *et al.* [45] reviewed the potential role that ARA and DHA play in protecting against some central nervous system injuries in preterm infants. Deficits of ARA and DHA may contribute to the complications related to prematurity [45]. The mechanism of action responsible for central nervous system injury is reduced vascular or endothelial integrity leading to hemorrhage or ischemia. ARA acts as an endothelial relaxation factor and plays a dominant role in endothelial membrane lipids. The inner cell membrane lipid of the endothelium is especially rich in ARA which provides for membrane properties, signaling and protein kinase C activation [281]. ARA is also a precursor for a range of small molecules that play a key role in cell trafficking, communication and vaso-regulation. As a result, any ARA or DHA deficiency in very preterm infants will be exacerbated after birth during a period of rapid growth. This deficiency may then lead to fragile, leaking vessels and rupture as seen in ROP [45].

The proportion of ARA the placenta delivers to the fetus ranges from 14% to 20% [45]. Infant formula for preterm infants only delivers ~0.4%–0.6% of ARA. For DHA, the placenta delivery to the fetus is ~6% whereas infant formula delivers ~0.3%. That is a 50-fold reduction in ARA and a >10-fold reduction in DHA compared with the infant's apparent physiological need. When plasma levels of ARA and DHA are followed from birth, they continue to decrease to about one third of that of the fetus. Crawford *et al.* [45] argue that higher intakes of ARA and DHA are needed to correct for deficiency during the first year of life.

To explore the impact that deficiency of ARA and DHA may have on immune cell function Moodley *et al.* [282] examined the fatty acid profile and main phosphoglyceride content of cord blood mononuclear cell (CBMC) membranes in healthy preterm infants (30 to 35 weeks) and term infants (37 to 40+ weeks). Results indicated that ARA was the dominant LCPUFA present in both PC and PE membrane fractions of CBMCs in both preterm and term infants. The proportions of ARA, DHA and other LCPUFA were significantly lower in PE and PC of preterm infants compared with those in term infants. The dominance of ARA was consistent with the process of biomagnification that preferentially selects ARA rather than other LCPUFA for transfer to the fetus. Preterm infants also had significantly lower absolute numbers of CD4+ leukocytes and CD4+ and CD8+ naïve T-cells. At birth, there is a period of transition from a sterile environment to one of higher infectious risk. The elevated levels of ARA in CBMCs concomitant with lower levels of other LCPUFA suggest that the acquisition of ARA is needed in preparation for a responsive immune system after birth. These findings indicate that in preterm infants a deficiency in the supply of ARA exists which may compromise their immune system [282].

Infants with mildly abnormal physical movements at 12 weeks of age are reported to have lower ARA content in erythrocyte membranes [283]. This abnormality occurred with maternal supplementation of DHA alone but was not seen when DHA was combined with ARA during pregnancy and lactation [283]. Mildly abnormal movements have been also observed during infancy and linked to increased prevalence of minor neurologic dysfunction and attention deficits at school age [284]. These findings imply that during early brain development of neonates, a supply of ARA is critical.

The effects that feeding preterm infants human milk (HM), infant formula without DHA and ARA (F) or formula with DHA (0.35%) and ARA (0.49%) have on isolated peripheral blood lymphocytes and lipid composition was evaluated by Field *et al.* [285]. Adding DHA and ARA to a preterm infant formula resulted in lymphocyte and cytokine production, phospholipid composition, and antigen maturity similar to those observed in infants fed human milk. These findings suggest that the addition of both DHA and ARA may improve the ability of the infant to respond to immune challenges in a manner similar to breastfed infants [285].

Several epidemiological studies have shown that individuals with learning disorders including attention deficit hyperactivity disorder (ADHD), dyslexia, and autism have signs of EFA deficiency or have lower than normal blood levels of DHA and ARA [286–289]. A meta-analysis of pooled data from RBC and plasma/serum samples indicated that ARA and DHA concentrations were significantly lower than normal in individuals with learning/developmental disorders [290]. In absolute amounts, the level of ARA was as severely depressed as DHA within RBC (both ~0.58 mg/100 mg of fatty acid below normal) but much lower than DHA within plasma/serum (−0.71 vs. −0.34). The reason for lower than normal blood levels of ARA in children with learning disorders is unknown but could be related to a low dietary intake of ARA relative to metabolic requirements or that ARA is not synthesized efficiently from precursor fatty acids, or not delivered or properly incorporated into the brain [290].

The effects of subnormal ARA on brain function seems to be independent of those associated with n-3 deficiency. In Japan where intakes of n-3 fatty acids are relatively high, the incidence of dyslexia in children is similar to that observed in Westernized countries (~6%) [291]. Therefore, although the Japanese population consumes sufficient amounts of n-3 fatty acids, there still may be insufficient intake of ARA to meet the needs for normal brain function during childhood [290]. The important role of ARA in normal growth and development requires as much research emphasis as DHA has received. ARA should be the focus of preclinical and clinical research for a detailed assessment of dietary requirements.

13. The Regulatory Requirements for ARA and DHA in Infant Formulas

A joint International Expert Consultation of the Food and Agricultural Organization of the United Nations (FAO) and the WHO was assembled in 1976 to review the literature on "The Role of Dietary Fats and Oils in Human Nutrition" [292]. The section dealing with infant growth and development indicated that the ideal recommendation for infant formulas would be to match the essential fatty acids found in human milk with respect to LCPUFA content [292]. The FAO further stated that LCPUFA were particularly important during fetal and infant growth when there is a high demand for the synthesis of cell structured lipid [292]. FAO issued a follow-up report in 1994 which provided additional supportive recommendations for adding both ARA and DHA to infant formulas. The FAO stated that "the n-6 and n-3 fatty acids have critical roles in the membrane structure and as precursors of eicosanoids, which are potent and highly reactive compounds. Various eicosanoids have widely divergent, and often opposing effects on, for example, smooth muscle cells, platelet aggregation, vascular parameters (permeability, contractility), and on the inflammatory processes and the immune system. Since they compete for the same enzymes and have different biological roles, the balance between the n-6 and the n-3 fatty acids in the diet can be of considerable importance" [293]. In a follow-up report in 2008–2010, the FAO/WHO Expert Consultancy on Fats and Fatty Acids further concluded that "There can be little doubt about the essentiality of DHA and ARA for the brain" [294].

A global standard for infant formula was established by the Codex Alimentarius Commission in 1981, and revised over the years [295]. The latest revision was issued in 2007 and the latest amendment was added in 2015 [296]. The standard includes details on essential composition of nutrients and a list of food additives that are allowed to be added. Quality control measures such as labeling, packaging, contaminants and hygiene are also specified. In the United States, standards for infant formula are the responsibility of the U.S. Food and Drug Administration (FDA). The U.S. Code of Federal Regulations Title 21, Part 106 specifies infant formula quality control procedures and Part 107 lists the nutrient requirements and other rules concerning labeling for infant formulas. Not surprisingly, the quality and safety standards for infant formulas are extremely high, exceeding most requirements for other food products [297].

In the European Union (EU), the legislation on infant formula and follow-on formulas was adopted in 2006 [298] and at the time of this writing is being revised. Before revising the legislation the European Commission requested the European Food Safety Authority (EFSA) Panel on Dietetic Products, Nutrition and Allergies to provide their scientific advice on the essential nutrient composition of infant and follow-on formulas [70,71]. In the first report of 2013, dedicated to nutrient requirements and dietary intakes of infants and young children in the EU, the EFSA Panel reviewed a variety of nutrients, including the levels of DHA and ARA. In the 2013 EFSA report, adequate intakes were defined as 100 mg/day of DHA and 140 mg/day of ARA from birth to six months of age. From 6 to 24 months of age, 100 mg/day of DHA were considered adequate. These recommendations were also supported by a global expert panel, based on a systematic review of the available scientific literature [299]. However, in the subsequent report of 2014, dedicated to essential composition of infant and follow-on formulae, the EFSA Panel advised that infant and follow-on formulas should contain relatively higher amounts of DHA (20–50 mg/100 kcal). Mandatory addition of ARA was not supported in this EFSA report. Still, the Panel noted that feeding an infant formula containing DHA alone resulted in lower concentration of ARA in erythrocytes compared with a control formula without DHA.

At an assumed mean fat content of 5.2 g 100 kcal in a typical infant formula, this means that the recommendation of higher levels of DHA would result in a DHA content of 0.38% to 0.96% of fatty acids, higher than the 0.2% to 0.3% of DHA currently found in most infant formulas available in the marketplace [2]. Notably, PUFA-supplemented commercially available infant formulas contain preformed ARA at levels equal to or higher than the DHA content. The ESFA Panel's advice of providing up to 1% DHA and no ARA is a unique approach and directly opposite to a consensus reached by international expert groups who have recommended that infant formulas for term infants should contain ARA at levels that range from 0.4% to 0.7% fatty acids (at a 1:1–2:1 ratio to DHA) based on the median worldwide range of ARA and DHA concentrations in breast milk [6–9].

14. Discussion

ARA is the principle LCPUFA in the inner cell membrane lipid of muscle, heart, vascular endothelium, adrenals, kidneys, liver, the placenta, and in almost all other organs [300]. ARA is essential for cell integrity. The cell membrane separates the interior structures of cells from the outside environment. It also controls the movement of substances in and out of the cell [300]. These membranes contain signalers, receptors, ion channels, antioxidant defense enzymes, and rafts. Changing any aspect of the composition of the cell membrane may alter its function [300]).

ARA has very different biological functions than DHA [300]. While DHA controls signaling membranes in the photoreceptor, brain and nervous system, ARA is indispensable in the vasculature and in specific aspects of immunity. ARA is important for brain growth during gestation and early infancy where it plays a critical role in cell division and signaling [11]. A potentially important aspect of ARA metabolism is its function as a precursor for leukotrienes, prostaglandins, and thromboxanes, collectively known as eicosanoids. Eicosanoids have numerous critical and specific functions occurring in almost every tissue of the body. Eicosanoids function to modulate the release of somatostatin, the principal hormone that stimulates cell proliferation and growth. Eicosanoids also have important roles in immunity and inflammation.

This review focused on the essentiality of ARA for infant growth and development. Animal studies demonstrated the importance of ARA for growth and maturation of neurons and myelin and the resolution of inflammation in models of NEC, influenza and EFA deficiency. These studies also provided compelling evidence that both preformed DHA and ARA are required for optimal cognitive and neurological development. The ratio of ARA and DHA added as supplements really matters. Brain tissue analysis of neonatal baboons fed formula with a high level of 0.96% DHA significantly reduced ARA levels in two regions of the brain indicating the importance of a proper balance of DHA and ARA [24].

For over 10 years, both DHA and ARA have been added to infant formulas worldwide in an attempt to match the nutrient supply and functional benefits achieved with human milk. The combination of ARA and DHA in infant formulas has been shown to be safe in many millions of infants globally. The DHA concentration in human milk is lower and more variable than for ARA and the level of ARA in human milk is more stable [5]. The relatively stability of the ARA level in human milk is biologically important because it provides preformed ARA consistently at a time when brain growth and development is most critical [300]. Although DHA is more variable than ARA it is always present in human milk and the balance between ARA and DHA can be as much as 2 to 1.

The biosynthetic capability for providing ARA and DHA for brain growth is low and preformed ARA and DHA are preferentially incorporated into the brain during gestation and early infancy [2,46]. Infant formulas devoid of ARA results in a dramatic decrease of up to 40% of ARA in plasma shortly after birth [223,230,238,239,300,301], especially in preterm infants who do not receive the third trimester's maternal supply of ARA and DHA. The finding that there is a decrease in ARA shortly after birth shows that biosynthetic capability is insufficient to meet the infant's demand [300]. The process of biomagnification and its resulting fatty acid profile further highlights the importance of ARA in infant growth [45]. In several clinical studies, the provision of high amounts of DHA/EPA without a concomitant supply of ARA has been associated with adverse effects on growth in premature infants [240–243].

EFSA [71] recently concluded that "there is no necessity to add ARA to infant formula even in the presence of DHA". This recommendation needs further explanation. One of the possible reasons for this recommendation is that it is generally believed that LA is converted into ARA in sufficient quantities, even though EFSA noted that feeding an infant formula containing DHA alone resulted in lower concentration of ARA in erythrocytes compared with a control formula without DHA. From the limited dietary intake data presented here for non-breastfed infants and young children (Table 1) living in developing and developed countries there is evidence that intakes of ARA from dietary sources are very low, much lower than the average amount of ARA available in human milk or infant formulas containing ARA and DHA. The composition of infant formulas and follow-on formulas should therefore not only be based on human milk composition but also on food/nutrient intake data to address the assumption that complementary foods fill nutrient gaps.

The EFSA Panel's advice of providing higher amounts of DHA (20–50 mg/100 kcal, 0.38% to 0.96% of fatty acids) without a concomitant supply of ARA is also questionable. As discussed here, DHA suppresses ARA concentration in membranes and its function. As a result, an infant formula with DHA and no ARA may result in a potential higher risk of morbidity due to the suppression of favorable eicosanoids that play a key role in cell trafficking, communication and vaso-regulation [45].

EFSA did not take into account the original FAO/WHO publications as well as the earlier 2008–2010 publication which strongly concluded "There can be little doubt about the essentiality of DHA and ARA for the brain" [294]. When infants are exclusively breastfed during the first 6 months of life, "there is evidence of a requirement for preformed ARA and DHA after 6 months of life" [294]. According to the 2010 FAO/WHO statement, DHA and ARA should be included in infant formula with DHA (from 0.2% to 0.5% of total fatty acids) and added ARA should be at least equal to the amount of DHA [294].

The clinical trials considered by EFSA were not designed to consider the specific physiological outcomes related to ARA. Most studies included both ARA and DHA. There were no clinical trials that evaluated the effects of ARA in the absence of DHA. The benefits of ARA + DHA supplementation cannot be ascribed to DHA alone but logically must be ascribed to the variables used in most of these studies, the combination of the two. The combination of ARA and DHA has shown benefits for cognitive development, visual function, and blood pressure well beyond the period of supplementation and into early childhood [249,302].

EFSA's lack of support of ARA in DHA-containing formulas relied almost exclusively on the meta-analysis of infant growth conducted by Makrides *et al.* [303]. However, the meta-analysis of Makrides *et al.* [303] was not comprehensive. The majority of subjects (*n* = 1050) included in the meta-analysis participated in 8 clinical trials using formula containing both DHA and ARA. Only 341 subjects in the 8 trials were provided infant formula with DHA/EPA without ARA. At 12 months of age, only 99 subjects were supplemented with DHA in the absence of ARA. Additionally, the analysis excluded studies that included preterm infants who are most vulnerable to growth faltering due to nutrition, and excluded studies in which DHA plus ARA supplementation was less than 3 months during which growth velocity is particularly sensitive to nutritional inadequacy. The reason for excluding these studies was not reported.

In the meta-analysis, Makrides *et al.* [303] noted that the results were inconclusive, *i.e.*, LCPUFA supplementation had no detrimental effect on growth. The importance of ARA as a structural and metabolically active lipid, was not addressed. Better visual and mental performance was attributed to the contribution of DHA. However, in one of the studies considered, DHA plus ARA improved mental function [265] compared with an unsupplemented control. In fact, in one study, DHA alone did not perform better than did the unsupplemented controls [72].

Clinical evidence to support the safe removal of ARA from infant formula and follow-on formula containing DHA is lacking. The human and nonhuman primate studies described herein question the EFSA recommendation to provide infant formula from birth with up to 1% of DHA without a proportional amount of ARA [2]. Any major change in infant formula composition should be subjected to a full preclinical and clinical evaluation of safety and nutritional adequacy before its introduction into the marketplace [2]. Without such an assessment, and in light of the universal presence of ARA in human milk and the numerous essential ARA functions for cell structure and function, the most judicious approach is to include ARA in DHA-containing infant formulas to promote optimal infant growth and development.

Acknowledgments: The corresponding author, Alan S. Ryan, has received funds from DSM Nutritional Products to cover the costs to publish this article.

Author Contributions: Kevin B. Hadley, Sheila Gautier and Norman Salem, Jr. conceived the structure of the review. Alan S. Ryan, Kevin B. Hadley, Stewart Forsyth, Sheila Gautier, and Norman Salem, Jr. were involved in drafting and writing of the manuscript, reviewing of scientific literature, and manuscript revision. All authors agreed on the final form of the manuscript.

Conflicts of Interest: The corresponding author, Alan S. Ryan received funds to help draft the manuscript. Kevin B. Hadley, Sheila Gautier and Norman Salem Jr. are employees of DSM Nutrition Products that manufactures and sells polyunsaturated fatty acids.

References

1. Martinez, M. Tissue levels of polyunsaturated fatty acids during early human development. *J. Pediatr.* **1992**, *120*, S129–S138. [CrossRef]
2. Koletzko, B.; Carlson, S.E.; van Goudoever, J.B. Should infant formula provide both omega-3 DHA and omega-6 arachidonic acid? *Ann. Nutr. Metab.* **2015**, *66*, 137–138. [CrossRef] [PubMed]
3. Bolling, K. Infant Feeding Survey, 2005. Available online: http://www.hscic.gov.uk/pubs/ifs2005 (accessed on 17 August 2015).
4. Centers for Disease Control and Prevention, Division of Nutrition, Physical Activity, and Obesity. Breastfeeding Report Card, 2014. Available online: http://www.cdc.gov/breastfeeding/data/reportcard.htm (accessed on 18 August 2015).
5. Brenna, J.T.; Varamini, B.; Jensen, R.G.; Diersen-Schade, D.A.; Boettcher, J.A.; Arterburn, L.M. Docosahexaenoic and arachidonic acid concentrations in human milk worldwide. *Am. J. Clin. Nutr.* **2007**, *85*, 1457–1464. [PubMed]
6. British Nutrition Foundation. *Unsaturated Fatty Acids: Nutritional and Physiological Significance*; Chapman & Hall: London, UK, 1992; pp. 152–163.
7. Food and Agricultural Organization of the United Nations/World Health Organization Joint Expert Consultation. Lipids in early development. In *Fats and Oils in Human Nutrition*; FAO Food and Nutrition Papers; FAO: Rome, Italy, 1994; Volume 57, pp. 49–55.
8. Simopoulos, A.P.; Leaf, A.; Salem, N., Jr. Workshop on the essentiality of and recommended dietary intakes for omega-6 and omega-3 fatty acids. *J. Am. Coll. Nutr.* **1999**, *18*, 487–489. [CrossRef] [PubMed]
9. Koletzko, B.; Baker, S.; Cleghorn, G.; Neto, U.F.; Gropalan, S.; Hernell, O.; Hock, Q.S.; Jirapinyo, P.; Lonnerdal, B.; Pencharz, P.; *et al.* Global standard for the composition of infant formula: Recommendations of an ESPAGHAN coordinated international expert group. *J. Pediatr. Gastroenterol. Nutr.* **2005**, *41*, 584–599. [CrossRef] [PubMed]

10. Lauritzen, L.; Hensen, H.S.; Jorgensen, M.H.; Michaelsen, K.F. The essentiality of long chain *n*-3 fatty acids in relation to development and function of the brain and retina. *Prog. Lipid Res.* **2001**, *40*, 1–94. [CrossRef]

11. Katsuki, H.; Okuda, S. Arachidonic acid as a neurotoxic and neurotrophic substance. *Prog. Neurobiol.* **1995**, *46*, 607–636. [CrossRef]

12. Crawford, M.A.; Broadhurst, C.L. The role of docosahexaenoic and the marine food web as determinants of evolution and hominid brain development: The challenges for human sustainability. *Nutr. Health* **2012**, *21*, 17–39. [CrossRef] [PubMed]

13. Bazan, N.G.; Reddy, T.S.; Bazan, H.E.P.; Birkle, D.L. Metabolism of arachidonic acid and docosahexaenoic acid in the retina. *Prog. Lipid Res.* **1886**, *25*, 595–606. [CrossRef]

14. Crawford, M.A.; Sinclair, A.J. Nutritional influences in the evolution of mammalian brain. In *Lipids, Malnutrition & the Developing Brain*; A Ciba Foundation Symposium: Amsterdam, The Netherlands, 1971; pp. 267–292.

15. Martinez, M. Polyunsaturated fatty acids in the developing human brain, red cells and plasma: Influence of nutrition and peroxisomal disease. In *Fatty Acids and Lipids: Biological Aspects*; Galli, C., Simopoulos, A.P., Tremoli, E., Eds.; Karger: Basel, Switzerland, 1994; Volume 75, pp. 70–78.

16. Dobbing, J.; Sands, J. Comparative aspects of the brain growth spurt. *Early Hum. Dev.* **1979**, *3*, 79–83. [CrossRef]

17. Su, H.-M.; Corso, T.N.; Nathanielsz, P.W.; Brenna, J.T. Linoleic acid kinetics and conversion to arachidonic acid in the pregnant and fetal baboon. *J. Lipid Res.* **1999**, *40*, 1304–1311. [PubMed]

18. Sanchez-Mejia, R.O.; Newman, J.W.; Toh, S.; Yu, G.; Zhou, G.Q.; Halabisky, B.; Cissé, M.; Scearce-Levie, K.; Cheng, I.H.; Gan, L.; *et al.* Phospholipase A2 reduction ameliorates cognitive deficits in a mouse model of Alzheimer's disease. *Nat. Neurosci.* **2008**, *11*, 1311–1318. [CrossRef] [PubMed]

19. Vijayaraghaven, S.; Huang, B.; Blumenthal, E.M.; Berg, D.L. Arachidonic acid as a possible negative feedback inhibitor of nicotinic acetylcholine receptors on neurons. *J. Neurosci.* **1995**, *15*, 3679–3687.

20. Williams, J.H.; Errington, M.L.; Lynch, M.A.; Bliss, T.V. Arachidonic acid induces a long term activity-dependent enhancement of synaptic transmission in the hippocampus. *Nature* **1989**, *341*, 739–742. [CrossRef] [PubMed]

21. Fukaya, T.; Gondaira, T.; Kashiyae, Y.; Kotani, S.; Ishikura, Y.; Fujikawa, S.; Kiso, Y.; Sakakibara, M. Arachidonic acid preserves hippocampal neuron membrane fluidity in senescent rats. *Neurobiol. Aging* **2007**, *28*, 1179–1186. [CrossRef] [PubMed]

22. Wang, Z.-J.; Liang, C.-L.; Li, G.-M.; Yu, C.-Y.; Yin, M. Neuroprotective effects of arachidonic acid against oxidative stress on rat hippocampal slices. *Chem. Biol. Interact.* **2006**, *163*, 207–217. [CrossRef] [PubMed]

23. Wijendran, V.; Lawrence, P.; Diau, G.-Y.; Boehm, G.; Nathanielsz, P.W.; Brenna, J.T. Significant utilization of dietary arachidonic acid is for brain adrenic acid in baboon neonates. *J. Lipid Res.* **2002**, *43*, 762–767. [PubMed]

24. Hsieh, A.T.; Anthony, J.C.; Diersen-Schade, D.A.; Rumsey, S.C.; Lawrence, P.; Li, C.; Nathanielsz, P.W.; Brenna, J.T. The influence of moderate and high dietary long chain polyunsaturated fatty acids (LCPUFA) on baboon neonate tissue fatty acids. *Pediatr. Res.* **2007**, *61*, 537–545. [CrossRef] [PubMed]

25. Yang, H.-J.; Sugiura, Y.; Ikegami, K.; Konishi, Y.; Setou, M. Axonal gradient of arachidonic acid-containing phosphatidylcholine and its dependence on actin dynamics. *J. Biol. Chem.* **2012**, *287*, 5290–5300. [CrossRef] [PubMed]

26. Bazan, N.G. The neuromessenger platelet-activation factor in plasticity and neurodegeneration. *Prog. Brain Res.* **1998**, *118*, 281–291. [PubMed]

27. Hattori, M.H.; Adachi, H.; Tsujimoto, M.; Arai, H.; Inoue, K. Miller-Dieker lissencephaly gene encodes a subunit of brain platelet-activation factor acetylhydrolase. *Nature* **1994**, *370*, 216–218. [CrossRef] [PubMed]

28. Darios, F.; Davletov, B. Omega-3 and omega-6 fatty acids stimulate cell membrane expansion by acting on syntaxin 3. *Nature* **2006**, *440*, 813–817. [CrossRef] [PubMed]

29. Darios, F.; Ruiperez, V.; Lopez, I.; Villanueva, J.; Gutierrez, L.M.; Davletov, B. α-synuclein sequesters arachidonic acid to modulate SNARE-mediated exocytosis. *EMBO Rep.* **2010**, *11*, 528–533. [CrossRef] [PubMed]

30. Smart, E.J.; Graf, G.A.; McNiven, M.A.; Sessa, W.C.; Engelman, J.A.; Scherer, P.E.; Okamoto, T.; Lisanti, M.P. Caveolins, liquid-ordered domains, and signal transduction. *Mol. Cell. Biol.* **1999**, *19*, 7289–7304. [CrossRef] [PubMed]

31. Pike, L.J.; Han, X.; Chung, K.-N.; Gross, R.W. Lipid rafts are enriched in arachidonic acid and plasmmenylethanolamine and their composition is independent of caveolin-1 expression: A quantitative electrospray ionization/mass spectrometric analysis. *Biochemistry* **2002**, *41*, 2075–2088. [CrossRef] [PubMed]

32. Pike, L. Lipid rafts: Bringing order to chaos. *J. Lipid Res.* **2003**, *44*, 655–667. [CrossRef] [PubMed]

33. Lee, H.-C.; Sasaki, J.; Kubo, T.; Matsuda, S.; Nakasaki, Y.; Hattori, M.; Tanaka, F.; Udagawa, O.; Kono, N.; Itoh, T.; *et al.* LPIAT1 regulates arachidonic acid content in phosphatidylinositol and is required for cortical lamination in mice. *Mol. Biol. Cell* **2012**, *23*, 4689–4697. [CrossRef] [PubMed]

34. Wolf, B.A.; Turk, J.; Sherman, W.R.; McDaniel, M.L. Intracellular Ca^{2+} mobilization of arachidonic acid. *J. Biol. Chem.* **1986**, *261*, 3501–3511. [PubMed]

35. Cao, Y.; Pearman, A.T.; Zimmermann, G.A.; McIntyre, T.M.; Prescott, S.M. Intracellular unesterified arachidonic acid signals apoptosis. *PNAS* **2000**, *97*, 11280–11285. [CrossRef] [PubMed]

36. Hicks, A.M.; DeLong, C.J.; Thomas, M.J.; Samuel, M.; Cui, Z. Unique molecular signatures of glycerophospholipid species in different rat tissues analyzed by tandem mass spectrometry. *Biochim. Biophys. Acta* **2006**, *71*, 1022–1029. [CrossRef] [PubMed]

37. Tanaka, T.; Iwawaki, D.; Sakamoto, M.; Takai, Y.; Morishige, J.-I.; Murakami, K.; Satouchi, K. Mechanisms of accumulation of aracidonate in phoshatidylinositol in yellowtail. *Eur. J. Biochem.* **2003**, *270*, 1466–1473. [CrossRef] [PubMed]

38. Jungalwala, F.B.; Evans, J.E.; McCluer, R.H. Compositional and molecular species analysis of phospholipids by high performance liquid chromatography couples with chemical ionization mass spectrometry. *J. Lipid Res.* **1984**, *25*, 738–749. [PubMed]

39. Szentpetery, Z.; Varnai, P.; Balla, T. Acute manipulation of Golgi phosphoinositides to assess their importance in cellular trafficking and signaling. *PNAS* **2010**, *107*, 8225–8230. [CrossRef] [PubMed]

40. Di Paolo, G.; De Camilli, P. Phosphoinositides in cell regulation and membrane dynamics. *Nature* **2006**, *44*, 12. [CrossRef] [PubMed]

41. Malaiyandi, L.M.; Honick, A.S.; Rintoul, G.L.; Wang, Q.L.; Reynolds, I.J. Zn^{2+} inhibits mitochondrial movement in neurons by phosphatidylinositol 3-kinase activation. *J. Neurosci.* **2005**, *25*, 9507–9514. [CrossRef] [PubMed]

42. De Vos, K.J.; Sable, J.; Miller, K.E.; Sheetz, M.P. Expression of phosphatidylinositol (4,5) bisphosphate-specific pleckstrin homology domains alters direction but not the level of axonal transport of mitochondria. *Mol. Biol. Cell* **2002**, *14*, 3636–3649. [CrossRef] [PubMed]

43. Caroni, P. New EMBO members' review: Actin cytoskeleton regulation through modulation of PI(4,5)P(2) rafts. *EMBO J.* **2001**, *20*, 4332–4336. [CrossRef] [PubMed]

44. Del Prado, M.; Villalpando, S.; Elizondo, A.; Rodriguez, M.; Demmelmair, H.; Koletzko, B. Contribution of dietary and newly formed arachidonic acid to human milk lipids in women eating a low-fat diet. *Am. J. Clin. Nutr.* **2001**, *74*, 242–247. [PubMed]

45. Crawford, M.A.; Golfetto, I.; Ghebremeskel, K.; Min, Y.; Moodley, T.; Poston, L.; Phylactos, A.; Cunnane, S.; Schmidt, W. The potential role for arachidonic and docosahaenoic acids in protection against some central nervous system injuries in preterm infants. *Lipids* **2003**, *38*, 303–315. [CrossRef] [PubMed]

46. Larque, E.; Ruiz-Palacios, M.; Koletzko, B. Placental regulation of fetal nutrient supply. *Curr. Opin. Clin. Nutr. Metab. Care* **2013**, *16*, 292–297. [CrossRef] [PubMed]

47. Koletzko, B.; Agostini, C.; Bergmann, R.; Ritzenthaler, K.; Shamir, R. Physiological aspects of human milk lipids and implications for infant feeding: A workshop report. *Acta Paediatr.* **2011**, *100*, 1405–1415. [CrossRef] [PubMed]

48. Sinclair, A.J.; Crawford, M.A. The accumulation of arachidonate and docosahaenoate in the developing rat brain. *J. Neurochem.* **1972**, *19*, 1753–1758. [CrossRef] [PubMed]

49. Makrides, M.; Neumann, M.; Byard, R.W.; Simmer, K.; Gibson, R.A. Fatty acid composition of brain, retina, and erythrocytes in breast- and formula-fed infants. *Am. J. Clin. Nutr.* **1994**, *60*, 189–194. [PubMed]

50. Kuipers, R.S.; Luxwolda, M.F.; Offringa, P.J.; Boersma, E.R.; Dijck-Brouwer, D.A.; Muskiet, F.A.J. Fetal intrauterine whole body linoleic, arachidonic, and docosahexaenoic acid contents and accretion rates. *Prostaglandins Leukot. Essent. Fat. Acids* **2011**, *86*, 13–20. [CrossRef] [PubMed]

51. Carver, J.D.; Benford, V.J.; Han, B.; Cantor, A.B. The relationship between age and the fatty acid composition of cerebral cortex and erythrocytes in human subjects. *Brain Res. Bull.* **2001**, *56*, 79–85. [CrossRef]

52. Salem, N.M.; Lin, Y.H.; Moriguchi, T.; Lim, S.Y.; Salem, N., Jr.; Hibbelin, J.R. Distribution of omega-6 and omega-3 polyunsaturated fatty acids in the whole rat body and 25 compartments. *Prostaglandins Leukot. Essent. Fat. Acids* **2015**, *100*, 13–20. [CrossRef] [PubMed]

53. DeMar, J.C., Jr.; DiMartino, C.; Baca, A.W.; Lefkowitz, W.; Salem, N., Jr. Effect of dietary docosahexaenoic acid on biosynthesis of docosahexaenoic acid from alpha-linolenic acid in young rats. *J. Lipid Res.* **2008**, *49*, 1963–1980. [CrossRef] [PubMed]

54. Tyburczy, C.; Kothapalli, K.S.D.; Park, W.J.; Blank, B.S.; Bradford, K.L.; Zimmer, J.P.; Butt, C.M.; Salem, N., Jr.; Brenna, J.T. Heart arachidonic acid is uniquely sensitive to dietary arachidonic acid and docosahexaenoic acid content in domestic piglets. *Prostaglandins Leukot. Essent. Fat. Acids* **2011**, *85*, 335–343. [CrossRef] [PubMed]

55. Axelrod, J. Receptor-mediated activation of phospholipase A2 and arachidonic acid release in signal transduction. *Biochem. Soc. Trans.* **1990**, *18*, 503–507. [CrossRef] [PubMed]

56. Piomelli, D. Eicosanoids in synaptic transmissions. *Crit. Rev. Neurobiol.* **1994**, *11*, 367–373.

57. Schoenheimer, R.; Rittenberg, D. Deuterium as an indicator in the study of intermediary metabolism V. The desaturation of fatty acids in the organism. *J. Biol. Chem.* **1936**, *113*, 505–510.

58. Nichaman, M.Z.; Olson, R.E.; Sweeley, C.C. Metabolism of linoleic acid-1-^{14}C in normolipidemic and hyperlipidemic humans fed linoleate diets. *Am. J. Clin. Nutr.* **1967**, *20*, 1070–1083. [PubMed]

59. Chambaz, J.; Ravel, D.; Manier, M.-C.; Pepin, D.; Mulliez, N.; Bereziat, G. Essential fatty acids interconversion in the human fetal liver. *Neonatology* **1985**, *47*, 136–140. [CrossRef]

60. El Boustani, S.; Descomps, B.; Monnier, L.; Warnant, J. *In vivo* conversion of dihommogamma linolenic acid into arachidonic acid in man. *Prog. Lipid Res.* **1986**, *25*, 67–71. [CrossRef]

61. Emken, E.A.; Adlof, R.O.; Rakoff, H.; Rohwedder, W.K. Metabolism of deuterium-labeled linolenic, linoleic, oleic, stearic and palmitic acid in human subjects. In Synthesis and Applications of Isotopically Labelled Compounds, Proceedings of the Third International Symposium, Innsbruck, Austria, 17–21 July 1988; Baillie, T.A., Jones, J.R., Eds.; Elsevier Science Publishers: Amsterdam, The Netherlands, 1988; pp. 713–716.

62. Emken, E.A.; Rohwedder, W.K.; Adlof, R.O.; Gulley, R.M. Metabolism in humans of cis-12, trans-15-octadecadienoic acid relative to palmitic, stearic, oleic and linoleic acids. *Lipids* **1987**, *22*, 495–504. [CrossRef] [PubMed]

63. Demmelmair, H.; von Schenck, U.; Behrendt, E.; Sauerwald, T.; Koletzko, B. Estimation of arachidonic acid synthesis in full-term neonates using natural variation of 13C content. *J. Pediatr. Gastroenterol. Nutr.* **1995**, *21*, 31–36. [CrossRef] [PubMed]

64. Salem, N., Jr.; Wegher, B.; Mena, P.; Uauy, R. Arachidonic and docosahexaenoic acids are biosynthesized from their 18-carbon precursors in human infants. *Proc. Natl. Acad. Sci. USA* **1996**, *93*, 49–54. [CrossRef] [PubMed]

65. Pawlosky, R.J.; Sprecher, H.W.; Salem, N., Jr. High sensitivity negative ion GC/MS method for detection of desaturated and chain-elongated products of deuterated linoleic and linolenic acids. *J. Lipid Res.* **1992**, *33*, 1711–1717. [PubMed]

66. Carnielli, V.P.; Wattimea, D.J.L.; Luijendijk, I.H.T.; Boerlage, A.; Degenhart, H.J.; Sauer, P.J.J. The very low weight premature infant is capable of synthesizing arachidonic and docosahexaenoic acids from linoleic and linolenic acids. *Pediatr. Res.* **1996**, *40*, 169–174. [CrossRef] [PubMed]

67. Pawlosky, R.J.; Lin, Y.H.; Llanos, A.; Mena, P.; Uauy, R.; Salem, N., Jr. Compartmental analysis of plasma ^{13}C- and ^{2}H-labelled *n*-6 fatty acids arising from oral administrations of ^{13}C-U-18:2*n*-6 and ^{2}H$_5$-20:3*n*-6 in newborn infants. *Pediatr. Res.* **2006**, *60*, 327–333. [CrossRef] [PubMed]

68. Sauerwald, T.U.; Hachey, D.L.; Jensen, C.L.; Chen, H.; Andersen, R.E.; Heird, W.C. Effect of dietary α-linolenic intake on incorporation of docosahexaenoic and arachidonic acids into plasma phospholipids of term infants. *Lipids* **1996**, *31*, S131–S135. [CrossRef] [PubMed]

69. Carnielli, V.P.; Simonato, M.; Verlato, G.; Luijendijk, I.; De Curtis, M.; Sauer, P.J.J.; Cogo, P.E. Synthesis of long-chain polyunsaturated fatty acids in preterm newborns fed formula with long-chain polyunsaturated fatty acids. *Am. J. Clin. Nutr.* **2007**, *86*, 1323–1330. [PubMed]

70. EFSA Panel on Dietetic Products. Scientific opinion on nutrient requirements and dietary intakes on infants and young children in the European Union. *EFSA J.* **2013**, *11*, 3408.

71. EFSA Panel on Dietetic Products, Nutrition and Allergies (NDA). Scientific opinion on the essential composition of infant and follow-on formulae. *EFSA J.* **2014**, *12*, 3760.

72. Birch, E.E.; Castañeda, Y.S.; Wheaton, D.H.; Birch, D.G.; Uauy, R.D.; Hoffman, D.R. Visual maturation of term infants fed long-chain polyunsaturated fatty acid-supplemented or control formula for 12 mo. *Am. J. Clin. Nutr.* **2005**, *81*, 871–879. [PubMed]
73. World Health Organization (WHO). Global Strategy on Infant and Young Child Feeding, 2002. Available online: http://www.who.int/nutrition/topics/infantfeeding _recommendation/en/ (accessed on 15 October 2015).
74. World Health Organization (WHO). Nutrient Adequacy of Exclusive Breastfeeding for the Term Infant during the First Six Months of Life, 2002. Available online: http://www.who.int/nutrition/publications/infantfeeding/9241562110/en/ (accessed on 15 October 2015).
75. American Academy of Pediatrics. Breastfeeding and the use of human milk. *Pediatrics* **2012**, *129*, e827. [CrossRef]
76. International Baby Food Action (IBFAN). The State of Breastfeeding in 33 Countries, 2010. Available online: https://www.google.co.uk/?gws_rd=ssl#q=IBFAN+33+countries (accessed on 15 October 2015).
77. U.S. Department of Agriculture, Agricultural Research Service. USDA National Nutrient Database for Standard Reference, Release 27. Nutrient Data Laboratory Home Page. 2014. Available online: http://www.ars.usda.gov/nutrientdata (accessed on 15 October 2015).
78. Centers for Disease Control and Prevention. Clinical Growth Charts, 2015. Available online: http://www.cdc.gov/growthcharts/cdccharts.htm (accessed on 19 November 2015).
79. Michaelsen, K.F.; Dewey, K.G.; Perez-Exposito, A.B. Food sources and intake of *n*-6 and *n*-3 fatty acids in low-income countries with emphasis on infants, young children (6–24 months), and pregnant and lactating women. *Mater. Child Nutr.* **2011**, *7* (Suppl. S2), 124–140. [CrossRef] [PubMed]
80. Agostoni, C. Docosahexaenoic acid (DHA): From the maternal-foetal dyad to the complementary feeding period. *Early Hum. Dev.* **2010**, *86* (Suppl. S1), 3–6. [CrossRef] [PubMed]
81. Prentice, A.M.; Paul, A.A. Fat and energy needs of children in developing countries. *Am. J. Clin. Nutr.* **2000**, *72*, 1253S–1265S. [PubMed]
82. Barbarich, B.N.; Willows, N.D.; Wang, L.; Clandinin, M.T. Polyunsaturated fatty acids and anthropometric indices of children in rural China. *Eur. J. Clin. Nutr.* **2006**, *60*, 1100–1107. [CrossRef] [PubMed]
83. PAHO/WHO. *Guiding Principles for Complementary Feeding of the Breastfed Child*; PAHO/WHO: Washington, DC, USA, 2003.
84. Joshi, N.; Agho, K.E.; Dibley, M.J.; Senarath, U.; Tiwari, K. Determinants of inappropriate complementary feeding practices in young children in Nepal: Secondary data analysis of Demographic and Health Survey 2006. *Mater. Child Nutr.* **2012**, *1*, 45–59. [CrossRef] [PubMed]
85. Dutta, T.; Sywulka, S.M.; Frongillo, E.A.; Lutter, C.K. Characteristics attributed to complementary foods by caregivers in four countries of Latin America and the Caribbean. *Food Nutr. Bull.* **2006**, *27*, 316–326. [CrossRef] [PubMed]
86. Agostoni, C.; Decsi, T.; Fewtrell, M.; Goulet, O.; Kolacek, S.; Koletzko, B.; Michaelsen, K.F.; Moreno, L.; Puntis, J.; Rigo, J.; *et al.* Complementary feeding: A commentary by the ESPGHAN Committee on Nutrition. *J. Pediatr. Gastroenterol. Nutr.* **2008**, *46*, 99–110. [CrossRef] [PubMed]
87. Schwartz, J.; Dube, K.; Alexy, U.; Kalhoff, H.; Kersting, M. PUFA and LC-PUFA intake during the first year of life: Can dietary practice achieve a guideline diet? *Eur. J. Clin. Nutr.* **2010**, *64*, 124–130. [CrossRef] [PubMed]
88. Schwartz, J.; Dube, K.; Sichert-Hellert, W.; Kannenberg, F.; Kunz, C.; Kalhoff, H.; Kersting, M. Modification of dietary polyunsaturated fatty acids via complementary food enhances *n*-3 long-chain polyunsaturated fatty acid synthesis in healthy infants: A double blinded randomised controlled trial. *Arch. Dis. Child.* **2009**, *94*, 876–882. [CrossRef] [PubMed]
89. Grote, V.; Verduci, E.; Scalioni, S.; Vecchi, F.; Contarini, G.; Giovannini, M.; Koletzko, B.; Agostoni, C. Breast milk composition and infant nutrient intakes during the first 12 months of life. *Eur. J. Clin. Nutr.* **2015**, *70*, 250–256. [CrossRef] [PubMed]
90. Sioen, I.; Matthys, C.; De Backer, G.; Van Camp, J.; De Henauw, S. Importance of seafood as nutrient source in the diet of Belgian adolescents. *J. Hum. Nutr. Diet.* **2007**, *20*, 580–589. [CrossRef] [PubMed]
91. Meyer, B.J.; Mann, N.J.; Lewis, J.L.; Milligan, G.C.; Sinclair, A.J.; Howe, P.R. Dietary intakes and food sources of omega-6 and omega-3 polyunsaturated fatty acids. *Lipids* **2003**, *38*, 391–398. [CrossRef] [PubMed]
92. Innis, S.M.; Vaghri, Z.; King, D.J. *n*-6 docosapentaenoic acid is not a predictor of low docosahexaenoic acid status in Canadian preschool children. *Am. J. Clin. Nutr.* **2004**, *80*, 768–773. [PubMed]

93. Lien, V.W.; Clamdinin, M.T. Dietary assessment of arachidonic acid and docosahexaenoic acid intake in 4–7 year-old children. *J. Am. Coll. Nutr.* **2009**, *28*, 7–15. [CrossRef] [PubMed]

94. Keim, S.A.; Branum, A.M. Dietary intake of polyunsaturated fatty acids and fish among US children 12–60 months of age. *Mater. Child Health Nutr.* **2015**, *11*, 987–998. [CrossRef] [PubMed]

95. U.S. Department of Agriculture, Agricultural Research Service. What We Eat in America. 2015. Available online: http://www.ars.usda.gov/Services/docs.htm?docid=13793# (accessed on 15 October 2015).

96. Birch, E.E.; Khoury, J.C.; Berseth, C.L.; Castaneda, Y.S.; Couch, J.M.; Bean, J.; Tamer, R.; Harris, C.L.; Mitmesser, S.H.; Scalabrin, D.M. The impact of early nutrition on incidence of allergic manifestations and common respiratory illnesses in children. *J. Pediatr.* **2010**, *156*, 902–906. [CrossRef] [PubMed]

97. Calder, P.C. Polyunsaturated fatty acids and inflammation: From molecular biology to the clinic. *Lipids* **2003**, *38*, 343–352. [CrossRef] [PubMed]

98. Calder, P.C. *n*-3 polyunsaturated fatty acids, inflammation, and inflammatory diseases. *Am. J. Clin. Nutr.* **2006**, *83*, 1505S–1519S. [PubMed]

99. Jones, P.J.H.; Kubow, S. Lipids, sterols, and their metabolites. In *Modern Nutrition in Health and Disease*; Shils, M.E., Shike, M., Ross, A.C., Caballero, B., Cousins, B., Eds.; Lippincott Williams & Wilkins: Philadelphia, PA, USA, 2006; pp. 92–122.

100. Ricciotti, E.; FitzGerald, G.A. Prostaglandins and inflammation. *Arterioscler. Thromb. Vasc. Biol.* **2011**, *31*, 986–1000. [CrossRef] [PubMed]

101. Reinhold, H.; Ahmadi, S.; Depner, U.B.; Layh, B.; Heindl, C.; Hamza, M.; Pahl, A.; Brune, K.; Narumiya, S.; Müller, U.; *et al.* Spinal inflammatory hyperalgesia is mediated by prostaglandin E receptors of the EP2 subtype. *J. Clin. Investig.* **2005**, *115*, 673–679. [CrossRef] [PubMed]

102. Noda, M.; Kariura, Y.; Pannasch, U.; Nishikawa, K.; Wang, L.; Seike, T.; Ifuku, M.; Kosai, Y.; Wang, B.; Nolte, C.; *et al.* Neuroprotective role of bradykinin because of the attenuation of pro-inflammatory cytokine release from activated microglia. *J. Neurochem.* **2007**, *101*, 397–410. [CrossRef] [PubMed]

103. Min, Y.; Crawford, M.A. Essential fatty acids. In *The Eicosanoids*; Curtis, P., Ed.; John Wiley & Sons, Ltd.: West Sussex, UK, 2004; pp. 257–276.

104. McCarthy, T.L.; Casinghino, S.; Mittanck, D.W.; Ji, C.H.; Centrella, M.; Rotwein, P. Promoter-dependent and -independent activation of insulin-like growth factor binding protein-5 gene expression by prostaglandin E_2 in primary rat osteoblasts. *J. Biol. Chem.* **1996**, *271*, 6666–6671. [PubMed]

105. Urade, Y.; Hayaishi, O. Prostaglandin D2 and sleep regulation. *Biochem. Biophys. Acta* **1999**, *1436*, 606–615. [CrossRef]

106. Ushikubi, F.; Sergi, E.; Sugimoto, Y.; Murata, T.; Matsuoka, T.; Kobayashi, T.; Hizaki, H.; Tuboi, K.; Katsuyama, M.; Ichikawa, A.; *et al.* Impaired febrile response in mice lacking the prostaglandin E receptor subtype EP3. *Nature* **1998**, *395*, 281–284. [PubMed]

107. Murata, T.; Ushikubi, F.; Matsuoka, T.; Hirata, M.; Yamasaki, A.; Sugimoto, Y.; Ichikawa, A.; Aze, Y.; Tanaka, T.; Yoshida, N.; *et al.* Altered pain perception and inflammatory response in mice lacking prostacyclin receptor. *Nature* **1997**, *388*, 678–682. [PubMed]

108. Astudillo, A.M.; Balgoma, D.; Balboa, M.A.; Balsinde, J. Dynamics of arachidonic acid mobilization by inflammatory cells. *Biochim. Biophys. Acta* **2012**, *1821*, 249–256. [CrossRef] [PubMed]

109. Bagga, D.; Wang, L.; Faris-Eisner, R.; Glaspy, J.A.; Reddy, S.T. Differential effects of prostaglandin derived from ω-6 and ω-3 polyunsaturated fatty acids on COX-2 expression and IL-6 secretion. *Proc. Natl. Acad. Sci. USA* **2003**, *100*, 1751–1756. [CrossRef] [PubMed]

110. Levy, B.D.; Clish, C.B.; Schmidt, B.; Gronert, K.; Serhan, C.N. Lipid mediator class switching during acute inflammation signals in resolution. *Nat. Immunol.* **2001**, *2*, 612–619. [CrossRef] [PubMed]

111. Samuelsson, B.; Dahlen, S.E.; Lindgren, J.A.; Rouzer, C.A.; Serhan, C.N. Leukotrienes and lipoxins—Structures, biosynthesis, and biological effects. *Science* **1987**, *237*, 1171–1176. [CrossRef] [PubMed]

112. Fredman, G.; Serhan, C.N. Specialized proresolving mediator targets for RvE1 and RvD1 in peripheral blood and mechanisms of resolution. *Biochem. J.* **2011**, *437*, 185–197. [CrossRef] [PubMed]

113. Kelley, D.S. Modulation of human and inflammatory responses by dietary fatty acids. *Nutrition* **2001**, *17*, 669–673. [CrossRef]

114. Calder, P.C.; Kew, S. The immune system: A target for functional foods? *Br. J. Nutr.* **2002**, *88* (Suppl. S2), S165–S176. [CrossRef] [PubMed]

115. Lentz, A.K.; Feezor, R.J. Principles of immunology. *Nutr. Clin. Pract.* **2003**, *18*, 451–460. [CrossRef] [PubMed]
116. Mahadevappa, V.G.; Holub, B.J. The molecular species composition of individual diacyl phospholipids in human platelets. *Biochim. Biophys. Acta* **1982**, *713*, 73–79. [CrossRef]
117. Kaushansky, K. Lineage-specific hematopoietic growth factors. *N. Engl. J. Med.* **2006**, *354*, 2034–2045. [CrossRef] [PubMed]
118. Semple, J.W.; Italiano, J.E., Jr.; Freedman, J. Platelets and the immune system. *Nature* **2011**, *11*, 264–274.
119. Tamagawa-Mineoka, R. Important roles of platelets as immune cells in the skin. *J. Dermatol. Sci.* **2015**, *77*, 93–101. [CrossRef] [PubMed]
120. Martin, C.R.; DaSilva, D.A.; Cluette-Brown, J.E.; DiMonda, C.; Hamill, A.; Bhutta, A.Q.; Coronel, E.; Wilschanski, M.; Stephens, A.J.; Driscoll, D.F.; *et al.* Decreased postnatal docosahexaenoic and arachidonic acid blood levels in premature infants are associated with neonatal morbidities. *J. Pediatr.* **2011**, *159*, 743–749. [CrossRef] [PubMed]
121. Lands, W.F.; LeTellier, P.R.; Rome, L.H.; Vanderhoek, J.Y. Inhibition of prostaglandin biosynthesis. *Adv. Biosci.* **1973**, *9*, 15–227.
122. Vane, J.R. Inhibition of prostaglandin synthesis as a mechanism of action for aspirin-like drugs. *Nature* **1971**, *231*, 232–235. [CrossRef]
123. Hormones. Available online: http://www.medicinenet.com/script/main/art.asp?articlekey=3783 (accessed on 6 February 2016).
124. McMurray, W.C. *A Synopsis of Human Biochemistry*; Harper and Row Publishers: New York, NY, USA, 1982; pp. 193–199.
125. Bowen, R.A. Hormone Chemistry, Synthesis and Elimination. Available online: http://www.vivo.colostate.edu/hbooks/pathphys/endocrine/basics/chem.html (accessed on 15 October 2015).
126. Thorner, M.O.; Vance, M.L.; Hartman, M.L.; Holl, R.W.; Evans, W.S.; Veldhuis, J.D.; Van Cauter, E.; Copinschi, G.; Bowers, C.Y. Physiological role of somatostatin on growth hormone regulation in humans. *Metabolism* **1990**, *39*, 40–42. [CrossRef]
127. Brochhausen, C.; Neuland, P.; Kirkpatrick, C.J.; Nusing, R.M.; Klaus, G. Cyclooxygenases and prostaglandin E_2 receptors in growth plate chondrocytes *in vitro* and *in situ*-prostaglandin E_2 dependent proliferation of growth plate chondrocytes. *Arthritis Res. Ther.* **2006**, *8*, R78. [CrossRef] [PubMed]
128. Boyan, B.D.; Sylvia, V.L.; Dean, D.D.; Del Toro, F.; Schwartz, Z. Differential regulation of growth plate chondrocytes by 1alpha,25-(OH)2D3 and 24R,25-(OH)2D3 involves cell-maturation-specific membrane-receptor-activated phospholipid metabolism. *Crit. Rev. Oral Biol. Med.* **2002**, *13*, 143–154. [CrossRef] [PubMed]
129. Specker, B.; Binkley, T. Randomized trial of physical activity and calcium supplementation on bone mineral content in 3- to 5-year-old children. *J. Bone Miner. Res.* **2003**, *418*, 885–892. [CrossRef] [PubMed]
130. Specker, B.L.; Mulligan, L.; Ho, M. Longitudinal study of calcium intake, physical activity, and bone mineral content in infants 6–18 months of age. *J. Bone Miner. Res.* **1999**, *14*, 569–576. [CrossRef] [PubMed]
131. Del Toro, F., Jr.; Sylvia, V.L.; Schubkegel, S.R.; Campos, R.; Dean, D.D.; Boyan, B.D.; Schwartz, Z. Characterization of prostaglandin E(2) receptors and their role in 24,25-(OH)(2)D(3)-mediated effects on resting zone chondrocytes. *J. Cell Physiol.* **2000**, *182*, 196–208. [CrossRef]
132. Boyan, B.D.; Sylvia, V.L.; Dean, D.D.; Pedrozo, H.; Del Toro, F.; Nemere, I.; Posner, G.H.; Schwartz, Z. 1,25-(OH)2D3 modulates growth plate chondrocytes via membrane receptor-mediated protein kinase C by a mechanism that involves changes in phospholipid metabolism and the action of arachidonic acid and PGE$_2$. *Steroids* **1999**, *64*, 129–136. [PubMed]
133. Schwartz, Z.; Sylvia, V.L.; Curry, D.; Luna, M.H.; Dean, D.D.; Boyan, B.D. Arachidonic acid directly mediates the rapid effects of 24,25-dihydroxyvitamin D3 via protein kinase C and indirectly through prostaglandin production in resting zone chondrocytes. *Endocrinology* **1999**, *140*, 2991–3002. [CrossRef] [PubMed]
134. Sylvia, V.L.; Schwartz, Z.; Curry, D.B.; Chang, Z.; Dean, D.D.; Boyan, B.D. 1,25(OH)2D3 regulates protein kinase C activity through two phospholipid-dependent pathways involving phospholipase A2 and phospholipase C in growth zone chondrocytes. *J. Bone Miner. Res.* **1998**, *13*, 559–569. [CrossRef] [PubMed]
135. Kosher, R.A.; Walker, K.H. The effect of prostaglandins on *in vitro* limb cartilage differentiation. *Exp. Cell Res.* **1983**, *145*, 145–153. [CrossRef]

136. Copray, J.C.; Jansen, H.W. Cyclic nucleotides and growth regulation of the mandibular condylar cartilage of the rat *in vitro*. *Arch. Oral Biol.* **1985**, *30*, 749–752. [CrossRef]

137. Li, T.F.; Zuscik, M.J.; Ionescu, A.M.; Zhang, X.; Rosier, R.N.; Schwarz, E.M.; Drissi, H.; O'Keefe, R.J. PGE$_2$ inhibits chondrocyte differentiation through PKA and PKC signaling. *Exp. Cell Res.* **2004**, *300*, 159–169. [CrossRef] [PubMed]

138. Raisz, L.G. Prostaglandins and bone: Physiology and pathophysiology. *Osteoarthr. Cartil.* **1999**, *7*, 419–421. [CrossRef] [PubMed]

139. Suzawa, T.; Miyaura, C.; Inada, M.; Maruyama, T.; Sugimoto, Y.; Ushikubi, F.; Ichikawa, A.; Narumiya, S.; Suda, T. The role of prostaglandin E receptor subtypes (EP1, EP2, EP3, and EP4) in bone resorption: An analysis using specific agonists for the respective EPs. *Endocrinology* **2000**, *141*, 1554–1559. [CrossRef] [PubMed]

140. Baylink, D.J.; Finkelman, R.D.; Mohan, S. Growth factors to stimulate bone formation. *J. Bone Min. Res.* **1993**, *8*, S565–S572. [CrossRef] [PubMed]

141. Paralkar, V.M.; Borovecki, F.; Ke, H.Z.; Cameron, K.O.; Lefker, B.; Grasser, W.A.; Owen, T.A.; Li, M.; DaSilva-Jardine, P.; Zhou, M.; *et al.* An EP2 receptor-selective prostaglandin E$_2$ agonist induces bone healing. *PNAS* **2003**, *100*, 6736–6740. [CrossRef] [PubMed]

142. Tanaka, M.; Sakai, A.; Uchida, S.; Tanaka, S.; Nagashima, M.; Katayama, T.; Yamaguchi, K.; Nakamura, T. Prostaglandin E$_2$ receptor (EP4) selective agonist (ONO-4819.CD) accelerates bone repair of femoral cortex after drill-hole injury associated with local upregulation of bone turnover in mature rats. *Bone* **2004**, *34*, 940–943. [CrossRef] [PubMed]

143. Jee, W.S.; Ueno, K.; Kimmel, D.B.; Woodbury, D.M.; Price, P.; Woodbury, L.A. The role of bone cells in increasing metaphyseal hard tissue in rapidly growing rats treated with prostaglandin E$_2$. *Bone* **1987**, *8*, 171–178. [CrossRef]

144. Agas, D.; Marchetti, L.; Hurley, M.M.; Sabbieti, D. Prostaglandin F2α: A bone remodeling mediator. *J. Cell. Physiol.* **2013**, *228*, 25–29. [CrossRef] [PubMed]

145. Galea, G.L.; Meakin, L.B.; Williams, C.M.; Hulin-Curtis, S.L.; Lanyon, L.E.; Poole, A.W.; Price, J.S. Protein kinase Cα (PKCα) regulates bone architecture and osteoblast activity. *J. Biol. Chem.* **2014**, *289*, 25509–25522. [CrossRef] [PubMed]

146. Zaman, G.; Sunters, A.; Galea, G.L.; Javaheri, B.; Saxon, L.K.; Moustafa, A.; Armstrong, V.J.; Price, J.S.; Lanyon, L.E. Loading-related regulation of transcription factor EGR2/Krox-20 in bone cells is ERK1/2 protein-mediated and prostaglandin, Wnt-signaling pathway-, and insulin-like growth factor-I axis-dependent. *J. Biol. Chem.* **2012**, *287*, 3946–3962. [CrossRef] [PubMed]

147. Kido, S.; Kuriwaka-Kido, R.; Umino-Miyatani, Y.; Endo, I.; Inoue, D.; Taniguchi, H.; Inoue, Y.; Imamura, T.; Matsumoto, T. Mechanical stress activates Smad pathway through PKCδ to enhance interleukin-11 gene transcription in osteoblasts. *PLoS ONE* **2010**, *5*, e13090. [CrossRef] [PubMed]

148. Nakura, A.; Higuchi, C.; Yoshida, K.; Yoshikawa, H. PkCα suppresses osteoblastic differentiation. *Bone* **2011**, *48*, 476–484. [CrossRef] [PubMed]

149. Weiler, H.A.; Fitzpatrick-Wong, S. Dietary long-chain polyunsaturated fatty acids minimize dexamethasone-induced reductions in arachidonic acid status but not bone mineral content in piglets. *Pediatr. Res.* **2002**, *51*, 282–289. [CrossRef] [PubMed]

150. Blanaru, J.L.; Kohut, J.R.; Fitzpatrick-Wong, S.C.; Weiler, H.A. Dose response of bone mass to dietary arachidonic acid in piglets fed cow milk-based formula. *Am. J. Clin. Nutr.* **2004**, *79*, 139–147. [PubMed]

151. Pash, J.M.; Canalis, E. Transcriptional regulation of insulin-like growth factor-binding protein-5 by prostaglandin E$_2$ in osteoblast cells. *Endocrinology* **1996**, *137*, 2375–2382. [PubMed]

152. Almaden, Y.; Canalejo, A.; Ballesteros, E.; Anon, G.; Rodriguez, M. Effect of high extracellular phosphate concentration on arachidonic acid production by parathyroid tissue *in vitro*. *J. Am. Soc. Nephrol.* **2000**, *11*, 1712–1718. [PubMed]

153. Klein-Nulend, J.; Burger, E.H.; Semeins, C.M.; Raisz, L.G.; Pilbeam, C.C. Pulsating fluid flow stimulates prostaglandin release and inducible prostaglandin G/H synthase mRNA expression in primary mouse bone cells. *J. Bone Miner. Res.* **1997**, *12*, 45–51. [CrossRef] [PubMed]

154. Weiler, H.A. Dietary supplementation of arachidonic acid is associated with higher whole body weight and bone mineral density in growing pigs. *Pediatr. Res.* **2000**, *47*, 692–697. [CrossRef] [PubMed]

155. Weiler, H.; Fitzpatrick-Wong, S.; Schellenberg, J.; McCloy, U.; Veitch, R.; Kovacs, H.; Kohut, J.; Kin Yuen, C. Maternal and cord blood long-chain polyunsaturated fatty acids are predictive of bone mass at birth in healthy term-born infants. *Pediatr. Res.* **2005**, *58*, 1254–1258. [CrossRef] [PubMed]

156. Akatsu, T.; Takahashi, N.; Udagawa, N.; Imamura, K.; Yamaguchi, A.; Sato, K.; Nagata, N.; Suda, T. Role of prostaglandins in interleukin-1-induced bone resorption in mice *in vitro*. *J. Bone Miner. Res.* **1991**, *6*, 183–189. [CrossRef] [PubMed]

157. Liu, X.H.; Kirschenbaum, A.; Yao, S.; Levine, A.C. Interactive effect of interleukin-6 and prostaglandin E_2 on osteoclastogenesis via the OPG/RANKL/RANK system. *Ann. N. Y. Acad. Sci.* **2006**, *1068*, 225–233. [CrossRef] [PubMed]

158. Zhang, X.; Schwarz, E.M.; Young, D.A.; Puzas, J.E.; Rosier, R.N.; O'Keefe, R.J. Cyclooxygenase-2 regulates mesenchymal cell differentiation into the osteoblast lineage and is critically involved in bone repair. *J. Clin. Investig.* **2002**, *109*, 1405–1415. [CrossRef] [PubMed]

159. Samoto, H.; Shimizu, E.; Matsuda-Honjyo, Y.; Saito, R.; Nakao, S.; Yamazaki, M.; Furuyama, S.; Sugiya, H.; Sodek, J.; Ogata, Y. Prostaglandin E_2 stimulates bone sialoprotein (BSP) expression through cAMP and fibroblast growth factor 2 response elements in the proximal promoter of the rat BSP gene. *J. Biol. Chem.* **2003**, *278*, 28659–28667. [CrossRef] [PubMed]

160. Cherian, P.P.; Cheng, B.; Gu, S.; Sprague, E.; Bonewald, L.F.; Jiang, J.X. Effects of mechanical strain on the function of Gap junctions in osteocytes are mediated through the prostaglandin EP2 receptor. *J. Biol. Chem.* **2003**, *278*, 43146–43156. [CrossRef] [PubMed]

161. Miyaura, C.; Inada, M.; Matsumoto, C.; Ohshiba, T.; Uozumi, N.; Shimizu, T.; Ito, A. An essential role of cytosolic phospholipase A2alpha in prostaglandin E_2-mediated bone resorption associated with inflammation. *J. Exp. Med.* **2003**, *197*, 1303–1310. [CrossRef] [PubMed]

162. Boswell, K.; Koskelo, E.-K.; Carl, L.; Glaze, S.; Hensen, D.J.; Williams, K.D.; Kyle, D.J. Preclinical evaluation of single-cell oils that are highly enriched with arachidonic acid and docosahexaenoic acid. *Food Chem. Toxicol.* **1996**, *34*, 585–593. [CrossRef]

163. Suarez, A.; del Carmen Ramirez, M.; Faus, M.J.; Gil, A. Dietary long-chain polyunsaturated fatty acids influence tissue fatty acid composition in rats at weaning. *J. Nutr.* **1996**, *126*, 887–897. [PubMed]

164. De la Presa-Owens, S.; Innis, S.M.; Rioux, F.M. Addition of triglycerides with arachidonic acid or docosahexaenoic acid to infant formula has tissue- and lipid class-specific effects on fatty acids and hepatic desaturase activities in formula-fed piglets. *J. Nutr.* **1998**, *128*, 1376–1384. [PubMed]

165. Baur, L.A.; O'Connor, J.; Pan, D.A.; Kriketos, A.D.; Storlien, L.H. The fatty acid composition of skeletal muscle membrane phospholipid: Its relationship with the type of feeding and plasma levels in young children. *Metabolism* **1998**, *47*, 106–112. [CrossRef]

166. Blaauw, B.; Del Piccolo, P.; Rodriguez, L.; Hernandez Gonzales, V.H.; Agata, L.; Solagna, F.; Mammano, F.; Pozzan, T.; Schiaffino, S. No evidence for inositol 1,4,5-triphosphate-dependent Ca^{2+} release in isolated fibers of adult mouse skeletal muscle. *J. Gen. Physiol.* **2012**, *140*, 235–241. [CrossRef] [PubMed]

167. Berthier, C.; Kutchukian, C.; Bouvard, C.; Okamura, Y.; Jacquemond, V. Depression of voltage-activated Ca^{2+} release in skeletal muscle by activation of a voltage-sensing phosphatase. *J. Gen. Physiol.* **2015**, *145*, 315–330. [CrossRef] [PubMed]

168. Ohizumi, Y.; Hirata, Y.; Suzuki, A.; Kobayashi, M. Two novel types of calcium release from skeletal sarcoplasmic reticulum by phosphatidylinositol 4,5 biphosphate. *Can. J. Physiol. Pharmacol.* **1999**, *77*, 276–285. [CrossRef] [PubMed]

169. Sandow, A. Excitation-contraction coupling in muscular response. *Yale J. Biol. Med.* **1952**, *25*, 176–201. [PubMed]

170. Melzer, W.; Herrmann-Frank, A.; Luttgau, H.C. The role of Ca^{2+} ions in excitation-contraction coupling of skeletal muscle fibres. *Biochim. Biophys. Acta* **1995**, *1241*, 59–116. [CrossRef]

171. Kobayashi, M.; Muroyama, A.; Ohizumi, Y. Phosphatidylinositol 4,5-bisphosphate enhances calcium release from sarcoplasmic reticulum of skeletal muscle. *Biochem. Biophys. Res. Commun.* **1989**, *29*, 1487–1491. [CrossRef]

172. Ghigo, A.; Perino, A.; Hirsch, E. Phosphoinositides and cardiac function. In *Phosphoinositides and Disease, Current Topics in Microbiology and Immunology*; Falasca, M., Ed.; Springer Science + Business Media: Dordrecht, The Netherlands, 2012; pp. 43–60.

173. Rodemann, H.P.; Goldberg, A.L. Arachidonic acid, prostaglandin E_2 and $F_{2\alpha}$ influence rates of protein turnover in skeletal and cardiac muscle. *J. Biol. Chem.* **1982**, *25*, 1632–1638.

174. Standley, R.A.; Liu, S.; Jemiolo, B.; Trappe, S.W.; Trappe, T.A. Prostaglandin E_2 induces transcription of skeletal mass regulators interleukin-6 and muscle RING finger-1 in humans. *Prostaglandins Leukot. Essent. Fat. Acids* **2013**, *88*, 361–364. [CrossRef] [PubMed]

175. Kuipers, R.S.; Luxwolda, M.F.; Dijck-Brouwer, J.; Muskiet, F.A.J. Intrauterine, postpartum and adult relationships between arachidonic acid (AA) and docosahexaenoic acid (DHA). *Prostaglandins Leukot. Essent. Fat. Acids* **2011**, *85*, 245–252. [CrossRef] [PubMed]

176. Luxwolda, M.F.; Kuipers, R.S.; Sango, W.S.; Kwesigabo, G.; Dijck-Brouwer, D.A.J.; Muskiet, F.A.J. A maternal erythrocyte DHA content of approximately 6 g% is the DHA status at which intrauterine DHA biomagnifications turns into bioattenuation and postnatal infant DHA equilibrium is reached. *Eur. J. Nutr.* **2012**, *51*, 665–675. [CrossRef] [PubMed]

177. Carlson, S.E.; Werkman, S.H.; Peoples, J.M.; Cooke, R.J.; Tolley, E.A. Arachidonic acid status correlates with first year of growth in preterm infants. *Proc. Natl. Acad. Sci. USA* **1993**, *90*, 1073–1077. [CrossRef] [PubMed]

178. Clandinin, M.T. Brain development and assessing the supply of polyunsaturated fatty acids. *Lipids* **1999**, *34*, 131–137. [CrossRef] [PubMed]

179. Clandinin, M.T.; Chappell, J.E.; Leong, S.; Heim, T.; Sayer, P.R.; Chance, G.W. Intrauterine fatty acid accretion in infant brain: Implications for fatty acid requirements. *Early Hum. Dev.* **1980**, *4*, 121–129. [CrossRef]

180. Cunnane, S. Problems with essential fatty acids: Time for a new paradigm? *Prog. Lipid Res.* **2003**, *42*, 544–568. [CrossRef]

181. Stoffel, W.; Holz, B.; Jenke, B.; Binczek, E.; Günter, R.H.; Kiss, C.; Karakesisoglou, I.; Thevis, M.; Weber, A.A.; Arnhold, S.; *et al.* Δ6-desaturase (FADS2) deficiency unveils role of ω3- and ω6-polyunsaturated fatty acids. *EMBO J.* **2008**, *27*, 2281–2292. [CrossRef] [PubMed]

182. Stroud, C.K.; Nara, T.Y.; Roqueta-Rivera, M.; Radlowski, E.C.; Lawrence, P.; Zhang, Y.; Cho, B.H.; Segre, M.; Hess, R.A.; Brenna, J.T.; *et al.* Disruption of FADS2 gene in mice impairs male reproduction and causes dermal and intestinal ulceration. *J. Lipid Res.* **2009**, *50*, 1870–1880. [CrossRef] [PubMed]

183. Mohrhauer, H.; Holman, R.T. The effect of dose level of essential fatty acids upon fatty acid composition of the rat liver. *J. Lipid Res.* **1963**, *4*, 151–159. [PubMed]

184. Prottey, C. Essential fatty acids and the skin. *Br. J. Dermatol.* **1976**, *94*, 579–587. [CrossRef] [PubMed]

185. Hansen, H.S.; Jensen, B. Essential function of linoleic acid esterified in acylglucosylceramide and acylceramide in maintaining the epiderma; water permeability barrier. Evidence from feeding studies with oleate, linoleate, arachidonate, columbinate and alpha-linolenate. *Biochem. Biophys. Acta* **1985**, *834*, 357–363. [CrossRef]

186. Hartop, P.J.; Prottey, C. Changes in transepidermal water loss and the composition of epidermal lecithin after application of pure fatty acid triglycerides to the skin of essential fatty acid-deficient rats. *Br. J. Dermatol.* **1976**, *95*, 255–264. [CrossRef] [PubMed]

187. Bertram, T.A. Gastrointestinal tract. In *Handbook of Toxicologic Pathology*; Haschek, W.M., Rousseaux, C.G., Wallig, M., Eds.; Academic Press: San Diego, CA, USA, 2002; pp. 121–186.

188. Miller, C.C.; Ziboh, V.A. Induction of epidermal hyperproliferation by topical *n*-3 polyunsaturated fatty acids on guinea pig skin linked to decreased levels of 13-hydroxyoctadecadienoic acid (13-Hode). *J. Investig. Dermatol.* **1990**, *94*, 353–358. [CrossRef] [PubMed]

189. Cho, H.P.; Nakamura, T.; Clarke, S.D. Cloning, expression, and nutritional regulation of the mammalian delta-6 desaturate. *J. Biol. Chem.* **1999**, *274*, 471–477. [CrossRef] [PubMed]

190. Williard, D.E.; Nwankwo, J.O.; Kaduce, T.L.; Harmon, S.D.; Irons, M.; Moser, H.W.; Raymond, G.V.; Spector, A.A. Identification of a fatty acid delta6-desaturase deficiency in human skin fibroblasts. *J. Lipid Res.* **2001**, *42*, 501–508. [PubMed]

191. Fan, Y-Y.; Monk, J.M.; Hou, T.Y.; Callway, E.; Vincent, L.; Weeks, B.; Yang, P.; Chapkin, R.S. Characterization of an arachidonic acid-deficient (Fads1 knockout) mouse model. *J. Lipid Res.* **2012**, *53*, 1287–1295.

192. Hatanaka, E.; Yasuda, H.; Harauma, A.; Watanabe, J.; Konishi, Y.; Nakamura, M.; Salem, N., Jr.; Moriguchi, T. The Effects of Arachidonic Acid and/or Docosahexaenoic Acid on the Brain Development Using Artificial Rearing of Delta-6-Desaturase Knockout Mice. In Proceedings of the Asian Conference of Nutrition, Yokohama, Japan, 14–18 May 2015.

193. Tian, C.; Fan, C.; Liu, X.; Xu, F.; Qi, K. Brain histological changes in young mice submitted to diets with different ratios of *n*-6/*n*-3 polyunsaturated fatty acids during maternal pregnancy and lactation. *Clin. Nutr.* **2011**, *30*, 659–667. [CrossRef] [PubMed]

194. Nguyen, L.N.; Ma, D.; Shui, G.; Wong, P.; Cazenave-Gassiot, A.; Zhang, X.; Wenk, M.R.; Goh, E.L.K.; Silver, D.L. Mfsd2a is a transporter for the essential omega-3 fatty acid docosahexaenoic acid. *Nature* **2014**, *509*, 503–506. [CrossRef] [PubMed]

195. Berger, J.H.; Charron, M.J.; Silver, D.L. Major Facilitator superfamily domain-containing protein 2a (MFSD2A) has roles in body growth, motor function, and lipid metabolism. *PLoS ONE* **2012**, *7*, e50629. [CrossRef] [PubMed]

196. Peterson, L.D.; Jeffrey, N.M.; Sanderson, P.; Newholme, E.A.; Calder, P.C. Eicosapentaenoic and docosahexaenoic acids alter rat spleen leukocyte fatty acid composition and prostaglandin E_2 production but have different effects on lymphocyte functions and cell-mediated immunity. *Lipids* **1998**, *33*, 171–180. [CrossRef] [PubMed]

197. Jolly, C.A.; Jiang, Y-H.; Chapkin, R.S.; McMurray, D.N. Dietary (*n*-3) polyunsaturated fatty acids suppress murine lymphoproliferation, interleukin-2 secretion, and the formation of diacylglycerol and ceramide. *J. Nutr.* **1997**, *127*, 37–43. [PubMed]

198. Kelley, D.S.; Taylor, P.C.; Nelson, G.J.; Schmidt, P.C.; Mackey, B.E.; Kyle, D. Effects of dietary arachidonic acid on human immune response. *Lipids* **1997**, *32*, 449–456. [CrossRef] [PubMed]

199. Blikslager, A.T.; Moeser, A.J.; Gookin, J.L.; Jones, S.L.; Odle, J. Restoration of barrier function in injured intestinal mucosa. *Physiol. Rev.* **2007**, *87*, 545–564. [CrossRef] [PubMed]

200. Ferrer, R.; Moreno, J.J. Role of eicosanoids on intestinal epithelial homeostatis. *Biochem. Pharmacol.* **2010**, *80*, 431–438. [CrossRef] [PubMed]

201. Jacobi, S.K.; Moeser, A.J.; Corl, B.A.; Harrell, R.J.; Bilksager, A.T. Dietary long-chain PUFA enhances acute repair of ischemia-injured intestine of suckling pigs. *J. Nutr.* **2012**, *142*, 1266–1271. [CrossRef] [PubMed]

202. Le, H.D.; Meisel, J.A.; de Meijer, V.E.; Fallon, E.M.; Gura, K.M.; Nose, V.; Bistrian, B.R.; Puder, M. Docosahexaenoic acid and arachidonic acid prevent essential fatty acid deficiency and hepatic steatosis. *J. Parenter. Enter. Nutr.* **2012**, *36*, 431–441. [CrossRef] [PubMed]

203. Bassaganya-Riera, J.; Guri, A.J.; Noble, A.M.; Reynolds, K.A.; King, J.; Wood, C.M.; Ashby, M.; Rai, D.; Hontecillas, R. Arachidonic acid- and docosahexaenoic acid-enriched formulas modulate antigen-specific T cell responses to influenza virus in neonatal piglets. *Am. J. Clin. Nutr.* **2007**, *85*, 824–836. [PubMed]

204. Weisinger, H.S.; Vingrys, A.J.; Sinclair, A.J. The effect of docosahexaenoic acid on the electroretinogram of the guinea pig. *Lipids* **1996**, *31*, 65–70. [CrossRef] [PubMed]

205. Champoux, M.; Hibbeln, J.R.; Shannon, C.; Majchrzak, S.; Suomi, S.J.; Salem, N., Jr.; Higley, J.D. Fatty acid formula supplementation and neuromotor development in rhesus monkey neonates. *Pediatr. Res.* **2002**, *51*, 273–281. [CrossRef] [PubMed]

206. Ikemoto, A.; Ohishi, M.; Sato, Y.; Hata, N.; Misawa, Y.; Fujii, Y.; Okuyama, H. Reversibility of *n*-3 fatty acid deficiency-induced learning behavior in the rat: Level of *n*-6 fatty acids as another factor. *J. Lipid Res.* **2001**, *42*, 1655–1663. [PubMed]

207. Wainwright, P.E.; Xing, H.-C.; Mutsaers, L.; McCutcheon, D.; Kyle, D. Arachidonic acid offsets the effects on mouse brain and behavior of a diet with a low (*n*-6):(*n*-3) ratio and very high levels of docosahexaenoic acid. *J. Nutr.* **1997**, *127*, 184–193. [PubMed]

208. Wainwright, P.E.; Xing, H.-C.; Ward, G.R.; Huang, Y.-S.; Bobik, E.; Auestad, N.; Montalto, M. Water maze performance is unaffected in artificially reared rats fed diets supplemented with arachidonic acid and docosahexaenoic acid. *J. Nutr.* **1999**, *129*, 1079–1089. [PubMed]

209. Wainwright, P.E.; Huang, Y.S.; Bulman-Fleming, B.; Dalby, B.; Mills, D.E.; Redden, P.; McCutcheon, D. The effect of dietary *n*-3/*n*-6 ration on brain development in the mouse: A dose response study with long-chain *n*-3 fatty acids. *Lipids* **1992**, *27*, 98–103. [CrossRef] [PubMed]

210. Min, Y.; Lowry, C.; Ghebremeskel, K.; Thomas, B.; Offley-Shore, B.; Crawford, M. Unfavorable effect of type 1 and type 2 diabetes on maternal and fetal essential fatty acid status: A potential marker of fetal insulin resistance. *Am. J. Clin. Nutr.* **2005**, *82*, 1162–1168. [PubMed]

211. Siddappa, A.M.; Georgieff, M.K.; Wewerka, S.; Worwa, C.; Nelson, C.A.; Deregnier, R.A. Iron deficiency alters auditory recognition memory in newborn infants of diabetic mothers. *Pediatr. Res.* **2004**, *55*, 1034–1041. [CrossRef] [PubMed]

212. DeBoer, T.; Wewerka, S.; Bauer, P.J.; Geogieff, M.K.; Nelson, C.A. Explicit memory performance in infants of diabetic mothers at 1 year of age. *Dev. Med. Child Neurol.* **2005**, *47*, 525–531. [CrossRef] [PubMed]

213. Holman, R.T.; Johnson, S.B.; Gerrand, J.M.; Mauer, S.M.; Kupcho-Sandberg, S.; Brown, D.M. Arachidonic acid deficiency in streptozotocin-induced diabetes. *Proc. Natl. Acad. Sci. USA* **1983**, *80*, 1375–2379. [CrossRef]

214. Hadders-Algra, M. Prenatal long-chain polyunsaturated fatty acid status: The importance of a balanced intake of docosahexaenoic acid and arachidonic acid. *J. Perinat. Med.* **2008**, *36*, 101–109. [CrossRef] [PubMed]

215. Clandinin, M.T.; Chappell, J.E.; Leong, S.; Heim, T.; Sayer, P.R.; Chance, G.W. Extrauterine fatty acid accretion in infant brain: Implications for fatty acid requirements. *Early Hum. Dev.* **1980**, *4*, 131–138. [CrossRef]

216. Zhao, J.; Bigio, M.R.; Weiler, H.A. Maternal arachidonic acid supplementation improves neurodevelopment in young adult offspring from rat dams with and without diabetes. *Prostaglandins Leukot Essent. Fat. Acids* **2011**, *84*, 63–70. [CrossRef] [PubMed]

217. Amusquivar, E.; Ruperez, F.J.; Barbas, C.; Herrera, E. Low arachidonic acid rather than α-tocopherol is responsible for the delayed postnatal development of offspring of rats fed fish oil instead of olive oil during pregnancy and lactation. *J. Nutr.* **2000**, *13*, 2855–2865.

218. Haubner, L.; Sullivan, J.; Ashmeade, T.; Saste, M.; Wiener, D.; Carver, J. The effects of maternal dietary docosahexaenoic acid intake on rat pup myelin and the auditory startle response. *Dev. Neurosci.* **2007**, *29*, 460–467. [CrossRef] [PubMed]

219. Elsherbiny, M.E.; Goruk, S.; Monckton, E.A.; Richard, C.; Brun, M.; Emara, M.; Field, C.J.; Godbout, R. Long-term effect of docosahexaenoic acid feeding on lipid composition and brain fatty acid-binding protein expression in rats. *Nutrients* **2015**, *7*, 8802–8817. [CrossRef] [PubMed]

220. Maekawa, M.; Takashima, N.; Matsumata, M.; Ikegami, S.; Kontani, M.; Hara, Y.; Kawashima, H.; Owada, Y.; Kiso, Y.; Yoshikawa, T.; *et al.* Arachidonic acid drives postnatal neurogenesis and elicits a beneficial effect on prepulse inhibition, a biological trait of psychiatric illnesses. *PLoS ONE* **2009**, *4*, e5085. [CrossRef] [PubMed]

221. Fleith, M.; Clandinin, T. Dietary PUFA for preterm and term infants: Review of clinical studies. *Crit. Rev. Food Sci. Nutr.* **2005**, *3*, 205–229. [CrossRef]

222. Jensen, C.L.; Prager, T.C.; Fraley, J.K.; Chen, H.; Anderson, R.E.; Heird, W.C. Effect of dietary linoleic/alpha-linolenic acid ratio on growth and visual function of term infants. *J. Pediatr.* **1997**, *131*, 200–209. [CrossRef]

223. Makrides, M.; Neumann, M.A.; Jeffrey, B.; Lien, E.L.; Gibson, R.A. A randomized trial of different ratios of linoleic to alpha-linolenic acid in the diet of term infants: Effect on visual function and growth. *Am. J. Clin. Nutr.* **2000**, *71*, 120–129. [PubMed]

224. Makrides, M.; Neumann, M.A.; Simmer, K.; Gibson, R.A. Erythrocyte fatty acids of term infants fed either breast milk, standard formula, or formula supplemented with long-chain polyunsaturates. *Lipids* **1995**, *30*, 941–948. [CrossRef] [PubMed]

225. Makrides, M.; Neumann, M.A.; Simmer, K.; Pater, J.; Gibson, R. Are long-chain polyunsaturated fatty acids essential nutrients in infancy? *Lancet* **1995**, *345*, 1463–1468. [CrossRef]

226. Makrides, M.; Neumann, M.A.; Simmer, K.; Gibson, R.A. Dietary long-chain polyunsaturated fatty acids do not influence growth in term infants: A randomized clinical trial. *Pediatrics* **1999**, *104*, 468–475. [CrossRef] [PubMed]

227. Scott, D.T.; Janowsky, J.S.; Carroll, R.E.; Taylor, J.A.; Auestad, N.; Montalto, M.B. Formula supplementation with long-chain polyunsaturated fatty acids: Are there developmental benefits? *Pediatrics* **1998**, *102*, e59. [CrossRef] [PubMed]

228. Gibson, R.A.; Neumann, M.; Makrides, M. The effects of diets rich in docosahexaenoic acid and/or gamma-linolenic acid on plasma fatty acid profiles in term infants. In *Lipids in Infant Nutrition*; Huang, Y.S., Sinclair, A., Eds.; AOCS Press: Champaign, IL, USA, 1998; pp. 19–28.

229. Simmer, K. Longchain polyunsaturated fatty acid supplementation in infants born at term. *Cochrane Database Syst. Rev.* **2001**, *4*. [CrossRef]

230. Uauy, R.D.; Hoffman, D.R.; Birch, E.E.; Birch, D.G.; Jameson, D.M.; Tyson, J.E. Safety and efficacy of omega-3 fatty acids in the nutrition of very low birth weight infants: Soy oil and marine oil supplementation of formula. *J. Pediatr.* **1994**, *124*, 612–620. [CrossRef]

231. Clandinin, M.T.; Van Aerde, J.E.; Parrott, A.; Field, C.J.; Euler, A.R.; Lien, E.L. Assessment of the efficacious dose of arachidonic and docosahexaenoic acids in preterm infant formula: Fatty acid composition of erythrocyte membrane lipids. *Pediatr. Res.* **1997**, *42*, 819–825. [CrossRef] [PubMed]

232. Vanderhoof, J.; Gross, S.; Hegyi, T.; Clandinin, T.; Porcelli, P.; DeCristofaro, J.; Rhodes, T.; Tsang, R.; Shattuck, K.; Cowett, R.; *et al.* Evaluation of a long-chain polyunsaturated fatty acid supplemented formula on growth, tolerance, and plasma lipids in preterm infants up to 48 weeks postconceptional age. *J. Pediatr. Gastr. Nutr.* **1999**, *29*, 318–326. [CrossRef]

233. Vanderhoof, J.; Gross, S.; Hegyi, T. A multicenter long-term safety and efficacy trial of preterm formula with long-chain polyunsaturated fatty acids. *J. Pediatr. Gastr. Nutr.* **2000**, *31*, 121–127. [CrossRef]

234. Food and Drug Administration. *Agency Response Letter. GRAS Notice No. GRN 000041*; U.S. Food and Drug Administration, Department of Health and Human Services: Washington, DC, USA, 2001.

235. Health Canada. Novel Food Decision, DHASCO and ARASCO Oils as Sources of Docosahexaenoic (DHA) and Arachidonic Acid (ARA) in Human Milk Substitutes, 2002. Available online: http://www.novelfoods.gc.ca (accessed on 19 October 2015).

236. Ryan, A.S.; Zeller, S.; Nelson, E.B. Safety evaluation of single cell oils and the regulatory requirements for use as food ingredients. In *Single Cell Oils. Microbial and Algal Oil*, 2nd ed.; Cohen, Z., Ratledge, C., Eds.; AOCS Press: Urbana, IL, USA, 2010; pp. 317–350.

237. Dobbing, J. Vulnerable periods in developing brain. In *Brain, Behavior, and Iron in the Infant Diet*; Dobbing, J., Ed.; Springer-Verlag: London, UK, 1990; pp. 1–25.

238. Uauy, R.D.; Birch, D.G.; Birch, E.E.; Hoffman, D.R.; Tyson, J.E. Effect of dietary essential ω-3 fatty acids on retinal and brain development in premature infants. In *Essential Fatty Acids and Eicosanoids*; Sinclair, A., Gibson, E., Eds.; American Oil Chemists' Society: Champaign, IL, USA, 1992; pp. 197–202.

239. Uauy, R.D.; Treen, M.; Hoffman, D.R. Essential fatty acid metabolism and requirements during development. *Semin. Perinatol.* **1989**, *13*, 118–130. [PubMed]

240. Carlson, S.E.; Crooke, R.J.; Werkman, S.H.; Tolley, E.A. First year growth of preterm infants fed standard compared to marine oil *n*-3 supplemented formula. *Lipids* **1992**, *27*, 901–907. [CrossRef] [PubMed]

241. Carlson, S.E.; Werkman, S.H. A randomized trial of visual attention of preterm infants fed docosahexaenoic acid until two months. *Lipids* **1996**, *31*, 85–90. [CrossRef] [PubMed]

242. Diersen-Schade, D.A.; Hansen, J.W.; Harris, C.L.; Merkel, K.L.; Wisont, K.D.; Boettcher, J.A. Docosahexaenoic acid plus arachidonic acid enhance preterm infant growth. In *Essential Fatty Acids and Eicosanoids: Invited Papers from the Fourth International Congress*; Riemersma, R.A., Armstrona, R., Kelly, W., Wilson, R., Eds.; AOCS Press: Champaign, IL, USA, 1998; pp. 123–127.

243. Ryan, A.S.; Montalto, M.B.; Groh-Wargo, S.; Mimouni, F.; Sentipal-Walerius, J.; Doyle, J.; Siegman, J.; Thomas, A.J. Effect of DHA-containing formula on growth of preterm infants to 59 weeks postmenstrual age. *Am. J. Hum. Biol.* **1999**, *11*, 457–467. [CrossRef]

244. Carlson, S.E.; Werkman, S.H.; Peeples, J.M.; Wilson, W.M. Long-chain fatty acids and early visual and cognitive development of preterm infants. *Eur. J. Clin. Nutr.* **1994**, *48*, S27–S30. [PubMed]

245. Werkman, S.H.; Carlson, S.E. A randomized trial of visual attention of preterm infants fed docosahexaenoic acid until nine months. *Lipids* **1996**, *31*, 91–97. [CrossRef] [PubMed]

246. Carlson, S.E.; Werkman, S.H.; Tolley, E.A. Effect of long-chain *n*-3 fatt acid supplementation on visual acuity and growth of preterm infants with and without bronchopulmonary dysplasia. *Am. J. Clin. Nutr.* **1996**, *63*, 687–697. [PubMed]

247. Root, A.W. Mechanisms of hormone action: General Principals. In *Clinical Pediatric Endocrinology*; Hung, W., Ed.; Mosby-Year Book: St. Louis, MO, USA, 1992; pp. 1–12.

248. Watkins, B.A.; Shen, C.-L.; Allen, K.G.D.; Siefert, M.F. Dietary (*n*-3) and (*n*-6) polyunsaturates and acetylsalicylic acid alter *ex vivo* PGE_2 biosynthesis, tissue IGF-I levels, and bone morphometry in chicks. *J. Bone Miner. Res.* **1996**, *11*, 1321–1332. [CrossRef] [PubMed]

249. Colombo, J.; Carlson, S.E.; Cheatham, C.L.; Fitzgerald-Gust Afson, K.M.; Kepler, A.; Doty, T. Long-chain polyunsaturated fatty acid supplementation in infancy reduces heart rate and positively affects distribution of attention. *Pediatr. Res.* **2011**, *70*, 406–410. [CrossRef] [PubMed]

250. Colombo, J.; Carlson, S.E.; Cheatham, C.L.; Shaddy, D.J.; Kerling, E.H.; Thodosoff, J.M.; Gustafson, K.M.; Brez, C. Long-term effects of LCPUFA supplementation on childhood cognitive outcomes. *Am. J. Clin. Nutr.* **2013**, *98*, 403–412. [CrossRef] [PubMed]

251. Alshweki, A.; Munuzuri, A.P.; Bana, A.M.; de Castro, J.; Andrade, F.; Aldamiz-Echevarria, L.; de Pipaon, M.S.; Fraga, J.M.; Couce, M.L. Effects of different arachidonic acid supplementation on psychomotor development in very preterm infants; a randomized trial. *Nutr. J.* **2015**, *14*, 101. [CrossRef] [PubMed]

252. Beyerlein, A.; Hadders-Algra, M.; Kennedy, K.; Fewtrell, M.; Singhal, A.; Rosenfeld, E.; Lucas, A.; Bouwstra, H.; Koletzko, B.; von Kries, R. Infant formula supplementation with long-chain polyunsaturated fatty acids has no effect on Bayley developmental scores at 18 months of age-IPD meta-analysis of 4 large clinical trials. *J. Pediatr. Gastroenterol. Nutr.* **2010**, *50*, 79–84. [CrossRef] [PubMed]

253. Innis, S.M.; Auestad, N.; Siegman, J.S. Blood lipid docosahexaenoic and arachidonic acid in term gestation infants fed formula with high docosahexaenoic, low eicosapentaenoic acid fish oil. *Lipids* **1996**, *31*, 617–625. [CrossRef] [PubMed]

254. Desci, T.; Keleman, B.; Minda, H.; Burus, I.; Kohn, G. Effect of type of early infant feeding on fatty acid composition of plasma lipid classes in full-term infants during the second 6 months of life. *J. Pediatr. Gastroenterol. Nutr.* **2000**, *30*, 547–551.

255. Hoffman, D.R.; Boettcher, J.A.; Diersen-Schade, D.A. Toward optimizing vision and cognition in term infants by dietary docosahexaenoic and arachidonic acid supplementation: A review of randomized clinical trials. *Prostaglandins Leukot. Essent. Fat. Acids* **2009**, *81*, 151–158. [CrossRef] [PubMed]

256. Ryan, A.S.; Entin, E.K.; Hoffman, J.P.; Kuratko, C.N.; Nelson, E.B. Role of fatty acids in the neurological development of infants. In *Nutrition in Infancy, Volume 2, Nutrition and Health*; Watson, R.R., Ed.; Springer Science + Business Media: New York, NY, USA, 2013; pp. 331–346.

257. Drover, J.R.; Hoffman, D.R.; Casteneda, Y.S.; Morale, S.E.; Garfield, S.; Wheaton, D.H.; Birch, E.E. Cognitive function in 18-month-old term infants of the DIAMOND study: A randomized, controlled trial with multiple dietary levels of docosahexaenoic acid. *Early Hum. Dev.* **2011**, *87*, 223–230. [CrossRef] [PubMed]

258. Makrides, M.; Gibson, R.A.; McPhee, A.J.; Collins, C.T.; Davis, P.G.; Doyle, L.W.; Simmer, K.; Colditz, P.B.; Morris, S.; Smithers, L.G.; et al. Neurodevelopment outcomes of preterm infants fed high-dose docosahexaenoic acid: A randomized controlled trial. *JAMA* **2009**, *301*, 175–182. [CrossRef] [PubMed]

259. Makrides, M.; Gibson, R.A.; McPhee, A.J.; Yelland, L.; Quinlivan, J.; Ryan, P. Effect of DHA supplementation during pregnancy on maternal depression and neurodevelopment of young children: A randomized controlled trial. *JAMA* **2010**, *304*, 1675–1683. [CrossRef] [PubMed]

260. Lucas, A.; Stafford, M.; Morley, R.; Abbott, R.; Stephenson, T.; MacFadyen, U.; Elias-Jones, A.; Clements, H. Efficacy and safety of long-chain polyunsaturated fatty acid supplementation of infant formula milk: A randomized trial. *Lancet* **1999**, *354*, 1948–1954. [CrossRef]

261. Fewtrell, M.S.; Morley, R.; Abbott, R.A.; Singhal, A.; Isaacs, E.B.; Stephenson, T.; MacFadyen, U.; Lucas, A. Double-blind, randomized trial of long-chain polyunsaturated fatty acid supplementation in formula fed to preterm infants. *Pediatrics* **2002**, *110*, 73–82. [CrossRef] [PubMed]

262. Henriksen, C.; Haugholt, K.; Lindgren, M.; Aurvåg, A.K.; Rønnestad, A.; Grønn, M.; Solberg, R.; Moen, A.; Nakstad, B.; Berge, R.K.; et al. Improved cognitive development among preterm infants attributable to early supplementation of human milk with docosahexaenoic acid and arachidonic acid. *Pediatrics* **2008**, *121*, 1137–1145. [CrossRef] [PubMed]

263. Westerberg, A.C.; Schei, R.; Henriksen, C.; Smith, L.; Veierød, M.B.; Drevon, C.A.; Iversen, P.O. Attention among very low birth weight infants following early supplementation with docosahexaenoic acid and arachidonic acid. *Acta Pediatr.* **2011**, *100*, 47–52. [CrossRef] [PubMed]

264. Clandinin, M.T.; Van Aerde, J.E.; Merkel, K.L.; Harris, C.L.; Springer, M.A.; Hansen, J.W.; Diersen-Schade, D.A. Growth and development of preterm infants fed infant formulas containing docosahexaenoic acid and arachidonic acid. *J. Pediatr.* **2005**, *146*, 461–468. [CrossRef] [PubMed]

265. Birch, E.E.; Garfield, S.; Hoffman, D.R.; Uauy, R.; Birch, D.G. A randomized controlled trial of early dietary supply of long-chain polyunsaturated fatty acids and mental development in term infants. *Dev. Med. Child Neurol.* **2000**, *42*, 174–181. [CrossRef] [PubMed]

266. Carlson, S.E.; Montalto, M.B.; Ponder, D.L.; Werkman, S.H.; Korones, S.B. Lower incidence of necrotizing enterocolitis in infants fed a preterm formula with egg phospholipids. *Pediatr. Res.* **1998**, *44*, 491–498. [CrossRef] [PubMed]

267. Seki, H.; Sasaki, T.; Ueda, T.; Arita, M. Resolvins as regulators of the immune system. *Sci. World J.* **2010**, *10*, 18–31. [CrossRef] [PubMed]

258. Das, U.N. Perinatal supplementation of long-chain polyunsaturated fatty acids, immune response and adult diseases. *Med. Sci. Monit.* **2004**, *10*, HY19–HY25. [PubMed]

269. D'Vas, N.; Meldrum, S.J.; Dunstan, J.A.; Lee-Pullen, T.F.; Metcalfe, J.; Holt, B.J.; Serralha, M.; Tulic, M.K.; Mori, T.A.; Prescott, S.L. Fish oil supplementation in early infancy modulates developing infant immune responses. *Clin. Exp. Allergy* **2012**, *42*, 1206–1216.

270. Khader, S.A.; Gaffen, S.L.; Kolls, J.K. Th17 cells at the crossroads of innate and adaptive immunity against infectious diseases at the mucosa. *Mucosal Immunol.* **2009**, *2*, 403–411. [CrossRef] [PubMed]

271. Muc, M.; Kreiner-Moller, E.; Larsen, J.M.; Birch, S.; Brix, S.; Bisgaard, H.; Lauritzen, L. Maternal fatty acid desaturase genotype correlates with infant immune responses at 6 months. *Br. J. Nutr.* **2015**, *114*, 891–898. [CrossRef] [PubMed]

272. Barakat, R.; Abou El-Ela, N.E.; Sharaf, S.; El Sagheer, O.; Selim, S.; Tallima, H.; Bruins, M.J.; Hadley, K.B.; El Ridi, R. Efficacy and safety of arachidonic acid for treatment of school-aged children in *Schistosoma mansoni* high-endemicity regions. *Am. J. Trop. Med. Hyg.* **2015**, *92*, 797–804. [CrossRef] [PubMed]

273. Standl, M.; Lattka, E.; Stach, B.; Koletzko, S.; Bauer, C.P.; von Berg, A.; Berdel, D.; Kramer, U.; Schaaf, B.; Roder, S.; *et al.* FADS1 FADS2 gene cluster, PUFA intake and blood lipids in children: Results from the GINIplus and LISAplus Study Group. *PLoS ONE* **2012**, *7*, e37780.

274. Makajima, H.; Hirose, K. Role of IL-23 and Th17 cells in airway inflammation in asthma. *Immune Netw.* **2010**, *10*, 1–4. [CrossRef] [PubMed]

275. Dong, C. Regulation and pro-inflammatory function of interleukin-17 family cytokines. *Immunol. Rev.* **2008**, *226*, 80–86. [CrossRef] [PubMed]

276. Sapone, A.; Lammers, K.M.; Casolaro, V.; CAmmarota, M.; Giulano, M.T.; De Rosa, M.; Stefanile, R.; Mazzarella, G.; Tolone, C.; Russo, M.I.; *et al.* Divergence of gut permeability and mucosal immune gene expression in two gluten-associated conditions: Celiac disease and gluten sensitivity. *BMC Med.* **2011**, *9*, 23. [CrossRef] [PubMed]

277. Pastor, N.; Soler, B.; Mitmesser, S.H.; Ferguson, P.; Lifschitz, C. Infants fed docosahexaenoic acid- and arachidonic acid-supplemented formula have decreased incidence of bronchiolitis/bronchitis the first year of life. *Clin. Pediatr.* **2006**, *45*, 850–855. [CrossRef] [PubMed]

278. Lapillone, A.; Pastor, N.; Zhuang, W.; Scalabrin, D.M.F. Infants fed formula with added long chain polyunsaturated fatty acids have reduced incidence of respiratory illnesses and diarrhea during the first year of life. *BMC Pediatr.* **2014**, *14*, 168. [CrossRef] [PubMed]

279. Birch, E.E.; Carlson, S.E.; Hoffman, D.R.; Fitzgerald-Gustafson, K.M.; Fu, V.L.; Drover, J.R.; Castañeda, Y.S.; Minns, L.; Wheaton, D.K.; Mundy, D.; *et al.* The DIAMOND (DHA Intake and Measurement of Neural Development) Study: A double-masked, randomized controlled clinical trial of the maturation of infant visual acuity as a function of the dietary level of docosahexaenoic acid. *Am. J. Clin. Nutr.* **2010**, *91*, 848–859. [CrossRef] [PubMed]

280. Foiles, A.M.; Kerling, E.H.; Wick, J.A.; Scalabrin, D.M.; Colombo, J.; Carlson, S.E. Formula with long chain polyunsaturated fatty acids reduces incidence of allergy in early childhood. *Pediatr. Allergy Immunol.* **2015**. [CrossRef] [PubMed]

281. Hindenes, J.O.; Nerdal, W.; Guo, W.; Di, L.; Small, D.M.; Holmsen, H. Physical properties of the transmembrane signal molecule, sn-1-stearoyl-2-arachidonylglycerol. Acyl chain segregation and its biochemical implications. *J. Biol. Chem.* **2000**, *275*, 6857–6867. [CrossRef] [PubMed]

282. Moodley, T.; Vella, C.; Djahanbakhch, O.; Branford-White, C.J.; Crawford, M.A. Arachidonic and docosahexaenoic acid deficits in preterm neonatal mononuclear cell membranes. Implications for the immune response at birth. *Nutr. Health* **2009**, *20*, 167–185. [CrossRef] [PubMed]

283. Van Goor, S.A.; Schaafsma, A.; Erwich, J.J.; Dijck-Brouwer, D.A.; Muskiet, F.A. Mildly abnormal general movement quality in infants is associated with high Mead acid and lower arachidonic acid shows a U-shaped relation with the DHA/AA ratio. *Prostaglandins Leukot. Essent. Fat. Acids* **2010**, *82*, 15–20. [CrossRef] [PubMed]

284. Groen, S.E.; de Blecourt, A.C.; Postema, K.; Hadders-Algra, M. General movements in early infancy predict neuromotor development at 9 to 12 years of age. *Dev. Med. Child Neurol.* **2005**, *47*, 731–738. [CrossRef] [PubMed]

285. Field, C.J.; Thompson, C.A.; Van Aerde, J.E.; Parrott, A.; Euler, A.; Lien, E.; Clandinin, M.T. Lower proportion of CD45R0+ cells and deficient interleukin-10 production by formula-fed infants, compared with human-fed, is correlated with supplementation of long-chain polyunsaturated fatty acids. *J. Pediatr. Gastroenterol. Nutr.* **2000**, *31*, 291–299. [CrossRef] [PubMed]

286. Richardson, A.J.; Calvin, C.M.; Clisby, C.; Schoenheimer, D.R.; Montgomery, P.; Hall, J.A. Fatty acid deficiency signs predict the severity of reading and related difficulties in dyslexic children. *Prostaglandins Leukot. Essent. Fat. Acids* **2000**, *63*, 69–74. [CrossRef] [PubMed]

287. Burgess, J.R.; Stevens, L.; Zhang, W.; Peck, L. Long-chain polyunsaturated fatty acids in children with attention-deficit hyperactivity disorder. *Am. J. Clin. Nutr.* **2000**, *71*, 327S–330S. [PubMed]

288. Chen, J.R.; Hsu, S.F.; Hsu, C.D.; Hwang, L.H.; Yang, S.C. Dietary patterns and blood fatty acid composition in children with attention-deficit hyperactivity disorder in Taiwan. *J. Nutr. Biochem.* **2004**, *15*, 467–472. [CrossRef] [PubMed]

289. Young, G.S.; Maharaj, N.J.; Conquer, J.A. Blood phospholipid fatty acid analysis of adults with and without attention deficit/hyperactivity disorder. *Lipids* **2004**, *39*, 117–123. [PubMed]

290. Morse, N.L. A meta-analysis of blood fatty acids in people with learning disorders with particular interest in arachidonic acid. *Prostaglandins Leukot. Essent. Fat. Acids* **2009**, *81*, 373–389. [CrossRef] [PubMed]

291. Yamada, J.; Banks, A. Evidence for and characteristics of dyslexia among Japanese children. In *Annals of Dyslexia*; Schatschneider, C., Compton, D., Eds.; Springer: New York, NY, USA, 1994; pp. 103–119.

292. FAO. *Dietary Fats and Oils in Human Nutrition*; FAO/WHO: Rome, Italy, 1978.

293. FAO/WHO. *Fats and Oils in Human Nutrition*; Report of a Joint FAO/WHO Expert Consultation, 19 to 26 October 1993; FAO/WHO: Rome, Italy, 1994.

294. FAO. *Fats and Fatty Acids in Human Nutrition*; FAO/WHO: Rome, Italy, 2010.

295. Codex Alimentarius Commission. *Standards for Infant Formula and Formulas for Special Medical Purposes Intended for Infants*; CODEX STAN 72-1981, Last Revised 2007; Codex Alimentarius Commission: Rome, Italy, 2007.

296. Codex Alimentarius Commission. Amendments, 2015. Available online: http://www.fao.org/fao-who-codexalimentarius/en (accessed on 26 January 2016).

297. Infant Formula Act. H.R.6940—An Act to Amend the Federal Food, Drug, and Cosmetic Act to Strengthen the Authority under that Act to Assure the Safety and Nutrition of Infant Formulas, and for Other Purposes. *Fed. Regist.* **1980**, *50*, 45106–45108.

298. European Commission. *Commission Directive 2006/141/EC of 22 December 2006 on Infant Formulae and Follow-on Formulae and Amending Directive 1999/21/EC*; L.401/1; Official Journal of the European Union: Brussels, Belgium, 2008.

299. Koletzko, B.; Boey, C.C.; Campoy, C.; Carlson, S.E.; Chang, N.; Guillermo-Tuazon, M.A.; Joshi, S.; Prell, C.; Quak, S.H.; Sjarif, D.R.; *et al.* Current information and Asian perspectives on long-chain polyunsaturated fatty acids in pregnancy, lactation, and infancy: Systematic review and practice recommendations from an early nutrition academy workshop. *Ann. Nutr. Metab.* **2014**, *65*, 49–80. [CrossRef] [PubMed]

300. Crawford, M.A.; Wang, Y.; Forsyth, S.; Brenna, J.T. The European Food Safety Authority recommendation for polyunsaturated fatty acid composition of infant formula overrules breast milk, puts infants at risk, and should be revised. *Prostaglandins Leukot. Essent. Fat. Acids* **2015**, *102–103*, 1–3. [CrossRef] [PubMed]

301. Leaf, A.A.; Leighfield, M.J.; Costeloe, K.L.; Crawford, M.A. Long chain polyunsaturated fatty acids and fetal growth. *Early Hum. Dev.* **1992**, *30*, 183–191. [CrossRef]

302. Forsyth, J.S.; Willatts, P.; Agostoni, C.; Bissenden, J.; Casaer, P.; Boehm, G. Long chain polyunsaturated fatty acid supplementation in infant formula and blood pressure in later childhood: Follow up of a randomized controlled trial. *Br. Med. J.* **2003**, *326*, 953. [CrossRef] [PubMed]

303. Makrides, M.; Gibson, R.A.; Udell, T.; Ried, K. Supplementation of infant formula with long-chain polyunsaturated fatty acids does not influence the growth of term infants. *Am. J. Clin. Nutr.* **2005**, *81*, 1094–1101. [PubMed]

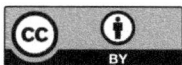

Review

The Effect of Low Dose Iron and Zinc Intake on Child Micronutrient Status and Development during the First 1000 Days of Life: A Systematic Review and Meta-Analysis

Nicolai Petry [1,*,†], **Ibironke Olofin** [1,†], **Erick Boy** [2], **Moira Donahue Angel** [2] and **Fabian Rohner** [1]

1   GroundWork, Fläsch 7306, Switzerland; ioo523@mail.harvard.edu (I.O.); fabian@groundworkhealth.org (F.R.)
2   Harvest Plus, International Food Policy Research Institute, Washington, DC 20006-1002, USA;
    E.Boy@cgiar.org (E.B.); m.angel@cgiar.org (M.D.A.)
*   Correspondence: nico@groundworkhealth.org; Tel.: +41-77-442-9175
†   Both authors have contributed equally to the work.

Received: 21 September 2016; Accepted: 24 November 2016; Published: 30 November 2016

Abstract: Adequate supply of micronutrients during the first 1000 days is essential for normal development and healthy life. We aimed to investigate if interventions administering dietary doses up to the recommended nutrient intake (RNI) of iron and zinc within the window from conception to age 2 years have the potential to influence nutritional status and development of children. To address this objective, a systematic review and meta-analysis of randomized and quasi-randomized fortification, biofortification, and supplementation trials in women (pregnant and lactating) and children (6–23 months) delivering iron or zinc in doses up to the recommended nutrient intake (RNI) levels was conducted. Supplying iron or zinc during pregnancy had no effects on birth outcomes. There were limited or no data on the effects of iron/zinc during pregnancy and lactation on child iron/zinc status, growth, morbidity, and psychomotor and mental development. Delivering up to 15 mg iron/day during infancy increased mean hemoglobin by 4 g/L ($p < 0.001$) and mean serum ferritin concentration by 17.6 µg/L ($p < 0.001$) and reduced the risk for anemia by 41% ($p < 0.001$), iron deficiency by 78% (ID; $p < 0.001$) and iron deficiency anemia by 80% (IDA; $p < 0.001$), but had no effect on growth or psychomotor development. Providing up to 10 mg of additional zinc during infancy increased plasma zinc concentration by 2.03 µmol/L ($p < 0.001$) and reduced the risk of zinc deficiency by 47% ($p < 0.001$). Further, we observed positive effects on child weight for age z-score (WAZ) ($p < 0.05$), weight for height z-score (WHZ) ($p < 0.05$), but not on height for age z-score (HAZ) or the risk for stunting, wasting, and underweight. There are no studies covering the full 1000 days window and the effects of iron and zinc delivered during pregnancy and lactation on child outcomes are ambiguous, but low dose daily iron and zinc use during 6–23 months of age has a positive effect on child iron and zinc status.

Keywords: Iron; zinc; iron status; zinc status; 1000 days window; infant and young child nutrition; fortification; biofortification

1. Introduction

Globally iron and zinc deficiencies are among the most widespread micronutrient deficiencies. While people of all ages are at risk, children and women of reproductive age are at elevated risk of experiencing concurrent deficiencies, especially in low-income countries [1,2]. Even mild deficiencies of one or both nutrients may contribute to increased morbidity and mortality [1]. The first 1000 days of life—the period from conception to the child's 2nd birthday—are most crucial, since some developmental and functional delays during this period are either irreversible or only partly reversible [3]. In utero exposure to iron deficiency has been associated with impaired brain maturation of the fetus [4,5], while during infancy and childhood, iron deficiency could lead to impaired cognitive and physical functionality and increased risk of mortality [1,6]. Zinc is essential for cellular differentiation and maturation and maternal zinc deficiency could lead to growth retardation and other developmental defects of the fetus [7]. Further, zinc deficient infants and young children are prone to infections and growth retardation [8].

The major cause of micronutrient malnutrition is a diet consisting mainly of staple foods and lacking in animal sources [9]. When compounded by exposure to environments laden with pathogens, there is a synergistic worsening of the malnutrition burden [10,11]. Although high dose supplementation has been successful in reducing the prevalence of micronutrient deficiencies, programs often only inadequately reach rural or marginalized populations; also high dose iron supplementation has been exposed to criticism in the past decade in malaria endemic areas [12]. Other interventions such as fortification and biofortification, delivering smaller amounts of micronutrients on a daily basis, might be more effective in reducing the prevalence of micronutrient deficiencies in populations at risk; yet, their effect on the infant during the first 1000 days of life starting from pregnancy until 23 months of age has hardly been investigated.

The objective of this work was thus to evaluate the potential of interventions delivering daily doses of iron and zinc in concentrations up to approximately the Recommended Nutrient Intake (RNI) in diets with low bioavailability [1] during the first 1000 days of life on child micronutrient status and health.

For this we used data from randomized and quasi-randomized trials of fortification, supplementation or biofortification interventions, in which iron and zinc were provided more than three times a week in concentrations up to approximately the (RNI) for women (iron: 45 mg/day; zinc 20 mg/day) and children 6–23 months (iron: 15 mg/day; zinc: 10 mg/day).

2. Materials and Methods

2.1. Search Strategy

We searched the WHO e-Library of Evidence for Nutrition Actions, the Cochrane Central library, Web of Science, and MEDLINE/PUBMED databases to identify systematic reviews and meta-analyses that investigated the effects of iron and zinc interventions (fortification, supplementation, or biofortification interventions) on nutritional, developmental and health outcomes of children. We restricted the search to reviews published from 2005 to 2015. The following search strategy was adapted for each database: (Fortification OR biofortification OR supplementation) AND (iron OR zinc OR multiple micronutrients OR micronutrient powder) AND (women OR children OR infants OR toddlers). For the relevant topics, 82 potentially useful reviews and meta-analyses published from 2005 to 2015 were identified, the most recent ones conducting their literature searches up until 2014. We searched their reference lists for suitable original studies. Additional searches for original studies published between 2011 and October 2015 were conducted in Web of Science and MEDLINE/PubMed using the following strategies for each age group of interest:

(a) Children: (Biofortification OR fortification OR supplementation) AND (iron OR zinc OR micronutrient powder OR multiple micronutrients) AND (children OR infants OR toddlers) AND (trial OR study OR survey OR assessment).
(b) Pregnant women: (Biofortification OR fortification OR supplementation) AND (pregnant women OR lactating women OR maternal) AND (iron OR zinc OR micronutrient powder OR multiple micronutrients) AND (trial OR study OR survey OR assessment).
(c) Lactating women: (Biofortification OR fortification OR supplementation) AND lactating women AND (zinc OR iron OR micronutrient powder OR multiple micronutrients OR breast milk) AND (trial OR study OR survey OR assessment).

2.2. Inclusion and Exclusion Criteria

Types of trials and interventions: Randomized controlled trials (RCTs) and quasi-experimental studies were included in the review. Studies were eligible if they assessed the impact of iron or zinc supplementation, fortification or biofortification interventions on the micronutrient status, growth or health outcomes of children (details below). Only studies where the daily iron and zinc dose did not exceed 15 mg and 10 mg, respectively for children and 45 mg and 21 mg, respectively for women, were included. We considered micronutrient powders and crushable tablets (foodlets) as fortification, since they are consumed as part of a normal meal. Furthermore, we included studies investigating the effects of iron or zinc supplements, as long as they were within the dose range we specified. We defined supplements as compounds, which are routinely consumed separately from a normal meal, including tablets, pills, drops, capsules, syrups, drinks, biscuits, and lipid-based supplement (LNS). Only studies administering the micronutrients >3 times a week were included.

Types of participants: For interventions administered to the mother, we included studies that provided interventions to pregnant women or lactating women, regardless of their health status. For interventions administered to children, we were interested in effects on young children, thus only studies where over 50% of participating children were 6–23 months old were included. Only studies involving apparently healthy children were considered, with the exception that studies including malnourished (underweight, stunted, wasted) children and children suffering from anemia or deficiencies of iron and zinc were included. We did not include therapeutic studies, such as short term zinc supplementation studies to treat acute diarrhea.

2.3. Study Design and Comparison Groups

The control groups of the included fortification trials either received unfortified foods or regular diets. Studies were also included if both the control and intervention groups received the same fortified foods, but either with different iron or zinc concentrations, or if the control group received an identical micronutrient compound given to the intervention group, but without iron or zinc. For supplementation, the control groups of the included trials either received no supplements, placebo, a lower concentration of iron or zinc or different micronutrients identical to intervention group preparations, except that they excluded zinc and/or iron.

Studies were only included in meta-analyses if the data for outcomes of interest were presented in a manner that allowed inclusion in the meta-analysis (i.e., data could only be used when presented as mean (SD or SE), mean (95% CI), median (95% CI), or median (range), but not when reported as median (IQR)). Where studies did not report on the average daily micronutrient intake, but instead stated the micronutrient concentration per 100 mL/100 g or the daily micronutrient intake in mg/kg body weight, we calculated the average intake as appropriate.

2.4. Outcome Measures

Only child outcomes were of interest, even when interventions were administered to pregnant or lactating women. For example, with regard to effects of prenatal iron supplementation on anemia, maternal anemia was not the focus of this analysis; rather, the infant/child anemia was of relevance even if the mother received the intervention.

Outcomes evaluated include: (1) hemoglobin (Hb) concentration (g/dL); (2) anemia (%; defined as Hb <110 g/L); (3) serum ferritin concentration (μg/L); (4) iron deficiency (%; defined as serum ferritin <10 μg/L or <12 μg/L); (5) iron deficiency anemia (%; defined as hb <105 g/L or <110 g/L and serum ferritin <10 μg/L or <12 μg/L); (6) serum or plasma zinc (μmol/L); (7) zinc deficiency (%; defined as serum zinc <10.7 μmol/L); (8) birth outcomes (birth weight in g; prevalence of low birth weight in %, defined as weight <2500 g); (9) infant anthropometric measures (height for age z-score (HAZ); weight for age z-score (WAZ); weight for height z-score (WHZ); stunting ($\leq$−2 HAZ scores), wasting ($\leq$−2 WHZ scores) underweight ($\leq$−2 WAZ scores)); (10) mental and motor development (Bayley mental development index (MDI); Bayley psychomotor development index (PDI)); (11) morbidity (diarrhea, fever and respiratory infection).

2.5. Data Synthesis and Statistical Analysis

From each eligible study, we extracted all data that would allow the estimation of the effects of interest. For example, for zinc studies, data were extracted for groups assigned to zinc alone compared with placebo, as well as data from groups assigned to more than one nutrient including zinc compared with a group assigned to the identical nutrient combination but excluding zinc. Where the total number of comparisons was sufficiently large, we examined the influence of combining such comparisons into one meta-analysis, and where possible, conducted sub-group analyses examining the possibility of nutrient interactions. Additionally, where studies had more than one group assigned to the nutrient of interest (for instance, different nutrient dosages) but only one suitable comparison group, we included such data as separate estimates for the meta-analysis. For that, we divided the comparison group into two groups (or more, when required) with smaller sample sizes, so the same children were not involved in more than one comparison. To examine if this decision affected the results, we conducted sensitivity analyses combining all relevant control groups of affected studies into a single comparison group, and combining all relevant intervention groups into a single group, for some outcomes. As results were very similar, we chose to continue analyses with the sub-groups. When studies reported outcomes at multiple time points, we selected only the results reported at the study end (or the latest time point) for the meta-analyses. Most studies were individually randomized trials, but where cluster randomized trials were eligible for inclusion, we estimated design effects to adjust for the influence of intra-cluster correlations on the precision of estimates as appropriate. To maximize the number of studies that could contribute to meta-analyses of continuous outcomes, we converted medians (reported with ranges) and geometric means (reported with standard deviations, standard errors or confidence intervals) to arithmetic means and standard deviations using methods developed by Hozo et al. [13] and Higgins et al. [14] and examined the effect that combining transformed and untransformed estimates had on pooled results. Studies were excluded from meta-analyses if published reports presented insufficient information for estimating desired effect estimates and variances.

For continuous outcomes, we estimated pooled mean differences or standardized mean differences and confidence intervals, as appropriate, while for categorical outcomes, we estimated pooled risk ratios and confidence intervals. Study-level effect estimates were pooled using the random effects meta-analysis method by DerSimonian and Laird [15]. We assessed heterogeneity among studies, and used the method proposed by Higgins et al. to measure the inconsistency (I^2) of effect estimates across studies [16]. Heterogeneity among study estimates was considered to be substantial if the I^2 exceeded 50%. For outcomes having at least 10 comparisons per variable of interest, we explored sources of heterogeneity by conducting pre-specified sub-group analyses and meta-regressions, to examine whether effects were modified by the study-level factors: micronutrient doses provided, type of intervention (whether fortification or supplementation), study quality and baseline micronutrient status. Funnel plots were constructed for visual assessment of the variability of individual study estimates and to evaluate the possibility of publication bias, and when appropriate, Egger's tests were used to examine if effect estimates varied with study sample size.

All analyses were conducted using the metafor package [17] of the R statistical program (R version 3.1.3 (2015-03-09), The R Foundation, Vienna, Austria, 2015).

2.6. Assessment of Quality and Risk of Bias

We assessed study quality in three areas—random sequence generation, adequacy of blinding of study participants and personnel and completeness of outcomes assessment—but did not exclude studies based on the assessment of quality. Studies were categorized as being of the 'highest quality' if interventions were randomly assigned, both participants and study personnel were adequately blinded to the intervention assignment, and if outcomes were assessed in at least 75% of the enrolled study population. Intermediate quality trials were randomized trials for which only one of the remaining two criteria was suboptimal, lowest quality trials were randomized trials for which both the remaining criteria were suboptimal, and quasi-experimental trials (although rarely included) were given the very lowest rating. The effect of pooling results from studies of different quality was examined in sub-group analyses where possible.

The quality of the evidence resulting from each analysis was assessed using the Grading of Recommendations Assessment, Development, and Evaluation (GRADE) method [18]. Domains included: risk of bias within studies (internal validity), inconsistency or heterogeneity of results across studies, indirectness or use of proxy populations, interventions or outcomes measures, imprecision (large variability and wide confidence intervals), number of studies and risk of publication bias. The evidence was judged as high quality if further research studies were unlikely to change the pooled estimate obtained; moderate quality if further research could alter the current estimate; low quality if further research was needed to confirm the magnitude and direction of the true effect; and very low quality if there was great uncertainty about the validity of the pooled estimate. It should be noted that because the GRADE method considers several domains and not just internal study validity, confidence in pooled estimates could be 'low' or 'very low' even if all studies that contributed to the estimate were well conducted.

3. Results

3.1. Literature Search

We identified and screened 4542 records, reviewed 326 full-texts for eligibility and finally included 90 studies in the review (Figure S1). Identified studies were supplementation or fortification studies—no biofortification studies qualified for inclusion. Thirty-three iron intervention studies and 47 zinc intervention studies involving children 6–23 months old met our inclusion criteria. Of the prenatal intervention studies that reported child outcomes, seven iron studies and 10 zinc studies met our inclusion criteria. Additionally, we identified one eligible study that delivered zinc to lactating women. The major reasons for excluding studies were: (a) micronutrient doses higher than our selected threshold; (b) ineligible ages, e.g., more than half of participating children over 23 months old and (c) dosing frequencies less than our threshold.

3.2. Effects of Low-Dose Iron Interventions during Pregnancy and Lactation on Child Outcomes

Six studies reported birth weights of infants [19–24] while five studies reported on the effects of iron on the prevalence of low birth weight (Table 1; [19,21–24]). Exclusively supplementation trials contributed to the analyses, delivering daily 18–30 mg of iron. We found that low dose iron interventions during pregnancy do not significantly change birth weights ($p = 0.17$; Figure S2) or the prevalence of low birth weight ($p = 0.23$; Figure S3) among the offspring. We did not identify any studies investigating the effects of prenatal iron interventions on child micronutrient status or child growth within the first two years of life. We identified a study by Li and colleagues [25] that investigated the effects of prenatal iron and folic acid compared with folic acid alone on PDI and MDI scores of children at 3, 6, and 12 months of age. No differences were detected between the iron/folic acid group and the folic acid only group. The main results of the meta-analysis of prenatal iron interventions are summarized in Table 1.

Table 1. Effects of prenatal iron interventions supplying ≤45 mg/day iron on birth weight and prevalence of low birth weight among offspring.

Variables	Mean Difference [1]	Relative Risk	Studies, Participants (*n*)	I^2 (%)	*p* Difference between Pooled Intervention and Control Groups
			Birth outcomes		
Birthweight (g)	38 (−16; 91)		6, 13,627	58.2	0.17
Low birth weight (%)		0.69 (0.38; 1.26)	5, 12,845	63.1	0.23

[1] 95% CI in parenthesis.

3.3. Iron Interventions in Children 6–23 Months of Age

The results of meta- analyses of iron intervention studies involving children are presented below and summarized in Tables 2 and 3.

Table 2. Effects of daily iron administration (≤15 mg/day) to children 6–23 months on levels of hemoglobin, anemia, serum ferritin, iron deficiency, and iron deficiency anemia [1].

Variables	Mean Difference [2]	Relative Risk	Studies, Participants (*n*)	I^2 (%)	*p* Difference between Pooled Intervention and Control Groups (Bold Font) and Subgroups (Regular Font)
Hb overall (g/dL)	4.1 (2.8; 5.3)		**30, 6569**	**81.5**	**<0.001**
Iron dose					
<6 mg/day	−0.7 (−6.1; 4.7)		2, 220	73.1	
6–8 mg/day	4.4 (2.1; 6.8)		7, 1864	83.9	
>8–10 mg/day	5.5 (3.4; 7.6)		13, 3068	83.8	0.12
11–15 mg/day	2.7 (1.2; 4.2)		4, 403	80.7	
Type of intervention					
Supplementation	5.6 (3.4; 7.7)		15, 3516	86.4	
Fortification [3]	2.6 (1.3; 3.9)		16, 3053	67.4	<0.01
RCT, quality rating					
highest	5.5 (3.3; 7.6)		12, 3403	87.1	
intermediate	3.2 (1.6; 4.8)		14, 2623	73.1	<0.05
lowest	1.3 (−2.9; 5.4)		4, 375	80.3	
Anemia overall		**0.59 (0.49; 0.70)**	**22, (5647)**	**73.8**	**<0.0001**
Iron dose					
6–8 mg/day		0.54 (0.44; 0.66)	7, 2089	18.4	
>8–10 mg/day		0.59 (0.45; 0.77)	9, 2575	85.2	0.32
11–15 mg/day		0.82 (0.51; 1.30)	3, 489	31.0	
Serum ferritin (µg/dL)	17.3 (13.5; 21.2)		**21, (4291)**	**95.1**	**<0.0001**
Iron dose					
<6 mg/day	5.8 (−14.8; 26.3)		2, 222	90.9	
6–8 mg/day	12.1 (2.6; 21.7)		5, 1261	96.4	<0.01
>8–10 mg/day	27.5 (16.0; 39.0)		9, 2068	96.4	
Type of intervention					
Supplementation	27.2 (18.2; 36.3)		8, 1747	90.1	
Fortification	11.3 (13.7; 21.4)		13, 2544	95.2	<0.001
RCT, quality rating					
highest	22.8 (15.2; 30.4)		9, 2351	93.0	
intermediate	11.4 (6.6; 16.1)		9, 1619	93.0	0.08
lowest	15.0 (7.0; 23.0)		3, 321	92.0	
Baseline ID prevalence					
Low (<15%)	27.0 (13.6; 40.4)		4, 276	60.5	
High (≥15%)	32.4 (8.9; 55.9)		4, 1226	98.3	0.76
Baseline mean serum ferritin [4]					
Low (<29.2 µg/L)	18.5 (11.7; 25.3)		9, 1352	76.4	
High (≥29.2 µg/L)	21.2 (11.5; 30.9)		8, 1698	94.0	0.99
ID overall		**0.22 (0.14; 0.35)**	**13, 3698**	**86.3**	**<0.0001**
IDA overall		**0.20 (0.11; 0.37)**	**8, 3464**	**64.2**	**<0.0001**

[1] Hb, hemoglobin, ID, iron deficiency; IDA, iron deficiency anemia; RCT, randomized controlled trial; [2] 95% CI in parenthesis; [3] Includes micronutrient powders and crushable tablets (foodlets); [4] Low is defined as below 50th percentile of all reported serum ferritin means; high is equal or above 50th percentile.

Effect on hemoglobin concentration: We identified 30 RCTs [26–55], contributing 43 comparisons, for evaluating the effect of up to 15 mg of additional iron daily on hemoglobin levels of children 6–23 months of age. In total, 6569 children contributed to the pooled estimate. The iron interventions led to significantly higher hemoglobin concentrations in children, compared with no iron (pooled mean difference 4.07 g/L (95% CI: 2.82, 5.33; Figure S4), although there was significant heterogeneity of results (I^2 82.5%; $p < 0.0001$). To examine the heterogeneity, we conducted meta-regression analyses and sub-group analyses investigating whether effect sizes were different for pre-specified sub-groups defined by the intervention dose (Figure S5), type of intervention (fortification vs. supplementation; Figure S6) and study quality (Figure S7). The increases in hemoglobin concentrations resulting from the intervention were significantly higher for supplementation trials than fortification trials ($p < 0.01$) and significantly lower as study quality worsened ($p < 0.05$). There was no significant difference in effect sizes by intervention dose ($p = 0.12$). Adjusting for these variables simultaneously did not substantially explain the observed heterogeneity (residual I^2 81%, $p < 0.0001$).

Effect on anemia prevalence: 22 RCTs involving a total of 5647 children contributed [26,27,29–32,34–39,43–45,47,48,51,52,54–56] to the meta-analysis. The iron interventions resulted in a 41% reduction in children's risk of anemia compared with no iron (pooled relative risk (RR) 0.59 (95% CI: 0.49, 0.70), Figure S8), although there was considerable heterogeneity of results, I^2: 73.8% (p value 0.0008). We investigated the influence of the intervention dose on effect sizes (Figure S9) and while it appears that interventions delivering 6–8 mg and >8–10 mg iron per day reduce the risk of anemia by 46% and 41%, respectively, intervention dose did not significantly explain the differences in study effect sizes ($p = 0.32$). This agrees with the results of sub-group analyses for hemoglobin outcomes, where the largest effect sizes were observed for iron interventions delivering between 6 mg and 10 mg per day (Figure S5).

Effect on serum ferritin: Twenty-one RCTs [26–28,31–34,36–38,40,42,44,45,48–54], contributing 25 comparisons, provided sufficient data for the meta-analysis of the effect of low dose iron interventions on serum ferritin concentrations in young children. In total, 4291 children contributed to the pooled estimate. After pooling the results, the iron intervention resulted in significantly higher serum ferritin concentrations compared with controls (mean difference 17.3 µg/L (95% CI: 13.1, 21.2; Figure S10), although there was significant heterogeneity, I^2 95.1% ($p < 0.001$). To understand the substantial heterogeneity in the results, we conducted meta-regression analyses and sub-group analyses investigating the influence of the dose (Figure S11), type of intervention (fortification vs. supplementation; Figure S12) and quality of interventions (Figure S13) on the effect size estimates. The effect sizes resulting from the intervention were significantly higher for higher doses ($p < 0.01$) and for supplementation trials compared with fortification trials ($p < 0.001$). Meta-regression results suggested that effects diminished as study quality worsened, although not significantly ($p = 0.08$). However, adjusting for dose, study quality, and intervention type simultaneously did not explain much of the observed heterogeneity (residual I^2 88%) and the change in effect size associated with increasing doses was no longer significant after adjusting for the quality of studies and type of intervention. We further examined the effect of baseline iron deficiency (categorized as low prevalence if <15% and high prevalence if ≥15%) on serum ferritin results. Only nine comparisons had information on baseline iron status. The pooled mean difference in serum ferritin for comparisons where baseline iron deficiency was high was not considerably different from the comparisons where baseline iron deficiency was low (Figure S14), and baseline iron deficiency did not explain the heterogeneity in serum ferritin results (p value = 0.76). Yet, with the limited number of studies, inadequate power could be a problem. In order to maximize the number of studies in the sub-group analysis, we created an 'in-house' measure of baseline iron status: from all reported mean serum ferritin concentrations, we took the 50th percentile (29.2 ug/L). Studies were categorized as having low iron status if mean serum ferritin was <29.2 and adequate if mean serum ferritin ≥29.2. This variable could be created for 21 comparisons. However, even so, we did not detect a significant effect of baseline iron status and it did not account for the observed heterogeneity of serum ferritin results (Figure S15; p value = 0.99). The created variable may be an inadequate surrogate for participants' baseline iron deficiency levels.

Effect on prevalence of ID and IDA: Thirteen trials [26,29,31,32,34,36,38,39,43,45,48,52,54] and eight trials [26,29,34–36,40,43,48] conducted mainly in Asia, provided 17 and 13 comparisons, respectively, that could be included in meta-analyses investigating the effect of the iron interventions on the risk of ID and IDA respectively among children 6–23 months old. The majority of trials defined ID as serum ferritin concentrations <12 µg/L or <10 µg/L while IDA was mainly defined as hemoglobin <110 g/L with serum ferritin concentrations <12 µg/L. The pooled relative risk from the random effects meta-analysis was 0.22 (95% CI: 0.14, 0.35), I^2: 86.3% (Figure S16) for ID and 0.20 (95% CI: 0.11, 0.37), I^2: 64.2% (Figure S17) for IDA, meaning that providing children 6–23 months old with up to 15 mg of iron daily significantly reduced their risk of ID and IDA by 78% (95% CI: 65% to 86% reduction) and 80% (95% CI: 63% to 89% reduction) respectively.

Effect on growth: Ten RCTs examined the effect of iron on WAZ [35–38,41,43,44,48,52]; nine studies each contributed to the meta-analyses of the iron effect on WHZ [35–38,42–44,48,52] and HAZ [35–38,41,43,44,48,52]. There was no significant effect of iron on WAZ (Figure S18; Table 3; $p = 0.69$), WHZ (Figure S19; Table 3; $p = 0.62$) or HAZ (Figure S20; Table 3; $p = 0.59$). Similarly, random effects meta-analysis indicated (Figures S21 and S22; Table 3) that there was no effect of iron on the risk for stunting [35–37,48] or wasting [35–37,48].

Effect on diarrhea, fever and respiratory infection: We identified eight eligible studies [27,38,42,44,48, 49,57,58], with a total of 11 comparisons, reporting on the impact of iron use on diarrhea, respiratory infection and/or fever. Given the variability of methods and outcome measures in the studies reviewed, it was not possible to conduct a meta-analysis without introducing a selection bias. The effect of iron alone was compared to placebo in seven RCTs, three compared the effect of iron and zinc to zinc alone, and one study compared the effect of MNP with and without iron on morbidity. Seven studies looked at the impact of iron on diarrhea, seven on respiratory infection and five on fever. None of the studies reported a beneficial effect of iron on any of the morbidities.

Effect on mental and motor development: Four eligible studies (five comparisons) reported children's Bayley mental development index (MDI; [27,36,51,54]) and Bayley psychomotor development index (PDI; [27,36,51,54]) scores. Children included in the analysis received daily 5–10 mg fortification or supplementation iron for 3–9 months. The analyses indicated that interventions delivering dietary doses of iron have no effect on mental development ($p = 0.6$; Figure S23; Table 3) and psychomotor development scores ($p = 0.5$; Figure S24; Table 3).

Table 3. Effects of daily iron administration (≤15 mg/day) to children 6–23 months on growth and mental and development outcomes [1].

Variables	Mean Difference [2]	Relative Risk	Studies, Participants (n)	I^2 (%)	p Difference between Pooled Intervention and Control Groups
		Growth			
WAZ	−0.01 (−0.08; 0.05)		10, 3511	12.5	0.69
WHZ	0.02 (−0.06; 0.09)		9, 3297	36.8	0.62
HAZ	−0.02 (−0.08; 0.04)		10, 3511	8.2	0.57
Stunting		1.09 (0.92; 1.29)	4, 2159	0	0.33
Wasting		1.11 (0.84; 1.47)	4, 1975	0	0.45
		Mental and motor development			
MDI	0.4 (−0.9; 1.7)		4, 1062	19.9	0.60
PDI	0.6 (−1.2; 2.4)		4, 1062	61.9	0.50

[1] HAZ, height for age z-score; MDI, Bayley mental development index; PDI, Bayley psychomotor development index; WAZ, weight for age z-score; WHZ, weight for height z-score; [2] 95% CI in parenthesis.

3.4. Zinc Interventions during Pregnancy and Lactation

Few data on the effect of maternal supplementation on infant outcomes are available during pregnancy and the lactation period for most of the outcomes of interest and thus a meta-analysis was only conducted for birth outcomes. Results of single studies investigating growth and micronutrient status are discussed in the section below.

3.4.1. Effect on Birth Weight and Prevalence of Low Birth Weight

The results of meta- analyses of studies conducted in pregnant women are summarized in Table 4.

Eight studies [59–66] and nine comparisons contributed to the meta-analysis for the effect of prenatal zinc use on birth weight, and six studies (seven comparisons) contributed to the meta-analysis of prenatal zinc and low birth weight prevalence [59,61–63,65,67]. We found that delivering up to 21 mg of zinc daily during pregnancy has no significant effect on birth weights of offspring ($p = 0.94$; Figure S25) or the prevalence of low birth weight ($p = 0.83$; Figure S26).

Table 4. Effects of administering ≤21 mg/day zinc to pregnant women on birth weights and prevalence of low birth weight among their offspring.

Variables	Mean Difference [1]	Relative Risk	Studies, Participants (*n*)	I^2 (%)	*p* Difference between Pooled Intervention and Control Groups
		Birth outcomes			
Birthweight (g)	1 (−32; 35)		8, 3457	0	0.94
Low birth weight		0.96 (0.67; 1.37)	6, 2518	0	0.83

[1] 95% CI in parenthesis.

3.4.2. Effect on Infant Growth and Micronutrient Status

Two studies examining child growth outcomes and one study examining the zinc status of children were identified. Prawirohartono et al. [60] looked at growth of infants whose mothers received either 20 mg zinc only, vitamin A only, 20 mg zinc and vitamin A or placebo during pregnancy. They monitored growth until 23 months of age. Zinc had a significant beneficial effect on HAZ at 6 months. No effects on any other growth parameters at any time point were observed. Iannotti et al. [68] administered 15 mg zinc daily to pregnant women from gestational week 16 until 1 month after delivery and measured infant growth from birth to 12 months of age. They did not assess any predefined outcomes, but observed differences between intervention and control group in weight, calf, chest, mid-upper arm circumferences, and skinfold thicknesses from age 6 month to 12 month; and no effect on length or head circumference.

Caulfield and colleagues [59] looked at the zinc status of neonates after zinc supplementation of pregnant women. Women were included at gestational ages of 10–24 weeks and received a daily dose of 15 mg zinc. They reported a significantly higher cord blood zinc concentration in neonates whose mothers received zinc supplementation, compared with controls.

Only one study was identified that investigated the effects of maternal zinc supplementation/ fortification during the lactation period on infant outcomes. The effect of maternal zinc supplementation on serum zinc concentration and growth in children after birth to 9 months of age was investigated by Salmenpera et al. [69]. They gave two different zinc doses (20 mg, 40 mg daily) to lactating women and compared the impact to a control group. Breast milk zinc concentration did not differ between groups at 0, 2, and 4 months after delivery, but was higher at 6 and 7.5 months in the group receiving 40 mg/day of zinc. When analyses were restricted to exclusively breastfed infants, no difference in serum zinc concentration was detected between intervention and control groups at any time point and maternal zinc supplementation had no effect on infant growth.

3.5. Zinc Interventions in Children 6–23 Months of Age

3.5.1. Effect on Serum or Plasma Zinc Concentrations and Zinc Deficiency

The main results of the meta-analyses of studies in children investigating the effect of zinc administration on serum zinc and zinc status are presented in Table 5.

Table 5. Effects of daily zinc administration (≤10 mg) to children 6–23 month on serum zinc and prevalence of zinc deficiency in children [1].

Variables	Mean Difference [2]	Relative Risk	Studies, Participants (*n*)	I^2 (%)	*p* Difference between Pooled Intervention and Control Groups (Bold Font) and Subgroups (Regular Font)
Serum zinc overall (μmol/L)	2.0 (1.2; 2.9)		23, 8848	96.1	<0.0001
Zinc dose					
<4 mg/day	0.81 (−0.07; 1.68)		1, 256	55.5	
4–<7 mg/day	0.9 (0.08; 1.71)		7, 1296	92.4	0.05
7–10 mg/day	3.0 (1.5; 4.5)		14, 6867	98.5	
Type of intervention					
Supplementation	2.4 (1.5; 3.4)		19, 7732	98.5	<0.05
Fortification [3]	0.3 (−0.1; 0.8)		6, 816	98.1	
Baseline ZD prevalence					
Low (<25%)	2.9 (0.2; 5.7)		4, 1231	97.8	0.15
High (≥25%)	2.8 (1.7; 3.9)		4, 2372	95.5	
Baseline mean serum zinc [4]					
Low (<10.75 μg/L)	2.4 (0.7; 4.2)		7, 5635	98.7	0.96
High (≥10.75 μg/L)	2.3 (0.7; 3.9)		9, 2200	96.9	
ZD overall		0.47 (0.32; 0.69)	12, 6666	92.2	<0.001

[1] RCT, randomized controlled trial; ZD, zinc deficiency; [2] 95% CI in parenthesis; [3] Includes micronutrient powders and crushable tablets (foodlets); [4] Low is defined as below 50th percentile of all reported serum zinc means; high is equal or above 50th percentile.

Twenty-three [36,43,48,59,70–88] RCTs (contributing 35 comparisons) provided sufficient information to be included in the meta-analysis summarizing the effect of up to 10 mg of additional zinc daily on the serum or plasma zinc concentrations of children 6–23 months old.

The pooled estimate suggests that the zinc interventions significantly increased serum or plasma zinc concentrations by 2.03 μmol/L compared with no zinc (95% CI 1.21, 2.85 μmol/L; $p < 0.0001$, Figure S27), but with significant heterogeneity (I^2 98%). Meta-regression analyses suggest that effect sizes were larger at higher doses ($p < 0.05$, Figure S28), and for supplementation compared with fortification trials ($p = 0.05$, Figure S29), while study quality did not significantly explain the heterogeneity. Dose, intervention type and study quality together did little to explain the heterogeneity of findings (residual I^2 97.9%). Subgroup analyses stratified by dose suggested that the strongest effect on serum zinc was obtained in studies delivering daily 7–10 mg (3.0 μmol/L; (95% CI 1.51, 4.48)). A small but significant effect was also detected in studies administering 4–<7 mg/day (0.9 μmol/L (95% CI 0.08, 1.71; Figure S28)). Stratification by intervention type revealed that the pooled effect size of fortification trials on serum zinc concentrations was small and not statistically significant (0.31 μmol/L (95% CI −0.12, 0.75; Figure S29), whereas supplementation showed a larger and significant difference (2.07 μmol/L (95% CI 1.5, 3.4).

Baseline zinc deficiency levels were reported for 12 comparisons with serum zinc as the outcome. We categorized baseline zinc deficiency as low prevalence if <25% and high prevalence if ≥25%. The pooled mean difference in serum zinc was similar regardless of baseline zinc deficiency status (Figure S30), and baseline zinc deficiency explains 8.4% of the heterogeneity in serum zinc results (*p* value = 0.15). In order to maximize the number of studies in the sub-group analysis, we created a measure of baseline zinc status: from all reported serum zinc means, we took the 50th percentile (10.75 μmol/L). Studies were categorized as having low zinc status if mean serum zinc was <10.75 μmol/L and adequate if mean serum zinc ≥10.75. This variable could be created for 25 comparisons. It did not explain any of the observed heterogeneity of serum zinc results (*p* value = 0.96; Figure S32). The created variable may be an inadequate surrogate for participants' baseline zinc deficiency levels.

For the effect of zinc interventions on the risk of zinc deficiency among children 6–23 months old, 12 RCTs [35,39,43,48,71,72,74,77,78,81,84,87], which provided 22 comparisons, contributed to the meta-analysis. Half defined zinc deficiency as serum or plasma zinc concentrations <10.7 µmol/L, while the others defined it using a cutoff of <~9.9 µmol/L.

The pooled relative risk from the random effects meta-analysis was 0.47 (95% CI 0.32, 0.69), I^2: 92%, meaning that providing children 6–23 months old with up to 10 mg of zinc daily significantly reduced their risk of zinc deficiency by 53% (95% CI 25% to 64% reduction; Figure S32).

3.5.2. Effect on Growth

Results of studies investigating effects of zinc interventions on child growth are summarized in Table 6.

Table 6. Effects of daily zinc administration (≤10 mg) to children 6–23 month on growth [1].

Variables	Mean Difference [2]	Relative Risk	Studies, Participants (*n*)	I^2 (%)	*p* Difference between Pooled Intervention and Control Groups
			Growth		
WAZ	0.05 (0.00; 0.10)		21, 7440	39.4	0.04
WHZ	0.04 (0.00; 0.08)		16, 6875	22.3	0.04
HAZ	0.00 (−0.04; 0.03)		20, 7340	9.2	0.80
Stunting		0.97 (0.90; 1.04)	6, 5443	0	0.39
Wasting		0.98 (0.79; 1.21)	6, 5441	32.0	0.82
Underweight		0.99 (0.90; 1.09)	5, 4793	10.7	0.83

[1] HAZ, height for age z-score; WAZ, weight for age z-score; WHZ, weight for height z-score; [2] 95% CI in parenthesis.

Twenty-one [36,37,43,48,74,75,78,83–86,88–97] studies (31 comparisons) contributed to meta-analyses of zinc effects on WAZ, and 20 studies yielding 30 comparisons [36,37,43,48,74,75, 78,82–86,88–92,94,95,97] reported HAZ outcomes. The WHZ meta-analysis included 16 studies [36,37, 43,48,74,75,78,82,84,85,88–92,97] with 25 comparisons. After pooling the studies, zinc interventions compared with placebo or no zinc slightly but significantly increased WAZ (mean difference: 0.05, 95% CI 0.0, 0.1) and WHZ (mean difference: 0.04, 95% CI 0.0, 0.08), while the HAZ result was not significant (mean difference: 0.00, 95% CI −0.04, 0.03; Figures S33–S35).

Fewer studies categorized children as stunted, wasted or underweight. Six studies with 10 comparisons [36,37,48,74,76,79] were included in the meta-analysis for the effect of zinc interventions on childhood stunting (HAZ <−2), five studies with eight comparisons [37,74,76,79] in the meta-analysis for childhood underweight, and six studies yielding 10 comparisons [36,37,48,74,76,79] in the meta-analysis for childhood wasting.

The zinc interventions were not associated with significant reductions in the risk of child stunting (RR 0.97, 95% CI 0.9, 1.04), wasting (RR 0.98, 95% CI 0.79, 1.21) or underweight (RR 0.99, 95% CI 0.90, 1.09; Figures S36–S38).

3.5.3. Effects on Diarrhea, Fever, and Respiratory Infections

In total, we identified 24 studies [48,57,70,71,73–77,79,82,85,87–91,93,97–103], with 33 comparisons, meeting our inclusion criteria and reporting on the impact of zinc on diarrhea, respiratory infections and fever. Twenty-one studies were individually randomized and three studies cluster randomized trials. We decided not to do a meta-analysis given the considerable variability of methods and outcome measures in the studies reviewed: more than half of the studies could not have been included in the analysis and thus, results might have been biased.

Similar to previous reviews, we found conflicting results for the effect of zinc intake on diarrhea, but not on respiratory infection and fever prevalence and/or incidence. Of the 16 studies [48,57,70,75,82,85,87,88,91,97,99,100,102–105] reporting on fever and/or respiratory infections, only 3 [82,91,104] found a positive effect of zinc intake. Out of the 24 studies investigating the effect of zinc on diarrhea, 11 studies [48,57,70,74–76,79,85,87,88,99] found no effect at all. Ten [71,73,89–91,93,97,100–102] reported a positive effect of zinc use on the prevalence and or incidence of diarrhea. Two [82,103] found a significant positive effect of zinc on diarrhea in the stunted sub-group, and Sazawal et al. [77] reported only a significant effect of zinc in children with low serum zinc concentrations and children older than 11 month of age. Age dependency has also been reported by Wuehler et al. [97], with a strong effect in the age group of 11.5–17.4 months and no effect in older children (17.5–30 months).

3.5.4. Effects on Mental and Motor Development

Three [57,106,107] eligible studies reported MDI and PDI scores and found no significant impact of zinc interventions on the two outcomes.

3.6. The Interaction of Iron and Zinc in Interventions in Children 6–23 Months of Age

3.6.1. Effect of Zinc on Serum Ferritin

Sub-group analyses of the 21 RCTs [26–28,31–34,36–38,40,42,44,45,48–54] reporting on the effect of iron interventions on serum ferritin indicated that iron has the strongest beneficial effect when it is the sole micronutrient administered (mean increase of 26.1 µg/L) and that it has a smaller, albeit significant, effect on serum ferritin when it is administered in combination with zinc (Figure 1).

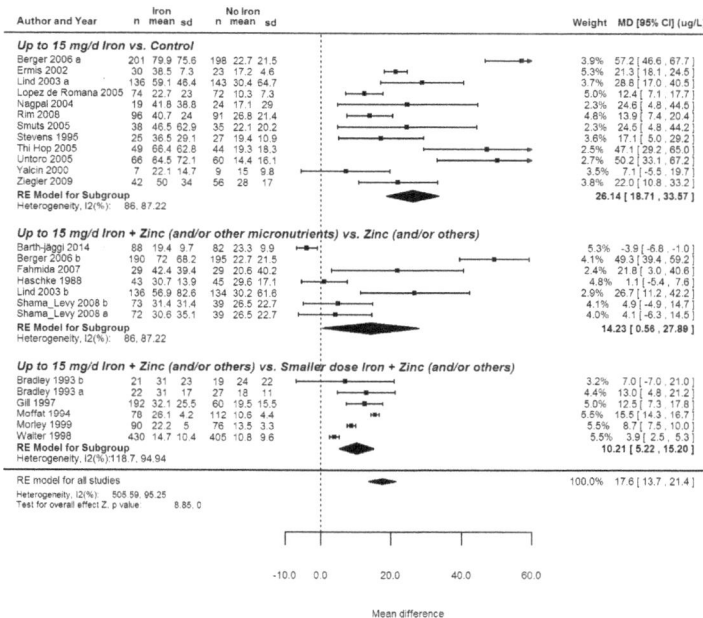

Figure 1. Forest plot summarizing the interactions of iron and zinc, supplying up to 15 mg of additional iron daily to children 6–23 months old on serum ferritin.

3.6.2. The Effect of Iron on Serum Zinc

We found 23 studies [36,43,48,59,70–88], with 35 comparisons, 14 of them comparing zinc alone to placebo, 17 of them comparing zinc in combination with iron to iron only and four of them comparing zinc and other micronutrients to other micronutrients. Sub-group analyses showed that if iron was part of the intervention, the effect of zinc on serum/plasma zinc concentrations was considerably lower (1.02 µmol/L, 95% CI 0.28, 1.76), compared to interventions delivering zinc alone (3.04 µmol/L, 95% CI 1.16, 4.92) and to interventions delivering zinc and other micronutrients, excluding iron (2.77 µmol/L, 95% CI 0.13, 5.42; Figure 2).

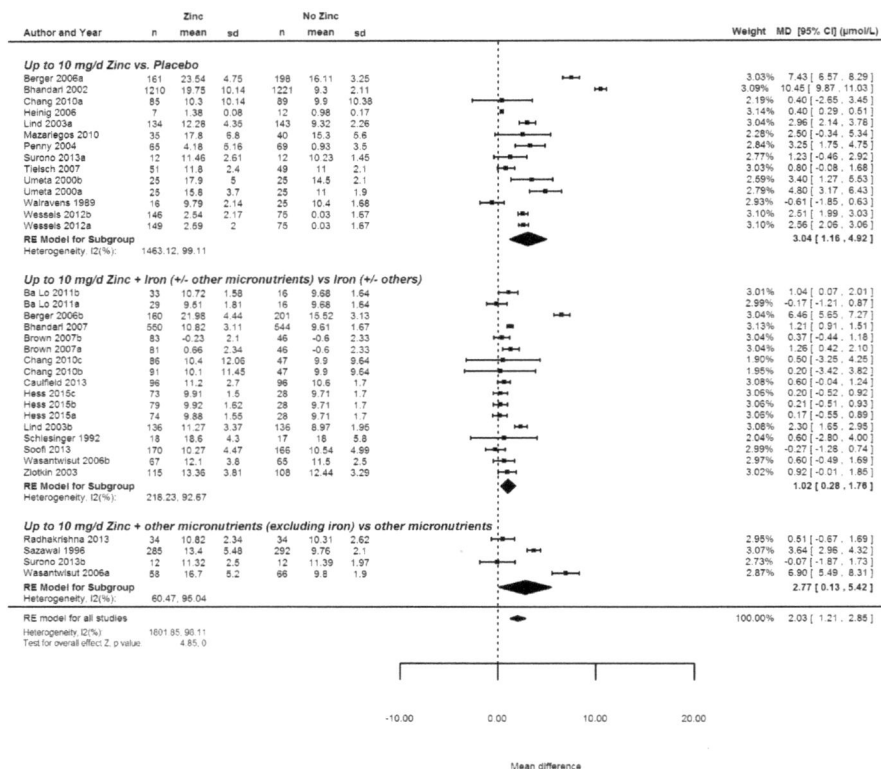

Author and Year	Zinc n	mean	sd	No Zinc n	mean	sd	Weight	MD [95% CI] (µmol/L)
Up to 10 mg/d Zinc vs. Placebo								
Berger 2006a	161	23.54	4.75	198	16.11	3.25	3.03%	7.43 [5.57, 8.29]
Bhandari 2002	1210	19.75	10.14	1221	9.3	2.11	3.09%	10.45 [9.87, 11.03]
Chang 2010a	85	10.3	10.14	89	9.9	10.38	2.19%	0.40 [-2.65, 3.45]
Heinig 2006	7	1.38	0.08	12	0.98	0.17	3.14%	0.40 [0.29, 0.51]
Lind 2003a	134	12.28	4.35	143	9.32	2.26	3.04%	2.96 [2.14, 3.78]
Mazariegos 2010	35	17.8	6.8	40	15.3	5.6	2.28%	2.50 [-0.34, 5.34]
Penny 2004	65	4.18	6.16	69	0.93	3.5	2.84%	3.25 [1.75, 4.75]
Surono 2013a	12	11.46	2.61	12	10.23	1.45	2.77%	1.23 [-0.46, 2.92]
Tielsch 2007	51	11.8	2.4	49	11	2.1	3.03%	0.80 [-0.08, 1.68]
Umeta 2000b	25	17.9	5	25	14.5	2.1	2.59%	3.40 [1.27, 5.53]
Umeta 2000a	25	15.8	3.7	25	11	1.9	2.79%	4.80 [3.17, 6.43]
Walravens 1989	16	9.79	2.14	25	10.4	1.68	2.93%	-0.61 [-1.85, 0.63]
Wessels 2012b	146	2.54	2.17	75	0.03	1.57	3.10%	2.51 [1.99, 3.03]
Wessels 2012a	149	2.59	2	75	0.03	1.67	3.10%	2.56 [2.06, 3.06]
RE Model for Subgroup								3.04 [1.16, 4.92]
Heterogeneity: I2(%):	1463.12, 99.11							
Up to 10 mg/d Zinc + Iron (+/- other micronutrients) vs Iron (+/- others)								
Ba Lo 2011b	33	10.72	1.58	16	9.68	1.64	3.01%	1.04 [0.07, 2.01]
Ba Lo 2011a	29	9.51	1.81	16	9.68	1.64	2.99%	-0.17 [-1.21, 0.87]
Berger 2006b	160	21.98	4.44	201	15.52	3.13	3.04%	6.46 [5.65, 7.27]
Bhandari 2007	550	10.82	3.11	644	9.61	1.67	3.13%	1.21 [0.91, 1.51]
Brown 2007b	83	-0.23	2.1	46	-0.6	2.33	3.04%	0.37 [-0.44, 1.18]
Brown 2007a	81	0.66	2.34	46	-0.6	2.33	3.04%	1.26 [0.42, 2.10]
Chang 2010c	86	10.4	12.06	47	9.9	9.64	1.90%	0.50 [-3.25, 4.25]
Chang 2010b	91	10.1	11.45	47	9.9	9.64	1.95%	0.20 [-3.42, 3.82]
Caulfield 2013	96	11.2	2.7	96	10.6	1.7	3.08%	0.60 [-0.04, 1.24]
Hess 2015c	73	9.91	1.5	28	9.71	1.7	3.05%	0.20 [-0.52, 0.92]
Hess 2015b	79	9.92	1.62	28	9.71	1.7	3.06%	0.21 [-0.51, 0.93]
Hess 2015a	74	9.88	1.55	28	9.71	1.7	3.06%	0.17 [-0.55, 0.89]
Lind 2003b	136	11.27	3.37	136	8.97	1.96	3.08%	2.30 [1.65, 2.95]
Schlesinger 1992	18	18.6	4.3	17	18	5.8	2.04%	0.60 [-2.80, 4.00]
Soofi 2013	170	10.27	4.47	166	10.54	4.99	2.99%	-0.27 [-1.28, 0.74]
Wasantwisut 2006b	67	12.1	3.8	65	11.5	2.5	2.97%	0.60 [-0.49, 1.69]
Zlotkin 2003	115	13.36	3.81	108	12.44	3.29	3.02%	0.92 [-0.01, 1.85]
RE Model for Subgroup								1.02 [0.28, 1.76]
Heterogeneity: I2(%):	216.23, 92.67							
Up to 10 mg/d Zinc + other micronutrients (excluding iron) vs other micronutrients								
Radhakrishna 2013	34	10.82	2.34	34	10.31	2.62	2.95%	0.51 [-0.67, 1.69]
Sazawal 1996	285	13.4	5.48	292	9.76	2.1	3.07%	3.64 [2.96, 4.32]
Surono 2013b	12	11.32	2.5	12	11.39	1.97	2.73%	-0.07 [-1.87, 1.73]
Wasantwisut 2006a	58	16.7	5.2	66	9.8	1.9	2.87%	6.90 [5.49, 8.31]
RE Model for Subgroup								2.77 [0.13, 5.42]
Heterogeneity: I2(%):	60.47, 95.04							
RE model for all studies							100.00%	2.03 [1.21, 2.85]
Heterogeneity: I2(%):	1601.85, 98.11							
Test for overall effect Z, p value:	4.85, 0							

X-axis (Mean difference): -10.00, 0.00, 10.00, 20.00

Figure 2. Forest plot summarizing the effect of interventions supplying up to 10 mg of additional zinc daily to children 6–23 months old, on serum or plasma zinc concentrations, stratified by micronutrient composition.

3.7. *Quality of the Evidence across Studies*

We used the GRADE approach to assess the quality of evidence across studies (Table S1). We considered that a publication bias or imprecision was unlikely for all outcomes. In contrast, the large heterogeneity, the lack of studies, and indirectness were considered important factors in the quality of evidence across studies. For indirectness of evidence we rated down in case ≥50% of the included studies was not food based interventions. For interventions delivering iron compared to a placebo group, the overall quality of evidence was found to be high for iron status (using serum ferritin concentration), ID and IDA; moderate for hemoglobin, HAZ, WAZ, and WHZ; low for anemia, stunting and wasting, whereas for birth weight, low birth weight, MDI and PDI the quality of evidence was very low. For interventions administering zinc compared to placebo the quality of evidence was moderate for birth weight, prevalence of low birth weight, zinc deficiency, zinc status (using serum zinc concentration), stunting, wasting, HAZ, WAZ, and WHZ, and low for underweight.

4. Discussion

We found that interventions delivering iron and zinc in concentrations up to the RNI during the 1000 days window from the prenatal period to the first 2 years of a child's life can have positive impacts on the iron and zinc status of young children. In particular, when interventions were conducted in children aged 6–23 months old, their hemoglobin levels, and iron and zinc status improved. For both nutrients, supplementation triggered a significantly stronger response than fortification even when doses were similar. For other outcomes assessed—birth weight, growth in childhood, psychomotor development—findings are less conclusive, partly due to the limited number of studies.

We show that low dose iron and zinc interventions providing no more than 45 mg/day of iron and 20 mg/day of zinc during pregnancy may not have an impact on children's birth weights and prevalence of low birth weight. Similar to our results, other meta-analyses found no effect of zinc on birth weight and prevalence of low birth weight [108,109]. Most of the studies included in those analyses did not meet our inclusion criteria because they gave higher doses of zinc than we were interested in. For iron, our results are also in accordance with a recent meta-analysis, which only observed beneficial effects at iron doses exceeding our threshold [110]. However, due to the scarcity of studies having follow-up data extending beyond the perinatal period, it is unclear if any growth advantages of routine iron and zinc ingestion during pregnancy could manifest later in infancy or early childhood.

We found that the use of iron in dietary doses (no more than 15 mg/day) during infancy and early childhood had positive effects on hemoglobin levels, anemia prevalence, and iron status (serum ferritin, ID and IDA prevalence), which agrees with a systematic review published in 2012 assessing the effect of micronutrient-fortified milk and cereal foods on infants and children [111] and a meta-analysis of supplementation trials in children 6–23 month of age, published in 2013 [112]. We did not find an effect of iron interventions on child growth or morbidity, suggesting that food-based iron interventions at doses investigated here have no beneficial impact on the occurrence of childhood morbidities. Limited effects of iron can be expected regarding mental and motor development until the age of 2 years (we focused on the Bayley's scales for mental and motor development due to more consistent reporting).

We conducted sub-group analyses stratified by type of intervention (fortification/ supplementation), intervention dose, a measure of baseline micronutrient status, as well as study quality. Sub-group analyses demonstrated that iron administered as fortificants significantly increased serum ferritin and hemoglobin levels, although to a lesser extent than supplements. This could be due to the presence of absorption inhibitors in fortified foods. For biofortification, the magnitude of the effect on iron and zinc status is unclear as to date no biofortification trials have been conducted with a focus on the 1000 days window. Yet, we would expect comparable effects as observed from fortification since both approaches deliver the micronutrients together with other dietary components. Sub-group analysis stratified by dose showed that daily iron doses as low as 6–8 mg increased serum ferritin levels. Larger effect sizes were observed for higher daily iron doses (8–10 mg), however, such doses might be difficult to attain for infants by dietary diversification or biofortification interventions alone. Surprisingly, baseline iron status did not explain much of the heterogeneity of the findings in our analysis. This is somewhat in contrast to previously published data [113,114] and could be ascribed to other factors influencing iron absorption and utilization in contexts of high exposure to inflammation [115]. But also, the categorization of studies into iron deficient versus iron sufficient population had to be done in a relatively crude manner.

We found that zinc supplementation at doses no higher than 10 mg/day increased the serum zinc concentrations of children and reduced the risk of suffering from zinc deficiency, whereas the effect of zinc administered in fortification trials, although in comparable concentrations as supplemental zinc, had no significant effect on serum zinc levels. We did not find any modification of the zinc intervention effects by child baseline zinc status. Sub-group analysis stratified by dose showed that daily zinc doses of 4–6 mg increased serum zinc by 0.9 µmol/L while larger effect sizes were observed for higher zinc doses 7–10 mg, which might be difficult to reach in children 6–23 months old through dietary means alone. Effects of zinc were significant for WHZ and WAZ, although the differences remained rather small, compared with controls. Zinc interventions probably do not have a measurable effect on the occurrence of respiratory infections and fever and effects on diarrhea are inconclusive.

Lastly, we found that, when zinc and iron were given together, their beneficial effects on serum zinc and serum iron levels were weaker than when each nutrient was given alone, suggesting that iron and zinc compete for absorption from the gut, a finding that has previously been posited [116].

Possible limitations of the review should be noted. First, many results exhibit large amounts of heterogeneity, which could not be explained by the factors we explored, and which are probably due to the differences in study design, the different types of interventions and reporting. Thus, the pooled estimates of some of the effects shown may be imprecise and results have to be interpreted with caution. Second, none of the studies meeting our inclusion criteria covered the full 1000 days window meaning that the impacts of the micronutrients could not be assessed holistically across the different life stages, but only in a compartmentalized manner. Thus, no statements can be made about whether a holistic approach covering the full 1000 days (iron and zinc interventions starting during pregnancy and continuing until 2 years of age) would have a synergistic or additive effect on certain outcome measures.

To illustrate this using ferritin levels and the Psychomotor Development Index, the absorption and utilization of dietary iron is affected by the subject's iron status [117,118]. Thus, if an iron intervention given to pregnant women suffering from moderate to severe dietary iron deficiency anemia has a positive effect on the fetus's iron status, infants born to such women would have a better iron status than control peers of the same age whose mothers received no iron [119]. Continuing the higher iron regime into infancy could actually decrease iron absorption/utilization by children in the intervention group, assuming they had benefited from exposure to prenatal use, while children in the prenatal control group who start receiving iron after birth may more efficiently absorb and utilize the little iron available. Taken together, it is possible that only small differences in iron status would be observed between the two groups at the age of two years. In contrast, with regard to the Psychomotor Development Index, one could imagine that a 1000-day intervention could lead to a synergistic effect, since some early neurodevelopmental constraints are partly irreversible [120]. Thus, a child exposed to prenatal iron would be primed for a better start early in life. Third, only few studies assessed the inflammatory status of the children and reported prevalence of inflammation and therefore it was not possible to stratify studies by level of inflammation. During inflammation the human body down regulates iron absorption, and thus studies with a high proportion of subjects suffering from inflammation would be expected to show less effects of iron on iron status. Also, in those populations, an effect of iron on hemoglobin and anemia prevalence could be masked by anemia of inflammation in the same subject.

To conclude, providing dietary or relatively low daily doses of iron and zinc to young children could be beneficial for their iron and zinc status, indicating that food based approaches can be useful tools to reduce the prevalence of iron and zinc deficiencies. However, it is questionable if an intervention would affect child outcomes throughout the whole 1000 days period, not least because of breast milk iron and zinc homeostasis [121–124]. More research assessing the impact of iron and zinc holistically over the different life stages (pregnancy, lactation, and early childhood) is required to understand the potential role of interventions provided throughout the 1000 days window.

Supplementary Materials: The following are available online at http://www.mdpi.com/2072-6643/8/12/773/s1.

Acknowledgments: Parts of data presented in this article were discussed during an expert consultation, organized by HarvestPlus on 31 March 2016, and we are thankful for all the comments from these participants.

Author Contributions: N.P., E.B., M.D.A. and F.R. designed the review. I.O. and N.P. conducted the analyses. N.P. wrote the first draft of the manuscript, and all authors contributed to the editing of the manuscript. All authors approved the final manuscript.

Conflicts of Interest: The review was funded by HarvestPlus. The authors declare no conflict of interest.

References

1. World Health Organization (WHO). *Guidelines for Food Fortification*; World Health Organization: Geneva, Switzerland, 2006. Available online: http://www.who.int/nutrition/publications/guide_food_fortification_micronutrients.pdf (accessed on 15 August 2016).

2. Murray, C.J.L.; Vos, T.; Lozano, R.; Naghavi, M.; Flaxman, A.D.; Michaud, C.; Ezzati, M.; Shibuya, K.; Salomon, J.A.; Abdalla, S.; et al. Disability-adjusted life years (DALYs) for 291 diseases and injuries in 21 regions, 1990–2010: A systematic analysis for the Global Burden of Disease Study 2010. *Lancet* **2012**, *380*, 2197–2223. [CrossRef]

3. Victora, C.G.; Adair, L.; Fall, C.; Hallal, P.C.; Martorell, R.; Richter, L.; Sachdev, H.S.; Study, M.C.U. Maternal and child undernutrition 2—Maternal and child undernutrition: Consequences for adult health and human capital. *Lancet* **2008**, *371*, 340–357. [CrossRef]

4. Black, M.M.; Quigg, A.M.; Hurley, K.M.; Pepper, M.R. Iron deficiency and iron-deficiency anemia in the first two years of life: Strategies to prevent loss of developmental potential. *Nutr. Rev.* **2011**, *69*, S64–S70. [CrossRef] [PubMed]

5. Black, M.M. Integrated strategies needed to prevent iron deficiency and to promote early child development. *J. Trace Elem. Med. Biol.* **2012**, *26*, 120–123. [CrossRef] [PubMed]

6. Oski, F.A. Iron-Deficiency in Infancy and Childhood. *N. Engl. J. Med.* **1993**, *329*, 190–193. [PubMed]

7. Christian, P.; Stewart, C.P. Maternal micronutrient deficiency, fetal development, and the risk of chronic disease. *J. Nutr.* **2010**, *140*, 437–445. [CrossRef] [PubMed]

8. Hess, S.Y.; Lonnerdal, B.; Hotz, C.; Rivera, J.A.; Brown, K.H. Recent advances in knowledge of zinc nutrition and human health. *Food Nutr. Bull.* **2009**, *30*, S5–S11. [CrossRef] [PubMed]

9. Bouis, H.E. Micronutrient fortification of plants through plant breeding: Can it improve nutrition in man at low cost? *Proc. Nutr. Soc.* **2003**, *62*, 403–411. [CrossRef] [PubMed]

10. Kau, A.L.; Ahern, P.P.; Griffin, N.W.; Goodman, A.L.; Gordon, J.I. Human nutrition, the gut microbiome and the immune system. *Nature* **2011**, *474*, 327–336. [CrossRef] [PubMed]

11. Muller, O.; Krawinkel, M. Malnutrition and health in developing countries. *CMAJ* **2005**, *173*, 279–286. [CrossRef] [PubMed]

12. Sazawal, S.; Black, R.E.; Ramsan, M.; Chwaya, H.M.; Stoltzfus, R.J.; Dutta, A.; Dhingra, U.; Kabole, I.; Deb, S.; Othman, M.K.; et al. Effects of routine prophylactic supplementation with iron and folic acid on admission to hospital and mortality in preschool children in a high malaria transmission setting: Community-based, randomised, placebo-controlled trial. *Lancet* **2006**, *367*, 133–143. [CrossRef]

13. Hozo, S.P.; Djulbegovic, B.; Hozo, I. Estimating the mean and variance from the median, range, and the size of a sample. *BMC Med. Res. Methodol.* **2005**, *5*, 13. [CrossRef] [PubMed]

14. Higgins, J.P.; White, I.R.; Anzures-Cabrera, J. Meta-analysis of skewed data: Combining results reported on log-transformed or raw scales. *Stat. Med.* **2008**, *27*, 6072–6092. [CrossRef] [PubMed]

15. DerSimonian, R.; Laird, N. Meta-analysis in clinical trials. *Contr. Clin. Trial.* **1986**, *7*, 177–188. [CrossRef]

16. Higgins, J.P.T.; Green, S. Reviews of Interventions 4.2.6. In *The Cochrane Library*; John Wiley & Sons, Ltd.: Chichester, UK, 2006; Volume 4.

17. Viechtbauer, W. Conducting Meta-Analyses in R with the metafor Package. *J. Stat. Softw.* **2010**, *36*, 1–48. [CrossRef]

18. Schünemann, H.; Brożek, J.; Guyatt, G.; Oxman, A. GRADE Handbook. Introduction to GRADE Handbook. GRADE Working Group, 2013. Available online: http://gdt.guidelinedevelopment.org/app/handbook/handbook.html (accessed on 28 November 2016).

19. Liu, J.M.; Mei, Z.G.; Ye, R.W.; Serdula, M.K.; Ren, A.G.; Cogswell, M.E. Micronutrient Supplementation and Pregnancy Outcomes Double-Blind Randomized Controlled Trial in China. *JAMA Intern. Med.* **2013**, *173*, 276–282. [CrossRef] [PubMed]

20. Ouladsahebmadarek, E.; Sayyah-Melli, M.; Taghavi, S.; Abbasalizadeh, S.; Seyedhejazie, M. The effect of supplemental iron elimination on pregnancy outcome. *Pak. J. Med. Sci.* **2011**, *27*, 641–645.

21. Makrides, M.; Crowther, C.A.; Gibson, R.A.; Gibson, R.S.; Skeaff, C.M. Efficacy and tolerability of low-dose iron supplements during pregnancy: A randomized controlled trial. *Am. J. Clin. Nutr.* **2003**, *78*, 145–153. [PubMed]

22. Siega-Riz, A.M.; Hartzema, A.G.; Turnbull, C.; Thorp, J.; McDonald, T.; Cogswell, M.E. The effects of prophylactic iron given in prenatal supplements on iron status and birth outcomes: A randomized controlled trial. *Am. J. Obstet. Gynecol.* **2006**, *194*, 512–519. [CrossRef] [PubMed]

23. Cogswell, M.E.; Parvanta, I.; Ickes, L.; Yip, R.; Brittenham, G.M. Iron supplementation during pregnancy, anemia, and birth weight: A randomized controlled trial. *Am. J. Clin. Nutr.* **2003**, *78*, 773–781. [PubMed]

24. Dawson, E.B.; Albers, J.; Mcganity, W.J. Serum Zinc Changes Due to Iron Supplementation in Teen-Age Pregnancy. *Am. J. Clin. Nutr.* **1989**, *50*, 848–852. [PubMed]

25. Li, Q.; Yan, H.; Zeng, L.X.; Cheng, Y.; Liang, W.F.; Dang, S.N.; Wang, Q.L.; Tsuji, I. Effects of Maternal Multimicronutrient Supplementation on the Mental Development of Infants in Rural Western China: Follow-up Evaluation of a Double-Blind, Randomized, Controlled Trial. *Pediatrics* **2009**, *123*, E685–E692. [CrossRef] [PubMed]

26. Walter, T.; Pino, P.; Pizarro, F.; Lozoff, B. Prevention of iron-deficiency anemia: Comparison of high- and low-iron formulas in term healthy infants after six months of life. *J. Pediatr.* **1998**, *132*, 635–640. [CrossRef]

27. Moffatt, M.E.; Longstaffe, S.; Besant, J.; Dureski, C. Prevention of iron deficiency and psychomotor decline in high-risk infants through use of iron-fortified infant formula: A randomized clinical trial. *J. Pediatr.* **1994**, *125*, 527–534. [CrossRef]

28. Ermis, B.; Demirel, F.; Demircan, N.; Gurel, A. Effects of three different iron supplementations in term healthy infants after 5 months of life. *J. Trop. Pediatr.* **2002**, *48*, 280–284. [CrossRef] [PubMed]

29. Geltman, P.L.; Meyers, A.F.; Mehta, S.D.; Brugnara, C.; Villon, I.; Wu, Y.A.; Bauchner, H. Daily multivitamins with iron to prevent anemia in high-risk infants: A randomized clinical trial. *Pediatrics* **2004**, *114*, 86–93. [CrossRef] [PubMed]

30. Walter, T.; Dallman, P.R.; Pizarro, F.; Velozo, L.; Pena, G.; Bartholmey, S.J.; Hertrampf, E.; Olivares, M.; Letelier, A.; Arredondo, M. Effectiveness of iron-fortified infant cereal in prevention of iron deficiency anemia. *Pediatrics* **1993**, *91*, 976–982. [PubMed]

31. Gill, D.G.; Vincent, S.; Segal, D.S. Follow-on formula in the prevention of iron deficiency: A multicentre study. *Acta Paediatr.* **1997**, *86*, 683–689. [CrossRef] [PubMed]

32. Haschke, F.; Pietschnig, B.; Vanura, H.; Heil, M.; Steffan, I.; Hobiger, G.; Schuster, E.; Camaya, Z. Iron intake and iron nutritional status of infants fed iron-fortified beikost with meat. *Am. J. Clin. Nutr.* **1988**, *47*, 108–112. [PubMed]

33. Ziegler, E.E.; Nelson, S.E.; Jeter, J.M. Iron status of breastfed infants is improved equally by medicinal iron and iron-fortified cereal. *Am. J. Clin. Nutr.* **2009**, *90*, 76–87. [CrossRef] [PubMed]

34. Rim, H.; Kim, S.; Sim, B.; Gang, H.; Kim, H.; Kim, Y.; Kim, R.; Yang, M. Effect of iron fortification of nursery complementary food on iron status of infants in the DPRKorea. *Asia Pac. J. Clin. Nutr.* **2008**, *17*, 264–269. [PubMed]

35. Dijkhuizen, M.A.; Wieringa, F.T.; West, C.E.; Martuti, S. Muhilal: Effects of iron and zinc supplementation in Indonesian infants on micronutrient status and growth. *J. Nutr.* **2001**, *131*, 2860–2865. [PubMed]

36. Lind, T.; Lonnerdal, B.; Stenlund, H.; Ismail, D.; Seswandhana, R.; Ekstrom, E.C.; Persson, L.A. A community-based randomized controlled trial of iron and zinc supplementation in Indonesian infants: Interactions between iron and zinc. *Am. J. Clin. Nutr.* **2003**, *77*, 883–890. [PubMed]

37. Fahmida, U.; Rumawas, J.S.; Utomo, B.; Patmonodewo, S.; Schultink, W. Zinc-iron, but not zinc-alone supplementation, increased linear growth of stunted infants with low haemoglobin. *Asia Pac. J. Clin. Nutr.* **2007**, *16*, 301–309. [PubMed]

38. Untoro, J.; Karyadi, E.; Wibowo, L.; Erhardt, M.W.; Gross, R. Multiple micronutrient supplements improve micronutrient status and anemia but not growth and morbidity of Indonesian infants: A randomized, double-blind, placebo-controlled trial. *J. Nutr.* **2005**, *135*, 639S–645S. [PubMed]

39. Wieringa, F.T.; Dijkhuizen, M.A.; West, C.E.; Thurnham, D.I.; Muhilal; Van der Meer, J.W.M. Redistribution of vitamin A after iron supplementation in Indonesian infants. *Am. J. Clin. Nutr.* **2003**, *77*, 651–657. [PubMed]

40. Shamah-Levy, T.; Villalpando, S.; Rivera-Dommarco, J.A.; Mundo-Rosas, V.; Cuevas-Nasu, L.; Jimenez-Aguilar, A. Ferrous gluconate and ferrous sulfate added to a complementary food distributed by the Mexican nutrition program Oportunidades have a comparable efficacy to reduce iron deficiency in toddlers. *J. Pediatr. Gastroenterol. Nutr.* **2008**, *47*, 660–666. [CrossRef] [PubMed]

41. Domellof, M.; Cohen, R.J.; Dewey, K.G.; Hernell, O.; Rivera, L.L.; Lonnerdal, B. Iron supplementation of breast-fed Honduran and Swedish infants from 4 to 9 months of age. *J. Pediatr.* **2001**, *138*, 679–687. [CrossRef] [PubMed]

42. Smuts, C.M.; Dhansay, M.A.; Faber, M.; van Stuijvenberg, M.E.; Swanevelder, S.; Gross, R.; Benade, A.J.S. Efficacy of multiple micronutrient supplementation for improving anemia, micronutrient status, and growth in south African infants. *J. Nutr.* **2005**, *135*, 653S–659S. [PubMed]

43. Wasantwisut, E.; Winichagoon, P.; Chitchumroonchokchai, C.; Yamborisut, U.; Boonpraderm, A.; Pongcharoen, T.; Sranacharoenpong, K.; Russameesopaphorn, W. Iron and zinc supplementation improved iron and zinc status, but not physical growth, of apparently healthy, breast-fed infants in rural communities of northeast Thailand. *J. Nutr.* **2006**, *136*, 2405–2411. [PubMed]

44. De Romana, G.L.; Cusirramos, S.; de Romana, D.L.; Gross, R. Efficacy of multiple micronutrient supplementation for improving anemia, micronutrient status, growth, and morbidity of Peruvian infants. *J. Nutr.* **2005**, *135*, 646S–652S.

45. Stevens, D.; Nelson, A. The Effect of Iron in Formula Milk after 6 Months of Age. *Arch. Dis. Child.* **1995**, *73*, 216–220. [CrossRef] [PubMed]

46. Virtanen, M.A.; Svahn, C.J.; Viinikka, L.U.; Raiha, N.C.; Siimes, M.A.; Axelsson, I.E. Iron-fortified and unfortified cow's milk: Effects on iron intakes and iron status in young children. *Acta Paediatr.* **2001**, *90*, 724–731. [CrossRef] [PubMed]

47. Nogueira Arcanjo, F.P.; Santos, P.R.; Costa Arcanjo, C.P.; Meira Magalhaes, S.M.; Madeiro Leite, A.J. Daily and Weekly Iron Supplementations are Effective in Increasing Hemoglobin and Reducing Anemia in Infants. *J. Trop. Pediatr.* **2013**, *59*, 175–179. [CrossRef] [PubMed]

48. Berger, J.; Ninh, N.X.; Khan, N.C.; Nhien, N.V.; Lien, D.K.; Trung, N.Q.; Khoi, H.H. Efficacy of combined iron and zinc supplementation on micronutrient status and growth in Vietnamese infants. *Eur. J. Clin. Nutr.* **2006**, *60*, 443–454. [CrossRef] [PubMed]

49. Barth-Jaeggi, T.; Moretti, D.; Kvalsvig, J.D.; Holding, P.A.; Njenga, J.; Mwangi, A.; Chhagan, M.; Lacroix, C.; Zimmermann, M.B. In-home fortification with 2.5 mg iron as NaFeEDTA does not reduce anaemia but increases weight gain: A randomised controlled trial in Kenyan infants. *Matern. Child Nutr.* **2015**, *11*, 151–162. [CrossRef] [PubMed]

50. Nagpal, J.; Sachdev, H.P.S.; Singh, T.; Mallika, V. A randomized placebo-controlled trial of iron supplementation in breastfed young infants initiated on complementary feeding: Effect on haematological status. *J. Health Popul. Nutr.* **2004**, *22*, 203–211. [PubMed]

51. Morley, R.; Abbott, R.; Fairweather-Tait, S.; MacFadyen, U.; Stephenson, T.; Lucas, A. Iron fortified follow on formula from 9 to 18 months improves iron status but not development or growth: A randomised trial. *Arch. Dis. Child.* **1999**, *81*, 247–252. [CrossRef] [PubMed]

52. Hop, L.T.; Berger, J. Multiple micronutrient supplementation improves anemia, micronutrient nutrient status, and growth of Vietnamese infants: Double-blind, randomized, placebo-controlled trial. *J. Nutr.* **2005**, *135*, 660S–665S.

53. Bradley, C.K.; Hillman, L.; Sherman, A.R.; Leedy, D.; Cordano, A. Evaluation of two iron-fortified, milk-based formulas during infancy. *Pediatrics* **1993**, *91*, 908–914. [PubMed]

54. Yalcin, S.S.; Yurdakok, K.; Acikgoz, D.; Ozmert, E. Short-term developmental outcome of iron prophylaxis in infants. *Pediatr. Int.* **2000**, *42*, 625–630. [CrossRef] [PubMed]

55. Engstrom, E.M.; Castro, I.R.; Portela, M.; Cardoso, L.O.; Monteiro, C.A. Effectiveness of daily and weekly iron supplementation in the prevention of anemia in infants. *Rev. Saude Publica* **2008**, *42*, 786–795. [CrossRef] [PubMed]

56. Massaga, J.J.; Kitua, A.Y.; Lemnge, M.M.; Akida, J.A.; Malle, L.N.; Ronn, A.M.; Theander, T.G.; Bygbjerg, I.C. Effect of intermittent treatment with amodiaquine on anaemia and malarial fevers in infants in Tanzania: A randomised placebo-controlled trial. *Lancet* **2003**, *361*, 1853–1860. [CrossRef]

57. Lind, T.; Lonnerdal, B.; Stenlund, H.; Gamayanti, I.L.; Ismail, D.; Seswandhana, R.; Persson, L.A. A community-based randomized controlled trial of iron and zinc supplementation in Indonesian infants: Effects on growth and development. *Am. J. Clin. Nutr.* **2004**, *80*, 729–736. [PubMed]

58. Dewey, K.G.; Domellof, M.; Cohen, R.J.; Landa Rivera, L.; Hernell, O.; Lonnerdal, B. Iron supplementation affects growth and morbidity of breast-fed infants: Results of a randomized trial in Sweden and Honduras. *J. Nutr.* **2002**, *132*, 3249–3255. [PubMed]

59. Caulfield, L.E.; Zavaleta, N.; Figueroa, A. Adding zinc to prenatal iron and folate supplements improves maternal and neonatal zinc status in a Peruvian population. *Am. J. Clin. Nutr.* **1999**, *69*, 1257–1263. [PubMed]

60. Prawirohartono, E.P.; Nystrom, L.; Ivarsson, A.; Stenlund, H.; Lind, T. The impact of prenatal vitamin A and zinc supplementation on growth of children up to 2 years of age in rural Java, Indonesia. *Public Health Nutr.* **2011**, *14*, 2197–2206. [CrossRef] [PubMed]

61. Castillo-Duran, C.; Marin, V.B.; Alcazar, L.S.; Iturralde, H.; Ruz, M.O. Controlled trial of zinc supplementation in Chilean pregnant adolescents. *Nutr. Res.* **2001**, *21*, 715–724. [CrossRef]

62. Mahomed, K.; James, D.K.; Golding, J.; Mccabe, R. Zinc Supplementation during Pregnancy—A Double-Blind Randomized Controlled Trial. *Br. Med. J.* **1989**, *299*, 826–830. [CrossRef]

63. Hafeez, A.; Mehmood, G.; Mazhar, F. Oral zinc supplementation in pregnant women and its effect on birth weight: A randomised controlled trial. *Arch. Dis. Child. Fetal Neonatal Ed.* **2005**, *90*, 170–171. [CrossRef] [PubMed]

64. Hunt, I.F.; Murphy, N.J.; Cleaver, A.E.; Faraji, B.; Swendseid, M.E.; Browdy, B.L.; Coulson, A.H.; Clark, V.A.; Settlage, R.H.; Smith, J.C. Zinc Supplementation during Pregnancy in Low-Income Teenagers of Mexican Descent—Effects on Selected Blood-Constituents and on Progress and Outcome of Pregnancy. *Am. J. Clin. Nutr.* **1985**, *42*, 815–828. [PubMed]

65. Hunt, I.F.; Murphy, N.J.; Cleaver, A.E.; Faraji, B.; Swendseid, M.E.; Coulson, A.H.; Clark, V.A.; Browdy, B.L.; Cabalum, M.T.; Smith, J.C. Zinc Supplementation during Pregnancy—Effects on Selected Blood-Constituents and on Progress and Outcome of Pregnancy in Low-Income Women of Mexican Descent. *Am. J. Clin. Nutr.* **1984**, *40*, 508–521. [PubMed]

66. Ross, S.M.; Nel, E.; Naeye, R.L. Differing effects of low and high bulk maternal dietary supplements during pregnancy. *Early Hum. Dev.* **1985**, *10*, 295–302. [CrossRef]

67. Prawirohartono, E.P.; Nystrom, L.; Nurdiati, D.S.; Hakimi, M.; Lind, T. The Impact of Prenatal Vitamin A and Zinc Supplementation on Birth Size and Neonatal Survival—A Double-Blind, Randomized Controlled Trial in a Rural Area of Indonesia. *Int. J. Vitam. Nutr. Res.* **2013**, *83*, 14–25. [CrossRef] [PubMed]

68. Iannotti, L.L.; Zavaleta, N.; Leon, Z.; Shankar, A.H.; Caulfield, L.E. Maternal zinc supplementation and growth in Peruvian infants. *Am. J. Clin. Nutr.* **2008**, *88*, 154–160. [PubMed]

69. Salmenpera, L.; Perheentupa, J.; Nanto, V.; Siimes, M.A. Low Zinc Intake during Exclusive Breast-Feeding Does Not Impair Growth. *J. Pediatr. Gastroenterol. Nutr.* **1994**, *18*, 361–370. [CrossRef] [PubMed]

70. Lo, N.B.; Aaron, G.J.; Hess, S.Y.; Dossou, N.I.; Guiro, A.T.; Wade, S.; Brown, K.H. Plasma zinc concentration responds to short-term zinc supplementation, but not zinc fortification, in young children in Senegal. *Am. J. Clin. Nutr.* **2011**, *93*, 1348–1355. [CrossRef] [PubMed]

71. Bhandari, N.; Bahl, R.; Taneja, S.; Strand, T.; Molbak, K.; Ulvik, R.J.; Sommerfelt, H.; Bhan, M.K. Substantial reduction in severe diarrheal morbidity by daily zinc supplementation in young north Indian children. *Pediatrics* **2002**, *109*, e86. [CrossRef] [PubMed]

72. Bhandari, N.; Taneja, S.; Mazumder, S.; Bahl, R.; Fontaine, O.; Bhan, M.K. Adding zinc to supplemental iron and folic acid does not affect mortality and severe morbidity in young children. *J. Nutr.* **2007**, *137*, 112–117. [PubMed]

73. Chang, S.; El Arifeen, S.; Bari, S.; Wahed, M.A.; Rahman, K.M.; Rahman, M.T.; Mahmud, A.B.A.; Begum, N.; Zaman, K.; Baqui, A.H.; Black, R.E. Supplementing iron and zinc: Double blind, randomized evaluation of separate or combined delivery. *Eur. J. Clin. Nutr.* **2010**, *64*, 153–160. [CrossRef] [PubMed]

74. Hess, S.Y.; Abbeddou, S.; Jimenez, E.Y.; Some, J.W.; Vosti, S.A.; Ouedraogo, Z.P.; Guissou, R.M.; Ouedraogo, J.B.; Brown, K.H. Small-Quantity Lipid-Based Nutrient Supplements, Regardless of Their Zinc Content, Increase Growth and Reduce the Prevalence of Stunting and Wasting in Young Burkinabe Children: A Cluster-Randomized Trial. *PLoS ONE* **2015**, *10*, e0122242. [CrossRef] [PubMed]

75. Mazariegos, M.; Hambidge, K.M.; Westcott, J.E.; Solomons, N.W.; Raboy, V.; Das, A.; Goco, N.; Kindem, M.; Wright, L.L.; Krebs, N.F. Neither a Zinc Supplement nor Phytate-Reduced Maize nor Their Combination Enhance Growth of 6-to 12-Month-Old Guatemalan Infants. *J. Nutr.* **2010**, *140*, 1041–1048. [CrossRef] [PubMed]

76. Radhakrishna, K.V.; Hemalatha, R.; Geddam, J.J.B.; Kumar, P.A.; Balakrishna, N.; Shatrugna, V. Effectiveness of Zinc Supplementation to Full Term Normal Infants: A Community Based Double Blind, Randomized, Controlled, Clinical Trial. *PLoS ONE* **2013**, *8*, e61486. [CrossRef] [PubMed]

77. Sazawal, S.; Black, R.E.; Bhan, M.K.; Jalla, S.; Bhandari, N.; Sinha, A.; Majumdar, S. Zinc supplementation reduces the incidence of persistent diarrhea and dysentery among low socioeconomic children in India. *J. Nutr.* **1996**, *126*, 443–450. [PubMed]

78. Schlesinger, L.; Arevalo, M.; Arredondo, S.; Diaz, M.; Lonnerdal, B.; Stekel, A. Effect of a Zinc-Fortified Formula on Immunocompetence and Growth of Malnourished Infants. *Am. J. Clin. Nutr.* **1992**, *56*, 491–498. [PubMed]

79. Soofi, S.; Cousens, S.; Iqbal, S.P.; Akhund, T.; Khan, J.; Ahmed, I.; Zaidi, A.K.M.; Bhutta, Z.A. Effect of provision of daily zinc and iron with several micronutrients on growth and morbidity among young children in Pakistan: A cluster-randomised trial. *Lancet* **2013**, *382*, 29–40. [CrossRef]

80. Surono, I.S.; Martono, P.D.; Kameo, S.; Suradji, E.W.; Koyama, H. Effect of probiotic L. plantarum IS-10506 and zinc supplementation on humoral immune response and zinc status of Indonesian pre-school children. *J. Trace Elem. Med. Biol.* **2014**, *28*, 465–469. [CrossRef] [PubMed]

81. Tielsch, J.M.; Khatry, S.K.; Stoltzfus, R.J.; Katz, J.; LeClerq, S.C.; Adhikari, R.; Mullany, L.C.; Black, R.; Shresta, S. Effect of daily zinc supplementation on child mortality in southern Nepal: A community-based, cluster randomised, placebo-controlled trial. *Lancet* **2007**, *370*, 1230–1239. [CrossRef]

82. Umeta, M.; West, C.E.; Haidar, J.; Deurenberg, P.; Hautvast, J.G.A.J. Zinc supplementation and stunted infants in Ethiopia: A randomised controlled trial. *Lancet* **2000**, *355*, 2021–2026. [CrossRef]

83. Walravens, P.A.; Hambidge, K.M.; Koepfer, D.M. Zinc Supplementation in Infants with a Nutritional Pattern of Failure to Thrive—A Double-Blind, Controlled-Study. *Pediatrics* **1989**, *83*, 532–538. [PubMed]

84. Zlotkin, S.; Arthur, P.; Schauer, C.; Antwi, K.Y.; Yeung, G.; Piekarz, A. Home-fortification with iron and zinc sprinkles or iron sprinkles alone successfully treats anemia in infants and young children. *J. Nutr.* **2003**, *133*, 1075–1080. [PubMed]

85. Brown, K.H.; de Romana, D.L.; Arsenault, J.E.; Peerson, J.M.; Penny, M.E. Comparison of the effects of zinc delivered in a fortified food or a liquid supplement on the growth, morbidity, and plasma zinc concentrations of young Peruvian children. *Am. J. Clin. Nutr.* **2007**, *85*, 538–547. [PubMed]

86. Penny, M.E.; Marin, R.M.; Duran, A.; Peerson, J.M.; Lanata, C.F.; Lonnerdal, B.; Black, R.E.; Brown, K.H. Randomized controlled trial of the effect of daily supplementation with zinc or multiple micronutrients on the morbidity, growth, and micronutrient status of young Peruvian children. *Am. J. Clin. Nutr.* **2004**, *79*, 457–465. [PubMed]

87. Wessells, K.R.; Ouedraogo, Z.P.; Rouamba, N.; Hess, S.Y.; Ouedraogo, J.B.; Brown, K.H. Short-term zinc supplementation with dispersible tablets or zinc sulfate solution yields similar positive effects on plasma zinc concentration of young children in Burkina Faso: A randomized controlled trial. *J. Pediatr.* **2012**, *160*, 129.e3–135.e3. [CrossRef] [PubMed]

88. Heinig, M.J.; Brown, K.H.; Lonnerdal, B.; Dewey, K.G. Zinc supplementation does not affect growth, morbidity, or motor development of US term breastfed infants at 4–10 months of age. *Am. J. Clin. Nutr.* **2006**, *84*, 594–601. [PubMed]

89. Alarcon, K.; Kolsteren, P.W.; Prada, A.M.; Chian, A.M.; Velarde, R.E.; Pecho, I.L.; Hoeree, T.F. Effects of separate delivery of zinc or zinc and vitamin A on hemoglobin response, growth, and diarrhea in young Peruvian children receiving iron therapy for anemia. *Am. J. Clin. Nutr.* **2004**, *80*, 1276–1282. [PubMed]

90. Gardner, J.M.M.; Powell, C.A.; Baker-Henningham, H.; Walker, S.P.; Cole, T.J.; Grantham-McGregor, S.M. Zinc supplementation and psychosocial stimulation: Effects on the development of undernourished Jamaican children. *Am. J. Clin. Nutr.* **2005**, *82*, 399–405. [PubMed]

91. Ninh, N.X.; Thissen, J.P.; Collette, L.; Gerard, G.; Khoi, H.H.; Ketelslegers, J.M. Zinc supplementation increases growth and circulating insulin-like growth factor I (IGF-I) in growth-retarded Vietnamese children. *Am. J. Clin. Nutr.* **1996**, *63*, 514–519. [PubMed]

92. Rivera, J.A.; Ruel, M.T.; Santizo, M.C.; Lonnerdal, B.; Brown, K.H. Zinc supplementation improves the growth of stunted rural Guatemalan infants. *J. Nutr.* **1998**, *128*, 556–562. [PubMed]

93. Sur, D.; Gupta, D.N.; Mondal, S.K.; Ghosh, S.; Manna, B.; Rajendran, K.; Bhattacharya, S.K. Impact of zinc supplementation on diarrheal morbidity and growth pattern of low birth weight infants in Kolkata, India: A randomized, double-blind, placebo-controlled, community-based study. *Pediatrics* **2003**, *112*, 1327–1332. [CrossRef] [PubMed]

94. Walravens, P.A.; Chakar, A.; Mokni, R.; Denise, J.; Lemonnier, D. Zinc supplements in breastfed infants. *Lancet* **1992**, *340*, 683–685. [CrossRef]

95. Olney, D.K.; Pollitt, E.; Kariger, P.K.; Khalfan, S.S.; Ali, N.S.; Tielsch, J.M.; Sazawal, S.; Black, R.; Allen, L.H.; Stoltzfus, R.J. Combined iron and folic acid supplementation with or without zinc reduces time to walking unassisted among Zanzibari infants 5-to 11-month old. *J. Nutr.* **2006**, *136*, 2427–2434. [PubMed]

96. Umeta, M.; West, C.E.; Verhoef, H.; Haidar, J.; Hautvast, J.G.A.J. Factors associated with stunting in infants aged 5–11 months in the Dodota-Sire District, rural Ethiopia. *J. Nutr.* **2003**, *133*, 1064–1069. [PubMed]

97. Wuehler, S.E.; Sempertegui, F.; Brown, K.H. Dose-response trial of prophylactic zinc supplements, with or without copper, in young Ecuadorian children at risk of zinc deficiency. *Am. J. Clin. Nutr.* **2008**, *87*, 723–733. [PubMed]

98. Sazawal, S.; Black, R.E.; Bhan, M.K.; Jalla, S.; Sinha, A.; Bhandari, N. Efficacy of zinc supplementation in reducing the incidence and prevalence of acute diarrhea—A community-based, double-blind, controlled trial. *Am. J. Clin. Nutr.* **1997**, *66*, 413–418. [PubMed]

99. Tielsch, J.M.; Khatry, S.K.; Stoltzfus, R.J.; Katz, J.; LeClerq, S.C.; Adhikari, R.; Mullany, L.C.; Shresta, S.; Black, R.E. Effect of routine prophylactic supplementation with iron and folic acid on preschool child mortality in southern Nepal: Community-based, cluster-randomised, placebo-controlled trial. *Lancet* **2006**, *367*, 144–152. [CrossRef]

100. Larson, C.P.; Nasrin, D.; Saha, A.; Chowdhury, M.I.; Qadri, F. The added benefit of zinc supplementation after zinc treatment of acute childhood diarrhoea: A randomized, double-blind field trial. *Trop. Med. Int. Health* **2010**, *15*, 754–761. [CrossRef] [PubMed]

101. Gupta, D.N.; Mondal, S.K.; Ghosh, S.; Rajendran, K.; Sur, D.; Manna, B. Impact of zinc supplementation on diarrhoeal morbidity in rural children of West Bengal, India. *Acta Paediatr.* **2003**, *92*, 531–536. [CrossRef] [PubMed]

102. Ruel, M.T.; Rivera, J.A.; Santizo, M.C.; Lonnerdal, B.; Brown, K.H. Impact of zinc supplementation on morbidity from diarrhea and respiratory infections among rural Guatemalan children. *Pediatrics* **1997**, *99*, 808–813. [CrossRef] [PubMed]

103. Chhagan, M.K.; Van den Broeck, J.; Luabeya, K.K.; Mpontshane, N.; Tucker, K.L.; Bennish, M.L. Effect of micronutrient supplementation on diarrhoeal disease among stunted children in rural South Africa. *Eur. J. Clin. Nutr.* **2009**, *63*, 850–857. [CrossRef] [PubMed]

104. Sazawal, S. Daily zinc supplements reduced the incidence and severity of acute lower respiratory infections in children in India. *Evid. Based Nurs.* **1999**, *2*, 12.

105. Ramakrishnan, U.; Gonzalez-Cossio, T.; Neufeld, L.M.; Rivera, J.; Martorell, R. Multiple micronutrient supplementation during pregnancy does not lead to greater infant birth size than does iron-only supplementation: A randomized controlled trial in a semirural community in Mexico. *Am. J. Clin. Nutr.* **2003**, *77*, 720–725. [PubMed]

106. Taneja, S.; Bhandari, N.; Bahl, R.; Bhan, M.K. Impact of zinc supplementation on mental and psychomotor scores of children aged 12 to 18 months: A randomized, double-blind trial. *J. Pediatr.* **2005**, *146*, 506–511. [CrossRef] [PubMed]

107. Castillo-Duran, C.; Perales, C.G.; Hertrampf, E.D.; Marin, V.B.; Rivera, F.A.; Icaza, G. Effect of zinc supplementation on development and growth of Chilean infants. *J. Pediatr.* **2001**, *138*, 229–235. [CrossRef] [PubMed]

108. Ota, E.; Mori, R.; Middleton, P.; Tobe-Gai, R.; Mahomed, K.; Miyazaki, C.; Bhutta, Z.A. Zinc supplementation for improving pregnancy and infant outcome. *Cochrane Database Syst. Rev.* **2015**, *2*, CD000230.

109. Chaffee, B.W.; King, J.C. Effect of Zinc Supplementation on Pregnancy and Infant Outcomes: A Systematic Review. *Paediatr. Perinat. Epidemiol.* **2012**, *26*, 118–137. [CrossRef] [PubMed]

110. Pena-Rosas, J.P.; De-Regil, L.M.; Garcia-Casal, M.N.; Dowswell, T. Daily oral iron supplementation during pregnancy. *Cochrane Database Syst. Rev.* **2015**, *7*, CD004736.

111. Eichler, K.; Wieser, S.; Ruthemann, I.; Brugger, U. Effects of micronutrient fortified milk and cereal food for infants and children: A systematic review. *BMC Public Health* **2012**, *12*, 506. [CrossRef] [PubMed]

112. Pasricha, S.R.; Hayes, E.; Kalumba, K.; Biggs, B.A. Effect of daily iron supplementation on health in children aged 4–23 months: A systematic review and meta-analysis of randomised controlled trials. *Lancet Glob. Health* **2013**, *1*, E77–E86. [CrossRef]

113. Cook, J.D.; Lipschit, D.A.; Miles, L.E.M.; Finch, C.A. Serum Ferritin as a Measure of Iron Stores in Normal Subjects. *Am. J. Clin. Nutr.* **1974**, *27*, 681–687. [PubMed]

114. Moretti, D.; Zimmermann, M.B.; Wegmuller, R.; Walczyk, T.; Zeder, C.; Hurrell, R.F. Iron status and food matrix strongly affect the relative bioavailability of ferric pyrophosphate in humans. *Am. J. Clin. Nutr.* **2006**, *83*, 632–638. [PubMed]

115. Petry, N.; Olofin, I.; Hurrell, R.F.; Boy, E.; Wirth, J.P.; Moursi, M.; Donahue Angel, M.; Rohner, F. The Proportion of Anemia Associated with Iron Deficiency in Low, Medium, and High Human Development Index Countries: A Systematic Analysis of National Surveys. *Nutrients* **2016**, *8*. [CrossRef] [PubMed]

116. De Brito, N.J.; Rocha, E.D.; de Araujo Silva, A.; Costa, J.B.; Franca, M.C.; das Gracas Almeida, M.; Brandao-Neto, J. Oral zinc supplementation decreases the serum iron concentration in healthy schoolchildren: A pilot study. *Nutrients* **2014**, *6*, 3460–3473. [CrossRef] [PubMed]

117. Cook, J.D.; Dassenko, S.A.; Lynch, S.R. Assessment of the role of nonheme-iron availability in iron balance. *Am. J. Clin. Nutr.* **1991**, *54*, 717–722. [PubMed]

118. Reddy, M.B.; Hurrell, R.F.; Cook, J.D. Estimation of nonheme-iron bioavailability from meal composition. *Am. J. Clin. Nutr.* **2000**, *71*, 937–943. [PubMed]

119. Singla, P.N.; Tyagi, M.; Shankar, R.; Dash, D.; Kumar, A. Fetal iron status in maternal anemia. *Acta Paediatr.* **1996**, *85*, 1327–1330. [CrossRef] [PubMed]

120. Beard, J. Iron deficiency alters brain development and functioning. *J. Nutr.* **2003**, *133*, 1468S–1472S. [PubMed]

121. Nakamori, M.; Ninh, N.X.; Isomura, H.; Yoshiike, N.; Hien, V.T.; Nhug, B.T.; Nhien, N.V.; Nakano, T.; Khan, N.C.; Yamamoto, S. Nutritional status of lactating mothers and their breast milk concentration of iron, zinc and copper in rural Vietnam. *J. Nutr. Sci. Vitaminol. (Tokyo)* **2009**, *55*, 338–345. [CrossRef] [PubMed]

122. Mahdavi, R.; Nikniaz, L.; Gayemmagami, S.J. Association between Zinc, Copper, and Iron Concentrations in Breast Milk and Growth of Healthy Infants in Tabriz, Iran. *Biol. Trace Elem. Res.* **2010**, *135*, 174–181. [CrossRef] [PubMed]

123. Domellof, M.; Lonnerdal, B.; Dewey, K.G.; Cohen, R.J.; Hernell, O. Iron, zinc, and copper concentrations in breast milk are independent of maternal mineral status. *Am. J. Clin. Nutr.* **2004**, *79*, 111–115. [PubMed]

124. Shashiraj; Faridi, M.M.A.; Singh, O.; Rusia, U. Mother's iron status, breastmilk iron and lactoferrin—Are they related? *Eur. J. Clin. Nutr.* **2006**, *60*, 903–908. [CrossRef] [PubMed]

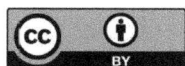

    MDPI

Article

Changes in Biochemical Parameters of the Calcium-Phosphorus Homeostasis in Relation to Nutritional Intake in Very-Low-Birth-Weight Infants

Viola Christmann [1,*], Charlotte J. W. Gradussen [1], Michelle N. Körnmann [1], Nel Roeleveld [2,3], Johannes B. van Goudoever [4,5] and Arno F. J. van Heijst [1]

1   Department of Paediatrics, Subdivision of Neonatology, Radboudumc Amalia Children's Hospital, Radboud University Medical Center, Nijmegen 6500HB, The Netherlands; charlotte.gradussen@radboudumc.nl (C.J.W.G.); michelle.kornmann@radboudumc.nl (M.N.K.); arno.vanheijst@radboudumc.nl (A.F.J.v.H.)
2   Department for Health Evidence, Radboud Institute for Health Science, Radboud University Medical Center, Nijmegen 6500HB, The Netherlands; nel.roeleveld@radboudumc.nl
3   Department of Paediatrics, Radboudumc Amalia Children's Hospital, Radboud University Medical Center, Nijmegen 6500HB, The Netherlands
4   Department of Paediatrics, VU university medical center Amsterdam, Amsterdam 1081HV, The Netherlands; h.vangoudoever@vumc.nl
5   Department of Paediatrics, Emma Children's Hospital-AMC Amsterdam, Amsterdam 1105AZ, The Netherlands
*   Correspondence: viola.christmann@radboudumc.nl; Tel.: +31-243-614-430

Received: 14 September 2016; Accepted: 24 November 2016; Published: 29 November 2016

Abstract: Preterm infants are at significant risk to develop reduced bone mineralization based on inadequate supply of calcium and phosphorus (Ca-P). Biochemical parameters can be used to evaluate the nutritional intake. The direct effect of nutritional intake on changes in biochemical parameters has not been studied. Our objective was to evaluate the effect of Ca-P supplementation on biochemical markers as serum (s)/urinary (u) Ca and P; alkaline phosphatase (ALP); tubular reabsorption of P (TrP); and urinary ratios for Ca/creatinin (creat) and P/creatinin in Very-Low-Birth-Weight infants on Postnatal Days 1, 3, 5, 7, 10, and 14. This observational study compared two groups with High ($n = 30$) and Low ($n = 40$) intake of Ca-P. Birth weight: median (IRQ) 948 (772–1225) vs. 939 (776–1163) grams; and gestational age: 28.2 (26.5–29.6) vs. 27.8 (26.1–29.4) weeks. Daily median concentrations of biochemical parameter were not different between the groups but linear regression mixed model analyses showed that Ca intake increased the uCa and TrP ($p = 0.04$) and decreased ALP ($p = 0.00$). Phosphorus intake increased sP, uP and uP/creat ratio and ALP ($p \leq 0.02$) and caused decrease in TrP ($p = 0.00$). Protein intake decreased sP ($p = 0.000$), while low gestational age and male gender increased renal excretion of P ($p < 0.03$). Standardized repeated measurements showed that biochemical parameters were affected by nutritional intake, gestational age and gender.

Keywords: blood; bone mineralization; minerals; monitoring; nutrition; renal tubular reabsorption; supplementation; urine

---

1. Introduction

Bone development is one of the key processes of intrauterine and postnatal growth [1]. Preterm infants are at significant risk to develop reduced bone mineral content based on inadequate supply of calcium and phosphorus (Ca-P) [2,3]. During normal pregnancies in healthy mothers, there is an active, placental transfer of Ca-P to the fetus leading to a high mineral accretion during the last trimester, while after birth the infant is dependent on nutritional supply of minerals [4,5].

In clinical practice, postnatally it is difficult to meet the high fetal needs, because of limited solubility of parenteral fluids, low content of Ca-P of human milk and impaired intestinal absorption through formula feeding [6–9]. Studies tried to define nutritional requirements, but, in clinical practice, it is often uncertain whether the nutritional intake of Ca-P provided to preterm infants is sufficient and is actually used for bone mineralization [10–12].

Assuming that biochemical parameters of Ca-P homeostasis within a normal range will lead to optimal bone mineralization, evaluation of electrolyte disturbances is standard of care in many neonatal units [13–28]. However, there is currently neither a consensus on the appropriateness of either parameter or the frequency of measurements [29,30]. A recent survey among U.S. neonatologists showed a great lack of consensus and variation in practices regarding definition and screening methods for metabolic bone disease [31]. Reference values in relation to adequate nutritional intake have not been developed. Urinary excretion of minerals in spot urine samples has been shown to be an easy tool for routine evaluation. Pohlandt proposed to aim for a small "surplus of minerals" in urine samples, while Aladangady et al. developed reference values for urinary Ca-P/creatinine ratios for preterm infants [17,23]. Staub et al. compared both methods with regard to an agreement between their results and found neither method to be superior [32]. None of the studies evaluated the direct effect of nutritional intake on biochemical parameter of Ca-P homeostasis. It is not sure whether biochemical parameters are able to indicate sufficiency of nutritional intake.

The aim of this study was to evaluate changes in biochemical parameters of the Ca-P homeostasis in blood and urine in relation to different nutritional intake during the first 14 days of life in Very Low Birth Weight (VLBW) infants. Our hypothesis was that the nutritional intake of calcium and phosphorus would have an effect on biochemical parameters of the calcium–phosphorus homeostasis.

2. Materials and Methods

2.1. Study Design and Randomization

The current study (Early Supplementation Study (ESS)) was part of the Early Nutrition Study (ENS), a multi-center double-blinded randomized controlled trial. While the ENS evaluated the effects of human milk on postnatal outcome, the primary objective of the ESS was bone mineralization in relation to early and late enteral supplementation of minerals [33]. The studies were approved by the Ethical Committee of the VU university medical center (Amsterdam, The Netherlands), 13 September 2013 (CMO file number: NL37296.029.11, Dutch Trial Registry: NTR 3225). Patients were distributed into three groups through two steps of randomization. The first step randomized eligible infants either into the early supplementation group (High) or the late supplementation group (Low) being part of the ENS. The second step of the randomization was only performed if infants were assigned to late supplementation and randomized them to either "ENS A" or "ENS B" as part of the ENS. Both randomization steps were performed before the first enteral nutrition was administered resulting in basically three groups.

2.2. Study Population

Participants for the ENS/ESS were recruited at the level III neonatal intensive care unit of the Radboud university medical center (Radboudumc), Nijmegen, The Netherlands. The inclusion criteria were a birth weight below 1500 grams and written informed consent of both parents. The exclusion criteria were maternal drugs and/or alcohol use during pregnancy, birth defects, congenital infection within 72 h after birth, perinatal asphyxia with a pH < 7.0 and any intake of cow's milk based products prior to randomization. For the current study, infants who died or were discharged before the end of the study period of 14 days were excluded from analysis.

2.3. Intervention and Nutritional Protocol

Parenteral nutrition (PN) was started directly within the first hour after birth. The PN solution consisted of 2.5 mmol/dL calcium-gluconate (calcium-gluconate 10%; B. Braun, Melsungen, Germany) and 1.6 mmol/dL sodium-glycerophosphate (Glycophos; Fresenius Kabi BV, Zeist, The Netherlands) and 2.25 grams/dL amino acids (Primene; Clintec, Brussels). Additional parenteral supplementation with 10% calcium-gluconate or sodium glycero-phosphate was administrated depending on biochemical parameters. Table A1 presents the standard protocol for PN. The decision to start additional supplementation was left to the attending neonatologist based on biochemical parameter as being a standard procedure of our department.

Enteral feeding was started on the first day of life with daily increments, while PN was gradually reduced to maintain a daily fluid intake within the protocol range. Late supplementation was assumed to provide a low intake of nutrients because "Group Low", comprising of group ENS A and ENS B, received no additional enteral supplementation or fortification of human milk during the first 10 days of life. Group ENS A received donor milk if mother's own milk (MOM) was not available. Group ENS B received preterm formula (Hero Baby Prematuur Start; Hero Kindervoeding, Breda, The Netherlands) if MOM was not available, containing 2.4 mmol/dL calcium, 1.7 mmol/dL phosphorus and 2.6 grams/dL proteins. The additional nutrition in ENS A and ENS B was blinded to all caretakers and parents. After 10 days, all infants received nutrition according to the standard protocol of the Radboudumc.

Early supplementation was assumed to provide a high intake (Group High). This group received enteral nutrition from Day 1 onwards according to the local protocol. They received additional enteral supplementation and human milk fortifier (Nutrilon Neonatal BMF; Nutricia, Zoetermeer, The Netherlands; BMF) by the time the enteral intake was 50 mL per day. The human milk fortifier added 1.65 mmol/dL calcium, 1.22 mmol/dL phosphorus and 0.8 grams/dL protein to human milk. They received preterm formula if MOM was not available. The decision to start additional enteral supplementation was left to the attending neonatologist based on biochemical parameter and postnatal growth as being a standard procedure of our department. The additional enteral supplementation could comprise of either a supplement of protein (Nutrilon Nenatal Protein Fortifier; Nutricia, Zoetermeer, The Netherlands) or a potassium phosphate (KPO_4) and calcium chloride ($CaCl_2$) suspension for enteral supplementation.

Group ENS A received 100% human milk during the first 10 days and reflected a group with low intake of minerals and protein, because human milk has a very low nutrient content. Group High reflected a high intake of nutrients, because human milk was enriched with minerals and protein as soon as possible. Group ENS B could be considered as intermediate depending on the amount of MOM or preterm formula an infant received, since preterm formula contained approximately the same amount of minerals as fortified human milk.

2.4. Biochemical Parameters of Bone Mineralization

For this study, blood and urine samples were analyzed according to the local protocol of the department. Samples were taken on Days 1, 3, 5, 7, 10 and 14 after birth. Urine was collected through spot samples [25]. The following parameters were analyzed: serum calcium (sCa), serum phosphorus (sP), serum alkaline phosphatase (ALP), urine calcium (uCa), urine phosphorus (uP), urine calcium/creatinin ratio (uCa/Creat), urine phosphorus/creatinin ratio (uP/Creat), and tubular reabsorption of phosphorus (TrP).

2.5. Data Registration and Handling

Patient characteristics, clinical course, growth and intake of all nutrients were recorded daily from the patient records and abstracted for this study. Amounts of enteral, parenteral and additional supplementation (parenteral and enteral) of all nutrients were calculated separately for each patient. The total intakes were calculated per kg per day per infant. The intake through human milk was calculated based on the reference of Gidrewicz et al. [34]. The calcium/phosphorus ratio was calculated per day by dividing the daily intake of calcium in mmol/kg through the daily intake of phosphorus in mmol/kg.

After closure of patient enrollment and de-blinding of the ENS, we performed a reallocation procedure for the intermediate group ENS B. Infants who received more than 90% MOM were considered to reflect a low intake of minerals and were allocated to group Low together with the infants of group ENS A. Infants who received more than 90% of preterm formula were considered to reflect a high intake of minerals and were allocated to High. Infants in between these extremes were not included in the analyses.

2.6. Statistical Analysis

The primary objective of the ESS was bone mineralization in relation to mineral supplementation, and the original power calculation was based on bone mineral content at term corrected age. For the evaluation of changes in biochemical parameters in relation to nutritional intake the power calculation was based on sP. In a previous evaluation of our nutritional protocol performed at our department, we found a mean 1.7 mmol/L of sP during the first week [35]. A concentration of 2.0 mmol/L was defined as target for optimal bone mineralization by Hellstern et al. [20]. Assuming an expected mean of 1.7 mmol/L, we determined that 24 infants were required in each group to find a difference of 0.3 mmol/L in sP between High and Low with $\alpha = 0.05$ (two-sided) and a power of $\beta = 0.80$.

The statistical analyses were performed using IBM SPSS statistics 22.0 for Windows (IBM SPSS Inc., Chicago, IL, USA). Differences in patient characteristics, nutritional characteristics and biochemical parameters between the High and Low group were determined using the Mann-Whitney U test or the chi-square test, depending on the variable under examination. Due to non-normality of the continuous variables, the data were presented as median (with interquartile range (IQR)), unless otherwise indicated. A *p*-value < 0.05 was considered statistically significant.

To account for repeated outcome measurements, we used a mixed model analysis to determine the effects of daily nutritional intake of calcium and phosphorus on each biochemical parameter. We included the total intake of Ca/P and protein, the percentage of enteral amount of Ca/P intake, and a number of clinical parameter that could affect the Ca/P homeostasis such as birth weight, gestational age, gender, caesarian section, multiple births, sepsis, and days of caffeine, furosemide, steroids, and sedation during the first two weeks as co-variables in the initial models. Necrotizing enterocolitis was not included as co-variable because of small numbers. Using manual backward selection, variables were kept in the model when they contributed statistically significantly with a *p*-value < 0.1.

3. Results

3.1. Patient Characteristics

Enrollment of patients occurred between January 2013 and December 2014. The distribution of the infants is presented in the consort diagram (Figure 1). Finally, 109 infants were randomized, eithe to Late Supplementation (Low; *n* = 72; distributed into Group ENS A (*n* = 40) and ENS B (*n* = 32) or Early Supplementation (High; *n* = 37).

The characteristics of all infants included in the three groups of the ENS/ESS study are presented in Table A2. After de-blinding of group Low, four infants of group ENS B were reallocated to High and 13 to Low so that Low and High consisted of 53 and 41 infants, respectively. Infants who died or were discharged before postnatal Day 14 (13 in Low, 11 in High) were excluded. Finally, data of 40 infants of Low and 30 of High were analyzed. The baseline patient characteristics, morbidity, medication and nutritional characteristics for these patients are presented in Table 1. Infant characteristics were well balanced between the groups Low and High and comparable to the original groups.

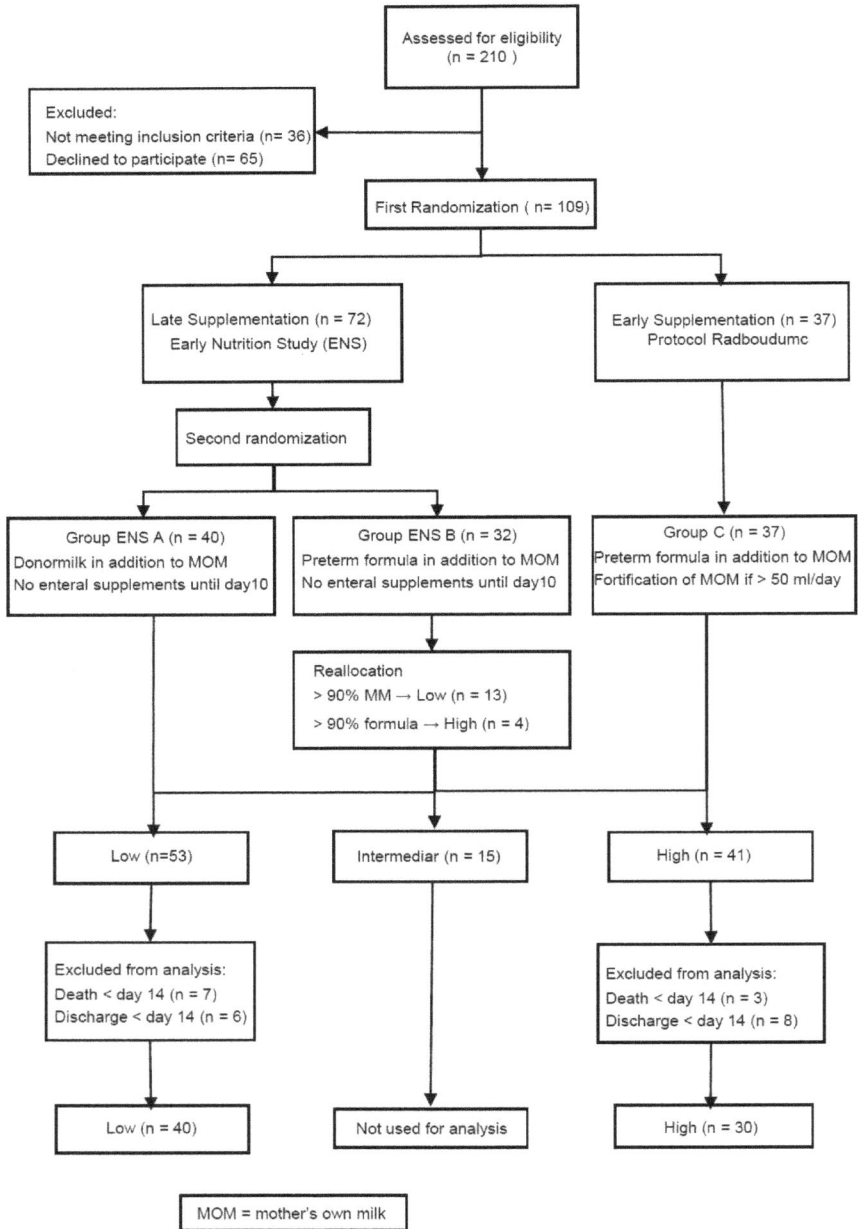

Figure 1. Consort diagram.

Table 1. Patient characteristics, morbidity, medication, and nutritional characteristics.

	Low (n = 40)	High (n = 30)	p-Value
Characteristics			
Birth weight, grams; median (IQR)	948 (772–1225)	939 (776–1163)	0.85
<1000 gram, n (%)	22 (55.0)	16 (53.3)	0.89
Gestational age, median (IQR)	28.2 (26.5–29.6)	27.8 (26.1–29.4)	0.76
SGA, n (%)	8 (20.0)	4 (13.3)	0.46
Male, n (%)	19 (47.5)	15 (50.0)	0.84
Singletons, n (%)	28 (70.0)	16 (53.3)	0.15
Cesarean section, n (%)	18 (45.0)	20 (66.7)	0.07
Apgar score (5 min), median (IQR)	7.0 (6.3–9.0)	7.5 (7.0–8.0)	0.71
Apgar score (5 min) <7, n (%)	10 (25.0%)	6 (20.0%)	0.62
Morbidity			
Sepsis, n (%)	8 (20.0%)	9 (30.0%)	0.33
NEC $\geq$ stage 2, n (%)	1 (2.5%)	2 (6.7%)	0.39
IVH Grade 3–4 n (%)	5 (12.5)	3 (10)	0.75
Medication			
Caffeïne; n (%)	39 (97.5%)	28 (93.3%)	0.39
Furosemide, n (%)	3 (7.5%)	4 (13.3%)	0.42
Corticosteroids	3 (7.5)	1 (3.3)	0.46
Sedation, n (%)	8 (20.0%)	9 (30.0%)	0.33
Nutritional characteristics			
PN, days, median (IQR)	11.0 (9.0–14.0)	12.0 (10.0–14.0)	0.10
150 mL/kg enteral, study day, median (IQR)	12.0 (9.8–17.0)	13.0 (10.5–20.0)	0.59
Start day of BMF, median (IQR)	11 (11.0–13.0)	7.9 (5.0–10.0)	0.00
Human milk in mL/kg/day *, median (IQR)	50.9 (24.0–82.2)	30.0 (8.5–54.6)	0.01
Formula in mL/kg/day *, median (IQR)	0.0 (0.0–0.2)	1.1 (0.1–7.3)	0.00
Nutritional intake			
Ca (total) W1, mmol/kg; median (IQR)	10.7 (9.9–12.0)	13.1 (11.1–14.6)	0.00
Ca (total) W2, mmol/kg; median (IQR)	16.4 (12.9–17.7)	21.7 (15.3–24.4)	0.00
P (total) W1, mmol/kg; median (IQR)	10.8 (9.3–12.4	12.3 (11.1–14.2)	0.00
P (total) W2, mmol/kg; median (IQR)	16.4 (12.9–19.6)	18.2 (16.0–22.1)	0.02
Prot (total) W1, grams/kg; median (IQR)	18.6 (15.9–21.1)	20.0 (16.9–23.4)	0.16
Prot (total) W2, grams/kg; median (IQR)	23.2 (21.0–26.6)	27.0 (24.1–30.6)	0.00

Low: no enteral supplementation of human milk before Day 11; High: standard protocol: enteral supplementation of human milk if intake was $\geq$50 mL/day; IQR: Interquartile range; SGA: small for gestational age: <p10; Sepsis: >72 h postnatally and positive blood culture, prevalence within the first 14 days; NEC: necrotizing enterocolitis according to Bell stage [36], prevalence within the first 14 days; IVH: Intraventricular hemorrhage (grade according to Papile) [37]; PN: parenteral nutrition; BMF: breast milk fortifier; *: during the intervention period; Ca: calcium; P: phosphorus; Prot: protein; W1: Week 1; W2: Week 2.

3.2. Nutritional Intake

The nutritional characteristics and intake of calcium, phosphorus and protein during Weeks 1 and 2 are presented in Table 1. The median and interquartile range (IQR) for the duration of PN was 12.0 (10.0–14.0) versus 11.0 (9.0–14.0) days for High versus Low, while the median day of reaching an enteral intake of 150 mL/kg was Day 13.0 (10.5–20.0) versus Day 12.0 (9.8–17.0), respectively. In accordance with the study protocol, Low received a higher amount of human milk. The median start day of BMF in groups High and Low was 7.9 (5.0–10.0) and 11.0 (11.0–13.0) respectively. As a result, High received a significant higher total intake of calcium and phosphorus during the first two weeks and of protein during Week 2 compared to Low. Table A3 presents the nutritional intake divided into four routes of administrations: parenteral, enteral and additional supplementation either par- or enteral. This shows that differences in intake were mainly based on differences in enteral intake. Further, both groups received additional parenteral supplementation of phosphorus, based on low sP concentrations.

Figure 2 presents the daily changes in nutritional intake during the first 14 days. Figure 2A,B,D demonstrate the total calcium, phosphorus and protein intake. High had a steady increase in intake during the study period, whereas Low showed a temporary decrease, and plateau at the end of the observational period, probably due to the decreasing amount of PN and increasing amount of unfortified human milk. Except for Day 1, both groups received a median total calcium, phosphorus and protein intake according to the ESPGHAN recommendations for parenteral and enteral nutrition [38,39]. The calcium/phosphorus ratios were highly variable. Both groups showed a decrease in the calcium/phosphorus ratio on Day 5 that lasted until Day 11 (Figure 2C), most likely caused by the transition from parenteral nutrition to enteral nutrition. For both groups, the ratio was below the recommendations of ESPGHAN on all days [38,39].

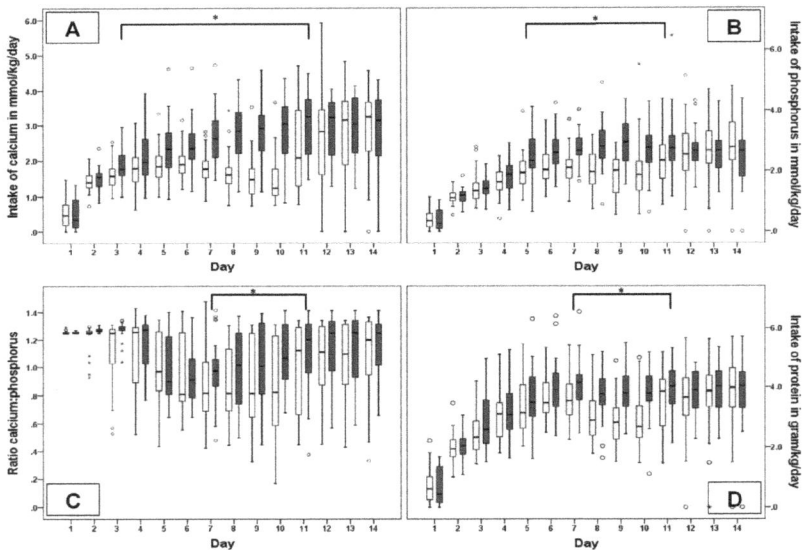

Figure 2. Nutritional intake during the first 14 days: white bars: Low; black bars: High; The horizontal black bars with * indicate the days on which the intake was statistically significant different. (**A**) Daily intake of calcium in mmol/kg/day; * = $p < 0.05$; (**B**) daily intake of phosphorus in mmol/kg/day; * = $p < 0.05$; (**C**) daily intake of protein in gram/kg/day; * = $p < 0.05$; and (**D**) ratio calcium intake to phosphorus intake; * = $p < 0.05$ Data are presented as median, interquartile range and upper and lower limits.

3.3. Biochemical Parameters

Table A4 summarizes the median daily values of both groups for all biochemical parameters. The median serum concentrations of Ca en P were within the normal range and only showed slight differences between the two groups and an overall increase during the study period [40]. Except for the first day, the median sP concentrations remained below our target of 2 mmol/L until Days 5 and 10 for High and Low, respectively. The median uCa and uP values were above the recommended surplus (uCa > 1.2 mmol/L, uP > 0.4 mmol/L) during the entire observational period [23]. The median TrP values were above the lower normal range of 85% until Day 5, and decreased thereafter, reflecting a higher loss of phosphorus. The median ALP values were within the normal range (80–330 U/L) until Day 5, but increased steadily thereafter [40]. In both groups, the uCa/Creat ratios were above the reference value (0.5 mmol/mmol) during the complete study period [32]. The uP/Creat ratios were below the reference value (4.0 mmol/mmol) until Day 5, but above the reference thereafter [32].

The results of the mixed model analyses are summarized in Table 2.

- The sCa concentration was not related to intake of Ca/P and was only marginally affected by a number of co-variables except for daily protein intake that caused an increase of 0.107 mmol/L per gram/kg protein.
- The sP concentration increased in relation to phosphorus intake (0.13 mmol/L per mmol/kg phosphorus) and birth weight (0.0004 mmol/L per gram birth weight), whereas protein intake (−0.13 mmol/L per gram/kg/day protein), gestational age (−0.05 mmol/L per week), furosemide (−0.11 mmol/L per day) and caffeine (−0.02 mmol/L per day) decreased in sP concentration.
- The urinary excretion of Ca seemed to increase in relation to Calcium intake (0.35 mmol/L per mmol/kg calcium), and increased in relation to protein (0.36 mmol/L per gram/kg protein) and being born by cesarean section (0.65 mmol/L if born by cesarean section), whereas it was not affected by the phosphorus intake.
- The urinary excretion of P increased in relation to daily phosphorus intake (3.18 mmol/L per mmol/kg phosphorus) and gender (1.88 mmol/L if infant was a boy), whereas P excretion lowered in relation to daily intake of protein (−1.18 mmol/L per mmol/kg protein), gestational age (−0.71 mmol/L per week) and caffeine (−0.29 mmol/L per day). Calcium intake did not affect the urinary P excretion.
- The TrP increased in relation the daily Calcium intake (3.10% per mmol/kg calcium) and gestational age (3.05% per week). The reabsorption of phosphorus lowered in relation to daily phosphorus intake (−6.21% per mmol/kg phosphorus), gender (−4.60% if infant was a boy), being born by cesarean section (−5.12%), and sepsis (−6.78%).
- The ALP increased in relation protein intake (30.54 U/L per mmol/kg) and daily intake of phosphorus (23.64 U/L per mmol/kg phosphorus). A decrease in ALP was related to calcium intake (−44.94 U/L per mmol/kg calcium), gestational age (−20.71 U/L per week) and the number of days of steroid use (−23.86 U/L per day).
- The uCa/creat ratio increased in relation to daily protein intake (0.54 L/L per gram/day protein) and sepsis (0.66 L/L), but it was not affected by the total calcium and phosphorus intake.
- The uP/creat ratio increased in relation to daily phosphorus intake (4.01 L/L per mmol/kg phosphorus), gender (2.31 L/L if infant was a boy), while the P/creat ratio seemed lower in relation to daily protein intake (−0.81 L/L per gram/kg protein), and decreased with gestational age (−0.94 L/L per week), and caffeine (−0.30 L/L per day).

Table 2. Mixed Model analysis: Effect of nutritional intake and clinical characteristics on biochemical parameter.

Dependant Variable	Covariates	Estimate	95% CI	*p*-Value
Serum Calcium	Total intake of Ca (mmol/kg/day)	0.004	−0.046–0.054	0.89
	Total intake of P (mmol/kg/day)	−0.036	−0.073–0.002	0.06
	Enteral intake of P (%)	0.001	−0.000–0.001	0.06
	Intake of protein (grams/kg /day)	0.107	0.075–0.139	0.00
	Gestational age (weeks)	0.027	0.013–0.042	0.00
	Singleton (yes)	0.081	0.021–0.140	0.01
	Sepsis (yes)	−0.092	−0.167–−0.019	0.02
	Sedation (days)	−0.007	−0.016–0.001	0.07
Serum Phosphorus	Total intake of Ca (mmol/kg/day)	0.0345	−0.0473–0.1164	0.41
	Total intake of P (mmol/kg/day)	0.1252	0.0586–0.1918	0.00
	Enteral intake of Ca (%)	0.0035	0.0023–0.0048	0.00
	Intake of protein (grams/kg/day)	−0.1274	−0.1825–−0.0723	0.00
	Birth weight (grams)	0.0004	0.0002–0.0006	0.00
	Gestational age (weeks)	−0.0479	−0.0701–−0.0258	0.00
	Gender (boy)	−0.0698	−0.1493–0.096	0.08
	Caffeine (days)	−0.0215	−0.0354–−0.0075	0.00
	Furosemide (days)	−0.1116	−0.2029–−0.0203	0.02

Table 2. *Cont.*

Dependant Variable	Covariates	Estimate	95% CI	*p*-Value
Urine Calcium	Total intake of Ca (mmol/kg/day)	0.35	0.01–0.70	0.05
	Total intake of P (mmol/kg/day)	−0.01	−0.29–0.27	0.94
	Enteral intake of Ca (%)	−0.02	−0.02−−0.01	0.00
	Intake of protein (grams/kg/day)	0.36	0.12–0.61	0.00
	Cesarean section (yes)	0.65	0.32–0.98	0.00
Urine Phosphorus	Total intake of Ca (mmol/kg/day)	−0.05	−1.56–1.45	0.94
	Total intake of P (mmol/kg/day)	3.18	2.06–4.30	0.00
	Enteral intake of P (%)	0.07	0.04–0.09	0.00
	Intake of protein (grams/kg/day)	−1.18	−2.20−−0.16	0.02
	Gestational age (weeks)	−0.71	−1.09−−0.33	0.00
	Gender (boy)	1.88	0.26–3.50	0.02
	Caffeine (days)	−0.29	−0.54−−0.01	0.04
Tubular reabsorption of P	Total intake of Ca (mmol/kg/day)	3.10	0.160–6.04	0.04
	Total intake of P (mmol/kg/day)	−6.21	−8.78−−3.65	0.00
	Enteral intake of P (%)	−0.09	−0.15−−0.03	0.01
	Gestational age (weeks)	3.05	1.92–4.17	0.00
	Gender (boy)	−4.60	−9.22–0.01	0.05
	Cesarean section (yes)	−5.12	−9.95−−0.29	0.04
	Sepsis (yes)	−6.78	−12.72−−0.85	0.03
	Furosemide (days)	4.75	−0.53–10.03	0.07
Alkaline Phosphatase	Total intake of Ca (mmol/kg/day)	−44.94	−69.51−−20.37	0.00
	Total intake of P (mmol/kg/day)	23.64	4.14–43.14	0.02
	Enteral intake of Ca (%)	2.07	1.69–2.45	0.00
	Intake of protein (grams/kg/day)	30.54	14.08–47.01	0.00
	Gestational age (weeks)	−20.71	−30.37−−11.05	0.00
	Postnatal steroids (days)	−23.86	−44.29−−3.43	0.02
Urine Ca/Crea ratio	Total intake of Ca (mmol/kg/day)	0.138	−0.292–0.568	0.53
	Total intake of P (mmol/kg/day)	0.139	−0.204–0.481	0.43
	Enteral intake of Ca (%)	−0.023	−0.029−−0.016	0.00
	Intake of protein (grams/kg/day)	0.497	0.206–0.787	0.01
	Sepsis (yes)	0.584	0.003–1.166	0.05
Urine P/Crea ratio	Total intake of Ca (mmol/kg/day)	−1.10	−2.51–0.31	0.12
	Total intake of P (mmol/kg/day)	4.01	2.97–5.05	0.00
	Enteral intake of P (%)	0.06	0.04–0.08	0.00
	Intake of protein (grams/kg/day)	−0.81	−1.76–0.14	0.10
	Gestational age (weeks)	−0.94	−1.32−−0.55	0.00
	Gender (boy)	2.31	0.72–3.89	0.01
	Sepsis (yes)	1.72	−0.24–3.68	0.09
	Caffeine (days)	−0.30	−0.56−−0.03	0.03

sCa: serum calcium (mmol/L); uCa: urine calcium (mmol/L); sP: serum phosphorus (mmol/L); uP: urine phosphorus (mmol/L); TrP: tubular reabsorption of phosphorus (%); ALP: Alkaline phosphatase (U/L); uCa/Crea ratio: urine calcium/creatinin ratio (mmol/mmol); uP/Crea ratio: urine phosphorus/creatinine ratio (mmol/mmol); 95% CI: 95% confidence interval; Co-variables initially included: daily nutritional intake of calcium, phosphorus, and protein, the enteral amount of calcium and phosphorus intake, caesarian section, multiple births, birth weight, gestational age, gender, necrotizing enterocolitis, sepsis, caffeine, furosemide, steroids and sedation.

4. Discussion

In this observational study of initially three randomized groups providing different nutritional intake to VLBW infants during the first 10 days of life, we found no differences between groups Low and High concerning the biochemical parameters of Ca-P homeostasis. However, the mixed model analysis showed that the intake of calcium was associated with increased urinary calcium excretion and tubular reabsorption of phosphorus and a decrease in the ALP, while the nutritional intake of phosphorus was associated with a decreased sCa and an increase in sP, uP and uP/creat ratio. The nutritional intake of calcium and phosphorus affected the TrP and ALP in opposite directions. Protein intake was greatly associated with a decrease in sP, uP and an increase in ALP, sCa, and uCa, while, in addition, gestational age and male gender affected especially the phosphorus metabolism.

VLBW infants belong to one of the most vulnerable patient groups for whom adequate postnatal nutritional intake has life-long consequences [41]. Therefore, intervention studies with different nutritional intakes could be seen as unethical in the light of the right of optimal treatment for every patient. On the other hand, in clinical practice a great variation in clinical guidelines has been reported, often based on rather low evidence [42]. While fortification of human milk is generally seen as necessary nowadays, there is also concern about possible risks of introducing cow-milk based products too early [43,44]. According to our local protocol, fortification is introduced early and additional mineral supplementation is provided based on laboratory results. The intention is to optimize postnatal growth and bone mineralization but the efficacy of our protocol has not been proven. The combination of the Early Nutrition Study and the Early Supplementation Study provided the opportunity to evaluate two different nutritional concepts within the range of nutritional guidelines and therefore within the ethical limits. On the other hand, all infants participating in the ESS, independent of group allocation, received the standard treatment according to the local practice, which frequently led to additional parenteral supplementation of nutrients in case of electrolyte disturbances or impaired growth. This practice may have ameliorated the differences between the groups and therefore affected the results. By reallocating infants from group ENS B to either group Low or High and excluding infants with intermediate intake from further analysis, we tried to maximize the differences in nutritional intake between the two remaining groups. The reallocation of infants did not change the baseline patient characteristics. The detailed analysis of nutritional intake showed that additional supplementation was not different between the groups and differences in intake were mainly based on enteral nutrition.

Even though the two groups had a maximum difference in nutritional intake, the comparison of daily concentrations of the biochemical parameters showed no differences between groups High and Low, probably by leveling out inter-individual differences on group level. In contrast, the linear mixed model analysis took into account both intra- and inter-individual fluctuations, and thereby enabled us to specify effects of various co-variables.

Despite an increasing intake of phosphorus, sP remained below our target concentration during the first week. Recently, a randomized trial, evaluating nutritional support according to current recommendations in VLBW infants, observed hypophosphatemia in relation to high protein intake [45]. Jamin et al. observed electrolyte disturbances, especially hypophosphatemia and hypokalemia, in low-birth weight piglets with a high protein diet [46]. Hypophosphatemia is the hallmark of the refeeding syndrome and a well-known complication in relation to parenteral nutrition of malnourished patients [47–49]. Bonsante et al. proposed the concept of Placental Incompletely Restored Feeding (PI-Refeeding) syndrome for electrolyte disturbances found in VLBW infants [50]. This syndrome is said to be caused by an imbalanced nutritional intake of amino acids and phosphorus. Amino acids and energy are needed to maintain an anabolic state of the cell, while phosphorus is necessary for a number of cellular functions, energy homeostasis as well as for bone mineralization. Phosphorus in blood will preferably be transferred to the cell regardless of bone mineral status. A higher intake of amino acids will enhance the need for phosphorus in growing cells, and in case of low concentrations of phosphorus in blood it will be released from bone. Simultaneously with the release of phosphorus, calcium will also be released from the bone because of an unfavorable Ca/P ratio and will consecutively be excreted in urine if the sP concentrations are too low. Our results are in agreement with this concept. According to the mixed model analyses, we found that an increasing amount of protein was associated with an increase in the sCa, uCa, ALP and uCa/Creat ratio, whereas it was associated with a decrease in sP, uP and the uP/Creat ratio. Remarkably, in our study, an increase in a sP concentration of 0.13 mmol/L occurred per 1 mmol/kg intake of phosphorus and a decrease of −0.13 mmol/L per 1 gram/kg protein intake, meaning that 1 gram/kg of protein intake should be accompanied by 1 mmol/kg of phosphorus in nutrition of VLBW infants to maintain adequate sP concentrations.

The role of ALP in bone mineralization is controversial, but an increase is usually associated with poor bone mineralization [30,51]. According to our results, an increasing intake of protein was associated with an increase in ALP. Again, following the above mentioned mechanisms higher protein intake enhanced the cellular need of phosphorus and thereby decreased the sP concentration and the availability of phosphorus for bone mineralization, leading to activation of ALP. We also found that an increased ALP was associated with increasing phosphorus intake, while one would expect lowering of ALP. An explanation for this phenomenon could be a relatively insufficient intake of calcium in combination with phosphorus intake, since an increasing calcium intake was associated with decrease in ALP concentrations. In this study, for both groups, the calcium/phosphorus ratio was below recommendations, meaning that relatively more phosphorus than calcium was administered.

Gestational age at birth seemed to be an important determinant for the phosphorus metabolism in our study, meaning that infants with a lower gestational age had a higher renal excretion of phosphorus, irrespective of nutritional intake. Immaturity of the kidneys at lower gestational age has been shown to cause impaired tubular reabsorption of phosphorus [15]. Renal losses of minerals may then compromise the effect of nutritional intake on bone mineralization. However, current recommendations for nutritional intake of calcium and phosphorus usually do not take into account differences in renal function based on gestational age.

Further, we found that male gender was related to low serum phosphorus concentrations, low tubular reabsorption and increased renal excretion of phosphorus and uP/creat ratio. We speculate a retardation in maturation of the renal function in male infants compared to females as is known for the development of the pulmonary function [52].

All parameters evaluated in this study are regularly used to monitor either electrolyte homeostasis or bone mineralization. Practices among units vary greatly, measurements may be performed at later age and greater intervals and not standardized or in combination, leading to inconsistent results and handling. An explanation for the inconsistency in results of other studies could be the underestimation of the effects of inter-relationships between various co-variates. In our opinion, these associations can only be discovered with standardized repeated measurements taking into account other clinical factors. To our knowledge, this is the first study evaluating changes in biochemical parameters of the calcium-phosphorus homeostasis based on standardized repeated measurements and daily changes in nutritional intake in a mixed model linear regression analysis including also clinical factors.

Our data show that standardized repeated measurements of blood and urine samples can provide useful information with regard to the Ca-P homeostasis. This does not result in a clear advice for nutritional intake. Nevertheless, this study is a first step and its importance lies in the description and quantification of changes in a more "physiological way" that will further enable us to develop new guidelines to improve bone mineral status in preterm infants. Notwithstanding, we confirmed the relationship between the intake of protein and phosphorus, and demonstrated the effect of renal immaturity and gender. Thus, a second step could be, to relate the current results to bone mineralization and provide recommendations for nutritional intake and a third step to develop a concept of target values for biochemical parameter so that these can be used to monitor nutritional intake to achieve optimal bone mineralization in daily practice.

This study had several limitations. The mixed model analysis assumes that the effects of the different variables are linear which has not been proven yet. In addition, the biochemical parameters may have been influenced by factors that were not taken into account in our analysis. Daily sampling of biochemical parameter would have been optimal, but this was judged unethical regarding the amount of blood volume needed. Nevertheless, measurements were performed in a standardized manner and therefore provided a good reflection of changes in blood and urine concentrations for the complete study period. Further, in comparison to other studies, both groups had relatively high daily intakes. This may partly explain the small variations in biochemical parameters. This study only investigated the biochemical parameters during the first 14 days of life. Maturational changes in renal function may alter the results; however, repeated measurements will indicate these changes and thereby can be used as guide for optimal supplementation of minerals.

5. Conclusions

In conclusion, standardized repeated measurements showed that biochemical parameters of Ca-P homeostasis seemed to be affected by nutritional intake of calcium and phosphorus as well as protein, while immaturity of kidneys was related to an increase in urinary excretion of minerals irrespective of nutritional intake. Further studies are needed to define target values to stabilize electrolyte balances and improve bone mineralization taking into account nutritional intake and gestational age of the patient.

Acknowledgments: This study was part of the "Early Nutrition Study" that was sponsored by Mead Johnson Nutrition, for which J.B.v.G. received a grant. The Early Supplementation Study was sponsored by Hero Kindervoeding, Breda, Netherlands, for which V.C. and A.v.H. received a grant. The sponsors had no role in the design and conduct of the study; collection, management, analysis, and interpretation of the data, the preparation of the manuscript and the decision to submit the manuscript for publication. All other authors declare that they do not have any conflict of interest and that they do not have anything to disclose. The first draft of the manuscript was written by V.C., who did not receive an honorarium or any other form of payment to produce the manuscript. All authors gratefully thank W.R.J.C. Jansen, research nurse of the Pediatric Drug Research Center Radboudumc, for the dedicated support in patient recruitment and data collection as well as T.A.J. Antonius, neonatologist at Radboudumc, for the development of the algorithm to calculate the nutritional intakes.

Author Contributions: V.C. is the primary researcher responsible for designing the study, analyzing and interpreting the data, and writing of the manuscript; C.G. and M.K. were responsible for data acquisition, analysis of the data and review of the manuscript; N.R. contributed to the analysis and interpretation of the data, and to writing and review of the manuscript; J.B.v.G. contributed in designing the study, interpretation of the data and review of the manuscript; and A.v.H. supervised the design, analyses and interpretation of the data, and writing of the manuscript. All authors listed on the manuscript have seen and approved the manuscript and take full responsibility for the manuscript.

Conflicts of Interest: The authors declare no conflict of interest. J.B.v.G. reports grants outside the submitted work from Mead Johnson Nutrition, during the conduct of the study, grants from Danone, grants and non-financial support from Hipp, personal fees and non-financial support from Nestle Institute and non-financial support from Baxter.

Appendix A

Table A1. Standard parenteral nutritional intake.

	Day 1	Day 2	Day 3	Day 4
Fluid mL/kg/day	80	100	125	150
CH grams/kg/day	8	9.6	11.7	13.8
AA grams/kg/day	0.75	1.5	2.25	3
Lipids grams/kg/day	1	2	3	3
EQ Kcal/kg/day	44	62	82	94
Calcium mmol/kg/day	0.75	1.5	2.25	3.00
Phosphorus mmol/kg/day	0.48	0.96	1.44	1.92

Parenteral nutritional intake based on standardized parenteral solutions [35,53]. For infants below 1000 grams, amino acids were additionally added according to current recommendations [12]. Amino acid solution: Primene (Baxter, the Netherlands); Lipid emulsion including vitamins: Clinoleic (20%; Baxter, The Netherlands) or SMOFlipid 20% (Fresenius Kabi; The Netherlands); CH: carbohydrates, AA: amino acids, EQ: energy quotient.

Table A2. Cohort characteristics of all patients included in the Early Supplementation Study.

Characteristics	Group ENS A (*n* = 40)	Group ENS B (*n* = 32)	Group C (*n* = 37)
GA, weeks; med (IQR)	28.2 (25.7–30.1)	28.3 (26.5–30.7)	27.9 (26.1–29.7)
Birth weight, grams; med (IQR)	967 (753–1245)	1012 (847–1199)	1006 (771–1220)
SGA; *n* (%)	9 (23)	8 (25)	6 (16)
Male; *n* (%)	21 (53)	20 (63)	18 (49)
Singletons; *n* (%)	25 (63)	24 (74)	25 (68)
Antenatal Steroids compl.; *n* (%)	36 (90)	31 (97)	31 (86)
Cesarean section; *n* (%)	19 (48)	20 (63)	25 (68)
Apgar score (5 min); med (IQR)	7.5 (6.3–9.0)	8.0 (7.0–9.0)	7.0 (7.0–8.0)
Apgar score (5 min) <7; *n* (%)	10 (25)	5 (16)	8 (22)
Mortality; *n* (%)	6 (15)	3 (9)	7 (19)
Morbidity			
IRDS	24 (60)	19 (59)	23 (62)
Days of MV; med (IQR)	1.5 (0.0–4.8)	1.0 (0.0–4.0)	1.0 (0.0–7.0)
Days of N-CPAP; med (IQR)	18.0 (6.5–38.8)	28.0 (7.0–40.8)	16.0 (6.0–36.5)

Table A2. *Cont.*

Characteristics	Group ENS A (*n* = 40)	Group ENS B (*n* = 32)	Group C (*n* = 37)
CLD; *n* (%)	12 (30)	14 (44)	10 (27)
PDA; *n* (%)	20 (50)	20 (63)	21 (57)
Ductal ligation; *n* (%)	4 (10)	2 (6.3)	1 (3)
IVH grade ≤ 2; *n* (%)	15 (38)	5 (16)	5 (14)
IVH grade ≥ 3; *n* (%)	2 (5)	7 (21)	4 (11)
Sepsis; *n* (%)	13 (33)	10 (32)	14 (38)
NEC; *n* (%)	4 (10)	5 (16)	3 (8)
Bell stage 2; *n*	2	3	1
Bell stage 3; *n*	2	2	2
Laparotomy; *n*	2	1	2
ROP; *n* (%)	4 (10)	1 (3)	5 (14)
ROP grade ≥ 3	1	0	1
Medication			
Caffeine; *n* (%)	38 (95)	30 (94)	33 (90)
Furosemide; *n* (%)	11 (28)	10 (31)	7 (19)
Diuretics (maintenance); *n* (%)	3 (8)	0	3 (8)
Corticosteroids; *n* (%)	1 (3)	2 (6)	4 (11)
Sedation; *n* (%)	13 (33)	11 (34)	15 (41)
Nutritional characteristics			
Days of PN; med (IQR)	10.0 (8.0–13.0)	10.5 (9.0–14.8)	10.5 (8.3–21.0)
120 mL/kg enteral, day; med (IQR)	9.0 (7.0–12.5)	9.0 (8.0–13.0)	9.0 (7.2–14.8)
150 mL/kg enteral, day; med (IQR)	12.0 (9.0–17.0)	11.0 (10.0–17.0)	12.0 (10.0–20.0)
Start day of BMF; med (IQR)	11.0 (11.0–12.7)	12.0 (11.0–14.0)	6.0 (4.0–8.0)

ENS A: donor milk in addition to mother's own milk (MOM) and no supplements with enteral feeding until Day 10; ENS B: preterm formula in addition to MOM and no supplements with enteral feeding until Day 10; Group C: preterm formula in addition to MOM and fortifier if intake ≥50 mL/day; med: median; IQR: inter quartile range; GA: gestational age; SGA: small for gestational age according to Fenton et al. [54]; IRDS: infant respiratory distress syndrome; MV: mechanical ventilation; N-CPAP: nasal continuous positive airway pressure; CLD: chronic lung disease defined as oxygen dependency at 36 weeks gestational age; PDA: patent ductus arteriosus with need for treatment; IVH: intra-ventricular hemorrhage; Sepsis: >72 h postnatally and positive blood culture; NEC: necrotizing enterocolitis with staging according to Bell [36]; ROP: retinopathy of prematurity; sedation: morphine and/or midazolam >24 h; PN: parenteral nutrition; BMF: breast milk fortifier.

Table A3. Nutritional intake of calcium and phosphorus by route of administration.

Nutritional Intake (mmol/kg/Week)	Low (*n* = 40) Median (IQR)	High (*n* = 30) Median (IQR)	*p*-Value
Ca (total) W1	10.7 (9.9–12.0)	13.1 (11.1–14.6)	0.00
Ca (total) W2	16.4 (12.9–17.7)	21.7 (15.3–24.4)	0.00
Ca (enteral) W1	1.7 (1.1–2.2)	3.3 (1.1–5.7)	0.00
Ca (enteral) W2	10.8 (6.2–16.0)	17.5 (2.3–22.8)	0.07
Ca (enteral suppl) W1	0.0 (0.0–0.0)	0.0 (0.0–0.0)	1.0
Ca (enteral suppl) W2	0.0 (0.0–0.0)	0.0 (0.0–0.0)	0.22
Ca (PN) W1	9.4 (8.0–10.2)	9.8 (7.9–11.5)	0.34
Ca (PN) W2	3.1 (0.7–7.9)	5.1 (1.9–10.9)	0.14
Ca (PNsuppl) W1	0.0 (0.0–0.0)	0.0 (0.0–0.0)	1.0
Ca (PNsuppl) W2	0.0 (0.0–0.0)	0.0 (0.0–0.0)	0.74
P (total) W1	10.8 (9.2–12.4)	12.3 (11.1–14.2)	0.00
P (total) W2	16.4 (12.9–19.6)	18.9 (16.0–22.1)	0.02
P (enteral) W1	1.0 (0.6–1.4)	2.1 (0.7–3.9)	0.00
P (enteral) W2	8.1 (5.0–12.0)	10.4 (1.7–17.2)	0.08
P (enteral suppl) W1	0.0 (0.0–0.0)	0.0 (0.0–0.9)	0.03
P (enteral suppl) W2	0.0 (0.0–0.0)	0.0 (0.0–1.4)	0.33
P (PN) W1	7.5 (6.4–8.2)	7.8 (6.3–9.2)	0.34
P (PN) W2	2.5 (0.6–6.3)	4.1 (1.5–8.7)	0.14
P (PN suppl) W1	2.4 (0.5–3.8)	1.8 (0.0–2.7)	0.16
P (PN suppl) W2	2.3 (0.0–4.2)	0.7 (0.0–4.3)	0.30

Low: no enteral supplementation of human milk before Day 11; High: standard protocol: enteral supplementation of human milk if intake was ≥50 mL/day; IQR: inter quartile range; Ca: calcium; P: phosphorus; total: som of all nutritional intake; enteral: enteral intake including standard fortification; enteral suppl: additional enteral supplementation; PN: parenteral intake; PN suppl: additional parenteral supplementation; W1: week 1; W2: week 2.

Table A4. Daily measurements of biochemical parameter of the calcium and phosphorus homeostasis.

		Day 1	Day 3	Day 5	Day 7	Day 10	Day 14
Serum Ca (mmol/L)	Low	2.2 (2.0–2.4)	2.4(2.2–2.5)	2.5 (2.4–2.7)	2.6 (2.4–2.7)	2.5 (2.4–2.7)	2.6 (2.4–2.8)
	High	2.2 (2.0–2.4)	2.4 (2.3–2.6)	2.5 (2.4–2.7)	2.4 (2.3–2.6)	2.5 (2.3–2.7)	2.6 (2.5–2.8)
	p-Value	0.94	0.17	0.34	0.15	0.69	0.17
Urine Ca (mmol/L)	Low	1.3 (1.0–1.9)	2.1 (1.5–3.4)	2.6 (2.0–3.9)	2.7 (1.6–3.8)	2.0 (1.6–3.3)	1.8 (1.4–3.5)
	High	1.5 (1.2–1.7)	3.3 (2.0–4.7)	3.1 (2.3–5.8)	2.5 (1.8–3.8)	2.7 (2.0–3.4)	2.3 (1.6–3.4)
	p-Value	0.66	0.03	0.06	0.84	0.21	0.50
Serum P (mmol/L)	Low	1.8 (1.7–2.2)	1.8 (1.5–2.0)	1.7 (1.5–2.0)	1.9 (1.8–2.2)	2.0 (1.8–2.2)	2.3 (2.1–2.4)
	High	2.1 (1.8–2.3)	1.8 (1.5–2.0)	1.6 (1.3–2.2)	2.1 (1.8–2.4)	2.1 (2.0–2.4)	2.2 (2.0–2.3)
	p-Value	0.22	0.88	0.71	0.21	0.08	0.16
Urine P (mmol/L)	Low	1.7 (0.3–3.8)	2.1 (0.7–5.5)	1.3 (0.7–3.5)	4.1 (0.7–6.8)	5.4 (2.2–8.2)	10.4 (6.8–18.4)
	High	2.3 (0.2–4.6)	2.6 (0.9–4.1)	3.1 (1.6–6.9)	5.4 (3.5–9.8)	7.4 (4.5–13.7)	9.5 (5.5–16.4)
	p-Value	0.68	0.98	0.04	0.02	0.04	0.46
Tubular reabsorption of P (%)	Low	94.0 (76.8–98.2)	86.5 (76.1–95.3)	92.2 (83.8–96.9)	83.1 (72.4–96.3)	80.8 (68.8–92.7)	75.9 (64.9–85.2)
	High	85.3 (76.4–98.1)	92.7 (73.3–95.7)	88.1 (80.8–95.1)	79.4 (51.9–87.6)	76.6 (59.1–83.2)	67.4 (53.9–82.4)
	p-Value	0.59	0.62	0.21	0.08	0.23	0.36
Alkaline Phosphatase (U/L)	Low	167.0 (138.0–236.0)	213.0 (182.0–291.0)	263.5 (202.3–368.5)	329 (261.3–455.0)	379 (311.0–503.0)	423.0 (301.8–506.0)
	High	203 (146.5–232.8)	244.0 (174.3–270.8)	275.5 (206.3–307.0)	304.5 (249.3–375.0)	342.0 (213.8–414.3)	380.0 (281.8–509.8)
	p-Value	0.76	0.94	0.76	0.22	0.10	0.66
uCa/Crea ratio (mmol/mmol)	Low	2.1 (1.3–3.5)	2.5 (1.8–3.1)	3.6 (2.3–5.2)	3.8 (2.3–6.2)	2.9 (1.8–4.1)	2.3 (1.6–3.7)
	High	1.7 (1.4–3.7)	2.7 (2.0–6.1)	4.0 (2.9–6.3)	3.0 (2.1–5.4)	3.8 (2.4–5.0)	3.4 (1.9–4.8)
	p-Value	0.98	0.30	0.35	0.49	0.21	0.14
uP/Crea ratio (mmol/mmol)	Low	1.6 (0.5–5.9)	2.8 (1.0–6.8)	1.9 (0.8–5.4)	5.1 (1.1–9.3)	7.2 (2.5–12.3)	11.2 (6.2–18.6)
	High	3.8 (0.5–6.7)	1.8 (1.1–5.8)	3.5 (1.6–6.1)	7.7 (5.0–10.9)	9.4 (7.0–16.5)	14.5 (9.3–18.7)
	p-Value	0.64	0.72	0.15	0.14	0.06	0.73

All data are presented as median and interquartile range; sCa: serum calcium (mmol/L); uCa: urine calcium (mmol/L); sP: serum phosphorus (mmol/L); uP: urine phosphorus (mmol/L); TrP: tubular reabsorption of phosphorus (%); ALP: Alkaline phosphatase (U/L); uCa/Crea ration: urine calcium/creatinine ration (mmol/mmol); uP/Cre ratio (mmol/mmol).

References

1. Rauch, F.; Schoenau, E. The developing bone: Slave or master of its cells and molecules? *Pediatr. Res.* **2001**, *50*, 309–314. [CrossRef] [PubMed]
2. Greer, F.R. Osteopenia of prematurity. *Annu. Rev. Nutr.* **1994**, *14*, 169–185. [CrossRef] [PubMed]
3. Harrison, C.M.; Johnson, K.; McKechnie, E. Osteopenia of prematurity: A national survey and review of practice. *Acta Paediatr.* **2008**, *97*, 407–413. [CrossRef] [PubMed]
4. Demarini, S. Calcium and phosphorus nutrition in preterm infants. *Acta Paediatr. Suppl.* **2005**, *94*, 87–92. [CrossRef] [PubMed]
5. Kovacs, C.S. Calcium, phosphorus, and bone metabolism in the fetus and newborn. *Early Hum. Dev.* **2015**, *91*, 623–628. [CrossRef] [PubMed]
6. Ribeiro Dde, O.; Lobo, B.W.; Volpato, N.M.; da Veiga, V.F.; Cabral, L.M.; de Sousa, V.P. Influence of the calcium concentration in the presence of organic phosphorus on the physicochemical compatibility and stability of all-in-one admixtures for neonatal use. *Nutr. J.* **2009**, *8*, 51. [CrossRef] [PubMed]
7. Rigo, J.; Pieltain, C.; Salle, B.; Senterre, J. Enteral calcium, phosphate and vitamin d requirements and bone mineralization in preterm infants. *Acta Paediatr.* **2007**, *96*, 969–974. [CrossRef] [PubMed]
8. Carnielli, V.P.; Luijendijk, I.H.; van Goudoever, J.B.; Sulkers, E.J.; Boerlage, A.A.; Degenhart, H.J.; Sauer, P.J. Feeding premature newborn infants palmitic acid in amounts and stereoisomeric position similar to that of human milk: Effects on fat and mineral balance. *Am. J. Clin. Nutr.* **1995**, *61*, 1037–1042. [PubMed]
9. Abrams, S.A.; Hawthorne, K.M.; Placencia, J.L.; Dinh, K.L. Micronutrient requirements of high-risk infants. *Clin. Perinatol.* **2014**, *41*, 347–361. [CrossRef] [PubMed]
10. Schanler, R.J.; Abrams, S.A.; Garza, C. Mineral balance studies in very low birth weight infants fed human milk. *J. Pediatr.* **1988**, *113*, 230–238. [CrossRef]
11. Lapillonne, A.A.; Glorieux, F.H.; Salle, B.L.; Braillon, P.M.; Chambon, M.; Rigo, J.; Putet, G.; Senterre, J. Mineral balance and whole body bone mineral content in very low-birth-weight infants. *Acta Paediatr. Suppl.* **1994**, *405*, 117–122. [CrossRef] [PubMed]
12. Rigo, J.; Senterre, J. Nutritional needs of premature infants: Current issues. *J. Pediatr.* **2006**, *149*, S80–S88. [CrossRef]
13. Bert, S.; Gouyon, J.B.; Semama, D.S. Calcium, sodium and potassium urinary excretion during the first five days of life in very preterm infants. *Biol. Neonate* **2004**, *85*, 37–41. [CrossRef] [PubMed]
14. Catache, M.; Leone, C.R. Role of plasma and urinary calcium and phosphorus measurements in early detection of phosphorus deficiency in very low birthweight infants. *Acta Paediatr.* **2003**, *92*, 76–80. [CrossRef] [PubMed]
15. De Curtis, M.; Rigo, J. Nutrition and kidney in preterm infant. *J. Matern. Fetal. Neonatal Med.* **2012**, *25*, 55–59. [CrossRef] [PubMed]
16. Boehm, G.; Wiener, M.; Schmidt, C.; Ungethum, A.; Ungethum, B.; Moro, G. Usefulness of short-term urine collection in the nutritional monitoring of low birthweight infants. *Acta Paediatr.* **1998**, *87*, 339–343. [CrossRef] [PubMed]
17. Aladangady, N.; Coen, P.G.; White, M.P.; Rae, M.D.; Beattie, T.J. Urinary excretion of calcium and phosphate in preterm infants. *Pediatr. Nephrol.* **2004**, *19*, 1225–1231. [CrossRef] [PubMed]
18. Giapros, V.I.; Papaloukas, A.L.; Andronikou, S.K. Urinary mineral excretion in preterm neonates during the first month of life. *Neonatology* **2007**, *91*, 180–185. [CrossRef] [PubMed]
19. Giles, M.M.; Fenton, M.H.; Shaw, B.; Elton, R.A.; Clarke, M.; Lang, M.; Hume, R. Sequential calcium and phosphorus balance studies in preterm infants. *J. Pediatr.* **1987**, *110*, 591–598. [CrossRef]
20. Hellstern, G.; Poschl, J.; Linderkamp, O. Renal phosphate handling of premature infants of 23–25 weeks gestational age. *Pediatr. Nephrol.* **2003**, *18*, 756–758. [CrossRef] [PubMed]
21. Hillman, L.S.; Rojanasathit, S.; Slatopolsky, E.; Haddad, J.G. Serial measurements of serum calcium, magnesium, parathyroid hormone, calcitonin, and 25-hydroxy-vitamin D in premature and term infants during the first week of life. *Pediatr. Res.* **1977**, *11*, 739–744. [CrossRef] [PubMed]
22. Mihatsch, W.A.; Muche, R.; Pohlandt, F. The renal phosphate threshold decreases with increasing postmenstrual age in very low birth weight infants. *Pediatr. Res.* **1996**, *40*, 300–303. [CrossRef] [PubMed]

23. Pohlandt, F. Prevention of postnatal bone demineralization in very low-birth-weight infants by individually monitored supplementation with calcium and phosphorus. *Pediatr. Res.* **1994**, *35*, 125–129. [CrossRef] [PubMed]

24. Senterre, J.; Salle, B. Renal aspects of calcium and phosphorus metabolism in preterm infants. *Biol. Neonate* **1988**, *53*, 220–229. [CrossRef] [PubMed]

25. Trotter, A.; Stoll, M.; Leititis, J.U.; Blatter, A.; Pohlandt, F. Circadian variations of urinary electrolyte concentrations in preterm and term infants. *J. Pediatr.* **1996**, *128*, 253–256. [CrossRef]

26. Trotter, A.; Pohlandt, F. Calcium and phosphorus retention in extremely preterm infants supplemented individually. *Acta Paediatr.* **2002**, *91*, 680–683. [CrossRef] [PubMed]

27. Abrams, S.A.; Schanler, R.J.; Garza, C. Relation of bone mineralization measures to serum biochemical measures. *Am. J. Dis. Child.* **1988**, *142*, 1276–1278. [CrossRef] [PubMed]

28. Acar, D.B.; Kavuncuoglu, S.; Cetinkaya, M.; Petmezci, E.; Dursun, M.; Korkmaz, O.; Altuncu, E.K. Assessment of the place of tubular reabsorption of phosphorus in the diagnosis of osteopenia of prematurity. *Turk Pediatri Ars.* **2015**, *50*, 45–50. [CrossRef] [PubMed]

29. Visser, F.; Sprij, A.J.; Brus, F. The validity of biochemical markers in metabolic bone disease in preterm infants: A systematic review. *Acta Paediatr.* **2012**, *101*, 562–568. [CrossRef] [PubMed]

30. Tinnion, R.J.; Embleton, N.D. How to use... alkaline phosphatase in neonatology. *Arch. Dis. Child. Educ. Pract. Ed.* **2012**, *97*, 157–163. [CrossRef] [PubMed]

31. Kelly, A.; Kovatch, K.J.; Garber, S.J. Metabolic bone disease screening practices among US Neonatologists. *Clin. Pediatr. (Phila.)* **2014**, *53*, 1077–1083. [CrossRef] [PubMed]

32. Staub, E.; Wiedmer, N.; Staub, L.P.; Nelle, M.; von Vigier, R.O. Monitoring of urinary calcium and phosphorus excretion in preterm infants: Comparison of 2 methods. *J. Pediatr. Gastroenterol. Nutr.* **2014**, *58*, 404–408. [CrossRef] [PubMed]

33. Corpeleijn, W.E.; de Waard, M.; Christmann, V.; van Goudoever, J.B.; Jansen-van der Weide, M.C.; Kooi, E.M.; Koper, J.F.; Kouwenhoven, S.M.; Lafeber, H.N.; Mank, E.; et al. Effect of Donor Milk on Severe Infections and Mortality in Very Low-Birth-Weight Infants: The Early Nutrition Study Randomized Clinical Trial. *JAMA Pediatr.* **2016**, *170*, 654–661. [CrossRef] [PubMed]

34. Gidrewicz, D.A.; Fenton, T.R. A systematic review and meta-analysis of the nutrient content of preterm and term breast milk. *BMC Pediatr.* **2014**, *14*, 216. [CrossRef] [PubMed]

35. Christmann, V.; de Grauw, A.M.; Visser, R.; Matthijsse, R.P.; van Goudoever, J.B.; van Heijst, A.F. Early postnatal calcium and phosphorus metabolism in preterm infants. *J. Pediatr. Gastroenterol. Nutr.* **2014**, *58*, 398–403. [CrossRef] [PubMed]

36. Bell, M.J.; Ternberg, J.L.; Feigin, R.D.; Keating, J.P.; Marshall, R.; Barton, L.; Brotherton, T. Neonatal necrotizing enterocolitis. Therapeutic decisions based upon clinical staging. *Ann. Surg.* **1978**, *187*, 1–7. [CrossRef] [PubMed]

37. Papile, L.A.; Burstein, J.; Burstein, R.; Koffler, H. Incidence and evolution of subependymal and intraventricular hemorrhage: A study of infants with birth weights less than 1500 gm. *J. Pediatr.* **1978**, *92*, 529–534. [CrossRef]

38. Koletzko, B.; Goulet, O.; Hunt, J.; Krohn, K.; Shamir, R.; Parenteral Nutrition Guidelines Working Group; European Society for Clinical Nutrition and Metabolism; European Society of Paediatric Gastroenterology, Hepatology and Nutrition (ESPGHAN); European Society of Paediatric Research. 1. Guidelines on paediatric parenteral nutrition of the European Society of Paediatric Gastroenterology, Hepatology and Nutrition (Espghan) and the European Society for Clinical Nutrition and Metabolism (ESPEN), Supported by the European Society of Paediatric Research (ESPR). *J. Pediatr. Gastroenterol. Nutr.* **2005**, *41*, S1–S87. [PubMed]

39. Agostoni, C.; Buonocore, G.; Carnielli, V.P.; De Curtis, M.; Darmaun, D.; Decsi, T.; Domellof, M.; Embleton, N.D.; Fusch, C.; Genzel-Boroviczeny, O.; et al. Enteral nutrient supply for preterm infants: Commentary from the European Society of Paediatric Gastroenterology, Hepatology and Nutrition Committee on Nutrition. *J. Pediatr. Gastroenterol. Nutr.* **2010**, *50*, 85–91. [CrossRef] [PubMed]

40. Fenton, T.R.; Lyon, A.W.; Rose, M.S. Cord blood calcium, phosphate, magnesium, and alkaline phosphatase gestational age-specific reference intervals for preterm infants. *BMC Pediatr.* **2011**, *11*, 76. [CrossRef] [PubMed]

41. Ehrenkranz, R.A.; Dusick, A.M.; Vohr, B.R.; Wright, L.L.; Wrage, L.A.; Poole, W.K. Growth in the neonatal intensive care unit influences neurodevelopmental and growth outcomes of extremely low birth weight infants. *Pediatrics* **2006**, *117*, 1253–1261. [CrossRef] [PubMed]

42. Klingenberg, C.; Embleton, N.D.; Jacobs, S.E.; O'Connell, L.A.; Kuschel, C.A. Enteral feeding practices in very preterm infants: An international survey. *Arch. Dis. Child. Fetal. Neonatal. Ed.* **2012**, *97*, F56–F61. [CrossRef] [PubMed]

43. Sullivan, S.; Schanler, R.J.; Kim, J.H.; Patel, A.L.; Trawoger, R.; Kiechl-Kohlendorfer, U.; Chan, G.M.; Blanco, C.L.; Abrams, S.; Cotten, C.M.; et al. An exclusively human milk-based diet is associated with a lower rate of necrotizing enterocolitis than a diet of human milk and bovine milk-based products. *J. Pediatr.* **2010**, *156*, 562–567; 562.e1–567.e1. [CrossRef] [PubMed]

44. Cristofalo, E.A.; Schanler, R.J.; Blanco, C.L.; Sullivan, S.; Trawoeger, R.; Kiechl-Kohlendorfer, U.; Dudell, G.; Rechtman, D.J.; Lee, M.L.; Lucas, A.; et al. Randomized trial of exclusive human milk versus preterm formula diets in extremely premature infants. *J. Pediatr.* **2013**, *163*, 1592.e1–1595.e1. [CrossRef] [PubMed]

45. Moltu, S.J.; Strommen, K.; Blakstad, E.W.; Almaas, A.N.; Westerberg, A.C.; Braekke, K.; Ronnestad, A.; Nakstad, B.; Berg, J.P.; Veierod, M.B.; et al. Enhanced feeding in very-low-birth-weight infants may cause electrolyte disturbances and septicemia—A randomized, controlled trial. *Clin. Nutr.* **2013**, *32*, 207–212. [CrossRef] [PubMed]

46. Jamin, A.; D'Inca, R.; Le Floc'h, N.; Kuster, A.; Orsonneau, J.L.; Darmaun, D.; Boudry, G.; Le Huerou-Luron, I.; Seve, B.; Gras-Le Guen, C. Fatal effects of a neonatal high-protein diet in low-birth-weight piglets used as a model of intrauterine growth restriction. *Neonatology* **2010**, *97*, 321–328. [CrossRef] [PubMed]

47. Mehanna, H.M.; Moledina, J.; Travis, J. Refeeding syndrome: What it is, and how to prevent and treat it. *BMJ* **2008**, *336*, 1495–1498. [CrossRef] [PubMed]

48. Walmsley, R.S. Refeeding syndrome: Screening, incidence, and treatment during parenteral nutrition. *J. Gastroenterol. Hepatol.* **2013**, *28*, 113–117. [CrossRef] [PubMed]

49. Ross, J.R.; Finch, C.; Ebeling, M.; Taylor, S.N. Refeeding syndrome in very-low-birth-weight intrauterine growth-restricted neonates. *J. Perinatol.* **2013**, *33*, 717–720. [CrossRef] [PubMed]

50. Bonsante, F.; Iacobelli, S.; Latorre, G.; Rigo, J.; De Felice, C.; Robillard, P.Y.; Gouyon, J.B. Initial amino acid intake influences phosphorus and calcium homeostasis in preterm infants—It is time to change the composition of the early parenteral nutrition. *PLoS ONE* **2013**, *8*, e72880. [CrossRef] [PubMed]

51. Lucas, A.; Brooke, O.G.; Baker, B.A.; Bishop, N.; Morley, R. High alkaline phosphatase activity and growth in preterm neonates. *Arch. Dis. Child.* **1989**, *64*, 902–909. [CrossRef] [PubMed]

52. Peacock, J.L.; Marston, L.; Marlow, N.; Calvert, S.A.; Greenough, A. Neonatal and infant outcome in boys and girls born very prematurely. *Pediatr. Res.* **2012**, *71*, 305–310. [CrossRef] [PubMed]

53. Christmann, V.; Visser, R.; Engelkes, M.; de Grauw, A.; van Goudoever, J.; van Heijst, A. The enigma to achieve normal postnatal growth in preterm infants—Using parenteral or enteral nutrition? *Acta Paediatr.* **2013**, *102*, 471–479. [CrossRef] [PubMed]

54. Fenton, T.R.; Kim, J.H. A systematic review and meta-analysis to revise the Fenton growth chart for preterm infants. *BMC Pediatr.* **2013**, *13*, 59. [CrossRef] [PubMed]

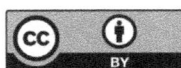

nutrients

MDPI

Article

Implementation of a Nutrition Program Reduced Post-Discharge Growth Restriction in Thai Very Low Birth Weight Preterm Infants

Suchada Japakasetr [1], **Chutima Sirikulchayanonta** [2,*], **Umaporn Suthutvoravut** [3], **Busba Chindavijak** [4], **Masaharu Kagawa** [5] and **Somjai Nokdee** [6]

1   Department of Nutrition, Faculty of Public Health, Mahidol University, Bangkok 10400, Thailand; scdj01@yahoo.com
2   College of Medicine, Rangsit University, Bangkok 10400, Thailand
3   Department of Pediatrics, Faculty of Medicine, Ramathibodi Hospital, Mahidol University, Bangkok 10400, Thailand; u_suthut@yahoo.com
4   Department of Pharmacy, Faculty of Pharmacy, Mahidol University, Bangkok 10400, Thailand; pybcd@mahidol.ac.th
5   Institute of Nutrition Sciences, Kagawa Nutrition University, Saitama Prefecture 350-0288, Japan; mskagawa@eiyo.ac.jp
6   Nursing Department, Buddhasothorn Hospital, Chachoengsao 24000, Thailand; somjainokdee@gmail.com
*   Correspondence: chutimabk@yahoo.com; Tel.: +66-2-354-4725

Received: 24 September 2016; Accepted: 8 December 2016; Published: 17 December 2016

Abstract: Very low birth weight (VLBW) preterm infants are vulnerable to growth restriction after discharge due to cumulative protein and energy deficits during their hospital stay and early post-discharge period. The current study evaluated the effectiveness of the preterm infant, post-discharge nutrition (PIN) program to reduce post-discharge growth restriction in Thai VLBW preterm infants. A prospective, non-randomized interventional cohort study was undertaken to assess the growth of 22 VLBW preterm infants who received the PIN program and compared them with 22 VLBW preterm infants who received conventional nutrition services. Infant's growth was recorded monthly until the infants reached six months' corrected age (6-moCA). Intervention infants had significantly greater body weights ($p = 0.013$) and head circumferences ($p = 0.009$). Also, a greater proportion of the intervention group recovered their weight to the standard weight at 4-moCA ($p = 0.027$) and at 6-moCA ($p = 0.007$) and their head circumference to the standard head circumference at 6-moCA ($p = 0.004$) compared to their historical comparison counterparts. Enlistment in the PIN program thus resulted in significantly reduced post-discharge growth restriction in VLBW preterm infants. Further research on longer term effects of the program on infant's growth and development is warranted.

Keywords: very low birth weight preterm infant; growth restriction; post-discharge; nutrition program

1. Introduction

Very low birth weight (VLBW) preterm infants are those born before 37 weeks gestation weighing less than 1500 g, and they comprise between 4% and 8% of neonatal live-births [1,2]. Survival of these small infants has significantly improved mainly due to the advancement of medical intervention in neonatal intensive care units (NICU) [2,3]. However, the extra-uterine growth restriction (EUGR), defined as a decrease in z-score greater than two standard deviations (SD) between birth to discharge [4], is common in the preterm population [5]. A recent cohort study estimated that a prevalence of being small for gestational age (SGA) among VLBW infants (birth weight 750–1500 g) born between 2005 and 2012 to be 44.4%–58.8% at discharge [6]. This may be caused by several health problems such as need for respiratory support, unstable glucose levels, early sepsis, risk of necrotizing enterocolitis and feeding intolerance during NICU stay. These concerns impact highly on the prescribed feeding regimen and result in unrecovered early protein and energy deficits accumulated during hospital admission [7]. Moreover, post-discharge growth restriction also usually occurs in these infants at 28%–40% until 18–22 months corrected age (moCA) [8]. These poor postnatal growths are potentially associated with developmental delay [8], obesity and related complications, such as cardiovascular disease, type II diabetes mellitus and hypertension during adulthood [4,8,9].

In order to compensate for these nutritional deficits and improve the EUGR, the initiation of aggressive parenteral nutrition (PN) in the first week of life and fortified human milk (HM) to this population has been suggested during their hospital stay [10–12]. Furthermore, enriching HM or formula is widely recommended to decrease post-discharge growth restriction and accelerate catch-up growth [10,13]. However, the HM feeding rate in preterm infants usually declines after discharge [14]. Enriched-nutrient formula (EF) is therefore supplemented to provide adequate intakes of energy and nutrients to meet the infant's needs [15–17].

In 2012, a preliminary study was performed at Buddhasothorn Hospital, Chachoengsao, Thailand. It investigated the nutritional care services and growth outcomes in 85 VLBW preterm infants at pre- and post-discharge. The findings revealed that the HM feeding rate was decreased from 87% at discharge to 7% at 6-moCA. After discharge, these infants received unfortified HM and/or standard term formula (TF). Moreover, 85% of VLBW preterm infants were below the standard growth at discharge and 43% remained as below the standard growth at 6-moCA.

In order to reduce post-discharge growth restriction in this population, the preterm infant, post-discharge nutrition (PIN) program was developed and implemented at Buddhasothorn hospital in early 2014. Based on recent recommendations [10,15,18], it focuses on providing an EF in addition to fortified HM with regular monitoring after discharge to ensure infant nutritional intakes. The aim of the present study was to compare growth outcomes in VLBW preterm infants who enlist in the PIN program with those who received conventional nutrition services.

2. Materials and Methods

A prospective non-randomized interventional cohort study was conducted at Buddhasothorn Hospital, located in Chachoengsao province, Thailand. The present study was approved by the Institutional Review Boards of the Faculty of Public Health, Mahidol University (COA. No. MUPH 2014-002), Buddhasothorn Hospital (COA. No.EC-CA 007/2556) and Chachoengsao provincial health office (COA. No. PH_CCO_REC 003/56). The current study used the subgroup of the study that registered as a clinical trial with the Thai clinical trials registration number of TCTR20160211001.

2.1. Participants

A total of 22 VLBW preterm infants who were admitted and discharged from the NICU between March 2014 and February 2015 and given the PIN program were invited to participate in the current study. Detailed verbal and written explanations were given to parents of VLBW preterm infants and informed written consent was obtained from the parents of each participant. These infants were compared with records of 22 VLBW preterm infants who were born and discharged from the NICU between January 2012 and December 2013. The intervention group was enlisted in the PIN program after discharge to 6-moCA whereas; the comparison group received a conventional nutrition service at post-discharge for the same period of time.

A sample size of 22 preterm infants for each group was determined based on a previous study using a power of 80% and a significance level of 5% to detect a program effect of an increase of 5% on the body weight with favorable outcomes at 6-moCA [19]. Inclusion criteria of the study include: (1) birth at $\leq$34 weeks gestation; (2) birth weight ranged between 750 and 1499 g; (3) no use of any medical feeding tube at discharge; and (4) residence in Chachoengsao. On the other hand, infants were excluded if they had: (1) severe respiratory problems; (2) serious congenital anomalies; (3) more than or equal to grade III periventricular or intraventricular hemorrhage; (4) surgical necrotizing enterocolitis; (5) gastrointestinal perforation; (6) severe retinopathy of prematurity; (7) severe birth asphyxia [6,19]; and also if (8) the mothers cannot communicate with researchers.

2.2. Recruitment Process of the Participants

Figure 1 describes the recruitment process of 22 VLBW preterm infants for both intervention and comparison group. The infants born in the comparison period were randomly assigned to the historical comparison group, stratified for sex and birth weight.

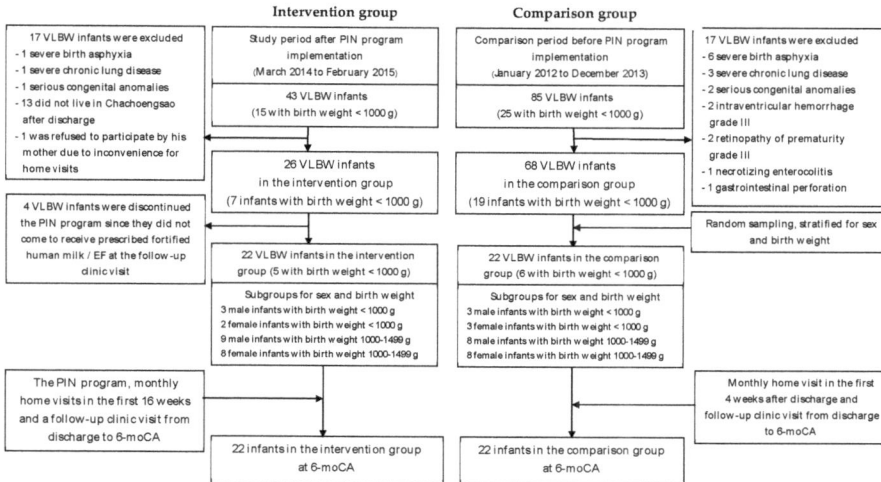

	Intervention group	Comparison group	
17 VLBW infants were excluded - 1 severe birth asphyxia - 1 severe chronic lung disease - 1 serious congenital anomalies - 13 did not live in Chachoengsao after discharge - 1 was refused to participate by his mother due to inconvenience for home visits	Study period after PIN program implementation (March 2014 to February 2015) 43 VLBW infants (15 with birth weight < 1000 g)	Comparison period before PIN program implementation (January 2012 to December 2013) 85 VLBW infants (25 with birth weight < 1000 g)	17 VLBW infants were excluded - 6 severe birth asphyxia - 3 severe chronic lung disease - 2 serious congenital anomalies - 2 intraventricular hemorrhage grade III - 2 retinopathy of prematurity grade III - 1 necrotizing enterocolitis - 1 gastrointestinal perforation
	26 VLBW infants in the intervention group (7 infants with birth weight < 1000 g)	68 VLBW infants in the comparison group (19 infants with birth weight < 1000 g)	
4 VLBW infants were discontinued the PIN program since they did not come to receive prescribed fortified human milk / EF at the follow-up clinic visit	22 VLBW infants in the intervention group (5 with birth weight < 1000 g)	22 VLBW infants in the comparison group (6 with birth weight < 1000 g)	Random sampling, stratified for sex and birth weight
	Subgroups for sex and birth weight 3 male infants with birth weight < 1000 g 2 female infants with birth weight < 1000 g 9 male infants with birth weight 1000-1499 g 8 female infants with birth weight 1000-1499 g	Subgroups for sex and birth weight 3 male infants with birth weight < 1000 g 3 female infants with birth weight < 1000 g 8 male infants with birth weight 1000-1499 g 8 female infants with birth weight 1000-1499 g	
The PIN program, monthly home visits in the first 16 weeks and a follow-up clinic visit from discharge to 6-moCA			Monthly home visit in the first 4 weeks after discharge and follow-up clinic visit from discharge to 6-moCA
	22 infants in the intervention group at 6-moCA	22 infants in the comparison group at 6-moCA	

Figure 1. Recruitment process of participants. VLBW = very low birth weight, PIN = preterm infant post-discharge nutrition, EF = enriched-nutrient formula, g = gram, moCA = months corrected age.

2.3. Nutritional Strategies Conducted for Both Groups during Hospital Admission

Until their discharge from hospital, both groups received parenteral and enteral nutrition. Infants in both groups received individualized PN formulation in the first few weeks of life. When the infant's clinical status was improved, trophic oral feeding was introduced until the full feedings of at least 120–150 mL/kg/day were achieved [20]. All preterm infants mainly received their mother's own milk. Mothers were instructed by NICU nurses to assess volume intake of breast milk by test-weighing procedure [21] before discharge. In order to increase energy density from 20 to 24 or 27 kcal/oz during NICU stay as recommended by recent studies [22–24], infants were given fortified HM that was prepared by adding preterm formula (PF) into expressed HM (calculated by definite formula) once their volume of feeding reached 100 mL/kg/day [20,25].

2.4. The PIN Program Conducted for the Intervention Group

The PIN program is a post-discharge nutritional plan of feeding fortified HM and/or EF for VLBW preterm infants from discharge to 6-moCA. It is based on a commentary by the European Society for Pediatric Gastroenterology, Hepatology, and Nutrition (ESPGHAN) committee on nutrition [22] and a nutrition care practice guideline developed by the Oregon Pediatric Nutrition Practice Group (OPNPG) [15]. The program was developed based on outcomes from focused group discussions of a multi-disciplinary team in the hospital. Four experts—including two pediatricians, one neonatologist, and one nurse—reviewed and approved the program. It was implemented as a routine nutritional service at Buddhasothorn hospital since January 2014. The program also includes education on mothers prior to their discharge such as benefits of breastfeeding to preterm infants [26], essential knowledge for lactating mothers [27,28], preparation method of fortified HM, feeding practices [29,30], and personal hygiene for their infant care after hospital discharge [29,30]. The contents of the education program were based on previous studies that recommended the importance of these variables [31,32].

2.4.1. Enriched Milk Intake

The fortified HM suggested in the program was prepared by adding a given calibrated spoon (0.42 g, contains 2.1 kcal) of a powdered preterm formula (PF) (Pre-Nan Abott, Bangkok, Thailand) per oz (30 cc) of expressed HM to prepare milk with energy density of 22 kcal/oz. All intervention infants received fortified HM at discharge. If its volume was less than 50% of daily total volume intake, EF (Enfalac catch up care, Mead Johnson, Bangkok, Thailand) was supplemented to meet the infant needs with a goal of energy including 85–120 kcal/kg/day and 1.5–2.5 g/kg/day of protein according to their corrected age [10,15,22].

Specific written instructions on the fortification of HM and reconstitution of EF powder as well as containers for the preparation and storage of reconstituted milk were provided to each parent. In addition, the written instructions were repeated verbally and parental understanding was confirmed by research personnel. Dietary intake records were given to parents at discharge to assess actual milk and complementary food intake of infants. At the follow-up clinic, the mothers or caregivers were asked for more detailed information of their records. Volume of fortified expressed HM, EF, and other fluid intakes were determined by measuring in oz according to the label on the milk bottle.

2.4.2. Introduction of Semi-Solid Foods

The introduction of semi-solid foods was commenced if: (1) they reached 4–6 months after birth; (2) body weight was not less than 5 kg; (3) they had no extrusion reflex; (4) they had well controlled neck and chair sitting posture; (5) they developed an ability to receive spoon feeding; and (6) they developed an ability to show desire or refusal of food [33–36]. Type and formula of semi-solid foods recommended in the PIN program was based on guidelines of complementary foods for Thai infant and toddlers by Thai Ministry of Public Health [36]. In the PIN program, Thai foods such as a pulp of Thai rice, pumpkin, egg yolk, some kinds of Thai vegetable, such as Coccinia grandis (dtam-leung) were recommended to the infants from 6 to 9 months after birth. In addition, half a teaspoon of vegetable oil per 250 g of semisolid foods was added to prevent fat soluble vitamin deficiencies [36].

2.4.3. Biochemical Blood Tests and Nutrient Supplementation

Biochemical blood profiles were also assessed monthly as a high-risk follow-up clinic. One mL of blood sample was taken at blood drawing unit from all infants and hematocrit (Hct), calcium (Ca), phosphorus (P), alkaline phosphatase (ALP), and blood urea nitrogen (BUN) were examined in order to monitor iron deficiency anemia [37], bone health [38], and nutritional status, including sufficiency of protein. All analyses were conducted at the laboratory unit in the hospital. However, the historical group did not conduct a regular biochemical blood tests after discharge at the follow-up clinic visit. As a result, with an exception of Hct, a nutritional status of historical group was unable to be compared with the intervention group during 1- to 6-moCA and therefore did not include in the results of the current study. Moreover, monthly home visits were performed to monitor HM fortification procedure and infant feeding practices [19].

All infants received 2 mg/kg/day of iron at discharge. When abnormal levels of biochemical markers were identified, special nutrient supplementations were prescribed by a pediatrician at a follow-up clinic as these follows:

- Hct < 35%: Increase dose of ferrous sulfate/fumarate solution from 2 to 4–5 mg/kg/day [17,37].
- Total Ca < 8.0 mg/dL: Supplement calcium suspension 100–140 mg/kg/day [15,17]

- Phosphorus < 5.5 mg/day and/or ALP > 450 IU/L: Supplement phosphate solution 60–90 mg/kg/day [15,17]
- BUN > 20 mg/dL: Consider substitution with unfortified HM and/or standard term formula (TF) [10].

The infants also received 0.5 mL/day of multivitamin drop (MVD) (1 mL of MVD—composed of 2000 international unit (IU) of vitamin A, 400 IU of vitamin D and other water soluble vitamins)—until infants received total daily milk intake of >32 oz (1000 mL) [15]. However, non-fortified HM and/or TF was substituted when infants cannot tolerate with fortified HM and/or EF, or had an excessive rate of weight gain, and also showed Ca, P, and BUN above their normal levels [10].

Estimated volume of breastfeeding was derived by test weighing procedure [21]. Energy and selected nutrients intakes (protein, vitamin A and D, calcium, phosphorus, zinc, and iron), at 2-, 4-, and 6-moCA were estimated using HM composition values from literatures [39,40] manufacturer label claims for PF, EF and TF, drug label of MVD and ferrous fumarate drop, commercial complementary feeding formula and complementary foods composition recommended by the Thai Ministry of Public Health [36].

A nutritionist explained to the mothers/caregiver about the procedure of recording actual amount of all milk feeding, complementary food intake, and nutrient supplementation before infant discharge and also re-checked their practices monthly at the follow-up clinic visit. These records were kept by mothers/caregivers at home and by a nutritionist during home visit and at a follow-up clinic visit.

2.5. The Conventional Nutrition Services Conducted for the Comparison Group

Prior to their infant discharge, parents in the comparison group received general education such as latching technique and observations of feeding intolerance without specific nutritional education. After discharge, infants received unfortified HM and/or TF. They were provided with 2–5 mg/kg/day of ferrous fumarate solution and 0.5–1 mL/day of MVD according to a decision of the in-charge pediatrician at a follow-up clinic. Hematocrit was also tested for all infants at every clinic visits; while the other chemical blood tests, including Ca, P, ALP and BUN were performed at some visits according to pediatricians' decisions.

Enteral intake data of the comparison group was also obtained from dietary intake recorded by mothers/caregivers and nutritional records by a nutritionist at a follow-up clinic as performed in the intervention group. Differences of the nutritional activities between the groups are described in Table 1.

Table 1. Comparisons of activities in the preterm infant post-discharge nutrition (PIN) program and conventional nutrition services.

The PIN Program Activities	Conventional Nutrition Activities
I. Pre-discharge activities	
Giving formal nutritional education to parents/caregivers	No formal nutritional education for parents/caregivers
II. Post-discharge activities	
Giving enriched-nutrient HM and/or EF to the infants from discharge to 6-moCA	Giving unfortified HM and/or TF from discharge to infant weaning
Using revised biochemical blood tests and nutrition supplements protocol	Using biochemical blood tests according to decisions by in-charge pediatricians
Using revised criteria to start and recommended types of semi-solid foods to preterm infants	Suggestions mainly about time to start semi-solid foods at six months after birth without other specific criteria to start semi-solid foods
Monthly home visit until preterm infants reached 6-moCA	Home visit only one time after hospital discharge

moCA = months corrected age; HM = human milk; EF = enriched-nutrient formula; TF = term formula.

2.6. Differences in Milk Formula between the Groups

The energy and nutrients values of fortified HM and EF used in the intervention group and unfortified HM [39,40] and TF used in the comparison group are shown in Table 2. Brands of TF formula were derived from nutritional records at a follow-up clinic in the historical group. Composition of TF is obtained from the average amount of ingredients from four commercial brands of TF in Thailand (S-26, Dumex Hi-Q, Lactogen and Enfalac A[+]) which contains equal energy density and protein per 100 mL, but are slightly different for the remaining nutrients.

The energy density of fortified HM and reconstituted formula of EF is 21.8 and 22.5 kcal/oz; while those of unfortified HM and TF is 19.7 and 20.1 kcal/oz, respectively. Fortified HM contains higher protein than unfortified HM and TF by 12.5% and 22.5%, respectively, but the remaining nutrients are equal to or less than TF. EF also contains higher protein, calcium, phosphorus, vitamin D and zinc by 42.9%, 79.2%, 70.6%, 33.8%, and 20.0%, respectively, and >100% of vitamin A and iron compared to those in TF.

Table 2. Composition of energy and selected nutrients in fortified human milk (HM) and enriched-nutrient formula (EF) in the intervention group versus unfortified HM and term formula (TF) in the comparison group.

Composition	Intervention Group		Comparison Group	
	Fortified HM	EF	Unfortified HM	TF
Energy (kcal)	72.60	75.00	65.60	67.00
Protein (g)	1.80	2.10	1.60	1.47
Vitamin A (IU)	122.40	343.30	72.00	160.83
Vitamin D (IU)	20.50	63.00	12.00	47.07
Calcium (mg)	38.03	82.00	29.00	45.77
Phosphorus (mg)	19.03	48.00	14.00	28.13
Zinc (mg)	0.63	0.72	0.53	0.60
Iron (mg)	0.25	1.37	0.13	0.63

HM = human milk, Fortified HM = expressed HM + preterm formula (PF: as a human milk fortifier), EF = enriched formula, TF = term formula, Milk composition is per 100 mL as provided by the literature and manufacturer, EF and TF were available cow milk protein-based formula.

The differences of feeding type and nutrient supplementation between the groups are summarized in Table 3.

Table 3. Comparisons of feeding type and nutrient supplementations for preterm infants after discharge between the intervention and comparison group.

	Intervention Group	Comparison Group
I. Feeding type		
1.1 Milk intake at discharge to 6-moCA	Fortified HM and/or EF with energy density of 22 kcal/oz	Unfortified HM and/or TF with energy density of 20 kcal/oz
1.2 Semi-solid foods	Recommended formula based on complementary food guideline for infants and toddlers by Thai MOPH	Commercial formula and/or any formula based on caregivers' decision
II. Nutrient supplementations		
2.1 At discharge		
Iron	2 mg/kg/day, increase to 4–5 mg/kg/day if Hct < 35%	2–5 mg/kg/day *
MVD	0.5 mL/day until infants had total daily milk intake of >32 oz	0.5–1 mL/kg/day *
Calcium suspension	100–140 mg/kg/day if total Ca < 8.0 mg/dL	90–120 mg/kg/day *
Phosphate solution	60–90 mg/kg/day if P < 5.5 mg/day and/or ALP > 450 IU/L	60–90 mg/kg/day *

* refers to dose of nutrient supplementation based on pediatricians' decisions, HM = human milk, EF = enriched formula, TF = term formula, moCA = months corrected age, MOPH = Ministry of Public Health, Hct = hematocrit, MVD = multivitamin drop, Ca = calcium, dL = deciliter, P = phosphorus, ALP = alkaline phosphatase.

2.7. Growth Assessments Conducted with Both Groups

Body weight, length and head circumference of infants in both groups were measured monthly, using revised anthropometric protocol for newborn by the same staff at the follow-up clinic. The hospital staff who perform growth measurement was trained and validated their measuring techniques every three months by the supervisor who is an expert in infant growth measurement. A digital balance (MS 2400; two decimals, maximum load 20 kg, maximum length measured 80 cm) was used for both weight and length measurements and a tape measure (Hochestmass 1.9 × 150 mm) was used for a head circumference measurement.

All data of the infants in the comparison group were recorded from patient charts during hospitalization and out-patient profiles at a follow-up clinic as secondary data until infants reached 6-moCA. Infant growth status was assessed by the Fenton [41] and WHO growth charts [42,43].

2.8. Statistical Analysis

Differences in energy and nutrient intakes between the groups were assessed by the Mann-Whitney *U* test. Comparisons of anthropometric variables between the two groups from 1- to 6-moCA were examined using multivariate of covariance (MANOVA) repeated measures. Mixed model analysis was used to adjust multiple measurements of each infant. The categorical data were compared using chi-squared test. Data analyses were conducted using PASW SPSS statistics (version 18.0, SPSS Inc., Chicago, IL, USA). All statistical analyses were examined with a significance level of 0.05.

3. Results

3.1. Baseline Characteristics of the Participants

Descriptive characteristics of infants were shown in Table 4. There were no statistically significant differences in baseline characteristics between the groups.

Table 4. Baseline characteristics of the intervention and comparison group.

Variables	Intervention Group (n = 22)	Comparison Group (n = 22)	p-Value
Sex, n (%)	Male, 13 (59.0)	Male, 11 (50.0)	0.763
GA at birth, week ± day	29 ± 12 day	30 ± 14 day	0.501
Twin, n (%)	3 (13.6)	6 (27.3)	0.457
Growth status at birth			
Birth weight, g	1192 ± 202	1151 ± 208	0.502
Length, cm	39.1 ± 2.6	38.4 ± 3.7	0.525
Head circumference, cm	26.1 ± 1.8	26.4 ± 1.9	0.626
SGA at birth			
Body weight, n (%)	1 (4.5)	2 (9.1)	1.000
Length, n (%)	1 (4.5)	1 (4.5)	1.000
Head circumference, n (%)	2 (9.1)	2 (9.1)	1.000
SGA at discharge			
Body weight, n (%)	19 (86.4)	20 (90.9)	1.000
Length, n (%)	10 (45.5)	14 (63.6)	0.364
Head circumference, n (%)	15 (68.2)	12 (54.5)	0.453
PMA at discharge, week ± day	37 ± 12 day	38 ± 20 day	0.199
LOS, days	52 ± 12	53 ± 17	0.895
Feeding type at discharge, n (%)			
Breast milk feeding	18 (81.8)	17 (77.3)	1.000
Mixed feeding	3 (13.6)	4 (18.2)	1.000
Standard formula	1 (4.5)	2 (9.1)	1.000
Growth status at term (40 weeks)			
Body weight, g	2631 ± 538	2426 ± 531	0.145
Length, cm	47.7 ± 2.7	46.9 ± 2.9	0.318
Head circumference, cm	33.1 ± 1.6	32.2 ± 2.3	0.470
Maternal age (years)	22.5 ± 4.8	25.3 ± 5.5	0.087

n = number of infant; GA = gestational Age; SGA = small of gestational age; PMA = postmenstrual age; LOS = length of hospital stay. Data are expressed as mean ± SD. The differences between the groups were determined by chi-squared test.

3.2. Human Milk Feeding and Introduction of Semi-Solid Foods

The volume of HM consumed (mL/kg/day) and proportion of HM volume per total volume of all milk feeds per day (%) among infants in the intervention group was greater than those of the comparison group ($p < 0.05$) at 6-moCA, but not 2-and 4-moCA. However, the total duration of HM feeding did not differ significantly between two groups. The length of time from birth to the introduction of semi-solids was also not significantly different (Table 5).

Table 5. Comparisons of exclusively human milk feeding, feeding duration and a timing of introducing semisolid foods between the groups.

	Intervention Group (*n* = 22) Median (Q1–Q3)	Comparison Group (*n* = 22) Median (Q1–Q3)	*p*-Value
Exclusively of HM feeding			
2-moCA			
HM intake, mL/kg/day	40.37 (5.51–111.14)	61.20 (3.05–139.55)	0.234
Proportion of HM volume per Total volume of milk feeds per day, %	35.50 (10.17–79.17)	48.50 (20.21–120.21)	0.381
4-moCA			
HM intake, mL/kg/day	24.67 (13.34–61.55)	27.45 (10.00–57.80)	0.761
Proportion of HM volume per Total volume of milk feeds per day, %	22.82 (15.09–61.09)	21.86 (16.33–56.33)	0.859
6-moCA			
HM intake, mL/kg/day	11.73 (3.16–13.51)	3.05 (1.12–11.43)	0.044 *
Proportion of HM volume per Total volume of milk feeds per day, %	11.82 (4.43–16.43)	2.27 (0.56–7.94)	0.041 *
Total HM feeding duration, weeks after birth	16.00 (10.00–26.00)	18.00 (12.00–24.00)	0.427
Time at introduction of semisolid foods, weeks after birth	20.00 (17.00–23.00)	21.00 (19.00–24.00)	0.625

n = number of infant, Q1 = the first quartile, Q3 = the third quartile, HM = human milk. moCA = months corrected age. Total HM feeding duration refers to duration of exclusively HM feeding and/or mixed feeding (HM feedings plus formula feedings). Differences between groups were assessed by Mann-Whitney *U* test. * refers to statistically significant differences.

3.3. Nutritional Intake

Table 6 shows differences in daily energy and nutrient intakes of both groups. The intervention group showed greater energy and nutrient intakes except in zinc and iron compared to the comparison group at 2-, 4- and 6-moCA. It was also found that a median iron intake in both groups were slightly greater than the daily recommendation for healthy term infants.

Table 6. Comparisons of daily energy and nutrient intakes of preterm infants between the groups.

Energy/Nutrient	Intervention Group (*n* = 22) Median (Q1–Q3)	Comparison Group (*n* = 22) Median (Q1–Q3)	*p*-Value	RDA
Energy, kcal/kg				
2-moCA	91.08 (89.27–93.46)	88.40 (85.85–91.74)	0.014	85–120
4-moCA	86.39 (82.15–88.22)	76.67 (72.65–78.16)	0.001	
6-moCA	82.07 (80.11–88.63)	69.22 (66.49–71.98)	<0.001	
Protein, g/kg				
2-moCA	2.87 (2.44–3.30)	2.21 (1.95–2.69)	0.024	1.5–2.5
4-moCA	2.48 (2.01–2.89)	2.07 (1.73–2.17)	0.037	
6-moCA	1.85 (1.67–2.25)	1.53 (1.39–1.63)	<0.001	
Vitamin A, IU/kg				
2-moCA	555.66 (294.81–779.81)	219.66 (165.33–357.06)	0.004	320–700
4-moCA	476.99 (301.20–665.91)	209.63 (185.04–238.95)	<0.001	
6-moCA	389.03 (227.10–521.58)	202.24 (191.11–221.02)	0.035	
Vitamin D, IU/kg				
2-moCA	107.98 (45.14–145.78)	50.00 (36.09–71.00)	0.007	60–160
4-moCA	91.19 (55.00–125.30)	42.72 (32.06–47.84)	<0.001	
6-moCA	73.23 (40.22–96.57)	40.78 (38.40–44.72)	<0.001	

Table 6. *Cont.*

Energy/Nutrient	Intervention Group (n = 22) Median (Q1–Q3)	Comparison Group (n = 22) Median (Q1–Q3)	p-Value	RDA
Calcium, mg/kg				
2-moCA	85.80 (63.95–88.95)	68.24 (63.17–69.86)	<0.001	60–120
4-moCA	94.64 (78.61–100.08)	54.20 (51.76–57.94)	<0.001	
6-moCA	66.01 (49.04–69.60)	48.75 (45.77–49.87)	0.016	
Phosphorus, mg/kg				
2-moCA	40.43 (31.31–59.31)	33.13 (30.00–36.92)	<0.001	35–60
4-moCA	71.31 (66.32–77.83)	32.29 (30.14–34.73)	<0.001	
6-moCA	44.35 (35.08–48.81)	30.30 (29.66–34.33)	0.018	
Zinc, mg/kg				
2-moCA	0.78 (0.70–0.84)	0.74 (0.70–0.78)	0.226	0.5–1
4-moCA	0.72 (0.64–0.79)	0.71 0.69–0.75)	0.451	
6-moCA	0.67 (0.59–0.72)	0.64 (0.59–0.69)	0.572	
Iron, mg/kg				
2-moCA	4.95 (4.30–5.72)	4.37 (3.99–5.16)	0.080	2–4
4-moCA	5.02 (3.64–5.47)	5.30 (4.16–5.49)	0.411	
6-moCA	4.73 (3.17–5.58)	4.51 (2.68–5.41)	0.231	

Q1 = the first quartile, Q3 = the third quartile, PIs = preterm infants, RDA = recommended dietary allowance, the upper limit is for PIs 37–40 weeks GA, the lower limit is for term infants at six months of age, no = number, moCA = months corrected age, IU = international unit.

3.4. Infant Growth Outcomes

Compared to the comparison group, the intervention group showed significantly greater body weight (p = 0.013) at 4- and 6-moCA and head circumference (p = 0.009) at 6-moCA (Figure 2). However, no significant difference in length and weight gain velocity were observed between two groups at any time point of age. Furthermore, a greater proportion of the intervention group reached body weight greater than −2SD (Z score) at 4-moCA (81.8% vs. 45.5%, p = 0.027) and 6-moCA (90.9% vs. 50.0%, p = 0.007) compared with their comparison counterpart. In addition, the intervention group reached head circumference greater than −2SD (Z score) at 6-moCA (95.5% vs. 54.5%, p = 0.004) compared to the comparison group (Table 7). On the other hand, no differences were observed for length. Also, there was no over-standard growth or growth with higher +2SD (Z score) for body weight, length, and head circumference in both groups. Moreover, there was no correlation between HM feeding duration and any growth outcomes.

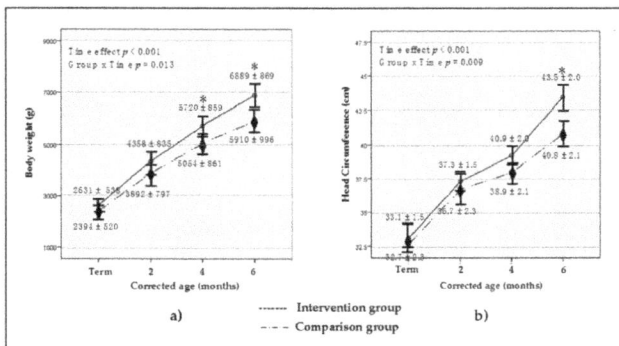

Figure 2. Anthropometric measurement of body weight, (**a**) and head circumference, (**b**) of the intervention and comparison group (n = 22). Data are reported as unadjusted mean ± SD. * denote a significant difference between groups at a specific time point with intervention greater than the comparison group (body weight at 4-moCA, p = 0.001, and 6-moCA, p < 0.001; head circumference at 6-moCA, p < 0.001).

Table 7. Comparisons of growth status of preterm infants between the groups.

Growth Status	*n* (%)		*p*-Value
	Intervention Group (*n* = 22)	Comparison Group (*n* = 22)	
2-moCA, higher−2SD (*Z* score) in			
Body weight	14 (63.6)	9 (40.9)	0.227
Length	15 (68.2)	8 (36.4)	0.069
Head circumference	17 (77.3)	10 (45.5)	0.062
4-moCA, higher−2SD (*Z* score) in			
Body weight	18 (81.8)	10 (45.5)	0.027 *
Length, *n* (%)	17 (77.3)	10 (45.5)	0.062
Head circumference, *n* (%)	18 (81.8)	11 (50.0)	0.055
6-moCA, higher−2SD (*Z* score) in			
Body weight	20 (90.9)	11 (50.0)	0.007 *
Length	17 (77.3)	11 (50.0)	0.116
Head circumference	21 (95.5)	12 (54.5)	0.004 *

moCA = months corrected age, −2SD (*Z* score) = −2SD line in *Z* score growth chart for newborn by World Health Organization. Data are expressed as number of cases (percentage). The difference between intervention and comparison group was determined by chi-square test. * refers to statistical significance.

4. Discussion

The current study found an increase in the proportion of infants who were underweight (after adjustment for gestational age) in both groups; 4.5% at birth and 86.3% at discharge for the intervention group and 9.1% at birth and 86.9% at discharge for the comparison group. The results may indicate that early protein and energy deficits were not recovered during hospital admission regardless of the groups. Our findings were consistent with previous studies [4,8,9,44,45] and the present study suggested a difficulty of preventing SGA among VLBW preterm infants during hospital admission.

The present study showed differences in anthropometric variables of fortified HM and/or EF fed versus HM alone and/or TF fed VLBW preterm infants from discharge to 6-moCA. The results indicated that the intervention group had significantly greater weight at 4- and 6-moCA and head circumference at 6-moCA compared to the comparison group. These results indicated the usefulness of the PIN program to compensate for energy and nutritional deficits which VLBW preterm infants experienced during their hospital stay and better recovery using fortified HM and/or EF. While there are controversies in beneficial effects of both fortified HM and enriched formula on growth parameters in preterm infants at post-discharge [7,18,46], the results from the current study were consistent with other studies that observed better recovery in infants who received energy and nutrient-enriched HM or formula at early hospital discharge [47–50].

In addition, the results showed significant differences in a proportion of infants reaching standard weight at 4- and 6-moCA, and head circumference at 6-moCA while no difference was observed at 2-moCA. This result showed that the PIN program may be effective in shortening the period of post-discharge growth restriction by 4-moCA without rapid acute effects. Casey, et al. [45] reported that achieving optimal catch-up growth during a post-natal period, especially by six months after term, will significantly result in better neurodevelopmental outcomes from 18 months to 6 years compared with those who achieved catch-up growth later. Considering suggestion by Casey, et al. [45], the PIN program that provides adequate nutrition to preterm infants during such a critical period may have beneficial impact on both short- and long-term health in this particular population.

Consistently, the nutrient intakes of infants with fortified HM and EF during study period were greater and more consistent with current dietary recommendations [15,23] than infants with unfortified HM and/or TF. These findings may attribute to the effect of enriching HM and formula to increase energy and protein intake. In addition, MVD, Ca, and P supplementation prescribed at a follow-up clinic according to the study protocol resulted in significantly higher intake of these nutrients. However, iron and zinc intakes did not differ between groups. This may be because of a similarity in iron and zinc supplementation practices in both groups. The results also showed a greater volume of human milk and the proportion of feed volume in the intervention group at 6-moCA. However, based on the obtained results, we interpreted the results as due to higher consumption of energy and protein that contained in enriched HM rather than increased volume.

While the PIN program included an education for mothers about benefits of breastfeeding before infant discharge, the present study did not show improvement in feeding duration between the groups and, in fact, was shorter than a previous study that reported a proportion and duration of exclusive HM feeding [20]. The results may indicate insufficient and inadequate lactation support of the PIN program to overcome problems that mothers experienced at post-discharge. Although the PIN program made more frequent home visits compared to the conventional service, the content including educational tools delivered prior to discharge and at each home visit should be adjusted as well as increasing involvement of lactation experts and frequencies of both on-site and distant counseling opportunities. In addition, the current study may indicate a presence of additional issues that prevent mothers from continuing HM feeding after discharge. As a result, further research may be warranted to evaluate factors that influence mothers to continue feeding HM to their child.

Study Limitations

Limitations of the current study included using the historical comparison group which contributed to slightly to differences in composition of TF formula intake. In addition, some data deviations might occur, such as an estimation of breast milk volume intake in some breastfed infants due to inadequate skill of test-weighing procedure in some mothers. Next, the currently applied inclusion and exclusion criteria also limited the extrapolation of the observations as documented in this cohort to all cases. Furthermore, except Hct, we cannot compare the nutritional status of biochemical blood test from 1- to 6-moCA. The main reason is that for the historical group, there were no regular biochemical blood tests after discharge at the follow-up clinic visit in the previous routine practice. The small sample size limits the interpretation and generalization of these results. Further studies are recommended in this area. Lastly, we use non-randomization to evaluate the program, resulting from a limitation of number of participants in a research setting.

5. Conclusions

Enlistment in a PIN program with enriched HM and formula feeding from hospital discharge to 6-moCA resulted in significantly reduced post-discharge growth restrictions for VLBW preterm babies compared to those who received unfortified HM and TF in conventional practices. Regular monitoring is needed to educate mothers or caregivers not to under- or overfeed their infants. Further lactation support and developed maternal education programs are needed to encourage continued HM feeding after discharge. Further studies are warranted with concurrent comparison groups and a longer follow-up period to analyze infant growth, neurodevelopment, and body composition.

Acknowledgments: We would like to thank the Director of Buddhasothorn Hospital for permission to conduct this study in the hospital and the NICU and hospital staff for coordination and assistance with providing the data. We also thank Dechavudh Nityasuddhi for attentive support and for his suggestions regarding statistical analysis. The study was partially funded by the Cerebos Health Research Foundation for Thai Society.

Author Contributions: S.J. was the principal investigator and carried out data collection. C.S. was responsible for overall supervision including the concept of the study, steps in the preterm infant nutrition program evaluation and data collection. S.J., C.S., U.S., B.C., M.K. and S.N. made contributions to the design of the study and the content validity of the nutrition program. U.S. invited and consulted with the experts on content validity of the protocol. S.N. provided substantial assistance with program implementation and research planning. J.S. was involved in the literature review and drafting of the manuscript. M.K. made contributions in coordination and program arrangements during S.J.'s Japan visit for conceptualization of the project proposal and assisted in editing the manuscript. C.S. revised the content and approved the final draft manuscript and all authors read and approved the final manuscript.

Conflicts of Interest: The authors declare no conflict of interest.

References

1. Afjeh, S.A.; Sabzehei, M.K.; Fallahi, M.; Esmaili, F. Outcome of very low birth weight infants over three years report from an Iranian center. *Iran. J. Pediatr.* **2013**, *23*, 579–587. [PubMed]
2. Fanaroff, A.A.; Stoll, B.J.; Wright, L.L.; Carlo, W.A.; Ehrenkranz, R.A.; Starh, A.R.; Bauer, C.R.; Donovan, E.F.; Korones, S.B.; Laptook, A.R.; et al. Trend in neonatal morbidity and mortality of very low birth weight infants. *Am. J. Obstet. Gynecol.* **2007**, *196*, 147–148. [CrossRef] [PubMed]
3. Ruegger, C.; Hegglin, M.; Adams, M.; The Swiss Neonatal Network. Population based trends in mortality, morbidity and treatment for very preterm and very low birthweight infants over 12 years. *BMC Pediatr.* **2012**, *12*. [CrossRef] [PubMed]
4. Euser, A.M.; de Wit, C.C.; Finken, M.J.; Rijken, M.; Wit, J.M. Growth of preterm born children. *Horm. Res. Paediatr.* **2008**, *70*, 319–328. [CrossRef] [PubMed]
5. De Curtis, M.; Rigo, J. Entrauterine growth restriction in very-low-birthweight infants. *Acta Pediatr.* **2004**, *93*, 1563–1568. [CrossRef]
6. Griffin, I.J.; Tancredi, D.J.; Bertino, E.; Lee, H.C.; Profit, J. Postnatal growth failure in very low birthweight infants born between 2005 and 2012. *Arch. Dis. Child. Fetal Neonatal Ed.* **2016**, *101*, F50–F55. [CrossRef] [PubMed]
7. McLeod, G.; Sherriff, J.; Patole, S. Post-discharge nutrition for high-risk preterm neonates. In *Nutrition for the Preterm Neonate: A Clinical Perspective*, 1st ed.; Patole, S., Ed.; Springer: Dordrecht, The Netherlands; Heidelberg, Germany; London, UK; New York, NY, USA, 2013; pp. 173–185.
8. Suppo, L.M.; Rugolo, S. Growth and developmental outcomes of the extremely preterm infant. *J. Pediatr.* **2005**, *81*, S101–S110.
9. Dusick, A.M.; Poindexter, B.B.; Ehrenkranz, R.A.; Lemons, J.A. Growth failure in the preterm infant: Can we catch up? *Semin. Perinatol.* **2003**, *27*, 302–310. [CrossRef]
10. Su, B.H. Optimizing nutrition in preterm infants. *Pediatr. Neonatol.* **2014**, *55*, 5–13. [CrossRef] [PubMed]
11. Morgan, C. Early amino acid administration in very preterm infants: Too little, too late or too much, too soon? *Semin. Fetal Neonatal Med.* **2013**, *18*, 160–165. [CrossRef] [PubMed]
12. Lee, B.S. Nutritional strategy of early amino acid administration in very low birth weight infants. *Korean J. Pediatr.* **2015**, *58*, 77–83. [CrossRef] [PubMed]
13. Yuen, D.E. Feeding premature infants after hospital discharge. *Paediatr. Child Health* **1998**, *3*, 307–308. [PubMed]
14. Menezes, M.A.; Garcia, D.C.; de Melo, E.V.; Cipolotti, R. Preterm newborns at Kangaroo Mother Care: A cohort follow-up from birth to six months. *Rev. Paul. Pediatr.* **2014**, *32*, 171–177. [CrossRef] [PubMed]
15. Authority, O.H. Nutrition Practice Care Guidelines for Preterm Infants in the Community. Available online: http://public.health.oregon.gov/HealthPeopleFamilies/wic/Documents/preterm.pdf (accessed on 16 January 2014).
16. Adamkin, D.H. *Nutritional Strategies for Very Low Birth Weight Infants*; Cambridge University Press: New York, NY, USA, 2009; pp. 101–108.
17. Dall'Agnola, A.; Beghini, L. Post-discharge supplementation of vitamins and minerals for preterm neonates. *Early Hum. Dev.* **2009**, *85*, S27–S29. [CrossRef] [PubMed]
18. Teller, I.C.; Embleton, N.D.; Griffin, I.J.; van Elberg, R.M. Post-discharge formula feeding in preterm infants: A systematic review mapping evedence about role of micronutrient enrichment. *Clin. Nutr.* **2016**, *35*, 791–801. [CrossRef] [PubMed]
19. Aimone, A.; Rovet, J.; Ward, W.; Jereries, A.; Campbell, D.M.; Asztalos, E.; Feldman, M.; Vaughan, J.; Westall, C.; Whyte, H.; et al. Growth and body composition of human milk-fed premature infants provided with extra energy and nutrients early after hospital discharge: 1-year follow-up. *J. Pediatr. Gastroenterol. Nutr.* **2009**, *49*, 456–466. [CrossRef] [PubMed]
20. Ors, R. The practical aspects of enteral nutrition in preterm infants. *J. Pediatr. Neonatal Individ. Med.* **2013**, *2*, 35–40.
21. Arthur, P.G.; Hartmann, P.E.; Smith, M. Measurement of the milk intake of breast-fed infants. *J. Pediatr. Gastroenterol. Nutr.* **1987**, *6*, 758–763. [CrossRef] [PubMed]

22. ESPGHAN Committee on Nutrition; Aggett, P.J.; Agostoni, C.; Axelsson, I.; De Curtis, M.; Goulet, O.; Hernell, O.; Koletzko, B.; Lafeber, H.N.; Michaelsen, K.F.; et al. Feeding preterm infants after hospital discharge. *J. Pediatr. Gastroenterol. Nutr.* **2006**, *42*, 596–603. [CrossRef] [PubMed]

23. Agostoni, C.; Buonocore, G.; Carnielli, V.P.; de Curtis, M.; Darmaun, D.; Decsi, T.; Domellof, M.; Embleton, N.D.; Fusch, C.; Genzel-Boroviczeny, O.; et al. Enteral nutrient supply for preterm infants: Commentary from the European Society of Paediatric Gastroenterology, Hepatology and Nutrition Committee on Nutrition. *J. Pediatr. Gastroenterol. Nutr.* **2010**, *50*, 85–91. [CrossRef] [PubMed]

24. Arslanoglu, S.; Bertino, E.; Coscia, A.; Tonetto, P.; Giuliani, F.; Moro, G.E. Update of adjustable fortification regimen for preterm infants: A new protocol. *J. Biol. Regul. Homeost. Agents* **2012**, *26*, 65–67. [PubMed]

25. Dutta, S.; Singh, B.; Chessell, L.; Wilson, J.; Janes, M.; McDonald, K.; Shahid, S.; Gardner, V.A.; Hjartarson, A.; Purcha, M.; et al. Guidelines for feeding very low birth weight infants. *Nutrients* **2015**, *7*, 423–442. [CrossRef] [PubMed]

26. Enrico, B.; Nicola, P.D.; Giuliani, F.; Peila, C.; Cester, E.; Vassia, C.; Pirra, A.; Tonetto, P.; Coscia, A. Benefits of human milk in preterm infant feeding. *J. Pediatr. Neonatal Individ. Med.* **2012**, *1*, 19–24.

27. Dewey, K.G. Energy and protein requirements during lactation. *Annu. Rev. Nutr.* **1997**, *17*, 19–36. [CrossRef] [PubMed]

28. Raiten, D.J.; Kalhan, S.C.; Hay, W.W., Jr. Maternal nutrition and optimal infant feeding practices: Executive summary. *Am. J. Clin. Nutr.* **2007**, *85*, S577–S583.

29. Turck, D. Safety Aspects in Preparation and Handling of Infant Food. *Ann. Nutr. Metab.* **2012**, *60*, 211–214. [CrossRef] [PubMed]

30. Agostoni, C.; Axelsson, I.; Goulet, O.; Koletzko, B.; Michaelsen, K.F.; Puntis, J.W.; Rigo, J.; Shamir, R.; Szajewska, H.; Turck, D.; et al. Preparation and handling of powdered infant formula: A commentary by the ESPGHAN Committee on Nutrition. *J. Pediatr. Gastroenterol. Nutr.* **2004**, *39*, 320–322. [CrossRef] [PubMed]

31. Thakur, S.K.; Roy, S.K.; Paul, K.; Khanam, M.; Khatun, W.; Sarker, D. Effect of nutrition education on exclusive breastfeeding for nutritional outcome of low birth weight babies. *Eur. J. Clin. Nutr.* **2012**, *66*, 376–381. [CrossRef] [PubMed]

32. Benzies, K.M.; Magill-Evans, J.E.; Hayden, K.A.; Ballantyne, M. Key components of early intervention programs for preterm infants and their parents: A systematic review and meta-analysis. *BMC Pregnancy Childbirth* **2013**, *13*, S10. [CrossRef] [PubMed]

33. Fanaro, S.; Borsari, G.; Vigi, V. Complementary feeding practices in preterm Infants: An observational study in a Cohort of Italian infants. *J. Pediatr. Gastroenterol. Nutr.* **2007**, *45*, S210–S214. [CrossRef] [PubMed]

34. Krebs, N.F.; Hambidge, K.M. Complementary feeding: Clinically relevant factors affecting timing and composition. *Am. J. Clin. Nutr.* **2007**, *85*, S639–S645.

35. Sanchez-Carrillo, C.; Padilla, B.; Marin, M.; Rivera, M.; Cercenado, E.; Vigil, D.; Sanchez-Luna, M.; Bouza, E. Contaminated feeding bottles: The source of an outbreak of *Pseudomonas aeruginosa* infections in a neonatal intensive care unit. *Am. J. Infect. Control* **2009**, *37*, 150–154. [CrossRef] [PubMed]

36. Suthutvoravut, U.; Tuntrachewathorn, S.; Khunsanong, S. *Manual of Complementary Feeding for Infants and Toddlers*; Beyond Enterprise: Bangkok, Thailand, 2009; pp. 5–36.

37. Anemia of Prematurity. Available online: http://emedicine.medscape.com/article/978238 (accessed on 23 August 2015).

38. Abrams, S.A. Calcium and vitamin D requirements of enterally fed preterm infants. *Pediatrics* **2013**, *131*, e1676–e1683. [CrossRef] [PubMed]

39. Gidrewicz, D.A.; Fenton, T.R. A systematic review and meta-analysis of the nutrient content of preterm and term breast milk. *BMC Pediatr.* **2014**, *14*, 216. [CrossRef] [PubMed]

40. Boyce, C.; Watson, M.; Lazidis, G.; Reeve, S.; Dods, K.; Simmer, K.; McLeod, G. Preterm human milk composition: A systematic literature review. *Br. J. Nutr.* **2016**, *116*, 1033–1045. [CrossRef] [PubMed]

41. Fenton, T.R.; Kim, J.H. A systematic review and meta-analysis to revise the Fenton growth chart for preterm infants. *BMC Pediatr.* **2013**, *13*, 59. [CrossRef] [PubMed]

42. Rao, S.C.; Tompkins, J.; World Health Organization. Growth curves for preterm infants. *Early Hum. Dev.* **2007**, *83*, 643–651. [CrossRef] [PubMed]

43. Bhatia, J. Growth curves: How to best measure growth of the preterm infant. *J. Pediatr.* **2013**, *162*, S2–S6. [CrossRef] [PubMed]

44. Cao, W.; Zhang, Y.H.; Zhao, D.Y.; Xia, H.P.; Zhu, T.W.; Xie, L.J. Risk factors for extrauterine growth restriction in preterm infants with gestational age less than 34 weeks. *Zhongguo Dang Dai Er Ke Za Zhi* **2015**, *17*, 453–458. [PubMed]

45. Casey, P.H. Growth of low birth weight preterm children. *Semin. Perinatol.* **2008**, *32*, 20–27. [CrossRef] [PubMed]

46. Young, L.; Embleton, N.D.; McCormick, F.M.; McGuire, W. Multinutrient fortification of human breast milk for preterm infants following hospital discharge. *Cochrane Database Syst. Rev.* **2013**, *28*, CD004866.

47. Young, L.; Morgan, J.; McCormick, F.M.; McGuire, W. Nutrient-enriched formula versus standard term formula for preterm infants following hospital discharge. *Cocharne Database Syst. Rev.* **2012**, *14*, CD004696.

48. Kuschel, C.A.; Harding, J.E. Multicomponent fortified human milk for promoting growth in preterm infants. *Cochrane Database Syst. Rev.* **2004**, *1*, CD000343.

49. Adamkin, D. Postdischarge nutritional therapy. *J. Perinat.* **2006**, *26*, S27–S30. [CrossRef] [PubMed]

50. Winston, W.K.; Koo, E.M.H. Posthospital discharge feeding for preterm infants: Effects of standard compared with enriched milk formula on growth, bone mass and body composition. *Am. J. Clin. Nutr.* **2006**, *84*, 1357–1364.

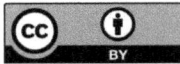

nutrients

MDPI

Article

Comparison of a Powdered, Acidified Liquid, and Non-Acidified Liquid Human Milk Fortifier on Clinical Outcomes in Premature Infants

Melissa Thoene [1,*], Elizabeth Lyden [2], Kara Weishaar [3], Elizabeth Elliott [3], Ruomei Wu [3], Katelyn White [3], Hayley Timm [3] and Ann Anderson-Berry [3]

1   Newborn Intensive Care Unit, Nebraska Medicine, 981200 Nebraska Medical Center, Omaha, NE 68198, USA
2   College of Public Health, University of Nebraska Medical Center, 984375 Nebraska Medical Center, Omaha, NE 68198-4375, USA; elyden@unmc.edu
3   Department of Pediatrics, University of Nebraska Medical Center, 981205 Nebraska Medical Center, Omaha, NE 68198-1205, USA; kara.weishaar@unmc.edu (K.W.); elizabeth.elliott@unmc.edu (E.E.); Ruomei.Wu@Creighton.edu (R.W.); katelyn.white@huskers.unl.edu (K.W.); hayley.timm@grmep.com (H.T.); alanders@unmc.edu (A.A.-B.)
*   Correspondence: mthoene@nebraskamed.com; Tel.: +1-402-559-4347

Received: 20 May 2016; Accepted: 18 July 2016; Published: 26 July 2016

Abstract: We previously compared infant outcomes between a powdered human milk fortifier (P-HMF) vs. acidified liquid HMF (AL-HMF). A non-acidified liquid HMF (NAL-HMF) is now commercially available. The purpose of this study is to compare growth and outcomes of premature infants receiving P-HMF, AL-HMF or NAL-HMF. An Institutional Review Board (IRB) approved retrospective chart review compared infant outcomes (born < 2000 g) who received one of three HMF. Growth, enteral nutrition, laboratory and demographic data were compared. 120 infants were included (P-HMF = 46, AL-HMF = 23, NAL-HMF = 51). AL-HMF infants grew slower in g/day (median 23.66 vs. P-HMF 31.27, NAL-HMF 31.74 ($p < 0.05$)) and in g/kg/day, median 10.59 vs. 15.37, 14.03 ($p < 0.0001$). AL-HMF vs. NAL-HMF infants were smaller at 36 weeks gestational age (median 2046 vs. 2404 g, $p < 0.05$). However AL-HMF infants received more daily calories ($p = 0.21$) and protein ($p < 0.0001$), mean 129 cal/kg, 4.2 g protein/kg vs. P-HMF 117 cal/kg, 3.7 g protein/kg , NAL-HMF 120 cal/kg, 4.0 g protein/kg. AL-HMF infants exhibited lower carbon dioxide levels after day of life 14 and 30 ($p < 0.0001$, $p = 0.0038$). Three AL-HMF infants (13%) developed necrotizing enterocolitis (NEC) vs. no infants in the remaining groups ($p = 0.0056$). A NAL-HMF is the most optimal choice for premature human milk-fed infants in a high acuity neonatal intensive care unit (NICU).

Keywords: human milk; fortifier; premature infant; enteral nutrition; growth; acidosis; necrotizing enterocolitis

---

1. Introduction

Premature infants have significantly increased nutrient needs compared to those born at term [1]. Nutrition-related goals for these infants must aim at promoting similar nutrient provision and growth as that achieved in utero. Providing human milk remains a preferable nutrient source over customized premature infant formulas, but alone remains inadequate to meet the high nutritional needs for rapid growth and development. Long term provision of unfortified human milk has been linked to suboptimal growth, poor bone mineralization, and multiple nutrient deficiencies of vitamins, minerals, and trace elements [1]. As a result, human milk fortifiers (HMF) are used to significantly enhance calorie, protein, vitamin, and mineral intake of the human milk fed premature infant.

Enteral macronutrient recommendations for premature infants vary according to size. The American Academy of Pediatrics on nutrition suggests 130–150 calories/kilogram (kg) and 3.8–4.4 g protein/kg/day for infants weighing <1000 g, and 110–130 calories/kg and 3.4–4.2 g protein/kg/day for infants weighing between 1000 and 1500 g [2]. Protein is highly emphasized as high adequate provision has been correlated with improved growth and neurodevelopment [3–6]. To achieve enteral protein goals, powdered or liquid protein modulars may be added alongside HMF to optimize overall nutrition.

Human milk fortifiers are available in many different compositions, specifically varying in protein type, protein amount, and form (powder vs. liquid). However if available, the Food and Drug Administration strongly recommends the use of liquid products over powder in the neonatal intensive care unit (NICU) setting in an effort to reduce contamination and infection risk [7]. Our unit originally used a powdered HMF, but transitioned to liquid form when they became commercially available. Previously, we published a study comparing two HMF used in our unit, one being a powder (P-HMF) and one being an acidified liquid (AL-HMF) [8]. Our results demonstrated that the acidified product, though sterile, caused more metabolic acidosis and poor growth in our population of premature infants. Infants receiving the AL-HMF also had a higher incidence of necrotizing enterocolitis (NEC), though we were not powered to find this. Our unit has now transitioned to using a non-acidified liquid fortifier (NAL-HMF). The purpose of this study is compare growth and clinical outcomes of infants receiving this new HMF to the previous two fortifier groups.

2. Patients and Methods

2.1. Participants and Data Collection

The institutional review board at the University of Nebraska Medical Center (Omaha, NE, USA) approved this study. Data was retrospectively collected from inpatient electronic medical records of all infants admitted to the NICU between August 2012 and July 2014 if they met the following criteria; birth weight (BW) < 2000 g, received at least 25% of enteral feedings as fortified human milk (with the NAL-HMF) during their NICU stay, and remained in the NICU at least 14 days. Exclusion criteria included infants with congenital abnormalities or conditions that inhibited growth, such as Trisomy 13. No infants were excluded based on clinical acuity, intrauterine growth restriction, APGAR score, or ventilator requirements.

Data on the P-HMF and AL-HMF groups was previously collected for infants admitted to the NICU between October 2009 and July 2011. The AL-HMF group contained a lower number of included infants due to this HMF being used for a limited time period. Six investigators familiar with the electronic medical record obtained all data for the NAL-HMF group in a similar manner as the original groups. Data was reviewed closely for accuracy and corrected if an electronic error occurred. Available data on each infant was included in the analysis and is displayed in the tables.

2.2. Demographics and Clinical Outcomes

Demographic information was collected for all infants including gender, gestational age at birth and discharge, and day of life (DOL) at discharge. Additional clinical outcomes were collected as available including presence of bronchopulmonary dysplasia (BPD) defined as oxygen requirement at 36 weeks estimated gestational age (EGA), retinopathy of prematurity (ROP) Stage 2 or greater, Grade 3 or 4 intraventricular hemorrhage (IVH), NEC, and death. Treatment requirements were also analyzed including need for intraventricular shunt, ROP procedure, and Dexamethasone use.

2.3. Growth and Nutrition

Infants were weighed daily on a gram (g) scale, and length and head circumference measurements (cm = centimeters) were taken weekly using a measuring tape by nursing staff. Percentile rankings from the Fenton growth chart were electronically plotted for each documented measurement. Weight, length, and head circumference measurements were recorded for infants at birth and 36 weeks EGA if still hospitalized. An EGA of 36 weeks was empirically selected as an equivalent point of analysis for growth prior to discharge.

Enteral feeding data collected included DOL enteral feedings were initiated and DOL full enteral feedings were reached. Full enteral feedings was defined as the infant receiving at least 140 milliliters (mL)/kilogram (kg)/day of fortified enteral feedings and no parenteral nutrition. Average calorie and protein intake measured in per kg/day was analyzed for infants who received at least 50% of their feedings as fortified human milk during NICU stay. Intake was analyzed from the start of full feedings until the HMF was discontinued or the infant received <50% of feedings as fortified milk. Growth as measured in g/day and g/kg/day was calculated for infants during the time of reaching full enteral feedings until they received <50% of feedings as fortified milk. Maximum caloric density of feedings was recorded for each infant. Number of days on caloric densities higher than the standard 24 calories/ounce was collected for infants requiring more to maintain growth chart percentiles for weight. Nutrient provision was captured by an electronic medical system (Intuacare), which contained protein references based on the caloric density of specified formulas or fortified human milk. Nursing staff recorded daily intake (in mL) of specified feedings, and daily calorie and protein per kilogram was electronically calculated using the daily recorded weight. The electronic system also calculated the percentage of human milk vs. infant formula received according to nursing documentation.

2.4. Comparison and Use of Human Milk Fortifiers

Comparison of ingredients and key HMF nutrients are listed in Table 1 according to online nutritional references [9–11].

Table 1. Comparison of primary nutrients and ingredients of the powdered, acidified liquid, and non-acidified liquid HMF.

24-Calorie-Per-Ounce Fortified Human Milk [9–11]			
Per 100 mL	**P-HMF**	**AL-HMF**	**NAL-HMF**
Protein (g)	2.35 g	3.2 g	2.34 g
Iron (mg)	0.46 mg	1.85 mg	0.46
Calcium (mg)	138 mg	141 mg	138
Phosphorus (mg)	78 mg	78 mg	77
Vitamin D (IU)	119 IU	200 IU	118
pH	—	4.7	—
Osmolality (mOsm/kg water)	385	326	385
Primary Fortifier Macronutrient Ingredients	nonfat milk, whey protein concentrate, corn syrup solids, medium-chain triglycerides (MCT oil)	water, whey protein isolate hydrolysate (milk), medium chain triglycerides (MCT oil), vegetable oil (soy and high oleic sunflower oils)	water, nonfat milk, corn syrup solids, medium-chain triglycerides (MCT oil), whey protein concentrate

– Information not available. P-HMF, powdered human milk fortifier; AL-HMF, acidified liquid HMF; NAL-HMF, non-acidified liquid HMF.

Enteral feeding are initiated in this NICU as soon as able following birth, within the first one to three days of life using maternal breast milk (MBM) as available or donor human milk (from the Milk Bank of Austin, Texas) at 20 mL/kg/day. Trophic feedings are continued for three to five days at the discretion of the attending neonatologist. Feedings are then advanced by 20 mL/kg/day and HMF is added when enteral volumes feedings reach 80–100 mL/kg. A protein modular is also added once caloric densities reach 24 calories/ounce to optimize protein intake to approximately 4 g/kg/day. The calories provided from the protein modular are accounted for in the calorie-per-ounce estimates. The P-HMF group received a powdered protein modular and the NAL-HMF group received a liquid protein modular. No additional protein modular was provided to infants receiving the AL-HMF due to higher protein content of the fortifier. All infants are transitioned off of donor human milk to 24 calorie/ounce high protein (3.5 g protein per 100 calories) premature infant formula at 14 days of life if a supplement to MBM is needed. We did not analyze differences in donor human milk use between groups because it is only used for a short period after birth and is provided to all infants in a similar manner. There were no other nutrition practice changes during the periods of different fortifier use. Our unit follows a written feeding protocol, so nutrition is managed closely and remains consistent among providers.

2.5. Laboratory Measurements

Lowest carbon dioxide (CO_2) lab values were collected after DOL 14 and 30 for all infants, if available. Values were not collected prior to eliminate values reflective of parenteral nutrition support and unfortified enteral feedings. Maximum blood urea nitrogen (BUN) while on full enteral feedings was additionally collected.

2.6. Data Analysis

The Kruskal Wallis test was used to compare continuous data between the three HMF groups. If the overall p-value was significant, indicating a significant difference between at least two of the three groups, the Dunn's post hoc test for three pair wise comparisons (i.e., Group 1 vs. 2, Group 1 vs. 3, Group 2 vs. 3) was performed. Associations of categorical variables were assessed with the Fisher's exact test. Time to weaning off oxygen distributions were estimated using the method of Kaplan and Meier and were compared using the log-rank test. A *p*-value < 0.05 was considered statistically significant.

To assess the difference in growth patterns between infants, a mixed effects model was used. We included random slopes and intercepts for each subject to capture individual growth pattern as well as fixed effects for group and day and a group day interaction term. A significant interacting of day and group indicated differing growth patterns based on group. Growth Velocity (GV) was calculated using the following equation [12]:

$$GV = [1000 \times \ln(Wn/W1)]/(D_n - D_1) \tag{1}$$

Where W_n refers to the weight on the last evaluated day; W_1 refers to the first weight; D_n refers to the last day of the time period evaluated and; D_1 refers to the first day of the time period evaluated.

3. Results

There were 46 infants in the P-HMF, 23 in the AL-HMF, and 51 in the NAL-HMF groups. There were no significant differences in gender (*p* = 0.6) or baseline characteristics as shown in Table 2. Clinical outcomes are displayed in Table 3. Laboratory, growth, and nutrition data are displayed in Table 4.

Table 2. Baseline characteristics of subjects by group.

Variable	P-HMF (Group 1)		AL-HMF (Group 2)		NAL-HMF (Group 3)		Overall *p*-Value
	n	Median	*n*	Median	*n*	Median	
EGA at Birth	46	29.15	22	31.00	51	29.60	0.15
Birth Weight (g)	46	1305	22	1481	51	1340	0.21
Weight at 36 Weeks EGA (g)	44	2179	18	2046	50	2404	0.0092 Group 2 vs. 3 *p* < 0.05
Birth Length (cm)	46	39	22	41	51	39	0.14
Length at 36 Weeks EGA (cm)	42	44.5	18	43.5	47	44	0.38
Birth HC (cm)	46	27	22	27.75	51	27.5	0.53
HC at 36 Weeks EGA (cm)	42	32.5	18	31.75	47	32.2	0.55

EGA = Estimated Gestational Age; HC = Head Circumference.

Table 3. Clinical outcomes of subjects by group.

Variable	P-HMF (Group 1) n = 46	AL-HMF (Group 2) n = 23	NAL-HMF (Group 3) n = 51	Overall *p*-Value
	n (%)	*n (%)*	*n (%)*	
NEC	0	3 (13%)	0	0.0056
ROP	16 (35%)	3 (13%)	4 (8%)	0.0030 Group 1 vs. 3, *p* = 0.006
ROP Procedure	3 (7%)	2 (9%)	1 (2%)	0.24
IVH (Grade 3 or 4)	3 (7%)	1 (5%)	4 (8%)	1.00
Intraventricular Shunt	0	0	0	N/A
Dexamethasone Treatment	9 (20%)	1 (5%)	7 (14%)	0.29
Death	0	0	1 (2%)	1.00
BPD	10/40 (25%)	4/18 (22%)	16/49 (33%)	0.65

Table 4. Laboratory, growth, and enteral nutrition data.

Variable	P-HMF (Group 1)		AL-HMF (Group 2)		NAL-HMF (Group 3)		Overall *p*-Value
	n	Median	*n*	Median	*n*	Median	
Mean Daily Calorie Provision (per kg)	42	117	18	129	48	120	0.21
Mean Daily Protein Provision (g/kg)	42	3.7	18	4.2	48	4.0	0.0001 Group 1 vs. 2 and Group 2 vs. 3, *p* <0.05
Day of Life Feedings Started	46	1	22	1	51	1	0.0019 Group 1 vs. 3 *p* < 0.05
Day of Life Full Feedings Achieved	46	12	22	10	51	9	0.0007 Group 1vs. 3 *p* < 0.05
Growth on HMF (g/day)	45	31.27	21	23.66	49	31.74	0.0001 Group 1 vs. 2 and Group 2 vs. 3, *p* < 0.05
Growth on HMF (g/kg/day)	45	15.37	21	10.59	49	14.03	<0.0001 Group 1 vs. 2 and Group 2 vs. 3, *p* < 0.05
BUN Maximum on Full Feedings	33	17	17	19	47	16	0.43
CO_2 Minimum after DOL 14	33	23	17	19	32	27	<0.0001 Group 1 vs. 3 and Group 2 vs. 3, 0.05
CO_2 Minimum after DOL 30	23	25	9	20	18	25.5	0.0038 Group 1 vs. 2 and Group 2 vs. 3, *p* < 0.05

3.1. Clinical Outcomes

All laboratory data analyzed for this study was collected for clinical purposes. Median lowest CO_2 levels while on full enteral feedings were significantly lower in the AL-HMF group compared to the other two groups after both DOL 14 and DOL 30 ($p < 0.0001$, $p = 0.0038$). Maximum BUN levels on full enteral feedings were similar among all groups and were not statistically significant.

The incidence of NEC was significantly higher in the AL-HMF group compared to the P-HMF and NAL-HMF groups (13% vs. 0% and 0%, $p = 0.0056$), though we were not powered to evaluate this variable. Incidence of ROP was significantly higher among the P-HMF than the NAL-HMF group (35% vs. 8%, $p = 0.003$). There were no differences in rates of BPD or IVH (Grade 3 or 4) among all groups.

3.2. Enteral Growth and Nutrition

Growth, as measured in both g/day and g/kg/day, was statistically significant between groups. More specifically, infants in the AL-HMF group grew slower than infants in the P-HMF and NAL-HMF groups. Median growth in g/day from start of full enteral feedings until 36 weeks EGA was 23.66, compared to 31.27 in the P-HMF and 31.74 in the NA-LHMF group ($p = 0.0001$). Median growth in g/kg/day was 10.59 in the AL-HMF group, compared to 15.37 and 14.03 respectively ($p < 0.0001$). Infants in the AL-HMF group were smaller at 36 weeks EGA compared to the NAL-HMF group (median 2046 g vs. 2404 g, $p = 0.0092$), though there were no differences in length or head circumference. There were no differences in Dexamethasone use among groups ($p = 0.15$) that may account for reduced growth. Infants in the NAL-HMF group started enteral feedings and achieved full enteral feedings faster than the P-HMF group ($p = 0.0019$, $p = 0.0007$), but these infants achieved similar growth.

Among infants receiving >50% of their feedings during NICU stay as fortified human milk , infants in the AL-HMF group received more protein at mean 4.2 g/kg/day compared to 3.7 and 4.0 g/kg/day in the P-HMF and NAL-HMF groups ($p < 0.0001$). These infants also received a higher mean calorie intake at 129 calories/kg, compared to 117 and 120 calories/kg, respectively, though this was not significant ($p = 0.21$).

There were no differences in maximum caloric density of enteral feedings ($p = 0.6$) or the number of days on feedings >24 calories/ounce ($p = 0.21$). Noted however, is that 48% of infants in the AL-HMF group received enteral feedings >24 calorie/ounce compared to 26% in the P-HMF group and 35% in the NAL-HMF group.

4. Discussion

Our previous research analyzing the P-HMF and AL-HMF suggested the P-HMF was the more optimal choice in promoting best clinical outcomes [8]. Now comparing data among all three fortifier groups, the NAL-HMF appears to be the most successful fortifier for use in a high acuity NICU population. Despite achieving adequate similar growth, the NAL-HMF is more desirable than the P-HMF due to its composition as a sterile liquid. When compared to the AL-HMF, the NAL-HMF promoted greater growth and was not associated with metabolic acidosis or NEC.

4.1. Growth and Enteral Nutrition

Appropriate growth was best achieved among the NAL-HMF and P-HMF groups when comparing both g/day and g/kg/day weight gain. Infants receiving the NAL-HMF attained the highest weight among all three groups at 36 weeks EGA, demonstrating most significance when compared to the AL-HMF group (median 2046 g vs. 2404 g, $p < 0.0092$). In further comparison of this, the median length and head circumference for both the acidified and non-acidified liquid group at this point plotted between the 25%–30% on the Fenton growth chart. By comparison of median weights at 36 weeks, the NAL-HMF group plotted around the 18% and the AL-HMF group plotted at the 5th. This demonstrates that infants receiving the NAL-HMF were able to achieve a more proportional weight-for-length ratio. Though we did not directly assess infant acuity level between groups, we do not suspect this to be a significant factor for decreased growth given the AL-HMF group having similar baseline characteristics as the other groups.

As growth remains a high priority, infants with suboptimal growth were fed enteral feedings with caloric densities >24 calories/ounce. Suboptimal growth was determined by clinical evaluation when an infant was unable to maintain growth percentiles for weight. Despite decreased growth, more infants in the AL-HMF (48%) group required increased caloric density of feedings compared to the P-HMF (26%) and NAL-HMF (35%) groups, $p = 0.6$. The AL-HMF group also received higher mean calorie intake compared to the other two groups. Had no infants been advanced to increased caloric densities, it is likely that the discrepancy of growth between the AL-HMF and the remaining two groups would have been of even greater significance. It may be theorized that additional enteral additives and higher caloric densities contributed to a higher incidence of NEC in the AL-HMF group. However, our previously low recorded rate of NEC at 3% is reflective of similar fortification practices to achieve desired growth [13]. Despite individual theories for these NEC occurrences, we must address why the additional additives were required in the first place to achieve adequate growth.

In additional to increased calories, infants in the AL-HMF group also received a higher mean protein intake compared to the other groups. Higher protein provisions have been linked to improved growth, yet these infants exhibited poor weight gain. We hypothesize that the acidification of the AL-HMF may be the explanatory factor in this conundrum. A study by Erickson et al. concluded that acidifying human milk resulted in 14% decrease in protein and a 56% decrease in lipase activity [14]. This may result in partial fat malabsorption and resulting poor energy intake. A recent study by Cibulskis and Armbrecht comparing infants receiving an acidified vs. powdered HMF did not report significant growth differences in weight, length, or head circumference between birth and discharge [15]. However, growth measured in g/day while on the HMF approached significance as infants receiving the acidified HMF grew slower (22.3 vs. 19.2 g/day, $p = 0.08$). In comparison, Moya et al. reported no discrepancies in weight gain when comparing infants $\leqslant$1250 g receiving either an acidified or powdered HMF, and further reported that infants receiving the acidified HMF had improved linear growth [16]. Limitations of this study, however, include that protein modulars were used infrequently among infants, so baseline protein provisions were higher in the acidified HMF group. This study also excluded infants with low APGAR scores and higher respiratory requirements so may not be applicable to the most fragile infants.

4.2. NEC

The only infants who developed NEC received the AL-HMF. Though not statistically powered to find NEC, the results raise concern from a clinical standpoint. Our feeding practices have remained consistent outside of which HMF was used, and we have documented low baseline rates of NEC on these feeding practices [13]. Feeding initiation and advancement remained fairly consistent across all three groups. While infants in the NAL-HMF group achieved full feedings more quickly, none developed NEC. Formula was utilized equally in all groups when MBM was limited and donor human milk was weaned.

The primary differences in enteral feedings between all fortifier groups are the acidity, high protein, and high iron content of the AL-HMF. Theoretically, infants receiving the AL-HMF had a reduced risk for cross-contamination due to the HMF composition as a sterile liquid and because additional enteral substrates (protein modular, iron) were not required. These infants also received lower osmolality feedings at baseline, and furthermore as additional supplements were not required due to the high iron and protein in the AL-HMF. A study by *Chan* suggests that a high iron-containing HMF compared to a low iron-containing HMF negates the antimicrobial effects of human milk against the growth of *E. coli*, Staphylococcus, Enterobacter, and Streptococcus [17]. Erickson et al. also noted a reduced white cell count by 76% in human milk acidified to a pH of 4.5, questioning if this decreases an infant's host defense [14]. The AL-HMF used in our study acidifies milk similarly to a pH of 4.7. We must consider if the protective effects of human milk were compromised in infants receiving the AL-HMF, making them more susceptible to infections. A limitation to this theory is that we did not analyze the incidence of sepsis between groups. As the cause of these NEC occurrences remains unknown, we can neither confirm nor exclude use of the AL-HMF as a primary contributor.

4.3. Acidosis

There was a higher incidence of metabolic acidosis in the AL-HMF group compared to the other two groups. As discussed in our previous study, premature infants are at risk for developing metabolic acidosis secondary to immature renal and metabolic processes [8]. There were no significant differences in baseline characteristics such as birth weight or gestational age to suggest any of the three groups included infants that were smaller or born more prematurely, and therefore more obviously susceptible to acidosis. We do not suspect protein provision as a contributor to acidosis. While infants receiving the AL-HMF received higher daily protein ($p < 0.001$), mean values remained within the reference ranges for very low birth weight infants of 3.4–4.4 g protein/kg/day [2]. BUN levels also remained similar among groups.

While the P-HMF and NAL-HMF do not have defined pH values as shown in Table 1, we suspect they have limited effects on the final pH of fortified milk, unlike the AL-HMF. Considering a similar baseline of other characteristics, we again hypothesize that the acidification of the AL-HMF contributed to this metabolic imbalance. Our results are concurrent with Cibulskis and Armbrecht who reported a higher incidence of metabolic acidosis (54% vs. 10%) in infants <32 weeks EGA or <1500 g receiving an acidified vs. powdered HMF [15]. Moya et al. also reported a lower pH at day of life 14 ($p = 0.004$) and lower carbon dioxide levels at both day of life 14 ($p < 0.001$) and 30 ($p = 0.021$) in infants ⩽1250 g receiving an acidified HMF [16].

Development of metabolic acidosis may also contribute to altered weight gain and poor nutritional consequences. A small study by Rochow et al. reported lower weight gain (median 9 vs. 21 g/kg/day, $p < 0.01$) in infants <34 weeks EGA who developed metabolic acidosis compared to those who remained unaffected [18]. It was also reported that infants who developed metabolic acidosis had a lower bone density at discharge. Likewise, an early study by Kalhoff et al. analyzed urinary excretion of minerals in premature infants, concluding that a higher amount of calcium and phosphorus is excreted during metabolic acidosis [19]. Resultantly, we suggest using a NAL-HMF to provide appropriate growth, without increasing risk for metabolic acidosis and suboptimal nutrient accretion.

4.4. Strengths and Limitations

This study is the first to quantify nutrition and growth outcomes of three HMF in a Level IIIc NICU. We did not exclude infants based on acuity, such as presence of IVH, need for high ventilatory settings, or low APGAR scores. Our high inclusion is more reflective of a standard NICU population, and therefore provides genuine outcomes for both high and moderate acuity infants. This is both relevant and applicable to current NICU settings. Nutrition is managed closely and consistently in our unit, and our current nutrition practices have been published demonstrating excellent growth and low baseline rates of NEC [13]. Additionally unique to our study is the use of protein modulars to provide infants similar protein provisions at baseline (approximately 4 g protein/kg/day when receiving 120 calories/kg/day), and reducing this as a significant confounding factor across fortifier groups.

Limitations of this study include that it is retrospective, and there is a limited number of subjects in the AL-HMF group due to its short term use. Additionally included is our reliance on electronic documentation for data collection, as we cannot quantify unrecorded or misrecorded data. However, the system does allow for review of daily entered data for each subject if needed. Evaluation of head circumference and length measurements may vary among nursing staff due to differences in measuring tape placement. Additionally, growth measurements were unavailable for infants discharged prior to 36 weeks EGA. Growth at 36 weeks EGA may also be partially reflective of formula use if MBM was no longer available. However, it may also provide indication of early growth failure while on MBM if growth percentiles are low or fall drastically from those at birth. The calculated provision for calories and protein in fortified human milk were estimated according to manufacturer information for each HMF. These may only serve as general estimates for our comparisons as the composition of human milk varies continuously. While standard NICU practices remain consistent, feedings may be advanced differently based on each infant's clinical status. Length of trophic feedings may also impact the day of life to achieving full enteral feedings. As in our previous study of the original two fortifiers, NEC was statistically significant despite our limited power to find this.

5. Conclusions

The NAL-HMF is an appropriate choice for use in a high level NICU. Caution should be taken when using an acidified HMF due to its potential effects on growth, tolerance, and metabolic acidosis.

Author Contributions: M.T. and A.A.-B. conceived and designed the study; M.T., K.W., E.E., R.W., K.W., and H.T. performed all required data collection for the study experiment; E.L. analyzed the data; M.T. and A.A.B. wrote the paper.

Conflicts of Interest: A. Anderson-Berry has received financial compensation as a speaker for Mead Johnson and Abbott Nutrition, as well as a monetary grant from Gerber Foundation. Mead Johnson, Abbott Nutrition, and the Gerber Foundation had no role in the funding or design of the study; in the collection, analyses, or interpretation of the data; in the writing of the manuscript, and in the decision to publish the results. The remaining authors declare no conflicts of interest.

References

1. Groh-Wargo, S.; Thompson, M.; Hovasi Cox, J.H. *Nutritional Care for High.-Risk Newborns*, 3rd ed.; Hartline, J.V., Ed.; Precept Press, Inc.: Chicago, IL, USA, 2000.
2. American Academy of Pediatrics. *Pediatric Nutrition Handbook*, 6th ed.; American Academy of Pediatrics: Washington, DC, USA, 2009; pp. 79–81.
3. Wagner, J.; Hanson, C.; Anderson-Berry, A. Considerations in meeting protein needs of the human milk-fed preterm infant. *Adv. Neonatal Care* **2014**, *14*, 281–289. [CrossRef] [PubMed]
4. Fenton, T.R.; Premji, S.S.; Al-Wassia, H.; Sauve, R.S. Higher versus lower protein intake in formula-fed low birth weight infants. *Cochrane Database Syst. Rev.* **2014**, *4*, CD003959. [CrossRef] [PubMed]
5. Ramel, S.E.; Gray, H.L.; Christiansen, E.; Boys, C.; Georgieff, M.K.; Demerath, E.W. Greater early gains in fat-free mass, but not fat mass, are associated with improved neurodevelopment at 1 year corrected age for prematurity in very low birth weight preterm infants. *J. Pediatr.* **2016**, *173*, 105–115. [CrossRef] [PubMed]
6. Yang, J.; Chang, S.S.; Poon, W.B. Relationship between amino acid and energy intake and long-term growth and neurodevelopmental outcomes in very-low-birth-weight infants. *JPEN J. Parenter. Enter. Nutr.* **2016**, *40*, 820–826. [CrossRef] [PubMed]
7. Taylor, C.J. Health Professionals Letter on *Enterobacter sakazakii* Infections Associated With Use of Powdered (Dry) Infant Formulas in Neonatal Intensive Care Units. US Department of Health and Human Services, 2002. Available online: http://www.fda.gov/Food/RecallsOutbreaksEmergencies/SafetyAlertsAdvisories/ucm111299.htm (accessed on 24 May 2016).
8. Thoene, M.; Hanson, C.; Lyden, E.; Dugick, L.; Ruybal, L.; Anderson-Berry, A. Comparison of the effect of two human milk fortifiers on clinical outcomes in premature infants. *J. Nutr.* **2014**, *6*, 261–275. [CrossRef] [PubMed]
9. Abbott Nutrition Similac Human Milk Fortifier. Available online: http://abbottnutrition.com/brands/products/similac-human-milk-fortifier (accessed on 29 January 2015).
10. Enfamil Human Milk Fortifier Acidified Liquid. Available online: http://www.enfamil.com/products/enfamil-human-milk-fortifier-acidified-liquid (accessed on 29 January 2015).
11. Abbott Nutrition Similac Human Milk Fortifier Concentrated Liquid. Available online: http://abbottnutrition.com/brands/products/similac-human-milk-fortifier-concentrated-liquid (accessed on 29 January 2015).
12. Patel, A.L.; Engstrom, J.L.; Meier, P.P.; Kimura, R.E. Accuracy of methods for calculating postnatal growth velocity for extremely low birth weight infants. *Pediatrics* **2005**, *116*, 1466–1473. [CrossRef] [PubMed]
13. Hanson, C.; Sundermeier, J.; Dugick, L.; Lyden, E.; Anderson-Berry, A.L. Implementation, process, and outcomes of nutrition best practices for infants <1500 g. *Nutr. Clin. Pract.* **2001**, *26*, 614–624.
14. Erickson, T.; Gill, G.; Chan, G.M. The effects of acidification on human milk's cellular and nutritional content. *J. Perinatol.* **2013**, *3*, 371–373. [CrossRef] [PubMed]
15. Cibulskis, C.C.; Armbrecht, E. Association of metabolic acidosis with bovine milk-based human milk fortifiers. *J. Perinatol.* **2015**, *35*, 115–119. [CrossRef] [PubMed]
16. Moya, F.; Sisk, P.M.; Walsh, K.R.; Berseth, C.L. A new liquid human milk fortifier and linear growth in preterm infants. *J. Pediatr.* **2012**, *130*, 928–935. [CrossRef] [PubMed]
17. Chan, G.M. Effects of powdered human milk fortifiers on the antibacterial actions of human milk. *J. Perinatol.* **2003**, *23*, 620–623. [CrossRef] [PubMed]

18. Rochow, N.; Jochum, F.; Redlich, A.; Korinekova, Z.; Linnemann, K.; Weitmann, K.; Boehm, G.; Müller, H.; Kalhoff, H.; Topp, H.; et al. Fortification of breast milk in VLBW infants: Metabolic acidosis is linked to the composition of fortifiers and alters weight gain and bone mineralization. *J. Clin. Nutr.* **2011**, *30*, 99–105. [CrossRef] [PubMed]

19. Kalhoff, H.; Diekmann, L.; Rudloff, S.; Manz, F. Renal excretion of calcium and phosphorus in premature infants with incipient late metabolic acidosis. *J. Pediatr. Gastroenterol. Nutr.* **2001**, *33*, 565–569. [CrossRef] [PubMed]

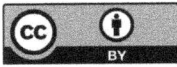

nutrients

MDPI

Article

Temporal Changes of Protein Composition in Breast Milk of Chinese Urban Mothers and Impact of Caesarean Section Delivery

Michael Affolter [1,*], Clara L. Garcia-Rodenas [1], Gerard Vinyes-Pares [2], Rosemarie Jenni [1], Iris Roggero [1], Ornella Avanti-Nigro [1], Carlos Antonio de Castro [1], Ai Zhao [3], Yumei Zhang [3], Peiyu Wang [4], Sagar K. Thakkar [1] and Laurent Favre [1]

[1] Nestlé Research Center, Nestec Ltd., Lausanne 1000, Switzerland; clara.garcia@rdls.nestle.com (C.L.G.-R.); rosemarie.jenni@rdls.nestle.com (R.J.); iris.roggero@rdls.nestle.com (I.R.); ornella.avanti-nigro@rdls.nestle.com (O.A.-N.); carlosantonio.decastro@rdls.nestle.com (C.A.d.C.); sagar.thakkar@rdls.nestle.com (S.K.T.); laurent.favre1@rdls.nestle.com (L.F.)

[2] Nestlé Research Center Beijing, Nestec Ltd., Beijing 100095, China; gerard.vinyespares@rd.nestle.com

[3] Department of Nutrition and Food Hygiene, School of Public Health, Peking University, Beijing 100191, China; xiaochaai@163.com (A.Z.); zhangyumei@hsc.pku.edu.cn (Y.Z.)

[4] Department of Social Medicine and Health Education, School of Public Health, Peking University, Beijing 100191, China; wpeiyu@bjmu.edu.cn

[*] Correspondence: michael.affolter@rdls.nestle.com; Tel.: +41-217-858-966; Fax: +41-217-859-486

Received: 16 June 2016; Accepted: 1 August 2016; Published: 17 August 2016

Abstract: Human breast milk (BM) protein composition may be impacted by lactation stage or factors related to geographical location. The present study aimed at assessing the temporal changes of BM major proteins over lactation stages and the impact of mode of delivery on immune factors, in a large cohort of urban mothers in China. 450 BM samples, collected in three Chinese cities, covering 8 months of lactation were analyzed for α-lactalbumin, lactoferrin, serum albumin, total caseins, immunoglobulins (IgA, IgM and IgG) and transforming growth factor (TGF) β1 and β2 content by microfluidic chip- or ELISA-based quantitative methods. Concentrations and changes over lactation were aligned with previous reports. α-lactalbumin, lactoferrin, IgA, IgM and TGF-β1 contents followed similar variations characterized by highest concentrations in early lactation that rapidly decreased before remaining stable up to end of lactation. TGF-β2 content displayed same early dynamics before increasing again. Total caseins followed a different pattern, showing initial increase before decreasing back to starting values. Serum albumin and IgG levels appeared stable throughout lactation. In conclusion, BM content in major proteins of urban mothers in China was comparable with previous studies carried out in other parts of the world and C-section delivery had only very limited impact on BM immune factors.

Keywords: breast milk; proteins; immune factors; Chinese mothers; CAESAREAN-section

1. Introduction

Evolution has shaped human breast milk (BM) composition to protect the infant against disease(s) and to supply their nutritional needs [1]. BM proteins are one of the major contributors to this dual role in early infancy. BM proteins are the primary source of amino acids required for body protein building and can facilitate nutrient digestion as well as increase their bioavailability. BM proteins can also act as immunologically active molecules able to confer passive protection against pathogens, to stimulate the infant's antimicrobial defences or to modulate the infant immune maturation and responses [2–4].

More than 2500 distinct protein sequences have been identified in BM [5]. The most abundant BM proteins include lactoferrin, α-lactalbumin, serum albumin and the β- and κ-casein fractions, collectively representing about 85% of total BM proteins [6]. Multiple biological activities have been proposed for lactoferrin, and possibly the best documented effect in the infants is protection against gastrointestinal infections [7]. Similarly, a multimeric α-lactalbumin-lipid complex (HAMLET) found in BM has potent pro-apoptotic effects on bacterial [8] and tumoral cells, while sparing healthy eukaryotic cells [9]. By contrast, serum albumin and caseins likely have a predominantly nutritional role as opposed to lactoferrin, and these proteins appear to be readily digested by the infant gastrointestinal proteases. Nevertheless, some biological activities have been proposed for the peptides produced during the digestion of these proteins [10]. For example, antibacterial activity has been found upon gastric digestion of β-casein in infants [11].

Immune factors are also important BM components, representing up to 10% of total proteins. Immunoglobulins (Ig) and members of the transforming growth factor (TGF)-β family are the most studied key partners of the immunological activity found in colostrum, transitional and mature milk, ensuring transfer of passive immunity from mother to offspring [12], as well as supporting the onset of gut homeostasis in the neonate [13–17]. IgA, or more precisely secretory IgA, is the major isotype found in BM, followed then by IgM and IgG. Its dynamic of secretion over lactation period has been investigated in several studies, showing high content in colostrum, followed by a rapid diminution during transition milk to then remain stable in mature milk [18,19]. The TGF-β family constitutes the most abundant cytokines of BM and consists of three isoforms, of which TGF-β2 predominates, followed by TGF-β1 [20]. Data on the changes of the secretion over lactation period of these two cytokines are more limited than for Igs, but tend to show overall similar patterns [21].

Infants born by Caesarean section (C-section) suffer from an associated increased risk of development later in life of immune-related diseases [22–24]. These alterations are commonly attributed to altered microbiota colonization patterns in those infants due to the absence of the initial inoculation of maternal vaginal and faecal microbiota [22]. However, potential impact of delivery mode on BM-related immune parameters may also be an important contributing factor. Indeed, data available from several studies indicate a delayed onset of lactation following C-section [25,26] preventing the new-born to gain prompt access to beneficial components of BM. In contrast, little is known about the impact of C-section delivery on BM composition and in particular on the milk immune factors. Current data from studies focusing on immunoglobulin content in colostrum samples do not allow us to draw a clear conclusion on a potential impact of the mode of delivery on the presence of these antibodies in the BM [4,27]. To our knowledge, no data are currently available on the effect of C-section delivery on major BM immune factors throughout transitional and mature milk.

Hence, the main objective of the present work was to assess the specific temporal changes of major proteins' content in BM across different stages of lactation, with a secondary interest in exploring the impact of the mode of delivery on BM immune factors. This work was performed in China, a country presenting one of the highest rates of C-section birth in the world [28], and is part of the larger Maternal Infant Nutrition Growth (MING) initiative, conducted in a large cohort of urban Chinese mothers [29].

2. Materials and Methods

2.1. Subjects

This study was part of MING, a cross-sectional study designed to investigate the dietary and nutritional status of pregnant women, lactating mothers, infants and young children up to three years of age living in urban areas of China. In addition, the BM composition of Chinese lactating mothers was characterized for major proteins and immune factors. The study was conducted between October 2011 and February 2012. A multi-stage BM sampling from lactating mothers in three cities (Beijing, Suzhou and Guangzhou) was performed for BM characterization. In each city, two hospitals with maternal and child care units were selected and, at each site, mothers at lactation period 0–240 days were randomly selected based on child registration information. Subjects included in the period 0–5 days were recruited at the hospital whereas the other subjects were requested by phone to join the study; if participation was dismissed a replacement was made. Response rate was 52%. Recruitment and BM sampling, as well as baseline data collection, were done on separate days.

A stratified BM sampling of 540 lactating mothers in six lactation periods of 0–4, 5–11 and 12–30 days, and 1–2, 2–4 and 4–8 months were obtained in MING study. Nevertheless, only 450 BM samples were analysed in the present study, as the 0–4 days stage could not be included due to the limited volume of BM collected during this period.

2.2. Inclusion and Exclusion Criteria

Eligibility criteria included women between 18 and 45 years of age with singleton pregnancy, apparently healthy, full-term infant and exclusively breastfeeding at least until 4 months post-partum. Exclusion criteria included gestational diabetes, hypertension, cardiac diseases, acute communicable diseases and postpartum depression. Lactating women who had nipple or lacteal gland diseases, who had been receiving hormonal therapy during the three months preceding recruitment, or who had insufficient skills to understand study questionnaires were also excluded.

2.3. Ethical and Legal Considerations

The study was conducted according to the guidelines in the Declaration of Helsinki. All of the procedures involving human subjects were approved by the Medical Ethics Research Board of Peking University (No. IRB00001052-11042, 15-11-2011). Written informed consent was obtained from all subjects participating in the study. The study was also registered in ClinicalTrials.gov with identifier NCT01971671.

2.4. Data Collection

All mothers completed a general questionnaire including socio-economic and lifestyle aspects. Self-reported weight during pre-pregnancy and at delivery, number of gestational weeks at delivery, and delivery method were also recorded. Additionally, a physical examination evaluated basic anthropometric parameters (height, weight, mid-arm circumference) blood pressure and haemoglobin.

Data collection was done through face-to-face interviews, on the day of BM sample collection. In addition, date of birth and gender information of the infant was collected after the data collection since the data was not included in the initial questionnaires. Subjects were contacted by phone and were asked to clarify these two aspects retrospectively.

2.5. Sample Characteristics

BM sampling was standardized for all subjects and an electric pump (Horigen HNR/X-2108ZB, Xinhe Electrical Apparatuses Co., Ltd., Beijing, China) was used to sample the BM. Samples were collected at the second feeding in the morning (9–11 a.m.) to avoid circadian influence on the outcomes. Single full breast was emptied and an aliquot of 40 mL BM for each time point was secured for characterization purposes. The rest of the BM was returned to the mother for feeding to the infant. Each sample was distributed in 5 mL freezing tubes, labelled with subject number, stored at $-80\,^{\circ}\text{C}$ and then shipped to the Nestlé Research Centre (Lausanne, Switzerland) for analyses within 6 months of collection.

2.6. Milk Sample Processing before Analyses

Frozen BM samples were skimmed by thawing to $4\,^{\circ}\text{C}$, high speed centrifugation ($2500\times g$ for 10 min at $4\,^{\circ}\text{C}$) and collection of the liquid fraction below the lipid phase. Each skimmed BM sample was then aliquoted in separate microtubes (Eppendorf AG, Hamburg, Germany) and frozen again until use. This aliquoting approach was put in place to avoid thawing-freezing cycles between the different analytical runs for the BM immune factors of interest as one aliquot was then dedicated to each analysis.

2.7. Measurement of Major Breast Milk Proteins

The following major BM proteins were measured in all 450 BM samples: α-lactalbumin, serum albumin, lactoferrin and all caseins. Due to the large number of samples, a classical approach using, for example, gel electrophoresis or HPLC separation did not provide sufficient throughput and speed. Therefore, an innovative microfluidic chip based quantitative method was specifically implemented and validated for BM protein analysis. The method was established on a LabChip GX-II instrument (Perkin Elmer, Waltham, MA, USA) allowing high-throughput analysis in a 96-well format. The principle of this technique is based on traditional SDS-PAGE protein separation but the whole procedure (separation, staining and detection) is integrated and fully automated in a microfluidic system. Results are provided in digital format (no gel staining or scanning, etc.). The general approach of this method was described previously [30] for bovine milk protein analysis and needed some slight adaptations for the BM sample analysis as described below.

2.7.1. Sample Preparation

BM sample preparation was performed according to the LabChip (Perkin Elmer, Waltham, MA, USA) protocol. A simple 5-fold dilution of BM with water (Merck Lichrosolv quality) was found to be sufficient prior to protein denaturation and derivatization steps. In contrast to the immune factor analysis by ELISA, BM defatting was not required for the LabChip analysis thus avoiding potential protein losses. All sample preparation and processing steps were performed in 96-well format using electronic multichannel pipettes (Eppendorf Xplorer, Eppendorf AG, Hamburg, Germany). The HT Protein Express protein chip and reagent kit (Perkin Elmer, Waltham, MA, USA) was used for all analyses and highest purity reagents were required for all buffer preparations. Pure human milk proteins (α-lactalbumin, serum albumin, lactoferrin from Sigma, St. Louis, MO, USA) and bovine milk proteins (α-, β- and κ-casein from Sigma, as human proteins not available) were used as standards to generate individual calibration curves for each protein. The purity of each standard protein, according to the certificate of analysis, was used to calculate the true concentration of the protein standard in solution. Reported limit of detection of the LabChip system is 5 ng/μL according to the manufacturer. Calibration concentrations of the individual protein standards ranged from 25 to 750 ng/μL for serum albumin, from 50 to 1500 ng/μL for α-lactalbumin and lactoferrin, and from 100 to 3000 ng/μL for caseins. Note that as the individual casein proteins could not be fully resolved on the LabChip system, all casein peaks were integrated as one peak and thus one value for total casein concentration in BM was obtained (sum of α-, β- and κ-casein). In order to monitor system performance, a quality control sample (pooled BM from Lee Biosolutions Inc., Maryland Heights, MO, USA) was analyzed every 20th sample. All samples were analyzed in triplicates using a volume of 25 μL of BM.

2.7.2. Method Validation

The method was validated for the determination of the four different proteins in human milk. For each protein (α-, β- and κ-caseins measured as total casein) the linear response of the LabChip detector was checked over the concentration range expected to be present in human milk samples. Each protein was analyzed at 8 different levels in triplicate. A quadratic regression was performed and linearity was assessed from the r^2 and the plot of residuals.

To determine the trueness and precision of the method a milk sample was selected and spiked with the protein standards at 3 levels (the levels were adapted for each protein to cover the concentration range expected in milk). The non-spiked sample and the spiked samples were analyzed in duplicate on 6 different days. The spike experiments were used to determine recoveries, data from the duplicate analyses were used to determine repeatability (r) and data from the between day analyses were used to determine intermediate reproducibility (iR).

2.8. Measurement of Selected Breast Milk Immune Factors

Concentrations of IgA, IgG, IgM, TGF-β1 and TGF-β2 in BM samples were measured using selected commercial ELISA quantification kits that were specifically validated for their usage in milk matrix background. In more detail, IgA and IgG contents of BM were measured with Human IgA and IgG ELISA Kits from Bethyl Laboratories Inc., USA (Montgomery, TX, USA) (catalogue numbers E80-102 and E80-104, respectively), following manufacturer instructions and with milk samples tested at 1:20,000 and 1:1000 dilutions, respectively. Kit performance with such dilution factors were for IgA and IgG, respectively: average intra-plate repeatability 5% and 4.5%; average inter-plate repeatability 10.1% and 7.2%; average recovery 87% and 98%. IgM content was measured with the Human IgM Ready-SET-Go from Affimetrix eBioscience, USA (Santa Clara, CA, USA) (catalogue number 88-50620) following manufacturer instructions and with milk samples tested at 1:300 dilution. Kit performance with this dilution factor was: average intra-plate repeatability 3.8%; average inter-plate repeatability 4%; average recovery 90%. Finally, TGF-β1 and TGF-β2 contents were measured with Quantikine ELISA Human TGF-β1 and TGF-β2 Immunoassay Kits from R&D Systems, USA (Minneapolis, MN, USA) (catalogue numbers DB100B and DB250, respectively), following manufacturer instructions and with milk samples tested respectively at 1:5 and 1:4 dilutions on the top of the already 1:1.4 dilution of the original samples linked to the acidification and pH neutralization steps mandatory to activate latent TFG-βs from BM samples to their measured immune-reactive forms. Kit performance with such dilution factors were for TGF-β1 and TGF-β2 respectively: average intra-plate repeatability 4% and 9.3%; average inter-plate repeatability 6.1% and 10.8%; average recovery 84% and 92%.

2.9. Data Analysis

A multiple linear regression was applied to analyze the effect of lactation stage on the levels of the individual proteins. This model was adjusted for the effects of maternal age and BMI, infant gender, mode of delivery and geographical location.

A multiple regression model to explain the protein and immune parameter concentration was applied. The distribution of the residuals were checked via Box-Cox transformation method and a logarithmic transformation seemed to be adequate for all immune parameters. The following model was used:

$$\log(\text{concentration}) = \text{timeframe} + \text{sex} + \text{delivery} + \text{city} + \text{mother's age} + \text{mother's BMI} + \varepsilon$$

The above model was the general model that was used to test for the effect of stage of lactation (timeframe) on immune parameter concentration taking in to consideration other variables such as gender, mode of delivery (natural vs. C-section) and geographic location (city). The term ε refers to a residual error (observed value–predicted value). With this model, contrast estimates were calculated comparing the successive timeframes (5–11 days vs. 12–30 days, 12–30 days vs. 1–2 months, etc.) to observe at which timeframes there were significant changes in nutrient concentration.

The same stage of lactation model was used in the subgroup of mothers delivering by C-section and also for natural delivery. In this case the model become simpler:

$$\log(\text{concentration}) = \text{timeframe} + \text{sex} + \text{city} + \text{mother's age} + \text{mother's BMI} + \varepsilon$$

A similar model was used to assess the impact of mode of delivery with the difference of taking into account the interaction effect of time with the variable in question. The following model was used so that a comparison of the delivery modes can be made for each timeframe:

$$\log(\text{concentration}) = \text{timeframe} \times \text{delivery} + \text{sex} + \text{city} + \text{mother's age} + \text{mother's BMI} + \varepsilon$$

The same methods were used for the proteins, but a normality assumption is made and therefore no logarithmic transformation was performed on the 4 protein nutrients.

3. Results

3.1. Subject Characteristics

In this cross-sectional study, nine different proteins were quantified in 450 BM samples collected at different stages from early to late lactation (8 months) in apparently healthy Chinese women from three different cities (i.e., Beijing, Guangzhou, and Suzhou). Figure 1 displays the recruitment flowchart from eligibility to sample analysis.

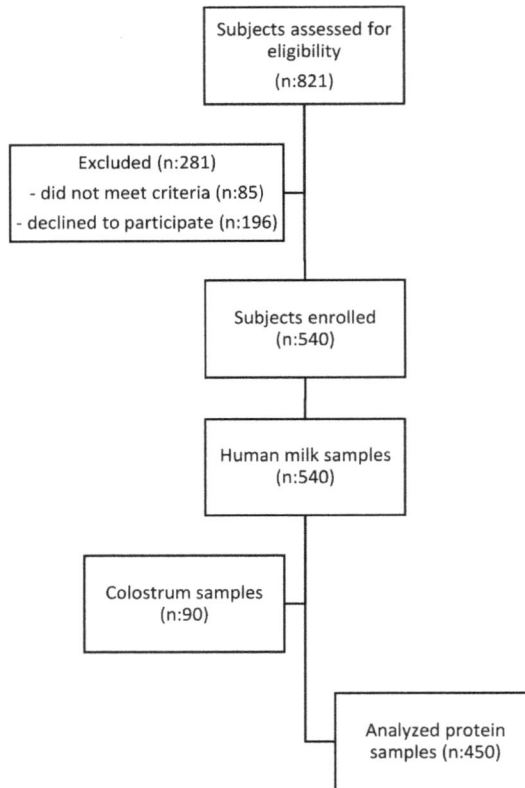

Figure 1. Study flow chart of subject recruitment.

Subject demographics and anthropometry are described in Table 1. Maternal age, weight, body mass index (BMI) and mode of delivery were significantly different among the lactation stage cohorts. No other significant differences were observed in maternal and infant characteristics analysed. Note that the significant differences were taken into consideration for the analyses of protein contents at the different lactation stages as the statistical model was adjusted for these potential confounding factors.

Table 1. Maternal and infant characteristics (adapted from [31]).

Study Population	5–11 Days	12–30 Days	1–2 Months	2–4 Months	4–8 Months
	(n = 90)	(n = 90)	(n = 90)	(n = 90)	(n = 90)
Mother					
Age (years), Mean (SD)	27 (4)	27 (3)	28 (4)	27 (4)	26 (4)
Height (cm), Mean (SD)	160 (4)	160 (5)	161 (5)	161 (5)	159 (5)
Weight (kg), Mean (SD)	60.7 (8.7)	60.8 (7.9)	61.9 (8.9)	58.4 (8.3)	56.2 (8.1)
BMI (kg/m^2), Mean (SD)	23.7 (3.3)	23.7 (2.8)	23.9 (3.1)	22.5 (2.9)	22.2 (3.1)
Gestational weight gain (kg), Mean (SD)	16.7 (7.4)	16.2 (6.0)	15.9 (5.7)	15.9 (5.9)	14.9 (7.6)
Postpartum weight loss (kg), Mean (SD)	9.1 (6.1)	8.6 (5.3)	9.8 (4.0)	10.0 (6.2)	10.6 (5.9)
Caesarean delivery, N (%)	39 (42)	43 (48)	53 (59)	35 (39)	35 (38)
Infant					
Males, N (%)	51 (57)	48 (53)	48 (53)	54 (60)	43 (48)
Gestational age at birth (weeks), Mean (SD)	39.3 (1.2)	39.2 (1.3)	39.2 (1.6)	39.4 (1.3)	39.5 (1.5)

3.2. Major Breast Milk Proteins

3.2.1. Analytical Method Performance

Each protein was quantified using an individual calibration curve (quadratic fitting, all $R^2 > 0.99$, LabChip GX-II software, v4.1, 2015), based on a dilution series of pure standard proteins. Figure 2A depicts a typical electropherogram trace of a BM sample measured with the LabChip GX II system. A calibration curve for α-lactalbumin is shown in Figure 2B which demonstrates the small variation of replicate measurements. Based on a simple 5-fold dilution of the BM samples, limit of detection was 50 ng/μL for α-lactalbumin and serum albumin, 100 ng/μL for caseins and 130 ng/μL for lactoferrin, respectively.

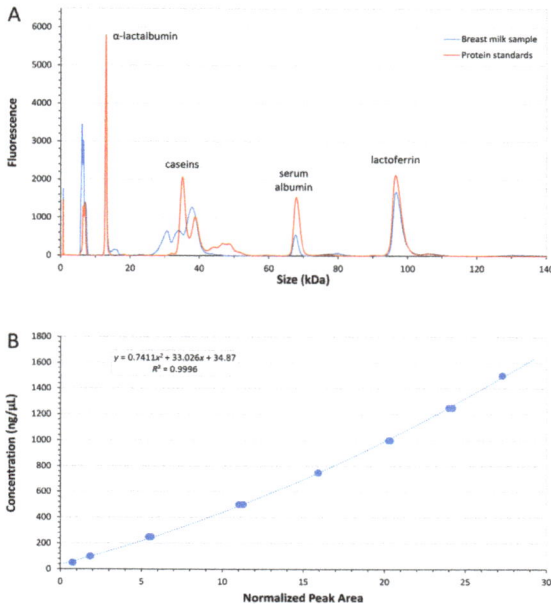

Figure 2. (**A**) Human breast milk protein separation on the LabChip GX II system. The electropherogram overlay depicts individual standard milk proteins (red) and a typical human breast milk sample trace (blue); (**B**) Calibration curve for α-lactalbumin (in duplicates, 50–1500 ng/μL, R^2 0.9996).

The method was fully validated. Recoveries of proteins, determined using spiking experiments (three spiking levels, analyzed in duplicate on six different days), were between 91.8% and 116.5%.

Relative repeatability (r%) for all proteins was <9.2% and relative intermediate reproducibility (iR%) was <26%. Measurement uncertainty was estimated using the simplified approach based on existing validation data proposed by Barwick [32]. The standard uncertainty (u) was determined at 11 ng/µL with relative standard uncertainty (u%) of 0.5%. Expanded uncertainty (U) was 19 ng/µL with relative expanded uncertainty (U%) of 1%.

3.2.2. Analysis of Major Breast Milk Proteins

The concentration of α-lactalbumin decreased from 3.27 to 2.28 g/L over the investigated lactation period (Table 2). With the exception of the two first stages, all subsequent stages showed a significant decrease ($p < 0.003$) in α-lactalbumin content, over time until eight months.

Table 2. Protein content of human breast milk from the different lactation stages (see also Figure S1).

Proteins	5–11 Days ($n = 90$)	12–30 Days ($n = 90$)	1–2 Months ($n = 90$)	2–4 Months ($n = 90$)	4–8 Months ($n = 90$)
Major breast milk proteins					
α-lactalbumin (g/L), Median (IQR)	3.27 (0.60)	3.16 (0.55)	2.84 [a] (0.55)	2.53 [a] (0.47)	2.28 [a] (0.63)
Lactoferrin (g/L), Median (IQR)	3.30 (2.11)	1.86 [a] (0.89)	1.24 [a] (0.53)	1.15 (0.46)	1.17 (0.47)
Serum albumin (g/L), Median (IQR)	0.48 (0.14)	0.48 (0.14)	0.42 (0.09)	0.44 (0.10)	0.42 (0.08)
Total caseins (g/L), Median (IQR)	5.84 (3.17)	6.57 [a] (2.15)	6.24 (2.25)	5.79 [a] (1.69)	5.60 (1.73)
Immune factors					
IgA (mg/L), Median (IQR)	1148 (1022)	615 [a] (494)	553 [a] (232)	557 (312)	564 (337)
IgM (mg/L), Median (IQR)	117 (168)	47 [a] (47)	35 [a] (31)	35 (29)	25 [a] (25)
IgG (mg/L), Median (IQR)	22 (13)	23 (12)	20 (14)	24 (15)	23 (14)
TGF-β1 (ng/L), Median (IQR)	1258 (1305)	685 [a] (482)	600 (356)	598 (379)	659 (410)
TGF-β2 (ng/L), Median (IQR)	5286 (10,444)	2322 [a] (3100)	1877 [a] (1890)	1920 [a] (2112)	2311 [b] (2868)

[a] $p < 0.05$ vs. previous stage; [b] $p < 0.05$ vs. previous 1–2 months stage.

The concentration of lactoferrin also decreased over full lactation period, from 3.30 to 1.17 g/L (Table 2). This decrease was constant during lactation until 1–2 months, with significant differences ($p < 0.000$) in lactoferrin content between the first three investigated stages, and then stabilizing until the eighth months.

The concentration of serum albumin during the lactation period ranged from 0.48 to 0.42 g/L (Table 2) and did not show any significant differences between stages.

The concentration of caseins during the lactation period followed a different pattern than the other proteins, showing a significant transient increase from 5.84 g/L at stage 1 to 6.57 g/L in Stage 2 and 6.24 g/L in Stage 3 before returning to starting values in later stages (Table 2).

3.3. Breast Milk Immune Factors

IgA and IgM contents reflected the temporal change pattern of most of the major BM proteins with significantly higher contents in early milk before rapidly decreasing over time, reaching a basal plateau after 1 month of infant's age (Table 2). IgG concentration did not follow the same pattern as it appeared stable throughout lactation (Table 2).

TGF-β1 and TGF-β2 BM contents proved to be also significantly higher in the very early milk (5–11 days period, Table 2). Then, while TGF-β1 concentration remained stable up to the end of the covered lactation period, TGF-β2 content continued to significantly decrease in the 1–2 months stage before significantly increasing again later back to 12–30 days levels.

Regarding impact of mode of delivery on immune factor contents in BM, even if occasional statistical significant differences or trends could be observed (see Figures 3 and 4), C-section delivery did not appear to consistently impact BM concentrations in immune factor.

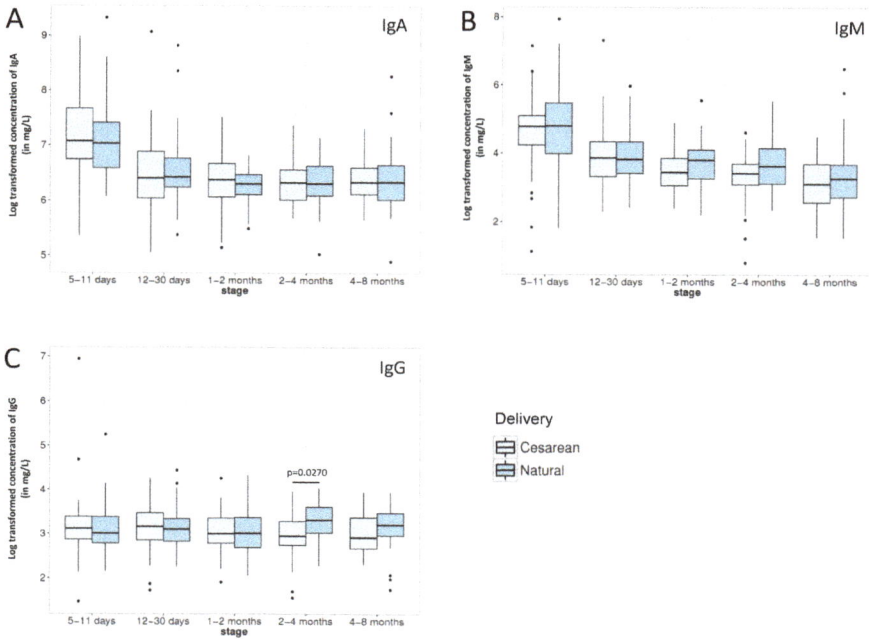

Figure 3. Comparison of (**A**) IgA; (**B**) IgM and (**C**) IgG immunoglobulin contents in breast milk from mothers delivering their infant either vaginally (Natural) or by Caesarean section for each lactation period of this study. Box plot represent medians with 25th and 75th percentile, min-max range and outliers. Statistical significance was set at $p < 0.05$ and significant p-values are indicated in the graphs.

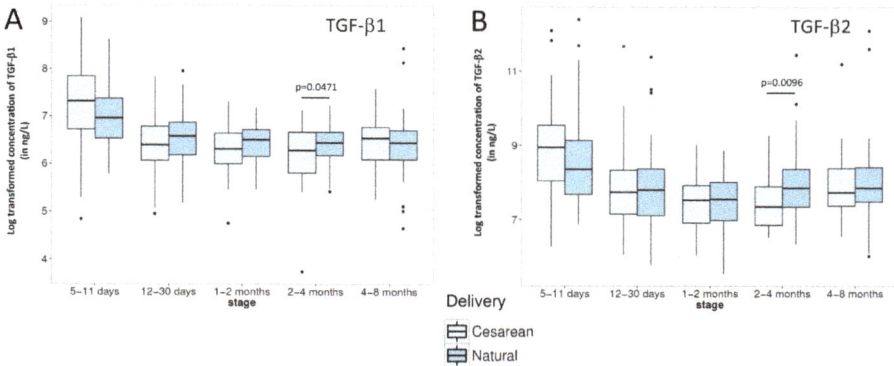

Figure 4. Comparison of (**A**) TGF-β1 and (**B**) TGF-β2 contents in breast milk from mothers delivering their infant either vaginally (Natural) or by Caesarean section for each lactation period of this study. Box plot represent medians with 25th and 75th percentile, min-max range and outliers. Statistical significance was set at $p < 0.05$ and significant p-values are indicated in the graphs.

4. Discussion

4.1. Major Breast Milk Proteins

Various separation techniques and approaches have been exploited to identify and quantify milk proteins. Traditionally, chromatographic or electrophoretic methods have been used to profile major BM proteins [33–35] whereas immuno-based approaches, i.e., ELISA or antibody arrays, were the method of choice for quantitative analysis of individual proteins [36–38]. More recently, targeted LC-MS techniques have been developed to separate and quantify specific milk proteins [39]. The low throughput nature of these methodologies is often the limiting factor for application to larger numbers of samples. In order to address the challenge to precisely quantify major BM proteins in a large number of individual samples, as in the case of the present study, an innovative microfluidic chip-based method was specifically implemented, validated and applied in a high-throughput approach.

Despite a small limitation in the quantification of individual caseins, we believe that the minimal sample preparation and the 96-well sample format ideally combines speed and robustness of the analysis process and thus paves the way for a new technological standard for the measurement of α-lactalbumin, lactoferrin, serum albumin and total caseins in future studies addressing BM protein composition.

α-lactalbumin was the most abundant whey protein in the Chinese mother's BM samples (Table 2), in agreement with previous data in the literature [19]. Even though its content decreased significantly over the first two months, it remained high in all lactation stages. The high levels of this protein in BM are likely key for the nutrition of the breast-fed infant. Contrary to other BM proteins, α-lactalbumin appears to be fully hydrolysed and absorbed in the infant intestine, thus to be a good source of nitrogen and indispensable amino acids [40]. This protein contributes as well to the balanced amino acid composition of BM and, in particular, to its high levels of tryptophan, which ultimately allows BM to cover the infant's amino acid requirements with limited amounts of protein [41]. High levels of tryptophan in this protein would be also associated with its protective effects against epileptic seizures in animal models [42]. Besides its nutritional role, the α-lactalbumin HAMLET complex found in BM has anti-tumoral [9] and bactericidal effects [8]. Furthermore, α-lactalbumin bears bioactive peptide sequences (e.g., mineral chelator or anti-microbial peptides) that may be released and transiently exert their activity (e.g., increased mineral absorption or prevention of infection) in the infant intestine. In line with this, Kelleher et al. [43] observed increased mineral absorption and Bruck et al. [44] inhibition of *E. coli*-induced diarrhoea in infant monkeys fed a formula supplemented with bovine α-lactalbumin.

The second most abundant whey protein in our samples was lactoferrin (Table 2) for which the observed concentration values and gradual decrease along lactation were similar to those previously reported [19,45]. The bioavailability of lactoferrin, thus its nutritional relevance as a source of amino acids and nitrogen to the infant, is not known. However, it has been found intact in infant faeces and resistant to digestion in an in vitro digestion model, which suggest that the nutritional role of lactoferrin may need reconsideration and further studies [40]. In contrast, multiple biological activities have been proposed for this protein [40] including infant protection against gastrointestinal infection and sepsis [7].

It is noteworthy that temporal changes trends of α-lactalbumin and lactoferrin along lactation are fully aligned with that of the total proteins measured in the same BM samples as previously reported [29].

Due to the complexity of the casein composition in BM and limitations in mass resolution of the new analytical method used in this study, caseins were not quantified individually but as total caseins (combining α-, β- and κ-casein concentrations, Table 2). This novel analytical approach, however, was potentially susceptible to introducing some bias in comparison to the more classical acid-precipitation based methodology. Interestingly, our results demonstrated that this was not the case as the increase of casein concentration at the beginning of lactation followed by a slight decrease at the later period was closely aligned with a previous report [46]. These results support the theory that casein and whey protein synthesis and/or secretion is regulated by different mechanisms in the mammary gland [47].

In contrast to the other major whey proteins, serum albumin concentration stayed mostly constant across the lactation stages. Comparison with literature data showed similar concentrations in our samples [19]. It is noteworthy that, contrary to other BM proteins that are synthesized by the mammary gland, serum albumin is transferred from the maternal blood [2]. To our knowledge, no specific biological activities have been attributed to this protein. It certainly contributes to the nutrition of the infant as it appears to be highly digestible [2].

4.2. Breast Milk Immune Factors

BM contents of immune factors at the different lactation stages (Table 2) were also in agreement with the previously published ranges [18,48–51], as well as with our own previous findings (unpublished data), indicating that BM from Chinese mothers does not differ from worldwide references in these bioactive components.

IgA and IgM BM contents were significantly high in early milk before rapidly decreasing over time, reaching a basal plateau after 1 month of infant's age, while IgG content was stable throughout lactation. These differences in production pattern between IgG and both other immunoglobulins resides in the fact that IgA and IgM are actively secreted in BM through the poly-immunoglobulin receptor expressed by mammary gland epithelial cells [12] while IgG is more passively appearing in BM through transudation from the systemic circulation, as already mentioned above for serum albumin.

While TGF-β1 contents of BM followed the same temporal changes that the majority of investigated proteins as previously described [21], variation of TGF-β2 concentration appeared to be slightly different, also with a strong decrease until the 1–2 months lactation stage but followed by an increase, reaching at 8 months the level observed in the second half of the first month of lactation (Table 2). Such type of fluctuating pattern of TGF-β2 BM content has already been observed in a previous study [49], however, to a smaller extent and at different time points. Whether this evolution of TGF-β2 has a physiological role for the infants remains to be determined. Indeed, studies mainly focusing on TFG-β1 and 2 demonstrated that milk-borne TGF-βs regulate inflammation [13], stimulation of IgA isotype switching in B cells [52], maintenance of intestinal epithelium barrier function [14], induction of oral tolerance [15], and consequently help to prevent allergic diseases [53,54].

It is noteworthy that C-section delivery did not appear to consistently impact BM content in the major immune factors measured in the present study. The high number of mothers participating in our study together with the high rate of C-section delivery thus allows increasing knowledge on the previously described limited impact of the mode of delivery on major immune BM proteins [4,27], while extending at the same time the former observations on colostrum to transitional and mature milk. Moreover, our data also tend to indicate that the increased risk of immune-related diseases associated with C-section delivery may not be associated with any alterations of major BM immune factors' composition. However, we cannot rule out a potential effect of the mode of delivery on the immune factor composition of the colostrum as our earliest milk samples were collected 5–11 days after delivery. In addition, the impact of delayed onset of lactation following C-section [25,26] on later infant health was not assessed in the present study and would deserve deeper investigation in order to further consolidate the above hypothesis.

The cross-sectional nature of our study limits the conclusions related to the stage-driven changes, which would have been best assessed by a longitudinal design. However, our statistical model adjusted for the maternal and infant baseline factors known or suspected to impact on milk nutrient composition [55]. Our results are also reinforced by the fact that they were remarkably consistent with those previously published.

5. Conclusions

This multi-centric cross-sectional study covering 8 months of lactation for 450 Chinese mothers demonstrated that their BM content in major proteins was comparable with previous studies carried out in other parts of the world, highlighting that key protein components of BM are conserved across geographic localization. Moreover, this study is to our knowledge the first one to address the effect of C-section delivery on major BM immune factors throughout transitional and mature milk, actually showing that C-section delivery had very limited impact on the maternal-to-offspring transmission of active immune competence.

Supplementary Materials: The following are available online at http://www.mdpi.com/2072-6643/8/8/504/s1, Figure S1: Comparison of major milk protein content for (A) α-lactalbumin; (B) lactoferrin; (C) serum albumin and (D) total casein for each lactation period. Box plot represent medians (n = 90 per lactation period) with 25th and 75th percentile, min-max range and outliers. Statistical significance was set at $p < 0.05$ and significant p-values are indicated in the graphs.

Acknowledgments: The authors would like to thank the funding sources of this work and Nestec Ltd. for covering the costs for publishing open access. Special acknowledgment to all participants who volunteered for this study, Lawrence Li for project support and guidance, Celia Ning for project management, Qiaoji Li for clinical project management, Emilie Ba for data management and Yindong Zheng for statistical guidance. Special acknowledgment to Jiaji Wang at Guangzhou Medical University and Liqiang Qin at Soochow University School of Public Health and their teams as well as the project staff at Peking University School of Public Health, for their tasks in recruitment and data collection. A special thank goes to Alexandre Panchaud who initiated the LabChip method development.

Author Contributions: M.A., L.F. and C.G. interpreted the results, drafted, reviewed and revised the initial manuscript. R.J. performed the LabChip experiments and data analysis. I.R. and O.A.-N. measured the breast milk immune factors and processed the results. C.A.d.C. performed the statistical analysis of all data, drafted, reviewed and revised the manuscript. S.T. contributed to the study design, breast milk sampling protocol and interpretation of the results. G.V.-P. contributed to the study design, drafted and reviewed the manuscript. Y.Z. and P.W. were the PI of MING study. Y.Z. and A.Z. were responsible of data collection and quality control. All authors approved the final manuscript as submitted.

Conflicts of Interest: This study was funded by Nestlé Nutrition Institute, China and Nestlé Research Centre, Beijing, China. M.A., C.G., G.V.-P., R.J., I.R., O.A.-N., C.A.d.C., S.T. and L.F. were all employees of Nestec Ltd. when this work was done. A.Z., Y.Z. and P.W. report grants from Nestle Research Center and Nestle Nutrition Institute China during the conduct of the study. The opinions expressed in the article are those of the authors alone and do not necessarily reflect the views or recommendations of their respective affiliations.

References

1. Vorbach, C.; Capecchi, M.R.; Penninger, J.M. Evolution of the mammary gland from the innate immune system? *Bioessays* **2006**, *28*, 606–616. [CrossRef] [PubMed]
2. Lonnerdal, B. Nutritional and physiologic significance of human milk proteins. *Am. J. Clin. Nutr.* **2003**, *77*, 1537S–1543S. [PubMed]
3. Lonnerdal, B. Bioactive proteins in breast milk. *J. Paediatr. Child. Health* **2013**, *49* (Suppl. 1), 1–7. [CrossRef] [PubMed]
4. Striker, G.A.; Casanova, L.D.; Nagao, A.T. Influence of type of delivery on A, G and M immunoglobulin concentration in maternal colostrum. *J. Pediatr.* **2004**, *80*, 123–128. [CrossRef]
5. Beck, K.L.; Weber, D.; Phinney, B.S.; Smilowitz, J.T.; Hinde, K.; Lonnerdal, B.; Korf, I.; Lemay, D.G. Comparative proteomics of human and macaque milk reveals species-specific nutrition during postnatal development. *J. Proteome Res.* **2015**, *14*, 2143–2157. [CrossRef] [PubMed]
6. Prentice, A. Constituents of human milk. *Food Nutr. Bull.* **1996**, *17*, 305–312.
7. Ochoa, T.J.; Pezo, A.; Cruz, K.; Chea-Woo, E.; Cleary, T.G. Clinical studies of lactoferrin in children. *Biochem. Cell Biol.* **2012**, *90*, 457–467. [CrossRef] [PubMed]
8. Hakansson, A.P.; Roche-Hakansson, H.; Mossberg, A.K.; Svanborg, C. Apoptosis-like death in bacteria induced by hamlet, a human milk lipid-protein complex. *PLoS ONE* **2011**, *6*, e17717. [CrossRef] [PubMed]
9. Hakansson, A.; Zhivotovsky, B.; Orrenius, S.; Sabharwal, H.; Svanborg, C. Apoptosis induced by a human milk protein. *Proc. Natl. Acad. Sci. USA* **1995**, *92*, 8064–8068. [CrossRef] [PubMed]

10. Wada, Y.; Lonnerdal, B. Bioactive peptides derived from human milk proteins—Mechanisms of action. *J. Nutr. Biochem.* **2014**, *25*, 503–514. [CrossRef] [PubMed]

11. Dallas, D.C.; Guerrero, A.; Khaldi, N.; Borghese, R.; Bhandari, A.; Underwood, M.A.; Lebrilla, C.B.; German, J.B.; Barile, D. A peptidomic analysis of human milk digestion in the infant stomach reveals protein-specific degradation patterns. *J. Nutr.* **2014**, *144*, 815–820. [CrossRef] [PubMed]

12. Brandtzaeg, P. The mucosal immune system and its integration with the mammary glands. *J. Pediatr.* **2010**, *156*, S8–S15. [CrossRef] [PubMed]

13. Kulkarni, A.B.; Karlsson, S. Transforming growth factor-beta 1 knockout mice. A mutation in one cytokine gene causes a dramatic inflammatory disease. *Am. J. Pathol.* **1993**, *143*, 3–9. [PubMed]

14. Planchon, S.M.; Martins, C.A.; Guerrant, R.L.; Roche, J.K. Regulation of intestinal epithelial barrier function by tgf-beta 1. Evidence for its role in abrogating the effect of a T cell cytokine. *J. Immunol.* **1994**, *153*, 5730–5739. [PubMed]

15. Gray, J.D.; Hirokawa, M.; Horwitz, D.A. The role of transforming growth factor beta in the generation of suppression: An interaction between CD8+ T and NK cells. *J. Exp. Med.* **1994**, *180*, 1937–1942. [CrossRef] [PubMed]

16. Mathias, A.; Pais, B.; Favre, L.; Benyacoub, J.; Corthesy, B. Role of secretory IgA in the mucosal sensing of commensal bacteria. *Gut Microbes* **2014**, *5*, 688–695. [CrossRef] [PubMed]

17. Rogier, E.W.; Frantz, A.L.; Bruno, M.E.; Wedlund, L.; Cohen, D.A.; Stromberg, A.J.; Kaetzel, C.S. Secretory antibodies in breast milk promote long-term intestinal homeostasis by regulating the gut microbiota and host gene expression. *Proc. Natl. Acad. Sci. USA* **2014**, *111*, 3074–3079. [CrossRef] [PubMed]

18. Lonnerdal, B.; Forsum, E.; Hambraeus, L. A longitudinal study of the protein, nitrogen, and lactose contents of human milk from swedish well-nourished mothers. *Am. J. Clin. Nutr.* **1976**, *29*, 1127–1133. [PubMed]

19. Jensen, R.G. *Handbook of Milk Composition*; Academic Press: San Diego, CA, USA, 1995.

20. Saito, S.; Yoshida, M.; Ichijo, M.; Ishizaka, S.; Tsujii, T. Transforming growth factor-beta (TGF-β) in human milk. *Clin. Exp. Immunol.* **1993**, *94*, 220–224. [CrossRef] [PubMed]

21. Agarwal, S.; Karmaus, W.; Davis, S.; Gangur, V. Immune markers in breast milk and fetal and maternal body fluids: A systematic review of perinatal concentrations. *J. Hum. Lact.* **2011**, *27*, 171–186. [CrossRef] [PubMed]

22. Neu, J.; Rushing, J. Cesarean versus vaginal delivery: Long-term infant outcomes and the hygiene hypothesis. *Clin. Perinatol.* **2011**, *38*, 321–331. [CrossRef] [PubMed]

23. Penders, J.; Gerhold, K.; Thijs, C.; Zimmermann, K.; Wahn, U.; Lau, S.; Hamelmann, E. New insights into the hygiene hypothesis in allergic diseases: Mediation of sibling and birth mode effects by the gut microbiota. *Gut Microbes* **2014**, *5*, 239–244. [CrossRef] [PubMed]

24. Sevelsted, A.; Stokholm, J.; Bonnelykke, K.; Bisgaard, H. Cesarean section and chronic immune disorders. *Pediatrics* **2015**, *135*, e92–e98. [CrossRef] [PubMed]

25. Dewey, K.G.; Nommsen-Rivers, L.A.; Heinig, M.J.; Cohen, R.J. Risk factors for suboptimal infant breastfeeding behavior, delayed onset of lactation, and excess neonatal weight loss. *Pediatrics* **2003**, *112*, 607–619. [CrossRef] [PubMed]

26. Evans, K.C.; Evans, R.G.; Royal, R.; Esterman, A.J.; James, S.L. Effect of caesarean section on breast milk transfer to the normal term newborn over the first week of life. *Arch. Dis. Child Fetal Neonatal Ed.* **2003**, *88*, F380–F382. [CrossRef] [PubMed]

27. Kulski, J.K.; Smith, M.; Hartmann, P.E. Normal and caesarian section delivery and the initiation of lactation in women. *Aust. J. Exp. Biol. Med. Sci.* **1981**, *59*, 405–412. [CrossRef] [PubMed]

28. Hellerstein, S.; Feldman, S.; Duan, T. China's 50% caesarean delivery rate: Is it too high? *BJOG* **2015**, *122*, 160–164. [CrossRef] [PubMed]

29. Yang, T.; Zhang, Y.; Ning, Y.; You, L.; Ma, D.; Zheng, Y.; Yang, X.; Li, W.; Wang, J.; Wang, P. Breast milk macronutrient composition and the associated factors in urban chinese mothers. *Chin. Med. J.* **2014**, *127*, 1721–1725. [PubMed]

30. Anema, S.G. The use of "lab-on-a-chip" microfluidic sds electrophoresis technology for the separation and quantification of milk proteins. *Int. Dairy J.* **2009**, *19*, 198–204. [CrossRef]

31. Austin, S.; De Castro, C.; Bénet, T.; Hou, Y.; Sun, H.; Thakkar, S.; Vinyes-Pares, G.; Zhang, Y.; Wang, P. Temporal change of the content of 10 oligosaccharides in the milk of chinese urban mothers. *Nutrients* **2016**, *8*, 346. [CrossRef] [PubMed]

32. Barwick, V.J.; Ellison, S.L.; Lucking, C.L.; Burn, M.J. Experimental studies of uncertainties associated with chromatographic techniques. *J. Chromatogr. A* **2001**, *918*, 267–276. [CrossRef]
33. Velona, T.; Abbiati, L.; Beretta, B.; Gaiaschi, A.; Flauto, U.; Tagliabue, P.; Galli, C.L.; Restani, P. Protein profiles in breast milk from mothers delivering term and preterm babies. *Pediatr. Res.* **1999**, *45*, 658–663. [CrossRef] [PubMed]
34. Kunz, C.; Lonnerdal, B. Human-milk proteins: Analysis of casein and casein subunits by anion-exchange chromatography, gel electrophoresis, and specific staining methods. *Am. J. Clin. Nutr.* **1990**, *51*, 37–46. [PubMed]
35. Ferreira, I.M.P.L. Chromatographic separation and quantification of major human milk proteins. *J. Liq. Chromatogr. Relat. Technol.* **2007**, *30*, 499–507. [CrossRef]
36. Broadhurst, M.; Beddis, K.; Black, J.; Henderson, H.; Nair, A.; Wheeler, T. Effect of gestation length on the levels of five innate defence proteins in human milk. *Early Hum. Dev.* **2015**, *91*, 7–11. [CrossRef] [PubMed]
37. Mehta, R.; Petrova, A. Biologically active breast milk proteins in association with very preterm delivery and stage of lactation. *J. Perinatol.* **2011**, *31*, 58–62. [CrossRef] [PubMed]
38. Collado, M.C.; Santaella, M.; Mira-Pascual, L.; Martinez-Arias, E.; Khodayar-Pardo, P.; Ros, G.; Martinez-Costa, C. Longitudinal study of cytokine expression, lipid profile and neuronal growth factors in human breast milk from term and preterm deliveries. *Nutrients* **2015**, *7*, 8577–8591. [CrossRef] [PubMed]
39. Altendorfer, I.; König, S.; Braukmann, A.; Saenger, T.; Bleck, E.; Vordenbäumen, S.; Kubiak, A.; Schneider, M.; Jose, J. Quantification of αs1-casein in breast milk using a targeted mass spectrometry-based approach. *J. Pharm. Biomed. Anal.* **2015**, *103*, 52–58. [CrossRef] [PubMed]
40. Lonnerdal, B. Infant formula and infant nutrition: Bioactive proteins of human milk and implications for composition of infant formulas. *Am. J. Clin. Nutr.* **2014**, *99*, 712S–717S. [CrossRef]
41. Lonnerdal, B.; Lien, E.L. Nutritional and physiologic significance of alpha-lactalbumin in infants. *Nutr. Rev.* **2003**, *61*, 295–305. [CrossRef] [PubMed]
42. Russo, E.; Scicchitano, F.; Citraro, R.; Aiello, R.; Camastra, C.; Mainardi, P.; Chimirri, S.; Perucca, E.; Donato, G.; De Sarro, G. Protective activity of alpha-lactoalbumin (ALAC), a whey protein rich in tryptophan, in rodent models of epileptogenesis. *Neuroscience* **2012**, *226*, 282–288. [CrossRef] [PubMed]
43. Kelleher, S.L.; Chatterton, D.; Nielsen, K.; Lonnerdal, B. Glycomacropeptide and alpha-lactalbumin supplementation of infant formula affects growth and nutritional status in infant rhesus monkeys. *Am. J. Clin. Nutr.* **2003**, *77*, 1261–1268. [PubMed]
44. Bruck, W.M.; Kelleher, S.L.; Gibson, G.R.; Nielsen, K.E.; Chatterton, D.E.; Lonnerdal, B. Rrna probes used to quantify the effects of glycomacropeptide and alpha-lactalbumin supplementation on the predominant groups of intestinal bacteria of infant rhesus monkeys challenged with enteropathogenic *Escherichia coli*. *J. Pediatr. Gastroenterol. Nutr.* **2003**, *37*, 273–280. [CrossRef] [PubMed]
45. Rai, D.; Adelman, A.S.; Zhuang, W.; Rai, G.P.; Boettcher, J.; Lonnerdal, B. Longitudinal changes in lactoferrin concentrations in human milk: A global systematic review. *Crit. Rev. Food Sci. Nutr.* **2014**, *54*, 1539–1547. [CrossRef] [PubMed]
46. Kunz, C.; Lonnerdal, B. Re-evaluation of the whey protein/casein ratio of human milk. *Acta Paediatr.* **1992**, *81*, 107–112. [CrossRef] [PubMed]
47. Lonnerdal, B.; Adkins, Y. Developmental changes in breast milk protein composition during lactation. In *Development of the Gastrointestinal Tract*; Sanderson, R., Walker, W., Eds.; B.C. Decker Inc.: Hamilton, ON, Canada, 1999; pp. 227–244.
48. Goldman, A.S.; Garza, C.; Nichols, B.L.; Goldblum, R.M. Immunologic factors in human milk during the first year of lactation. *J. Pediatr.* **1982**, *100*, 563–567. [CrossRef]
49. Hawkes, J.S.; Bryan, D.L.; James, M.J.; Gibson, R.A. Cytokines (IL-1β, IL-6, TNF-α, TGF-β1, and TGF-β2) and prostaglandin E2 in human milk during the first three months postpartum. *Pediatr. Res.* **1999**, *46*, 194–199. [CrossRef] [PubMed]
50. Oddy, W.H.; Halonen, M.; Martinez, F.D.; Lohman, I.C.; Stern, D.A.; Kurzius-Spencer, M.; Guerra, S.; Wright, A.L. Tgf-beta in human milk is associated with wheeze in infancy. *J. Allergy Clin. Immunol.* **2003**, *112*, 723–728. [CrossRef]
51. Urwin, H.J.; Zhang, J.; Gao, Y.; Wang, C.; Li, L.; Song, P.; Man, Q.; Meng, L.; Froyland, L.; Miles, E.A.; et al. Immune factors and fatty acid composition in human milk from river/lake, coastal and inland regions of China. *Br. J. Nutr.* **2013**, *109*, 1949–1961. [CrossRef] [PubMed]

Nutrients **2016**, *8*, 504

52. Van, V.P.; Punnonen, J.; de Vries, J.E. Transforming growth factor-beta directs iga switching in human B cells. *J. Immunol.* **1992**, *148*, 2062–2067.

53. Kalliomaki, M.; Ouwehand, A.; Arvilommi, H.; Kero, P.; Isolauri, E. Transforming growth factor-beta in breast milk: A potential regulator of atopic disease at an early age. *J. Allergy Clin. Immunol.* **1999**, *104*, 1251–1257. [CrossRef]

54. Penttila, I.A. Milk-derived transforming growth factor-beta and the infant immune response. *J. Pediatr.* **2010**, *156*, S21–S25. [CrossRef] [PubMed]

55. Stam, J.; Sauer, P.J.; Boehm, G. Can we define an infant's need from the composition of human milk? *Am. J. Clin. Nutr.* **2013**, *98*, 521S–528S. [CrossRef] [PubMed]

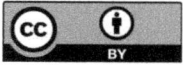

nutrients

MDPI

Article

Amino Acid Composition of Breast Milk from Urban Chinese Mothers

Clara L. Garcia-Rodenas [1,*], Michael Affolter [1], Gerard Vinyes-Pares [2], Carlos A. De Castro [1], Leonidas G. Karagounis [1], Yumei Zhang [3], Peiyu Wang [4] and Sagar K. Thakkar [1]

[1] Nestlé Research Center, Nestec Ltd., Lausanne 1000, Switzerland; michael.affolter@rdls.nestle.com (M.A.); carlosantonio.decastro@rdls.nestle.com (C.A.D.C.); leonidas.karagounis@rdls.nestle.com (L.G.K.); sagar.thakkar@rdls.nestle.com (S.K.T.)

[2] Nestlé Health Sciences, Nestec Ltd., Epalinges 1066, Switzerland; gerard.vinyespares@nestle.com

[3] Department of Nutrition and Food Hygiene, School of Public Health, Peking University, Beijing 100191, China; zhangyumei@hsc.pku.edu.cn

[4] Department of Social Medicine and Health Education, School of Public Health, Peking University, Beijing 100191, China; wpeiyu@bjmu.edu.cn

* Correspondence: clara.garcia@rdls.nestle.com; Tel.: +41-217-858-254

Received: 4 August 2016; Accepted: 23 September 2016; Published: 28 September 2016

Abstract: Human breast milk (BM) amino acid (AA) composition may be impacted by lactation stage or factors related to geographical location. The present cross-sectional study is aimed at assessing the temporal changes of BMAA over lactation stages in a large cohort of urban mothers in China. Four hundred fifty BM samples, collected in three Chinese cities covering eight months of lactation were analyzed for free (FAA) and total (TAA) AA by o-phthalaldehyde/ fluorenylmethylchloroformate (OPA/FMOC) derivatization. Concentrations and changes over lactation were aligned with previous reports. Both the sum and the individual TAA values significantly decreased during the first periods of lactation and then generally leveled off. Leucine and methionine were respectively the most and the least abundant indispensable amino acids across all the lactation stages, whereas glutamic acid + glutamine (Glx) was the most and cystine the least abundant dispensable AA. The contribution of FAA to TAA levels was less than 2%, except for free Glx, which was the most abundant FAA. In conclusion, the AA composition of the milk from our cohort of urban Chinese mothers was comparable to previous studies conducted in other parts of the world, suggesting that this is an evolutionary conserved trait largely independent of geographical, ethnic, or dietary factors.

Keywords: breast milk; amino acids; lactation period; cross-sectional study

1. Introduction

Evolution has shaped the composition of breast milk to ensure optimal development of healthy term offspring. However, breast milk composition is not constant and appears to be affected by multiple factors, including lactation stage, mothers' genetic background and diet, gestational age at delivery, or geographical location [1].

Breast milk protein is a key nutrient supporting body growth and organ development during the first few months of life by providing nitrogen and indispensable amino acids (IAA) required for body protein building and by stimulating the secretion of growth-promoting hormones (i.e., insulin, insulin-like growth factor (1-IGF1)). Potent insulinotropic amino acids such as the branched chain amino acids—Leucine, Lysine, and Threonine—can be particularly important in this context. However, emerging evidence suggests that the relatively low levels of protein and insulinotropic amino acids in breast milk may be protective against the development of metabolic disorders later in infant life [2]. Because body weight, body composition, growth rate, and volume of milk intake are known to change with an infant's age [3,4], infant requirements in terms of both protein and individual amino acid composition also varies along the different stages of lactation [3].

Most amino acids in breast milk are found as constituents of protein chains, but there is also a certain amount of free amino acids (FAA), which usually account for less than 10% of the total amino acid (TAA) levels [5,6]. Although still poorly explored, emerging evidence suggests specific physiological roles of the FAA fraction, such as appetite control [7]. Many studies have analyzed the TAA content in human milk, but they often characterize a limited number of samples, do not account for the important lactation-stage associated changes, or both. The number of studies on FAA is even more limited. In their systematic review of breast milk amino acid composition studies from different continents, Zhang et al. [8] report geographical differences in the content of some TAA and FAA, although data from some regions of the world is relatively limited. In particular, studies looking at breast milk protein quality in China are scarce, with only two small studies reporting on the average TAA composition of one to six months [9] and 7–180 days [10] postpartum milk. To our knowledge, no data on TAA and FAA content in milk from Chinese mothers along lactation is available to date.

The objective of this cross-sectional study was to assess the temporal changes of FAA and TAA in milk secreted during the different stages of lactation in a large cohort of Chinese mothers from three different cities in urban China.

2. Materials and Methods

2.1. Subjects

This study was part of the Maternal, Infant and Nutrition Growth study (MING), a cross-sectional study designed to investigate the dietary and nutritional status of pregnant women, lactating mothers, and young children aged from birth up to three years living in urban areas of China [11]. In addition, the human milk composition of the lactating mothers was characterized. The study was conducted between October 2011 and February 2012. A multi-stage milk sampling from lactating mothers in three cities (Beijing, Suzhou, and Guangzhou) was performed for breast milk characterization. In each city, two hospitals with maternal and child care units were randomly selected; at each site, mothers at lactation periods from 0 to 240 days were randomly selected based on child registration information. Subjects included in the 0–5-day period were recruited at the hospital, whereas the other subjects were invited by telephone to join the study; if participation was dismissed, a replacement was found. Response rate was 52%. Recruitment, milk collection, and baseline data collection were completed on separate days.

Stratified milk sampling of 540 lactating mothers in six lactation periods of 0 to 4, 5 to 11, and 12 to 30 days, and 1–2, 2–4, and 4–8 months, was obtained in the MING study. Nevertheless, only 450 milk samples were analyzed in the amino acid study, as the 0- to 4-day stage could not be included due to the limited volume of milk collected during this period.

Eligibility criteria included women between 18 and 45 years of age giving birth to a single, healthy, full-term infant and exclusively breastfeeding until at least 4 months after birth. Exclusion criteria included gestational diabetes, hypertension, cardiac diseases, acute communicable diseases, and postpartum depression. Lactating women who had nipple or lacteal gland diseases, who had been receiving hormonal therapy during the three months preceding recruitment, or who had insufficient skills to understand study questionnaires were also excluded.

The study was conducted according to the guidelines in the Declaration of Helsinki. All of the procedures involving human subjects were approved by the Medical Ethics Research Board of Peking University (No. IRB00001052-11042). Written informed consent was obtained from all subjects participating in the study. The study was registered at ClinicalTrials.gov (NCT01971671).

2.2. Data Collection

All subjects responded to a general questionnaire including socio-economic and lifestyle aspects of the mother. The self-reported weight at delivery, the number of gestational weeks at delivery, and the delivery method were also recorded. Additionally, a physical examination (height, weight, mid-arm circumference, blood pressure, and hemoglobin levels) was also carried out.

Data collection was done through face-to-face interviews on the day of milk sample collection. The infant's date of birth and gender information was collected retrospectively by phone interview.

2.3. Sample Collection

Breast milk sampling was standardized for all subjects and performed with an electric pump (Horigen HNR/X-2108ZB, Xinhe Electrical Apparatuses Co., Ltd., Beijing, China). Samples were collected at the second feeding in the morning (9–11 a.m.) to avoid circadian influence on the outcomes. Single full breast was emptied, and an aliquot of 40 mL was secured for characterization purposes. The rest of the milk was returned to the mother for infant feeding. One-milliliter aliquots of each sample were transported on dry ice to a laboratory and stored at −80 °C until further analysis.

2.4. Amino Acid Analysis

All samples were analyzed by Eurofins Technology Service (Suzhou) Co. Ltd., Suzhou, China.

TAA content was determined according to a validated o-phthalaldehyde/fluorenylmethylchloroformate (OPA/FMOC) derivatization procedure described by Blankenship et al. [12]. Briefly, protein-bound amino acids were converted to the free state by acid hydrolysis in 6 M of hydrochloric acid at 110 °C for 22 h with a phenol antioxidant in the absence of oxygen. The digests were derivatized with ortho-phthalaldehyde (OPA), mecaptopropionic acid (MCP), and 9-fluorenylmethyl chloroformate (FMOC-Cl) under alkaline conditions prior to injection. Separation and quantification of the amino acid derivatives were performed by high-performance liquid chromatography HPLC with a UV/diode array and fluorescence detection. The limit of detection (LOD) was 1 mg/100 g and the limit of quantification (LOQ) was 5 mg/100 g. Average repeatability was 12%, and reproducibility between duplicate determinations was 18% for the 18 measured amino acids with recoveries ranging from 64.9% to 129.6%.

FAA content was determined according to the same OPA/FMOC method, but without the acid hydrolysis step. All samples were analyzed in duplicate.

2.5. Statistical Analysis

Multiple linear regression was applied to analyze the effect of the lactation period on the levels of TAA and FAA. This model was adjusted for the effects of maternal age and body mass index (BMI), infant gender, mode of delivery, and geographical location. Comparisons were made regarding each subsequent lactation period (5–11 days vs. 12–30 days, 12–30 days vs. 1–2 months, 1–2 months vs. 2–4 months, and 2–4 months vs. 4–8 months) by calculating contrast estimates produced by the model.

For the socio-demographic and anthropometric data, analysis of variance was applied for the continuous variable in question and the lactation period in order to check if there was at least 1 period that was different than the others. For factor variables, an independence test was performed in order to detect differences in distribution among the different period.

All statistical analyses were performed with the statistical software R (version 3.0.1; R Foundation, Vienna, Austria).

3. Results

3.1. Subject Characteristics

In this cross-sectional study, TAA and FAA were quantified in 450 breast milk samples collected at different stages from early to late lactation in healthy urban Chinese women. The recruitment flowchart from eligibility to sample analysis is illustrated in Figure 1.

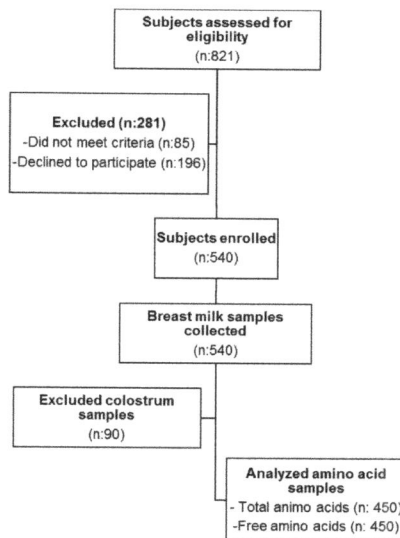

Figure 1. Study flow chart.

Subject demographics and anthropometry are described in Table 1. Maternal age, weight, BMI, and mode of delivery were significantly different among the lactation stage cohorts. No other significant differences were observed in maternal and infant characteristics analyzed.

Table 1. Maternal and infant characteristics.

| | Lactation Period | | | | | |
| | 5–11 Days | 12–30 Days | 1–2 Months | 2–4 Months | 4–8 Months | |
	(*n* = 90)	(*n* = 90)	(*n* = 90)	(*n* = 90)	(*n* = 90)	*p* Value
MOTHER						
Age (years), Mean (SD)	27 (4)	27 (3)	28 (4)	27 (4)	26 (4)	0.005
Height (cm), Mean (SD)	160 (4)	160 (5)	161 (5)	161 (5)	159 (5)	0.102
Weight (kg), Mean (SD)	60.7 (8.7)	60.8 (7.9)	61.9 (8.9)	58.4 (8.3)	56.2 (8.1)	<0.001
BMI (kg/m²), Mean (SD)	23.7 (3.2)	23.7 (3.0)	23.9 (3.1)	22.5 (2.9)	22.2 (3.1)	<0.001
Gestational weight gain (kg), Mean (SD)	16.7 (7.4)	16.2 (6.0)	15.9 (5.7)	15.9 (5.9)	14.9 (7.6)	0.419
Postpartum weight loss (kg), Mean (SD)	9.1 (6.1)	8.6 (5.3)	9.8 (4.0)	10.0 (6.2)	10.6 (5.9)	0.119
Non-Smoker, *n* (%)	90 (100)	89 (99)	90 (100)	86 (98)	89 (100)	0.176
Cesarean delivery, *n* (%)	39 (42)	43 (48)	53 (59)	35 (39)	35 (38)	0.004
Household income (RMB/month)						
<2000 RMB, *n* (%)	20 (22)	17 (19)	24 (27)	26 (29)	31 (34)	
2000–4000 RMB, *n* (%)	37 (41)	45 (50)	41 (46)	40 (44)	41 (46)	
>4000 RMB, *n* (%)	30 (33)	22 (24)	23 (26)	22 (24)	18 (20)	
Unknown, *n* (%)	1 (1)	6 (7)	2 (2)	0 (0)	0 (0)	0.206
INFANT						
Males, *n* (%)	51 (57)	48 (53)	48 (53)	54 (60)	43 (48)	0.865
Gestational age at birth (weeks), Mean (SD)	39.3 (1.2)	39.2 (1.3)	39.2 (1.6)	39.4 (1.3)	39.5 (1.5)	0.684

3.2. Total Amino Acids

The levels of TAA were compared across different lactation stages after adjusting for maternal age and BMI as well as for mode of delivery, infant gender, and geographical location.

The sum of TAA in milk samples significantly decreased with increasing lactation stage until the 2–4-month milk, which did not differ significantly from that at 4–8 months (Figure 2A). Median values ranged between 1608 mg/100 g and 1053 mg/100 g in the 5–11-day and the 2–4-month samples, respectively.

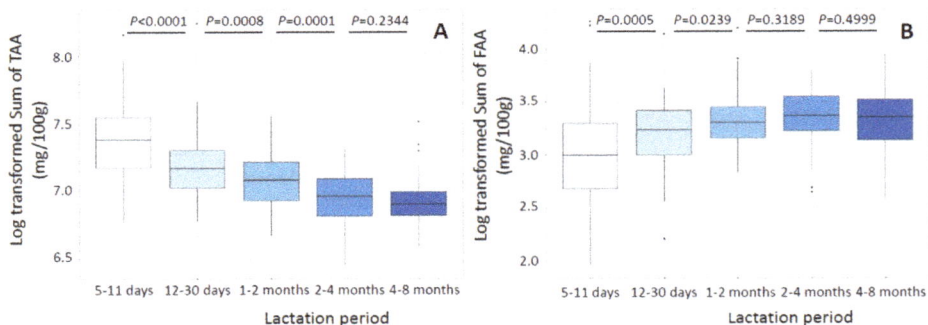

Figure 2. Box plot of the log-transformed sum of total (TAA, (**A**)) and of free (FAA, (**B**)) amino acids in milk from the different lactation periods. $n = 90$ milk samples per lactation period. Statistically significant differences between two periods were set at $p < 0.05$.

Concentrations of total IAA are reported in Table 2. Leucine and methionine were respectively the most and the least abundant IAA in our sample set across all the lactation stages. The levels of all IAA were highest in the early milk samples and then decreased with increasing lactation period until 2–4 months. Some differences of lower magnitude were still perceived between the two latest lactation stages; in particular, the levels of Leucine, lysine, and methionine were higher and the levels of histidine and phenylalanine were lower in 2–4-month than in 4–8-month milk.

Table 2. Total amino acid content (mg/100 g) of milk from the different lactation periods.

	Lactation Period				
	5–11 Days	12–30 Days	1–2 Months	2–4 Months	4–8 Months
IAA [†]					
Histidine	51.2 (19.9)	44.5 [§] (14.1)	36.5 [§] (12.6)	34.9 [§] (7.2)	25.0 [§] (6.8)
Isoleucine	81.0 (23.4)	71.6 [§] (15.4)	64.6 [§] (16.8)	54.0 [§] (11.6)	53.8 (10.7)
Leucine	153.7 (63.2)	133.7 [§] (35.1)	130.3 (33.5)	108.1 [§] (24.9)	122.6 [§] (38.8)
Lysine	112.0 (31.0)	93.8 [§] (23.1)	78.8 [§] (18.9)	63.4 [§] (13.1)	67.9 [§] (13.1)
Methionine	21.8 (11.7)	16.7 [§] (6.6)	13.0 [§] (9.0)	9.2 [§] (6.1)	11.8 [§] (7.1)
Phenylalanine	64.4 (35.9)	52.4 [§] (18.3)	40.4 [§] (13.6)	37.6 [§] (10.8)	28.4 [§] (9.0)
Threonine	85.1 (28.1)	66.9 [§] (14.6)	58.0 [§] (13.3)	50.0 [§] (8.7)	48.6 (11.3)
Valine	97.9 (34.3)	81.1 [§] (16.7)	72.1 [§] (21.0)	59.7 [§] (16.0)	60.9 (12.7)
DAA [†]					
Alanine	70.9 (23.0)	55.9 [§] (14.3)	45.9 [§] (15.7)	38.7 [§] (10.9)	38.6 (9.1)
Arginine	106.5 (36.6)	90.8 [§] (22.8)	77.0 [§] (24.5)	64.6 [§] (21.3)	65.3 (16.7)
Asx [‡]	132.9 (84.1)	115.5 [§] (54.4)	106.9 (40.0)	97.2 (56.8)	83.8 [§] (24.6)
Cystine	25.4 (12.5)	17.7 [§] (6.3)	12.5 [§] (5.2)	12.3 (3.4)	9.9 [§] (5.5)
Glx [‡]	248.1 (193.7)	220.1 [§] (92.4)	216.3 (59.3)	188.6 (105.2)	182.8 [§] (30.8)
Glycine	46.3 (15.2)	34.5 [§] (9.7)	27.6 [§] (10.5)	23.6 [§] (7.0)	23.5 (6.8)
Proline	140.2 (42.4)	117.7 [§] (26.5)	110.6 [§] (25.4)	95.3 [§] (20.9)	94.5 (17.2)
Serine	77.8 (27.0)	59.0 [§] (14.1)	47.9 [§] (9.8)	42.9 [§] (8.1)	41.7 (8.0)
Tyrosine	72.5 (30.4)	57.7 [§] (14.1)	44.1 [§] (19.5)	41.4 (13.9)	37.1 [§] (10.3)
SUM	1608.3 (589.5)	1296.5 [§] (368.4)	1188.1 [§] (341.7)	1053.2 [§] (291.9)	992.4 (175.9)

[†] IAA = indispensable amino acids; DAA = dispensable amino acid; [‡] Asx = sum of aspartic acid + asparagine; Glx = sum of glutamic acid + glutamine. Medians (inter-quartile ranges) of $n = 90$ samples per lactation period are shown. A median with a "[§]" superscript is significantly different from the median of the previous lactation period ($p < 0.05$).

Regarding dispensable amino acids (DAA) (Table 2) Glx (sum of glutamic acid + glutamine) was the most and cystine the least abundant amino acids. Again, the highest concentration for all DAA was recorded in the earliest milk (i.e., 5–11 days), and a subsequent decrease was observed in most DAA across the intermediate time points until reaching similar levels at the two latest lactation stages. In contrast, stable levels were observed for Glx and Asx (sum of aspartic acid + asparagine) between the 12–30-day and 2–4-month milk. A further decrease occurred in the 4–8-month samples.

3.3. Free Amino Acids

The levels of FAA were compared across the different lactation stages after adjusting for maternal age and BMI as well as for mode of delivery, infant gender, and geographical location.

In contrast to TAA, the sum of the individual FAA content was lower in the first compared with the latest lactation stages, with median values ranging between 20.1 mg/100 g of milk at 5–11 days and 29.0 mg/100 g of milk at 2–4 months (Figure 2B).

Concentrations of the individual FAA are reported in Table 3. Glx was the most abundant in FAA across the data set, and its concentration was higher in mature milk than in early-stage milk. In the latest lactation stages, it contributed up to more than 70% of the FAA mass. Similarly to Glx, levels of alanine, cystine, glycine, and serine were lowest in the early-stage milk. Opposite changes were observed in free IAA, of which highest concentrations were generally found in early-stage samples. The only exception was threonine, which remained stable across the lactation periods.

Table 3. Free AA content (mg/100 g) of milk from the different lactation periods.

	Lactation Period				
	5–11 Days	**12–30 Days**	**1–2 Months**	**2–4 Months**	**4–8 Months**
IAA [†]					
Histidine	0.29 (0.21)	0.42 [§] (0.23)	0.33 [§] (0.15)	0.33 (0.19)	0.28 (0.10)
Isoleucine	0.17 (0.11)	0.19 (0.13)	0.13 [§] (0.10)	0.13 (0.07)	0.15 [§] (0.07)
Leucine	0.33 (0.20)	0.4 (0.2)	0.34 [§] (0.14)	0.33 (0.14)	0.34 (0.15)
Lysine	0.61 (0.51)	0.56 [§] (0.28)	0.46 [§] (0.20)	0.42 [§] (0.23)	0.54 [§] (0.28)
Methionine	0.11 (0.07)	0.13 (0.13)	0.10 [§] (0.07)	0.07 [§] (0.06)	0.12 [§] (0.05)
Phenylalanine	0.31 (0.17)	0.40 (0.17)	0.32 [§] (0.17)	0.33 (0.17)	0.30 (0.12)
Threonine	0.69 (0.38)	0.69 (0.36)	0.70 (0.36)	0.78 (0.34)	0.85 (0.38)
Valine	0.58 (0.27)	0.70 [§] (0.30)	0.61 [§] (0.21)	0.59 (0.21)	0.59 (0.18)
DAA [†]					
Alanine	1.26 (0.81)	1.75 [§] (0.79)	2.07 [§] (0.67)	1.93 (0.68)	1.85 (0.46)
Arginine	0.46 (0.49)	0.42 [§] (0.28)	0.25 [§] (0.22)	0.25 (0.19)	0.25 (0.13)
Asx [‡]	0.47 (0.36)	0.52 (0.30)	0.54 (0.35)	0.55 (0.38)	0.58 (0.40)
Cystine	0.32 (0.13)	0.49 [§] (0.21)	0.46 (0.17)	0.49 (0.21)	0.50 (0.15)
Glx [‡]	10.89 (9.89)	15.09 [§] (8.74)	18.03 [§] (7.17)	20.22 [§] (7.28)	19.36 (8.07)
Glycine	0.51 (0.29)	0.62 [§] (0.23)	0.68 [§] (0.25)	0.64 (0.28)	0.76 [§] (0.28)
Proline	0.56 (0.33)	0.40 [§] (0.28)	0.54 (0.29)	0.40 (0.31)	0.45 [§] (0.44)
Serine	0.72 (0.43)	0.85 [§] (0.36)	0.91 [§] (0.40)	1.11 [§] (0.63)	1.11 (0.43)
Taurine	2.26 (2.65)	1.91 (1.78)	1.94 (1.31)	1.87 (1.42)	2.03 (1.12)
Tyrosine	0.38 (0.26)	0.40 (0.20)	0.28 [§] (0.17)	0.25 (0.14)	0.28 [§] (0.13)
SUM	20.1 (12.5)	25.5 [§] (10.4)	27.4 [§] (8.0)	29.0 (9.7)	28.6 (10.7)

[†] IAA = indispensable amino acids; DAA = dispensable amino acid; [‡] Asx = sum of aspartic acid + asparagine; Glx = sum of glutamic acid + glutamine. Medians (inter-quartile ranges) of $n = 90$ samples per lactation period are shown. A median with a "[§]" superscript is significantly different from the median of the previous lactation period ($p < 0.05$).

The contribution of FAA to TAA levels was less than 2% for most amino acids studied. A major exception was free Glx, which, on average, contributed to around 8% of the total Glx concentration. The ratio of free to total Glx gradually increased across the increasing lactation stages, from less than 5% at 5–11 days up to more than 10% at 4–8 months.

Of note is that compared with the TAA (Table 2) inter-individual variability in FAA values was very high (Table 3).

4. Discussion

Amino acids are an essential component in infant nutrition, and their levels in breast milk are believed to be optimal to support healthy growth during the first months of life. Because of this, the amino acid intake from human milk is considered to match infant requirements, and the breast milk amino acid content is used to estimate the protein quality and quantity in breast milk substitutes [3]. Therefore, a reliable evaluation of the amino acid composition in breast milk is important.

The concentration of the sum of TAA—a good proxy of the true protein content—at the different lactation stages was, in our samples, remarkably similar to that reported in transitional, mature, and late milk in a recent systematic review of studies from Africa, Asia, Europe, and North America [8]. A limitation in our study, however, is the lack of colostrum samples. This said, although colostrum is important for the protection of the neonate, the amount of amino acids provided by the colostrum protein is likely limited due to the low secreted volumes as well as to the relatively low digestibility of the major colostrum proteins [13]. Similar to the results reported in the systematic review by Zhang et al. [8], the sum of TAA was greater in the early stage of lactation, slowly declining in concentration as lactation progressed, reaching generally stable levels after 2–4 months. These changes are consistent with the protein content results of the MING study reported elsewhere [11] and with the well-known evolution of the protein content in breast milk, i.e., high during the early lactation stages, and sharply decreasing during the transitional milk period to level off in mature milk [13]. It has been proposed that these changes in the amino acid content of the milk match the infant requirements for growth, which is fast during the neonatal period sharply decreasing during the first months of life [14]. Declining protein concentrations may also prevent amino acid overfeeding as milk volume intake per unit body weight increases along lactation [3,4]. Of note, protein concentration in human milk is remarkably low compared with that from most other mammals. Low protein intake during infancy is believed to protect the individual against obesity and metabolic disease later in life, possibly related to optimal appetite and hormonal programming [15].

The levels of individual TAA's in the different lactation stages of the MING cohort were also close to those reported by Zhang et al. [8]. The only amino acid showing a consistently lower value in our samples was cystine. However, cystine is known to be particularly sensitive to the acid treatment used for protein hydrolysis in our samples [16], and the cystine levels that we report here may underestimate the real values.

Globally, the individual TAA levels showed similar temporal patterns as the sum of TAA. However, whereas a strong decrease between early, transitional, and mature milk was observed for some amino acids such as methionine, cystine, and glycine, this drop was less substantial for Glx levels, which were comparable in transitional and mature milk. This observation is consistent with the fact that besides the variations in protein content, changes in the quality of the protein occur along lactation. Specifically, a significant decline in the concentration of the sulfur amino acid-rich and glycine-rich whey proteins but stable levels of the Glx-rich casein were found in our milk samples [17] and are usually reported [18], resulting in a whey to casein ratio that increases throughout lactation [13] and, as observed in our samples, in an evolving amino acid profile.

As expected from previous reports [6], the contribution of FAA to the TAA mass was less than 3% in all lactation periods. Because of this, the contribution of the FAA to the nutritional requirements of the infant is expected to be low. The physiological importance of FAA for infants is not yet well understood. It has been proposed that FAA are more rapidly absorbed, leading to accelerated appearance in the systemic circulation and thus reaching the peripheral organs faster than the protein-bound amino acids [6,8]. However, to our knowledge, the absorption kinetics of free and protein-bound amino acids in breast milk has never been compared, and the physiological relevance of a potentially faster delivery to the peripheral tissue of the small FAA load delivered by milk remains speculative.

Free Glx was very abundant in our samples, contributing to around 70% of the FAA mass and reaching up to 10% of the total Glx levels in the later lactation periods. Similar observations have also previously been reported where both glutamic acid and glutamine were shown to be the most abundant FAA in human milk throughout the first trimester of lactation [19]. Specifically, the authors of [19] reported a 2.5- and 20-fold increase in glutamic acid and glutamine FAA concentrations, respectively, with progressing lactation. It should be noted that, similar to our findings, these FAAs represented more than 50% of total FAAs at three months [19]. Total Glx was also the most concentrated TAA in our samples, suggesting an important role of this amino acid on the mammary gland metabolism, on infant nutrition, or both, despite the fact that glutamic acid and glutamine are considered DAA that can be synthesized by the body [20]. More specifically, the transamination of glutamic acid by the mucosal intestinal cells yields alanine, which enters the gluconeogenic pathway. In addition, both glutamic acid and glutamine from the lumen act as major energy substrates for the intestinal cells [21,22]. In the neonatal pig for instance, the gastrointestinal tract uses dietary glutamine and glutamate as its key respiratory fuel. In humans, trials with very low birth weight infants and critically ill adult patients highlight the central role of glutamic acid and glutamine in protecting intestinal growth and integrity [23–25], therefore suggesting glutamic acid and glutamine as important molecules in milk for the immature infant gut. More recent results from Ventura et al. [7] also suggest a role of Glutamate on the satiety status of the lactating infant.

Similar to Glx, free alanine, cystine, glycine, and serine also increased along the lactation periods in our samples. Intriguingly, similar findings were reported in the systematic review by Zhang et al. [8], indicating a consistent pattern in stage-associated changes independent of ethnic or geographic factors. This consistency is outstanding in light of the important inter-individual FAA variability in our study, the inter-study variability observed in the report by Zhang et al., and even the intra-individual changes reported by others in transitional and mature breast milk [26]. However, the physiological significance of the concentration rise of these DAA through lactation is not clear. Furthermore, understanding the physiological relevance of the increased inter-individual variability observed in FAA needs to be elucidated.

An important limitation in our study is that our analytical method did not permit to quantify the concentration of tryptophan. Yet the IAA tryptophan is usually the limiting amino acid in infant formula; thus, its concentration in breast milk is often used to estimate the protein quality and to adjust the level of the protein in the formula. Another limitation is the cross-sectional nature of the study that weakens the conclusions related to the stage-driven changes, which would have been best assessed by a longitudinal design. However, our statistical model adjusted for the maternal and infant baseline factors that were known or suspected to impact milk nutrient composition [1], including maternal weight and mode of delivery, which differed between the lactation period cohorts. Our results are also reinforced by the fact that they were remarkably consistent with those previously published.

5. Conclusions

In conclusion, the amino acid composition of the milk from our cohort of urban Chinese mothers was comparable to human milk data from previously reported studies carried out in other parts of the world, suggesting that amino acid composition in breast milk is an evolutionary conserved trait largely independent of geographical, ethnical, or dietary factors.

Acknowledgments: The authors would like to thank the funding sources of this work and Nestec Ltd. for covering the costs for publishing open access. Special acknowledgment to the participants who volunteered for this study: Lawrence Li for project support and guidance, Celia Ning for project management, Qiaoji Li for clinical project management, and Emilie Ba for data management. Special acknowledgment to Jiaji Wang at Guangzhou Medical University, Liqiang Qin at Soochow University School of Public Health and their teams, as well as the project staff at Peking University School of Public Health for their tasks in recruitment and data collection. The Nestlé Research Center and the Nestlé Nutrition Institute China sponsored the study.

Author Contributions: C.L.G.R., L.G.K., and M.A. interpreted the results, drafted, reviewed, and revised the initial manuscript. G.V.P. contributed to the study design, drafted, reviewed, and revised the initial manuscript. S.K.T. contributed to the study design, the breast milk sampling protocol, and the interpretation of the results.

Y.Z. and P.W. contributed to study design and performed field collection. C.D.C. performed the statistical analysis and reviewed and revised the initial manuscript. All authors read and approved the final manuscript.

Conflicts of Interest: This study was funded by Nestlé Nutrition Institute, China and Nestlé Research Centre, Beijing, China. C.L.G.R., M.A., L.G.K., G.V.P., and S.K.T. were all employees of Nestec Ltd. when this work was completed. Y.Z. and P.W. report grants from Nestle Research Center and Nestle Nutrition Institute China during the conduct of the study.

References

1. Stam, J.; Sauer, P.J.; Boehm, G. Can we define an infant's need from the composition of human milk? *Am. J. Clin. Nutr.* **2013**, *98*, 521S–528S. [CrossRef] [PubMed]
2. Michaelsen, K.F.; Greer, F.R. Protein needs early in life and long-term health. *Am. J. Clin. Nutr.* **2014**, *99*, 718S–722S. [CrossRef] [PubMed]
3. World Health Organization; Food and Agriculture Organization of the United Nations; United Nations University. *Joint FAO/WHO/UNU Expert Consultation on Protein and Amino Acid Requirements in Human Nutrition*; WHO technical report series; WHO Press: Geneva, Switzerland, 2007; Volume 935, pp. 1–265.
4. Da Costa, T.H.; Haisma, H.; Wells, J.C.; Mander, A.P.; Whitehead, R.G.; Bluck, L.J. How much human milk do infants consume? Data from 12 countries using a standardized stable isotope methodology. *J. Nutr.* **2010**, *140*, 2227–2232. [CrossRef] [PubMed]
5. Svanberg, U.; Gebre-Medhin, M.; Ljungqvist, B.; Olsson, M. Breast milk composition in Ethiopian and Swedish mothers. III. Amino acids and other nitrogenous substances. *Am. J. Clin. Nutr.* **1977**, *30*, 499–507. [PubMed]
6. Carratu, B.; Boniglia, C.; Scalise, F.; Ambruzzib, A.M.; Sanzinia, E. Nitrogenous components of human milk: Non-protein nitrogen, true protein and free amino acids. *Food Chem.* **2003**, *81*, 357–362. [CrossRef]
7. Ventura, A.K.; Beauchamp, G.K.; Mennella, J.A. Infant regulation of intake: The effect of free glutamate content in infant formulas. *Am. J. Clin. Nutr.* **2012**, *95*, 875–881. [CrossRef] [PubMed]
8. Zhang, Z.; Adelman, A.S.; Rai, D.; Boettcher, J.; Lönnerdal, B. Amino acid profiles in term and preterm human milk through lactation: A systematic review. *Nutrients* **2013**, *5*, 4800–4821. [CrossRef] [PubMed]
9. Zhao, X.; Xu, Z.; Wang, Y.; Sun, Y. Studies of the relation between the nutritional status of lactating mothers and milk composition as well as the milk intake and growth of their infants in Beijing. Pt. 4. The protein and amino acid content of breast milk. *Acta Nutr. Sin.* **1989**, *11*, 227–232.
10. Ding, M.; Li, W.; Zhang, Y.; Wang, X.; Zhao, A.; Zhao, X.; Wang, P.; Sheng, Q.H. Amino acid composition of lactating mothers' milk and confinement diet in rural North China. *Asia Pac. J. Clin. Nutr.* **2010**, *19*, 344–349. [PubMed]
11. Yang, T.; Zhang, Y.; Ning, Y.; You, L.; Ma, D.; Zheng, Y.; Yang, X.; Li, W.; Wang, J.; Wang, P. Breast milk macronutrient composition and the associated factors in urban Chinese mothers. *Chin. Med. J. (Engl.)* **2014**, *127*, 1721–1725. [PubMed]
12. Blankenship, D.T.; Krivanek, M.A.; Ackermann, B.L.; Cardin, A.D. High-sensitivity amino acid analysis by derivatization with O-phthalaldehyde and 9-fluorenylmethyl chloroformate using fluorescence detection: Applications in protein structure determination. *Anal. Biochem.* **1989**, *178*, 227–232. [CrossRef]
13. Lonnerdal, B. Nutritional and physiologic significance of human milk proteins. *Am. J. Clin. Nutr.* **2003**, *77*, 1537S–1543S. [PubMed]
14. Dupont, C. Protein requirements during the first year of life. *Am. J. Clin. Nutr.* **2003**, *77*, 1544S–1549S. [PubMed]
15. Hassiotou, F.; Geddes, D.T. Programming of appetite control during breastfeeding as a preventative strategy against the obesity epidemic. *J. Hum. Lac.* **2014**, *30*, 136–142. [CrossRef] [PubMed]
16. Peace, R.W.; Gilani, G.S. Chromatographic determination of amino acids in foods. *J. AOAC Int.* **2005**, *88*, 877–887. [PubMed]
17. Affolter, M.; Garcia-Rodenas, C.L.; Vinyes-Pares, G.; Jenni, R.; Roggero, I.; Avanti-Nigro, O.; de Castro, C.A.; Zhao, A.; Zhang, Y.; Wang, P.; et al. Temporal Changes of Protein Composition in Breast Milk of Chinese Urban Mothers and Impact of Caesarean Section Delivery. *Nutrients* **2016**, *8*, E504. [CrossRef] [PubMed]
18. Sindayikengera, S.; Xia, W.S. Nutritional evaluation of caseins and whey proteins and their hydrolysates from Protamex. *J. Zhejiang Univ. Sci. B* **2006**, *7*, 90–98. [CrossRef] [PubMed]

19. Agostoni, C.; Carratu, B.; Boniglia, C.; Lammardo, A.M.; Riva, E.; Sanzini, E. Free glutamine and glutamic acid increase in human milk through a three-month lactation period. *J. Pediatr. Gastroenterol. Nutr.* **2000**, *31*, 508–512. [CrossRef] [PubMed]

20. Reeds, P.J. Dispensable and indispensable amino acids for humans. *J. Nutr.* **2000**, *130*, 1835S–1840S. [PubMed]

21. Reeds, P.J.; Burrin, D.G. Glutamine and the bowel. *J. Nutr.* **2001**, *131*, 2505S–2508S. [PubMed]

22. Rezaei, R.; Wang, W.; Wu, Z.; Dai, Z.; Wang, J.; Wu, G. Biochemical and physiological bases for utilization of dietary amino acids by young pigs. *J. Anim. Sci. Biotechnol.* **2013**, *4*, 7. [CrossRef] [PubMed]

23. Van der Hulst, R.R.; van Kreel, B.K.; von Meyenfeldt, M.F.; Brummer, R.J.; Arends, J.W.; Deutz, N.E.; Soeters, P.B. Glutamine and the preservation of gut integrity. *Lancet* **1993**, *341*, 1363–1365. [CrossRef]

24. Roig, J.C.; Meetze, W.H.; Auestad, N.; Jasionowski, T.; Veerman, M.; McMurray, C.A.; Neu, J. Enteral glutamine supplementation for the very low birthweight infant: Plasma amino acid concentrations. *J. Nutr.* **1996**, *126*, 1115S–1120S. [PubMed]

25. Burrin, D.G.; Stoll, B. Key nutrients and growth factors for the neonatal gastrointestinal tract. *Clin. Perinatol.* **2002**, *29*, 65–96. [CrossRef]

26. Sánchez, C.L.; Cubero, J.; Sánchez, J.; Franco, L.; Rodríguez, A.B.; Rivero, M.; Barriga, C. Evolution of the circadian profile of human milk amino acids during breastfeeding. *J. Appl. Biomed.* **2013**, *11*, 59–70. [CrossRef]

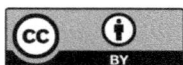

nutrients

MDPI

Article

Does Human Milk Modulate Body Composition in Late Preterm Infants at Term-Corrected Age?

Maria Lorella Giannì [1,*], **Dario Consonni** [2], **Nadia Liotto** [1], **Paola Roggero** [1], **Laura Morlacchi** [1], **Pasqua Piemontese** [1], **Camilla Menis** [1] and **Fabio Mosca** [1]

[1] Fondazione I.R.C.C.S. Ca Granda Ospedale Maggiore Policlinico, Neonatal Intensive Care Unit, Department of Clinical Science and Community Health, University of Milan, Via Commenda 12, 20122 Milano, Italy; nadia.liotto@unimi.it (N.L.); paola.roggero@unimi.it (P.R.); lally.morly@hotmail.it (L.M.); pasquina.piemontese@mangiagalli.it (P.P.); camilla.menis@studenti.unimi.it (C.M.); fabio.mosca@unimi.it (F.M.)

[2] Fondazione IRCCS Ca' Granda Ospedale Maggiore Policlinico, Epidemiology Unit, Via San Barnaba 8, 20122 Milan, Italy; dario.consonni@unimi.it

* Correspondence: maria.gianni@unimi.it; Tel.: +39-2-5503-2483; Fax: +39-2-5503-2436

Received: 26 July 2016; Accepted: 18 October 2016; Published: 23 October 2016

Abstract: (1) Background: Late preterm infants account for the majority of preterm births and are at risk of altered body composition. Because body composition modulates later health outcomes and human milk is recommended as the normal method for infant feeding, we sought to investigate whether human milk feeding in early life can modulate body composition development in late preterm infants; (2) Methods: Neonatal, anthropometric and feeding data of 284 late preterm infants were collected. Body composition was evaluated at term-corrected age by air displacement plethysmography. The effect of human milk feeding on fat-free mass and fat mass content was evaluated using multiple linear regression analysis; (3) Results: Human milk was fed to 68% of the infants. According to multiple regression analysis, being fed any human milk at discharge and at term-corrected and being fed exclusively human milk at term-corrected age were positively associated with fat-free mass content($\beta = -47.9$, 95% confidence interval (CI) $= -95.7$; -0.18; $p = 0.049$; $\beta = -89.6$, 95% CI $= -131.5$; -47.7; $p < 0.0001$; $\beta = -104.1$, 95% CI $= -151.4$; -56.7, $p < 0.0001$); (4) Conclusion: Human milk feeding appears to be associated with fat-free mass deposition in late preterm infants. Healthcare professionals should direct efforts toward promoting and supporting breastfeeding in these vulnerable infants.

Keywords: human milk; late preterm infants; body composition

1. Introduction

Late preterm birth, defined as a birth that occurs between 34 0/7 and 36 6/7 weeks of gestation, accounts for the majority of all preterm births [1]. Late preterm infants show increased mortality and morbidity compared with full-term newborn infants [2]. It has been reported that the first months of the postnatal life of late preterm infants are characterized by rapid postnatal catch-up growth, and as a result, at term-corrected age, late preterm infants achieve a weight either comparable to or higher than full-term newborns [3,4]. Evidence indicates that early body composition development in these infants is accompanied by a major deposition of fat mass so that, at term-corrected age, increased adiposity irrespective of the percentile at birth has been found. Unlike very preterm infants, however, late preterm infants appear not to develop a fat-free mass deficit [4].

It has long been recognized that early life represents a critical time window in terms of metabolic programming [5]. Indeed, increased adiposity early on may contribute to negative health outcomes later [6], whereas fat-free mass accretion has been positively associated with faster brain processing [7].

Considering the key role played by body composition development in modulating later health outcomes [6], identification of the determinants of body composition may help in tailoring nutritional interventions in infancy. Mode of feeding in early life has been reported to affect body composition development [8]. Human milk is recommended as the normal and unequalled method for feeding both preterm and term infants [9].

While some authors have investigated the determinants of body composition, including human milk feeding, in very preterm infants at the time of hospital discharge [10,11], there is a paucity of data on early determinants of body composition in late preterm infants who are recognized to be undergoing a critical period of development [12]. Huang et al. [8] have conducted a systematic review and meta-analysis, including infants born before completion of the 37th week of gestational age, to investigate whether body composition at term-corrected age differs between breastfed and formula-fed infants. However, late preterm infants were relatively underrepresented in the investigation. The aim of the present study was to investigate whether human milk consumption in early life could modulate body composition development at term-corrected age in late preterm infants.

2. Materials and Methods

2.1. Design and Setting

We conducted an observational cohort study. Approval was obtained from the institutional review board of Fondazione Istituto di Ricovero e Cura a Carattere Scientifico Cà Granda Ospedale Maggiore Policlinico (code number 506_2015, date of approval: 22 May 2015) and written informed consent from the infants' parents.

2.2. Sample

All consecutive newborns admitted to the authors' institution between July 2015 and May 2016 were screened for eligibility. The inclusion criteria were gestational age from 34 0/7 to 36 6/7, Caucasian parentage and clinical stability at term-corrected age. The exclusion criteria were presence of congenital disease; chromosomal abnormalities; cardiac, brain, renal, endocrine, gastrointestinal or infectious disease; respiratory distress syndrome, defined as the need for any respiratory support for longer than seven days; and pre-pregnancy maternal body mass index >30.

2.3. Nutritional Practices

Infants were fed on demand. Mothers were encouraged either to breastfeed their infant or express their milk according to their infant's clinical condition. According to our internal nutritional procedure, human milk was not fortified [13]. When human milk was unavailable or insufficient, formula feeding was started. Infants born at 34 weeks gestational age and infants born small for gestational age (SGA) at 35–36 weeks gestational age were fed a post-discharge formula (range of protein content: 2–2.4 g/100 mL; range of energy content: 73–82 kcal/100 mL) up to the maximum corrected age of 40 weeks. Late preterm infants, born adequate for gestational age (AGA), at 35–36 weeks of gestational age, were fed a regular-term formula (range of protein content: 1.3–1.7 g/100 mL; range of energy content: 66–68 kcal/100 mL).

2.4. Data Collection

Infants were enrolled at birth. At enrolment, basic subject characteristics such as gestational age at birth, anthropometrics parameters at birth and at discharge (weight, length and head circumference), gender, being a twin, and being adequate for gestational age or small for gestational age were recorded prospectively. Gestational age was based on the last menstrual period and first trimester ultrasonogram. Term-corrected age was calculated from the chronologic age, that is the time elapsed after birth, reduced by the number of weeks the infant was born before the expected date of delivery, that is, 40 weeks of gestation [14]. Infants with birth weight in the <10th or ≥10th percentile for gestational age, based on Fenton's growth chart [15], were, respectively, classified as having weight that was SGA or AGA. The feeding status at discharge (any human milk, including exclusively human milk or exclusively formula) and length of hospital stay were also collected. Specifically, infants fed any extent of human milk, irrespective of the quantity or the exclusivity, were categorized as fed any human milk [9]. After discharge, the parents were asked to report in a diary the mode of feeding from discharge up to term-corrected age (40 weeks ± 2 days).

2.5. Growth and Body Composition Assessment

Anthropometric measurements were assessed at birth, at discharge and at term-corrected age (40 weeks ± 2 days). Body weight, length and head circumference were measured according to standard procedures [16]. The weight of each baby was measured on an electronic scale accurate to 0.1 g (PEA POD Infant Body Composition System; Cosmed, Concord, CA, USA). Body length was measured to the nearest 1 mm on a Harpenden neonatometer (Holtain, Crymych, UK). Head circumference was measured to the nearest 1 mm using non-stretch measuring tape. All measurements were assessed by trained medical staff of the author's institution. The late preterm infants' growth (weight, length and head circumference) z-scores were then calculated using the z-score calculator provided by the University of Calgary, Calgary, Alberta, Canada [17]. Body composition was assessed at term-corrected age using an air-displacement plethysmograph (PEA POD Infant Body Composition System; COSMED, Concord, CA, USA). A detailed description of the PEA POD's physical design, operating principles, validation, and measurement procedures is provided elsewhere [18,19]. Briefly, the PEA POD assesses fat mass and fat-free mass by direct measurements of body mass and volume and the application of a classic densitometric model where percentage of body fat is calculated using body density and pre-determined fat and fat-free mass density values. Body fat was defined as body weight minus fat-free mass. A constant fat mass density value of 0.9007 g/mL [20,21] is used. Fat-free mass density values are calculated as the sum of the contribution of the various components in the fat-free mass compartment. Age- and sex-specific fat-free mass density values extrapolated from data by Fomon et al. are used [22].

2.6. Statistical Analysis

All descriptive data are expressed as the mean ± SD or n (%). The associations between neonatal characteristics (anthropometric measurements at birth and at term-corrected age, feeding status at discharge and at term-corrected age), fat mass and fat-free mass content at term-corrected age were assessed using univariate linear regression analysis. Multiple linear regression models, including variables that resulted to be significant at univariate analysis, were used to identify the determinants of fat mass and fat free mass content at term-corrected age. In order to avoid collinearity, with regard to anthropometric parameters, we included only weight at term-corrected age as independent variable since it was most closely correlated with fat-free mass and fat mass content at term-corrected age in the univariate analysis. Weight was expressed as z-scores, in order to take into account gestational age. All statistical analyses were performed using SPSS (SPSS, version 12; SPSS, Chicago, IL, USA) and Stata (StataCorp. 2013, Stata Statistical Software: Release 13. StataCorp LP, College Station, TX, USA).

3. Results

A total of 284 late preterm infants were enrolled. The flow chart of the study is reported in Figure 1. The mean hospital stay was 8.9 ± 5.05 days. The mean postmenstrual age at discharge was 36.6 ± 0.8 weeks. The mean chronological age at term-corrected age was 33.1 ± 3.6 days.

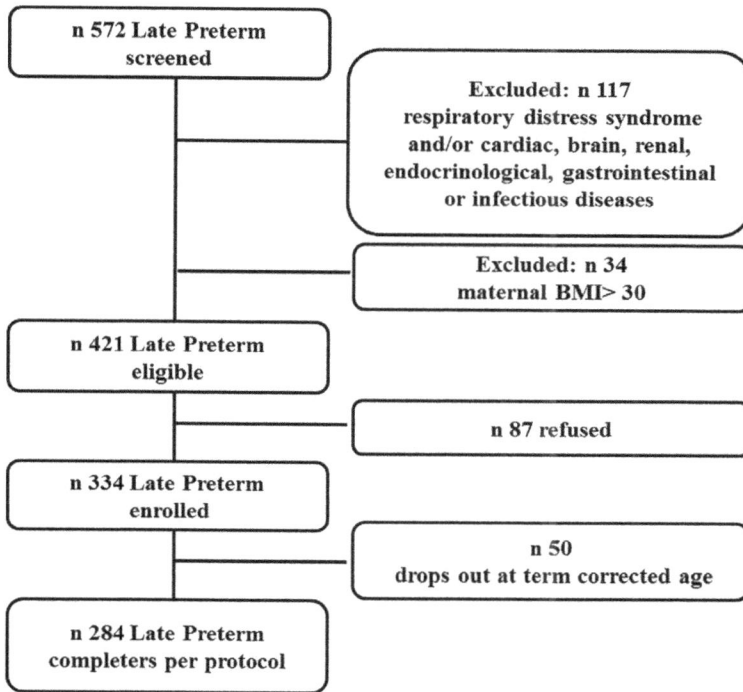

Figure 1. Flow chart of the study.

The basic characteristics of the subjects at birth are shown in Table 1.

Table 1. Basic subject characteristics at birth.

	Late Preterm Infants (n = 284)	Males (n = 147)	Females (n = 137)
Gestational age (weeks)	35.3 ± 0.8	35.2 ± 0.9	35.4 ± 0.7
Birth weight (g)	2413 ± 387	2427 ± 404	2397 ± 369
Length (cm)	45.3 ± 2.4	45.3 ± 2.6	45.3 ± 2.2
Head circumference (cm)	31.9 ± 1.4	31.9 ± 1.6	31.9 ± 1.2
Weight z-scores	−0.23 ± 0.87	−0.27 ± 0.8	−0.28 ± 0.8
Length z-scores	−0.33 ± 0.91	−0.31 ± 0.9	−0.28 ± 0.8
Head circumference z-scores	−0.09 ± 0.88	−0.06 ± 0.9	−0.01 ± 0.8
Small for gestational age n (%)	42 (15)	18 (12)	24 (18)
Twins n (%)	119 (42)	50 (34)	69 (50)

Data are presented as the mean (SD) or n (%).

Mode of feeding, anthropometric parameters and body composition in the enrolled late preterm infants at discharge and at term-corrected age are reported in Tables 2 and 3, respectively.

In the univariate analysis, anthropometric parameters at birth and at term-corrected age, gestational age, being male and being fed human milk at discharge and at term-corrected age were all positively associated with fat-free mass content at term-corrected age, whereas being born small for gestational age and being a twin were negatively associated. With regard to fat mass, anthropometric parameters at birth and at term-corrected age and being exclusively fed human milk at discharge were positively associated with fat mass content at term-corrected age, whereas being born small for gestational age was negatively associated (Table 4).

Table 2. Mode of feeding and anthropometric parameters of the enrolled late preterm infants at discharge.

	Late Preterm Infants (*n* = 284)	Males (*n* = 147)	Females (*n* = 137)
Exclusive human milk *n* (%)	97 (34)	53 (36)	44 (32)
Exclusive formula *n* (%)	91 (32)	35 (24)	56 (41)
Any human milk *n* (%)	193 (68)	112 (77)	81 (59)
Weight (g)	2270 ± 497	2317 ± 442	2200 ± 428
Length (cm)	45.1 ± 2.7	45.1 ± 3.4	45.1 ± 2.2
Head circumference (cm)	31.9 ± 1.4	31.9 ± 1.5	31.8 ± 1.1
Weight z-scores	−0.92 ± 0.8	−0.95 ± 0.8	−0.94 ± 0.8
Length z-scores	−0.70 ± 0.9	−0.85 ± 1.0	−0.53 ± 0.8
Head circumference z-scores	−0.38 ± 0.7	−0.51 ± 0.8	−0.30 ± 0.7

Table 3. Mode of feeding, anthropometric parameters and body composition of the enrolled late preterm infants at term-corrected age.

	Late Preterm Infants (*n* = 284)	Males (*n* = 147)	Females (*n* = 137)
Exclusive human milk *n* (%)	88 (31)	54 (37)	34 (25)
Exclusive formula *n* (%)	134 (47)	68 (46)	66 (48)
Any human milk *n* (%)	150 (53)	79 (54)	71 (52)
Weight (g)	3396 ± 504	3380 ± 526	3240 ± 521
Length (cm)	49.4 ± 2.3	49.7 ± 2.5	49.1 ± 2.2
Head circumference (cm)	35.1 ± 1.6	35.3 ± 2.0	34.7 ± 1.3
Weight z-scores	−0.31 ± 1.1	−0.38 ± 1.1	−0.23 ± 1.0
Length z-scores	−0.56 ± 1.0	−0.59 ± 1.1	−0.53 ± 0.9
Head circumference z-scores	0.14 ± 0.9	0.25 ± 0.9	−0.02 ± 0.9
Fat mass %	14.7 ± 4.7	14.2 ± 4.5	15.3 ± 4.9
Fat free mass %	85.2 ± 4.8	85.8 ± 4.6	84.7 ± 4.9
Fat mass (g)	510 ± 2.1	493.8 ± 204	527.6 ± 219
Fat free mass (g)	2878 ± 392	2934.2 ± 408	2817.1 ± 366

Table 4. Univariate linear regression analysis for associations of infant characteristics, anthropometric parameters and mode of feeding with fat-free mass and fat mass at term-corrected age.

Parameters	Fat-Free Mass at Term-Corrected Age (g)			Fat Mass at Term-Corrected Age (g)		
	β	95% Confidence Interval	*p*	β	95% Confidence Interval	*p*
Gestational age (weeks)	64.5	8.1; 120.9	0.025	−5.7	−36.5; 25.0	0.713
Being male (yes vs. no)	117.0	26.1; 207.8	0.012	−33.8	−83.2; 15.7	0.180
Being small for gestational age (no vs. yes)	−401.9	−522.3; −281.5	<0.0001	−128.5	−196.8; 60.3	<0.0001
Weight z-score at birth	280.9	238.1; 323.7	<0.0001	92.5	65.4; 119.6	<0.0001
Length z-score at birth	175.0	129; 220.9	<0.0001	60.8	34.5; 87.1	<0.0001
Head circumference z-score at birth	156.4	107.3; 205.4	<0.0001	57.5	29.9; 85.0	<0.0001
Weight z-score at term-corrected age	307.1	283.9; 330.2	<0.0001	140.3	124.1; 156.6	<0.0001
Length z-score at term-corrected age	246.4	212.4; 280.4	<0.0001	103.6	82.7; 124.4	<0.0001
Head circumference z-score at term-corrected age	232.5	191.3; 273.6	<0.0001	87.5	62.8; 112.1	<0.0001
Being twin (no vs. yes)	−187.6	−289.6; −85.6	<0.0001	−32.8	−89.8; 24.8	0.256
Being exclusively human milk fed vs. exclusively formula fed at discharge	−333	−483.6; −183.5	<0.0001	−99.1	−179.1; −19.1	0.016
Being fed any human milk vs. exclusively formula fed at discharge	−223	−337.9; −109.0	<0.0001	−43.6	−110.0; 22.9	0.197
Being exclusively human milk fed vs. exclusively formula fed at term-corrected age	−226	−344.6; 109.1	<0.0001	17.8	−48.1; 83.8	0.594
Being fed any human milk vs. exclusively formula fed at term-corrected age	−227	−327.8; −126.2	<0.0001	−7.8	−65.0; 49.4	0.788

At multiple regression analysis, when including mode of feeding at discharge, being male, weight z-score at term-corrected age and being fed any human milk at discharge were positively associated with fat-free mass content at term-corrected age (Tables 5 and 6).

Table 5. Multiple linear regression analysis for associations of gender, weight z-score at term-corrected age, being a twin and being exclusively fed human milk at discharge with fat-free mass at term-corrected age (R^2 = 0.88, p < 0.0001).

Model	Fat-Free Mass Content at Term-Corrected Age (g)		
	β	95% Confidence Interval	p
Intercept	3008.4	2898.5; 3118.3	<0.0001
Male (yes vs. no)	80.6	20.6; 140.6	0.009
Being a twin (no vs. yes)	−7.9	−73.4; 57.6	0.8
Weight z-score at term-corrected age	361.2	327.9; 394.6	<0.0001
Mode of feeding at discharge (being exclusively human milk fed vs. being exclusively formula fed)	−39.6	−102.4; 23.2	0.214

Table 6. Multiple linear regression analysis for associations of gender, weight z-score at term-corrected age, being a twin and being fed any human milk at discharge with fat-free mass at term-corrected age (R^2 = 0.85, p < 0.0001).

Model	Fat-Free Mass Content at Term-Corrected Age (g)		
	β	95% Confidence Interval	p
Intercept	3037.2	2961.2; 3113.1	<0.0001
Male (yes vs. no)	68.0	24.2; 111.7	0.002
Being a twin (no vs. yes)	−38.7	−82.3; 4.7	0.08
Weight z-score at term-corrected age	347.7	325.2; 370.2	<0.0001
Mode of feeding at discharge (being fed any human milk vs. being exclusively formula fed)	−47.9	−95.7; −0.18	0.049

With regard to fat mass content, the weight z-score at term-corrected age was positively associated with its content at term-corrected age, whereas the mode of feeding was not significantly associated (Table 7).

Table 7. Multiple linear regression analysis for associations of weight z-score at term-corrected age, and being exclusively human milk fed at discharge with fat mass at term-corrected age (R^2 = 0.63, p < 0.0001).

Model	Fat Mass Content at Term-Corrected Age (g)		
	β	95% Confidence Interval	p
Intercept	517.7	430.8; 604.5	<0.0001
Weight z-score at term-corrected age	164.9	137.8; 192.0	<0.0001
Mode of feeding at discharge (being exclusively human milk fed vs. being exclusively formula fed)	27.2	−27.0; 81.5	0.321

In the multiple regression analysis, when including the mode of feeding at term-corrected age, being male, the weight z-score at term-corrected age and being fed either exclusively or any human milk at term-corrected age were positively associated with fat-free mass content at term-corrected age (Tables 8 and 9).

Table 8. Multiple linear regression analysis for associations of gender, weight z-score at term-corrected age, being a twin and being fed exclusively human milk at term-corrected age with fat-free mass at term-corrected age ($R^2 = 0.88$, $p < 0.0001$).

Model	Fat-Free Mass Content at Term-Corrected Age (g)		
	β	95% Confidence Interval	*p*
Intercept	3098.2	3018.1; 3178.3	<0.0001
Male (yes vs. no)	84.3	41.1; 127.4	<0.0001
Being a twin (no vs. yes)	23.4	−23.6; 70.4	0.32
Weight z-score at term-corrected age	355.0	332.8; 377.2	<0.0001
Mode of feeding at term-corrected age (being exclusively human milk fed vs. being exclusively formula fed)	−104.1	−151.4; −56.7	<0.0001

Table 9. Multiple linear regression analysis for associations of gender, weight z-score at term-corrected age, being a twin and being fed any human milk at term-corrected age with fat-free mass at term-corrected age ($R^2 = 0.86$, $p < 0.0001$).

Model	Fat-Free Mass Content at Term-Corrected Age (g)		
	β	95% Confidence Interval	*p*
Intercept	3088.1	3023.3; 3152.9	<0.0001
Male (yes vs. no)	75.0	34.8; 115.2	<0.0001
Being a twin (no vs. yes)	1.5	−41.2; 44.2	0.94
Weight z-score at term-corrected age	354.5	333.7; 375.3	<0.0001
Mode of feeding at term-corrected age (being fed any human milk vs. being exclusively formula fed)	−89.6	−131.5; −47.7	<0.0001

4. Discussion

The findings of this study indicate that the consumption of human milk is associated with fat-free mass deposition in late preterm infants. It must be taken into account that the strength of this relationship appears to become stronger towards the achievement of term-corrected age, suggesting a potential cumulative effect of human milk consumption on body composition development.

Fat-free mass content has been recognized to positively modulate central nervous system development because greater fat-free mass gains during the hospital stay have been associated with improved cognitive and motor scores at one year of corrected age in very-low-birth-weight infants [23]. In addition, higher fat-free mass content in former preterm infants at four months of corrected age was found to be associated with shorter brain speed processing [7]. On the other hand, the consumption of human milk at term-corrected age was found to be negatively associated with fat mass deposition. Considering that late preterm infants are at risk for developing increased adiposity at term-corrected age [3,4], which in turn could represent a risk factor for developing metabolic syndrome later in life, it could be speculated that human milk exerts a potentially protective effect in late preterm infants against obesity risk.

The present results are consistent with previous data published in the literature. Larcade et al. [11] reported that the number of days very preterm infants were fed human milk during their hospital stay positively correlated with fat-free mass content at discharge. Accordingly, Huang et al. [8] conducted a meta-analysis investigating the effect of breastfeeding and formula feeding on the body composition of 642 preterm infants (<37 weeks of gestational age). The authors found significantly lower fat mass in breastfed infants in comparison to formula-fed infants (mean difference 0.24; 95% CI 0.17,

Nutrients **2016**, *8*, 664

0.31 kg) at term-corrected age. These results differ from those reported by Gale et al. [24] who found significantly higher fat mass content in healthy, full-term, breastfed infants at three to four months of age in comparison to formula-fed infants. However, it must be taken into account that preterm infants, including those born between 34 and 36 weeks of gestation, still need to complete their organ development and present a lack of both fat-free mass and fat mass at birth because premature birth interrupts the physiologic development of body composition [25]. Furthermore, it has been demonstrated that the early postnatal growth of late preterm infants is characterized by a major deposition of fat mass so that at term-corrected age, late preterm infants show a higher fat mass content than term infants [3,4]. Hence, the promotion of fat-free mass accretion by consumption of human milk may represent a physiological compensatory mechanism aimed at recovering body composition, promoting neurodevelopment and protecting preterm infants from potential unbalanced nutritional intake provided by infant formulas.

In the present study, not surprisingly, weight *z*-scores at birth and at term-corrected age were positively associated with fat-free mass at term-corrected age. Indeed, the fat-free mass compartment accounts for the majority of the weight [25]. In addition, the finding that weight *z*-scores at term-corrected age are positively associated with fat mass content at term-corrected age can be explained by the fact that the early postnatal growth of late preterm infants is characterized by a major deposition of fat mass [4]. Consistently with previous data reported in the literature [26], being male was positively associated with fat-free mass content at term-corrected age.

While this study is of clinical interest, it presents some limitations. First of all, the data collected in the present study refer to late preterm infants not affected by comorbidities, so that their effect on body composition development has not been assessed. Furthermore, body composition was evaluated only at one time point, and as a result, the effect of human milk feeding over time has not been investigated. The main strength of the paper is represented by the fact that body composition data have been collected from a large number of late preterm infants.

5. Conclusions

The findings from this study indicate that human milk feeding appears to be associated with early fat-free mass deposition in late preterm infants. On the basis of the present results, health care professionals should direct efforts toward promoting and supporting breastfeeding in these vulnerable infants. Future research is desirable to explore the effect of comorbidities and the persistence of the effect of human milk consumption on body composition development in late preterm infants.

Author Contributions: M.L.G. conceived and designed the study and wrote the article; D.C. analyzed the data and contributed to the discussion of the results; N.L. analyzed the data and contributed to the discussion of the results; P.R. was responsible for database management; L.M., P.P. and C.M. collected the data; F.M. provided suggestions concerning the content and concept of the article.

Conflicts of Interest: The authors declare no conflict of interest.

References

1. Dong, Y.; Yu, J.L. An overview of morbidity, mortality and long-term outcome of late preterm birth. *World J. Pediatr.* **2011**, *7*, 199–204. [CrossRef] [PubMed]
2. Engle, W.A. Morbidity and mortality in late preterm and early term newborns: A continuum. *Clin. Perinatol.* **2011**, *38*, 493–516. [CrossRef] [PubMed]
3. Giannì, M.L.; Roggero, P.; Liotto, N.; Amato, O.; Piemontese, P.; Morniroli, D.; Bracco, B.; Mosca, F. Postnatal catch-up fat after late preterm birth. *Pediatr. Res.* **2012**, *72*, 637–640. [CrossRef] [PubMed]
4. Giannì, M.L.; Roggero, P.; Liotto, N.; Taroni, F.; Polimeni, A.; Morlacchi, L.; Piemontese, P.; Consonni, D.; Mosca, F. Body composition in late preterm infants according to percentile at birth. *Pediatr. Res.* **2016**, *79*, 710–715. [CrossRef] [PubMed]

5. Koletzko, B.; Brands, B.; Chourdakis, M.; Cramer, S.; Grote, V.; Hellmuth, C.; Kirchberg, F.; Prell, C.; Rzehak, P.; Uhl, O.; et al. The Power of Programming and the EarlyNutrition project: Opportunities for health promotion by nutrition during the first thousand days of life and beyond. *Ann. Nutr. Metab.* **2014**, *64*, 187–196. [CrossRef] [PubMed]

6. Roy, S.M.; Spivack, J.G.; Faith, M.S.; Chesi, A.; Mitchell, J.A.; Kelly, A.; Grant, S.F.; McCormack, S.E.; Zemel, B.S. Infant BMI or weight-for-length and obesity risk in early childhood. *Pediatrics* **2016**, *137*. [CrossRef] [PubMed]

7. Pfister, K.M.; Gray, H.L.; Miller, N.C.; Demerath, E.W.; Georgieff, M.K.; Ramel, S.E. Exploratory study of the relationship of fat-free mass to speed of brain processing in preterm infants. *Pediatr. Res.* **2013**, *74*, 576–583. [CrossRef] [PubMed]

8. Huang, P.; Zhou, J.; Yin, Y.; Jing, W.; Luo, B.; Wang, J. Effects of breast-feeding compared with formula-feeding on preterm infant body composition: A systematic review and meta-analysis. *Br. J. Nutr.* **2016**, *116*, 132–141. [CrossRef] [PubMed]

9. American Academy of Pediatrics. Section on Breastfeeding. Breastfeeding and the use of human milk. *Pediatrics* **2012**, *129*, e827–e841.

10. Simon, L.; Frondas-Chauty, A.; Senterre, T.; Flamant, C.; Darmaun, D.; Rozé, J.C. Determinants of body composition in preterm infants at the time of hospital discharge. *Am. J. Clin. Nutr.* **2014**, *100*, 98–104. [CrossRef] [PubMed]

11. Larcade, J.; Pradat, P.; Buffin, R.; Leick-Courtois, C.; Jourdes, E.; Picaud, J.C. Estimation of fat-free mass at discharge in preterm infants fed with optimized feeding regimen. *J. Pediatr. Gastroenterol. Nutr.* **2016**. [CrossRef] [PubMed]

12. Kugelman, A.; Colin, A.A. Late preterm infants: Near term but still in a critical developmental time period. *Pediatrics* **2013**, *132*, 741–751. [CrossRef] [PubMed]

13. Giannì, M.L.; Roggero, P.; Piemontese, P.; Liotto, N.; Orsi, A.; Amato, O.; Taroni, F.; Morlacchi, L.; Consonni, D.; Mosca, F. Is nutritional support needed in late preterm infants? *BMC Pediatr.* **2015**, *15*, 194. [CrossRef] [PubMed]

14. Engle, W.A.; American Academy of Pediatrics Committee on Fetus and Newborn. Age terminology during the perinatal period. *Pediatrics* **2004**, *114*, 1362–1364. [PubMed]

15. Fenton, T.R. A new growth chart for preterm babies: Babson and Benda's chart updated with recent data and a new format. *BMC Pediatr.* **2003**, *16*, 3–13. [CrossRef] [PubMed]

16. Agostoni, C.; Grandi, F.; Scaglioni, S.; Giannì, M.L.; Torcoletti, M.; Radaelli, G.; Fiocchi, A.; Riva, E. Growth pattern of breastfed and non breastfed infants with atopic dermatitis in the first year of life. *Pediatrics* **2000**, *106*, E73. [CrossRef] [PubMed]

17. Two Apps Are Available Based on the 2013 Fenton Growth Charts. Available online: http://ucalgary.ca/fenton (accessed on 1 July 2016).

18. Roggero, P.; Giannì, M.L.; Amato, O.; Piemontese, P.; Morniroli, D.; Wong, W.W.; Mosca, F. Evaluation of air-displacement plethysmography for body composition assessment in preterm infants. *Pediatr. Res.* **2012**, *72*, 316–320. [CrossRef] [PubMed]

19. Urlando, A.; Dempster, P.; Aitkens, S. A new air displacement plethysmograph for the measurement of body composition in infants. *Pediatr. Res.* **2003**, *53*, 486–492. [CrossRef] [PubMed]

20. Going, S.B. Hydrodensitometry and air displacement plethysmography. In *Human Body Composition*, 2nd ed.; Heymsfield, S.B., Lohman, T.G., Wang, Z., Eds.; Human Kinetics: Champaign, IL, USA, 2005; pp. 17–34.

21. Brozek, J.; Grande, F.; Anderson, J.T.; Keys, A. Densitometric analysis of body composition: Revision of some quantitative assumptions. *Ann. N. Y. Acad. Sci.* **1963**, *11*, 113–340.

22. Fomon, S.J.; Haschke, F.; Ziegler, E.E.; Nelson, S.E. Body composition of reference children from birth to age 10 years. *Am. J. Clin. Nutr.* **1982**, *35*, 1169–1175. [PubMed]

23. Ramel, S.E.; Gray, H.L.; Christiansen, E.; Boys, C.; Georgieff, M.K.; Demerath, E.W. Greater early gains in fat-free mass, but not fat mass, are associated with improved neurodevelopment at 1 year corrected age for prematurity in very low birth weight preterm infants. *J. Pediatr.* **2016**, *173*, 108–115. [CrossRef] [PubMed]

24. Gale, C.; Logan, K.M.; Santhakumaran, S.; Parkinson, J.R.; Hyde, M.J.; Modi, N. Effect of breastfeeding compared with formula feeding on infant body composition: A systematic review and meta-analysis. *Am. J. Clin. Nutr.* **2012**, *95*, 656–669. [CrossRef] [PubMed]

25. Micheli, J.L.; Pfister, R.; Junod, S.; Laubscher, B.; Tolsa, J.F.; Schutz, Y.; Calame, A. Water, energy and early postnatal growth in preterm infants. *Acta Paediatr. Suppl.* **1994**, *405*, 35–42. [CrossRef] [PubMed]
26. Simon, L.; Borrego, P.; Darmaun, D.; Legrand, A.; Rozé, J.C.; Chauty-Frondas, A. Effect of sex and gestational age on neonatal body composition. *Br. J. Nutr.* **2013**, *109*, 1105–1108. [CrossRef] [PubMed]

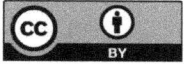

nutrients

MDPI

Article

Temporal Changes of Human Breast Milk Lipids of Chinese Mothers

Francesca Giuffrida [1,*], Cristina Cruz-Hernandez [1], Emmanuelle Bertschy [1], Patric Fontannaz [1], Isabelle Masserey Elmelegy [1], Isabelle Tavazzi [1], Cynthia Marmet [1], Belén Sanchez-Bridge [1], Sagar K. Thakkar [1], Carlos Antonio De Castro [1], Gerard Vinyes-Pares [2], Yumei Zhang [3] and Peiyu Wang [4]

[1]   Nestlé Research Center, Nestec Ltd., Vers-chez-les-Blanc, P.O. Box 44, 1000 Lausanne 26, Switzerland; cristina.cruz-hernandez@rdls.nestle.com (C.C.-H.); emmanuelle.bertschy@rdls.nestle.com (E.B.); patric.fontannaz@rdls.nestle.com (P.F.); isabelle.masserey-elmlegy@rdls.nestle.com (I.M.E.); isabelle.tavazzi@rdls.nestle.com (I.T.); cynthia.marmet@rdls.nestle.com (C.M.); belen.sanchez-bridge@rdls.nestle.com (B.S.-B.); sagar.thakkar@rdls.nestle.com (S.K.T.); carlosantonio.decastro@rdls.nestle.com (C.A.D.C.)
[2]   Nestlé Research Center Beijing, Building E-F, No. 5 Dijin Road, Haidian District, Beijing 100091, China; gerard.vinyespares@nestle.com
[3]   Department of Nutrition and Food Hygiene, School of Public Health, Peking University Health Science Center, Beijing 100191, China; zhangyumei@bjmu.edu.cn
[4]   Department of Social Medicine and Health Education, School of Public Health, Peking University Health Science Center, Beijing 100191, China; wpeiyu@bjmu.edu.cn
*   Correspondance: francesca.giuffrida@rdls.nestle.com; Tel.: +41-21-785-8084

Received: 15 August 2016; Accepted: 7 November 2016; Published: 10 November 2016

Abstract: Fatty acids (FA), phospholipids (PL), and gangliosides (GD) play a central role in infant growth, immune and inflammatory responses. The aim of this study was to determine FA, PL, and GD compositional changes in human milk (HM) during lactation in a large group of Chinese lactating mothers (540 volunteers) residing in Beijing, Guangzhou, and Suzhou. HM samples were collected after full expression from one breast and while the baby was fed on the other breast. FA were assessed by direct methylation followed by gas chromatography (GC) analysis. PL and GD were extracted using chloroform and methanol. A methodology employing liquid chromatography coupled with an evaporative light scattering detector (ELSD) and with time of flight (TOF) mass spectrometry was used to quantify PL and GD classes in HM, respectively. Saturated FA (SFA), mono-unsaturated FA (MUFA), and PL content decreased during lactation, while polyunsaturated FA (PUFA) and GD content increased. Among different cities, over the lactation time, HM from Beijing showed the highest SFA content, HM from Guangzhou the highest MUFA content and HM from Suzhou the highest n-3PUFA content. The highest total PL and GD contents were observed in HM from Suzhou. In order to investigate the influence of the diet on maternal milk composition, a careful analyses of dietary habits of these population needs to be performed in the future.

Keywords: FA; phospholipids; gangliosides; breast milk; chromatography

1. Introduction

Human milk (HM) is considered the optimal form of nourishment for infants during the first six months of life [1] and among its macronutrients, the lipid fraction is crucial, representing approximately 50% of the energy supplied to the newborn infant [2]. Lipids (2%–5%) occur in milk in the form of fat globules mainly composed of triacylglycerols (TAG) (~98% of total lipids) surrounded by a structural membrane composed of phospholipids (PL) (0.8%), cholesterol (0.5%), enzymes, proteins, glycosphingolipids (e.g., gangliosides (GD)), and glycoproteins [3,4].

The majority of fatty acids (FA), approximately 98%, are esterified to a glycerol backbone to form TAG and about 0.2%–2% is found in molecules, such as cholesterol, PL, and GD. In HM, saturated FA (SFA) content ranges from 20% to 70% of total FA, mono-unsaturated FA (MUFA) from 23% to 55%, polyunsaturated FA (PUFA) from 6% to 36%, and long chain polyunsaturated FA (LCPUFA) from 0.3% to 8%. Among PUFA, linoleic (LA, 18:2n-6) and alpha linolenic acids (ALA, 18:3n-3) are essential because they are not synthesized in the human body and they are precursors of arachidonic (ARA, 20:4n-6) and docosahexaenoic (DHA, 22:6n-3) FA that are associated with normal brain development, especially in early life [5].

PL are mainly distributed into five classes: phosphatydylinositol (PtdIns), phosphatydylethanolamine (PtdEtn), phosphatydylserine (PtdSer), phosphatidylcholine (PtdCho), and sphingomyelin (CerPCho). PtdIns, PtdEtn, PtdSer, and PtdCho consist of a glycerol esterified with FA in the *sn*-1 and *sn*-2 positions. A phosphate residue with different organic groups (inositol, serine, ethanolamine, or choline) is present in the *sn*-3 position. CerPCho consists of a sphingoid base backbone to which an amide-linked long-chain FA can be attached, leading to the ceramides (*N*-acyl-sphingoid bases) [6]. In the case of CerPCho the primary hydroxyl group of the sphingoid base is linked to phosphorylcholine. Therefore, PL are a source of FA and choline, the precursors of the neurotransmitter acetylcholine, which acts by regulating the transduction signal and serves as a source of methyl groups in intermediate metabolism, being considered essential for optimum development of the brain [7,8].

GD are glycosphingolipids formed by a hydrophobic ceramide and a hydrophilic oligosaccharide chain. This chain may contain *N*-acetylneuraminic acid (sialic acid) or, less commonly, *N*-glycoloylneuraminic acid (Neu5Gc), where a glycol group is bound to the C5 amino group. It has been reported that sialic acid is involved in many biological and pathological phenomena, either recognizing or masking the recognition of several ligands, such as selectins or pathogens [9]. Recently, Gurnida et al. [10] concluded that nutritional supplementation with a milk lipid preparation rich in GD appears to have beneficial effects on cognitive development in healthy infants aged 0–6 months.

Traditionally, lactation has been viewed in three stages: colostrum (day 1–5 postpartum), transitional milk (day 6–15 postpartum), and mature milk (after day 15 postpartum). It has been showed that FA, PL, and GD content in HM change during lactation stages [4,11–19] and factors, such as maternal diet. may influence HM short chain FA [20,21], PUFA composition [22–24], and gangliosides content [25].

The objective of this study was to determine, for the first time, the FA, PL, and GD content in HM of Chinese mothers, follow its temporal change along lactation, and evaluate if the geographical region within China would affect HM lipid composition. This study is part of the larger initiative: the Maternal Infant Nutrition Growth (MING) study [26].

2. Materials and Methods

2.1. Subjects

This study was part of MING, a cross-sectional study designed to investigate the dietary and nutritional status of pregnant women, lactating mothers, and young children aged from birth up to three years living in urban areas of China [26]. In addition, the HM composition of Chinese lactating mothers was characterized. The study was conducted between October 2011 and February 2012. A multi-stage milk sampling from lactating mothers in three cities (Beijing, Suzhou, and Guangzhou) was performed for breast milk characterization. In each city, two hospitals with maternal and child care units were selected and, at each site, mothers at lactation period 0–240 days were randomly selected based on eligibility criteria. Subjects included in the period 0–5 days were recruited at the hospital, whereas the other subjects were requested by phone to join the study; if participation was dismissed a replacement was made. The response rate was 52%. Recruitment and milk, as well as baseline

183

data collection, were done in separate days. A stratified milk sampling of 540 lactating mothers in six lactation periods of 0–4, 5–11, and 12–30 days, and 1–2, 2–4, and 4–8 months was obtained in the MING study.

2.2. Inclusion and Exclusion Criteria

Eligibility criteria included women between 18–45 years of age giving birth to a single, healthy, full-term infant and exclusive breastfeeding at least until four months of age. Exclusion criteria included gestational diabetes, hypertension, cardiac diseases, acute communicable diseases, and postpartum depression. Lactating women who had nipple or lacteal gland diseases, who had been receiving hormonal therapy during the three months preceding recruitment, or who had insufficient skills to understand study questionnaires were also excluded.

2.3. Ethical and Legal Considerations

The study was conducted according to the guidelines in the Declaration of Helsinki. All of the procedures involving human subjects were approved by the Medical Ethics Research Board of Peking University (No. IRB00001052-11042). Written informed consent was obtained from all subjects participating in the study. The study was also registered in ClinicalTrials.gov with the number identifier NCT01971671.

2.4. Data Collection

All subjects responded to a general questionnaire including socio-economic and lifestyle aspects of the mother. Self-reported weight at delivery, number of gestational weeks at delivery, and delivery method were also recorded. Additionally, a physical examination evaluated basic anthropometric parameters (height, weight, mid-arm circumference) blood pressure, and hemoglobin. Data collection was done through face-to-face interviews the day of HM sample collection. In addition, the date of birth and gender information of the baby was collected after the data collection, since the data was not included in the initial questionnaires. Subjects were contacted by phone and were asked to clarify these two aspects retrospectively.

2.5. HM Sampling

Breast milk sampling was standardized for all subjects and an electric pump (Horigen HNR/X-2108ZB, Xinhe Electrical Apparatuses Co., Ltd., Beijing, China) was used to sample the milk. Samples were collected at the second feeding in the morning (9:00–11:00 a.m.) to avoid circadian influence on the outcomes. A single full breast was emptied and aliquots of 10 mL for colostrum and 40 mL for the remaining time points was secured for characterization purposes. The rest of the milk was returned to the mother for feeding to the infant. Each sample was distributed in freezing tubes, labelled with subject number, and stored at $-80\,^{\circ}C$ until analysis. Figure 1 shows the study flowchart for the subjects' recruitment.

2.6. Analytical Methods

2.6.1. FA Quantification

FA profile was determined by preparing the methyl esters of FA (FAMEs). A direct transesterification of HM was performed with methanolic chloridric acid solution, as described by Cruz-Hernandez et al. [27]. Briefly, into a 10 mL screw cap glass test tube, milk (250 μL) was added and mixed with 300 μL of internal standard FAME 11:0 solution (3 mg/mL) and 300 μL of internal standard TAG 13:0 solution (3 mg/mL). After addition of 2 mL of methanol, 2 mL of methanolic chloridric acid (3 N), and 1 mL of hexane, the tubes were heated at $100\,^{\circ}C$ for 90 min. To stop the reaction 2 mL of water were added and after centrifugation ($1200\times g$ for 5 min) the upper phase (hexane) was transferred into gas chromatography vials. The analysis of FAMEs was performed by GC using a CP-Sil 88 capillary column (100 m, 0.25 mm i.d. 0.25 μm film thickness) and their identification by comparison of retention time with authentic standards (GC standard Nestlé 36 from NuCheck-Prep, Elysan, MN, USA).

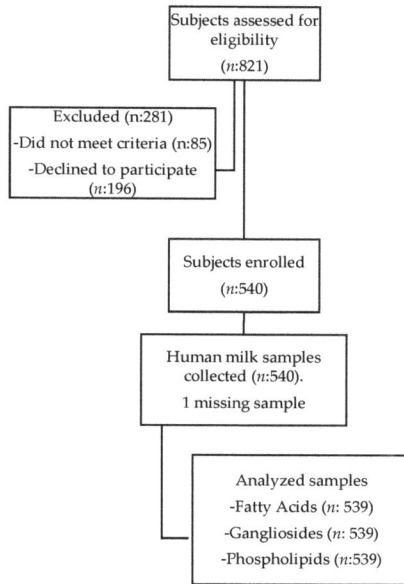

Figure 1. Study flowchart for subject recruitment.

2.6.2. Phospholipid Quantification

PL were quantified as previously described by Giuffrida et al. [28]. Briefly, 250 mg of maternal milk was mixed with 250 mg of water and 9.5 mL of chloroform/methanol (2/1 v/v). After addition of 10 μL of phosphatydilglycerol internal standard solution (5 mg/mL), the sample solution was put into an ultrasonic bath at 40 °C for 15 min. After centrifugation (1000 relative centrifugal force (RCF), for 10 min), the sample solution was filtered through 0.2 μm PTFE filters; the filtrate was mixed with 2 mL of potassium chloride solution (8.8 g/L) and centrifuged (1000 RCF for 10 min). The organic phases were evaporated to dryness and the residual lipids were redissolved in 150 μL of chloroform/methanol (9/1 v/v), filtered through 4 mm polyvinylidene fluoride (PVDF) membrane filters analyzed by high performance liquid chromatography coupled with evaporative light scattering detector (HPLC-ELSD). PL classes were separated by normal-phase HPLC using 2 Nucleosil 50-5, 250 × 3 mm, 5 μm (Macherey-Nagel, Easton, PA, USA) equipped with pre-column Nucleosil 50-5, 8 × 3 mm, 5 μm (Macherey-Nagel, Easton, PA, USA). All chromatography was performed at 55 °C. Solvent A contained ammonium formiate 3 g/L and solvent B of acetonitrile/methanol (100/3 v/v). Gradient conditions for PL analysis were as follows: time = 0 min 1% solvent A; time = 19 min 30% solvent A; time = 21 min 30% solvent A; time = 24 min 1% solvent A; with a flow rate 1 mL/min. Injection volume was 0.01 mL. The best signal and resolution was achieved at the following ELSD conditions: evap. = 90 °C; neb = 40 °C, flow rate of N_2 = 1 L/min.

2.6.3. Gangliosides Quantification

GD were quantified as previously described by Giuffrida et al. [2]. Briefly, HM (0.2 mL) was dissolved in water (1 mL) and mixed with 4 mL methanol/chloroform (2/1). After centrifugation

(3000× *g*, for 10 min), the upper liquid phase was quantitatively transferred into a 15 mL centrifuge tube. The residue was mixed with water (1 mL), 2 mL of methanol/chloroform (2/1), shaken, put into an ultrasonic bath at 25 °C for 10 min, centrifuged (3000× *g*, for 10 min), and upper liquid phases polled together; the volume was adjusted to 12 mL with methanol 60% and pH to 9.2 by adding Na2HPO4 30 mmol/L (0.2 mL). The extract solution was loaded on an Oasis HLB VAC RC SPE cartridges (30 mg, 15 mL, Waters) previously conditioned with methanol (2 mL) and methanol 60% (2 mL). The sample was passed through the cartridge at maximum flow rate 2–3 mL /min. The sorbent was washed with 2 mL of methanol 60% and dried by vacuum suction for a few seconds; the analyte was eluted with methanol (2 mL). Solvent was evaporated to dryness under a nitrogen flow at 30 °C and the residual lipids were re-dissolved in 0.2 mL of methanol 70% and analysed by liquid chromatography (LC) coupled with quadrupole time of flight (QTOF), using an Aquity BEH C18 column (1.7 μm; 150 × 2.1 mm i.d.; Waters). All chromatography was performed at 50 °C. Solvent A was composed of water/methanol/ammonium acetate (1 mmol/L) (90/10/0.1 *v*/*v*/*v*) and solvent B of methanol/ammonium acetate (1 mmol/L) (100/0.1 *v*/*v*). Gradient conditions were as follows: time = 0 min 10% solvent A; time = 0.2 min 10% solvent A; time = 8.2 min 5% solvent A; time = 12.2 min 5% solvent A; time = 12.4 min 0% solvent A; time = 18.4 min 0% solvent A; time = 18.6 min 10% solvent A; time = 21 min 10% solvent A. Flow rate was 0.2 mL/min. Injection volume was 0.01 mL for GD3 and 0.005 mL for GM3. The mass spectrometer was equipped with an electrospray ionization (ESI) ion source. The ESI mass spectra were recorded in the negative ion mode under the following conditions: ion spray voltage (IS) −4000 V, temperature of the source 400 °C, declustering potential (DP) −40 V, ion source gases one and two at 40 and 35 psi, respectively, curtain gas at 15 psi, collision energy −40 V. GD3 and GM3, were monitored by transitions of the precursor ions to the *m*/*z* 290. Quantification was performed by the standard addition method.

3. Results

3.1. Demographics and Anthropometrics of Study Subjects

In the current study we analyzed HM from 539 mothers (Figure 1), collected in a cross-sectional design over eight months postpartum. Milk obtained for analyses was a single, whole breast milk sample to have a comprehensive view on nutrient content. The details of the demographics and anthropometrics of the study subjects are outlined in Table 1. Groups of mothers, which delivered either a male or a female infant, were comparable for their age and anthropometric and demographic characteristics. Gestational age at birth (average 39 weeks) were also comparable between groups. The details of demographics and anthropometrics of the study subjects for the time period 0–4 days are not available.

Table 1. Maternal descriptive characteristics.

	5–11 Days	12–30 Days	1–2 Months	2–4 Months	4–8 Months
	(*n* = 90)	(*n* = 90)	(*n* = 90)	(*n* = 90)	(*n* = 90)
Mother					
Age (years), Mean ± SD	27 ± 4	27 ± 3	28 ± 4	27 ± 4	26 ± 4
Natural delivery	27 ± 4	27 ± 3	28 ± 5	26 ± 4	26 ± 4
Caesarean delivery	28 ± 3	27 ± 4	29 ± 4	28 ± 4	27 ± 4
Height (cm), Mean ± SD	160 ± 4	160 ± 5	161 ± 5	161 ± 5	159 ± 5
Weight (kg), Mean ± SD	60.7 ± 8.7	60.8 ± 7.9	61.9 ± 8.9	58.4 ± 8.3	56.2 ± 8.1
BMI (kg/m²), Mean ± SD	23.7 ± 3.3	23.7 ± 2.8	23.9 ± 3.1	22.5 ± 2.9	22.2 ± 3.1
Gestational weight gain(kg), Mean ± SD	16.7 ± 7.4	16.2 ± 6.0	15.9 ± 5.7	15.9 ± 5.9	14.9 ± 7.6
Postpartum weight loss (kg), Mean ± SD	9.1 ± 6.1	8.6 ± 5.3	9.8 ± 4.0	10.0 ± 6.2	10.6 ± 5.9
Gestational age at birth (weeks), Mean ± SD	39.3 ± 1.2	39.2± 1.3	39.2 ± 1.6	39.4 ± 1.3	39.5 ±1.5

SD: standard deviation.

3.2. FA

FA were determined by gas chromatography coupled with flame ionization detector (GC-FID), as previously described by Cruz-Hernandez et al. [27] and the results are listed in Table 2.

In our study total SFA content increased significantly from colostrum (35.7% of total FA) to transitional milk (38.9% of total FA) and decreased in mature milk (36.2% of total FA), with palmitic acid (16:0) being the most abundant FA and decreasing significantly ($p < 0.05$) from 23.2% in colostrum to 19.8% of total FA in mature milk (Table 2). Stearic acid (18:0) content was constant along the lactation period, i.e., colostrum, transitional, and mature milk, at about 5% of total FA, and medium-chain (MC) FA (10:0–14:0) content was low in colostrum (6.8% of total FA) compared to transitional (13.1% of total FA), and mature milk (11.0% of total FA) (Table 2). Arachidic (20:0) and lignoceric acids (24:0) were constant along the lactation time at about 0.2 and 0.1% of total FA, respectively. No significant differences ($p > 0.05$) on total SFA content were observed among cities in colostrum, and transitional milk (Table 2). SFA content was significant lower ($p < 0.05$) in mature milk from Suzhou (34.5% of total FA). Palmitic (22.5%, 19.4%, and 18.5% of total FA in colostrum, transitional, and mature milk, respectively) and stearic (4.9%, 4.5%, and 4.8% of total FA in colostrum, transitional and mature milk, respectively) FA also showed the lowest content in mature milk from Suzhou.

In the total population the MUFA content of HM decreased from 40.7% in colostrum to 36.9% of total FA in mature milk, with oleic acid (18:1n-9) being the most abundant FA and decreasing along the lactation time from 34.2% in colostrum to 31.9% of total FA in transitional and mature milk. Other MUFA (i.e., 17:1n-7, 20:1n-9, 22:1n-9. and 24:1n-9) also decreased over the lactation period (Table 2). The highest level of total MUFA content was found in colostrum (43.1% of total FA), transitional (39.3% of total FA), and mature milk (38.3% of total FA) from Guangzhou (Table 2). The lowest level of total MUFA content was found in colostrum (38.4% of total FA), transitional (34.7% of total FA), and mature milk (34.3% of total FA) from Beijing (Table 2). HM samples obtained from mothers in Guangzhou contained the highest level of Oleic acid whereas milk obtained from mothers in Beijing contained the lowest level, respectively: colostrum (37.1% vs. 32.6% of total FA), transitional (34.0% vs. 30.3% of total FA), and mature milk (33.4% vs. 30.1% of total FA).

In the total population, total PUFA n-6 increased from 21.7% in colostrum to 24.1% of total FA in mature milk with linoleic acid (18:2n-6) being the most abundant FA and increasing along the lactation time from 18.9% in colostrum to 22.8% of total FA in mature milk. ARA (20:4n-6) content decreased from 0.9% to 0.5% of total FA from colostrum to mature milk. Beijing and Suzhou showed higher total PUFAn-6 content in colostrum (23.3% and 22.8% of total FA, respectively), transitional (22.5% and 22.9% of total FA, respectively), and mature milk (26.6% and 25.3% of total FA, respectively) than Guangzhou (Table 2).

Total PUFA n-3 in HM from total population slightly increased from 1.4% in colostrum to 1.9% of total FA in mature milk with linolenic acid (18:3n-3) being the most abundant and increasing along the lactation time from 0.9% in colostrum to 1.5% of total FA in mature milk. DHA (22:6n-3) slightly decreased over lactation period from 0.5% in colostrum to 0.3% of total FA in mature milk, and EPA (20:5n-3) was present in a small amount (<0.1% of total FA in colostrum, transitional, and mature milk). The highest level of total PUFA n-3 content was found in colostrum (1.8% of total FA), transitional (2.1% of total FA), and mature milk (2.4% of total FA) from Suzhou (Table 2), which, as a consequence, showed the lowest n-6 to n-3 ratio (12.7% in colostrum, 10.9% in transitional milk, and 10.5% of total FA in mature milk).

Table 2. Median fatty acid composition of HM expressed as g/100 g of total FA.

FA (g/100 g)	Total Population			Guangzhou			Beijing			Suzhou		
	Colostrum (0–5 Days) n = 113	Transitional (6–15 Days) n = 81	Mature (16 Days–8 Months) n = 345	Colostrum (0–5 Days) n = 38	Transitional (6–15 Days) n = 22	Mature (16 Days–8 Months) n = 120	Colostrum (0–5 Days) n = 45	Transitional (6–15 Days) n = 21	Mature (16 Days–8 Months) n = 113	Colostrum (0–5 Days) n = 30	Transitional (6–15 Days) n = 38	Mature (16 Days–8 Months) n = 112
10:0	0.5 ± 0.4	1.5 ± 0.5 †	1.6 ± 0.4 ‡	0.4 ± 0.4	1.4 ± 0.5	1.5 ± 0.5	0.6 ± 0.5	1.5 ± 0.4	1.6 ± 0.4	0.5 ± 0.4	1.6 ± 0.5	1.6 ± 0.4
12:0	2.6 ± 1.6	6.1 ± 2.3 †	5.2 ± 1.9	2.3 ± 1.5	5.5 ± 2.1	5.0 ± 2.1	2.6 ± 1.7	6.5 ± 1.7	5.3 ± 1.6	2.7 ± 1.7	6.3 ± 2.6	5.3 ± 1.9
14:0	3.8 ± 1.7	5.5 ± 2.2 †	4.2 ± 1.7 ‡	3.6 ± 1.8	5.2 ± 1.9	4.1 ± 2.0	3.8 ± 1.7	5.8 ± 1.4	4.3 ± 1.4	4.0 ± 1.7	5.2 ± 2.7	4.0 ± 1.7
16:0	23.2 ± 1.9	20.5 ± 2.3 †	19.8 ± 2.6 ‡	23.9 ± 1.9	21.5 ± 2.1	20.6 ± 2.6	22.8 ± 2.2	21.5 ± 2.2	19.8 ± 2.2	22.5 ± 1.3	19.4 ± 2.2	18.5 ± 2.6
16:1n-7	5.2 ± 1.0	2.2 ± 0.7 †	2.0 ± 0.6	1.7 ± 1.0	2.4 ± 0.8	2.2 ± 0.7	2.2 ± 0.6	1.7 ± 0.6	2.0 ± 0.5	1.8 ± 0.8	2.2 ± 0.5	2.0 ± 0.6
18:0	5.2 ± 1.0	5.0 ± 0.8	5.1 ± 1.1	5.5 ± 1.2	5.3 ± 0.7	5.4 ± 1.2	5.1 ± 0.9	5.4 ± 0.7	5.1 ± 1.0	4.9 ± 0.9	4.5 ± 0.8	4.8 ± 1.0
18:1n-9	34.2 ± 3.2	31.9 ± 3.6 †	31.9 ± 3.6	37.1 ± 2.8	34.0 ± 2.2	33.4 ± 3.3	32.6 ± 2.9	30.3 ± 2.9	30.1 ± 2.9	34.0 ± 2.5	31.0 ± 4.1	31.7 ± 3.7
18:1n-7	2.5 ± 0.4	2.2 ± 0.5 †	1.9 ± 0.3 ‡	2.7 ± 0.5	2.2 ± 0.4	2.0 ± 0.3	2.3 ± 0.4	2.0 ± 0.3	1.7 ± 0.2	2.4 ± 0.3	2.3 ± 0.6	1.9 ± 0.3
18:2n-6	18.9 ± 3.6	19.7 ± 3.8 †	22.8 ± 4.9 ‡	15.7 ± 2.8	18.0 ± 3.4	19.7 ± 4.3	20.2 ± 3.5	20.2 ± 3.6	25.1 ± 3.9	19.9 ± 3.0	21.0 ± 3.9	23.8 ± 5.2
18:3n-3	0.9 ± 0.4	1.4 ± 0.6 †	1.5 ± 0.9 ‡	0.7 ± 0.3	1.0 ± 0.5	1.0 ± 0.6	0.9 ± 0.4	1.1 ± 0.7	1.6 ± 1.1	1.2 ± 0.3	1.7 ± 0.6	2.0 ± 0.8
18:3n-6	0.05 ± 0.07	0.09 ± 0.06 †	0.14 ± 0.06 ‡	<0.05	0.1 ± 0.1	0.1 ± 0.1	0.1 ± 0.1	0.1 ± 0.1	0.2 ± 0.1	<0.05	0.1 ± 0.1	0.1 ± 0.1
20:0	0.2 ± 0.1	0.2 ± 0.05	0.2 ± 0.1	0.2 ± 0.1	0.2 ± 0.1	0.2 ± 0.1	0.2 ± 0.1	0.2 ± 0.1	0.2 ± 0.1	0.2 ± 0.1	0.1 ± 0.1	0.2 ± 0.1
20:1n-9	0.9 ± 0.3	0.5 ± 0.2 †	0.4 ± 0.2	1.0 ± 0.3	0.5 ± 0.2	0.4 ± 0.1	0.7 ± 0.3	0.5 ± 0.1	0.3 ± 0.1	0.9 ± 0.4	0.5 ± 0.2	0.6 ± 0.3
20:2n-6	1.2 ± 0.4	0.6 ± 0.3 †	0.4 ± 0.1 ‡	1.1 ± 0.4	0.5 ± 0.3	0.4 ± 0.1	1.1 ± 0.4	0.8 ± 0.3	0.4 ± 0.1	1.3 ± 0.4	0.6 ± 0.2	0.4 ± 0.1
20:3n-6	0.7 ± 0.2	0.5 ± 0.2 †	0.4 ± 0.1 ‡	0.6 ± 0.2	0.4 ± 0.1	0.3 ± 0.2	0.8 ± 0.3	0.6 ± 0.2	0.4 ± 0.1	0.7 ± 0.2	0.5 ± 0.1	0.4 ± 0.1
20:5n-3	0.04 ± 0.05	0.05 ± 0.06 †	0.05 ± 0.07	<0.05	0.10 ± 0.1	<0.05	<0.05	<0.05	0.1 ± 0.1	0.1 ± 0.1	<0.05	0.1 ± 0.1
22:1n-9	0.2 ± 0.2	0.1 ± 0.1	0.1 ± 0.3	0.2 ± 0.1	0.1 ± 0.1	0.1 ± 0.1	0.2 ± 0.2	0.1 ± 0.1	0.1 ± 0.1	0.3 ± 0.3	0.1 ± 0.2	0.1 ± 0.5
20:4n-6 (ARA)	0.9 ± 0.3	0.7 ± 0.2 †	0.5 ± 0.1 ‡	0.9 ± 0.2	0.7 ± 0.2	0.5 ± 0.2	1.1 ± 0.4	0.8 ± 0.2	0.5 ± 0.2	0.9 ± 0.2	0.7 ± 0.2	0.6 ± 0.1
24:0	0.2 ± 0.1	0.1 ± 0.1 †	0.1 ± 0.1	0.2 ± 0.1	0.1 ± 0.1	0.1 ± 0.1	0.3 ± 0.2	0.1 ± 0.1	0.1 ± 0.1	0.2 ± 0.1	0.1 ± 0.1	0.1 ± 0.1
24:1n-9	0.4 ± 0.3	0.5 ± 0.2 †	0.3 ± 0.2 ‡	0.4 ± 0.2	0.4 ± 0.4	0.3 ± 0.2	0.4 ± 0.3	0.5 ± 0.1	0.2 ± 0.1	0.4 ± 0.3	0.4 ± 0.2	0.3 ± 0.2
22:6n-3 (DHA)	0.5 ± 0.3	0.5 ± 0.2 †	0.3 ± 0.2 ‡	0.7 ± 0.3	0.4 ± 0.4	0.3 ± 0.2	0.5 ± 0.2	0.5 ± 0.1	0.2 ± 0.1	0.5 ± 0.2	0.4 ± 0.2	0.3 ± 0.2
Total SFA	35.7 ± 3.9	38.9 ± 4.1 †	36.2 ± 4.7 ‡	36.1 ± 4.0	39.2 ± 3.8	36.9 ± 4.8	35.4 ± 3.9	41.0 ± 3.0	36.4 ± 3.9	35.0 ± 3.7	37.2 ± 4.8	34.5 ± 4.9
Total MUFA	40.7 ± 3.8	37.7 ± 4.3 †	36.2 ± 4.7 ‡	43.1 ± 3.3	39.3 ± 3.0	38.3 ± 3.6	38.4 ± 4.1	34.7 ± 3.5	34.3 ± 4.5	39.8 ± 2.6	36.2 ± 4.8	36.4 ± 4.4
MCFA	6.8 ± 2.4	13.1 ± 3.3	11.0 ± 2.6	6.3 ± 2.3	12.1 ± 3.5	10.6 ± 2.8	7.0 ± 2.2	13.8 ± 2.2	11.2 ± 2.3	7.2 ± 2.4	13.1 ± 3.8	10.9 ± 2.6
Total PUFA n-6	21.7 ± 3.6	21.6 ± 3.8	24.1 ± 5.0	18.3 ± 2.8	19.7 ± 3.4	21.1 ± 4.3	23.3 ± 3.6	22.5 ± 3.6	26.6 ± 3.9	22.8 ± 3.0	22.9 ± 3.9	25.3 ± 5.2
Total PUFA n-3	1.4 ± 0.5	1.9 ± 0.7	1.9 ± 0.9	1.4 ± 0.4	1.5 ± 0.6	1.3 ± 0.6	1.4 ± 0.4	1.6 ± 0.7	1.9 ± 1.1	1.8 ± 0.4	2.1 ± 0.6	2.4 ± 0.8
n-6 to n-3 ratio	14.4 ± 3.7	11.8 ± 3.7 †	12.5 ± 5.5	13.1 ± 3.7	13.1 ± 3.9	16.5 ± 5.6	16.6 ± 3.0	14.1 ± 3.9	13.8 ± 5.6	12.7 ± 3.8	10.9 ± 2.9	10.5 ± 4.0
ARA to DHA ratio	1.8 ± 0.7	1.6 ± 0.5	2.2 ± 0.9 ‡	1.3 ± 0.5	1.8 ± 0.6	1.9 ± 1.0	2.2 ± 0.7	1.6 ± 0.5	2.3 ± 0.8	1.8 ± 0.4	1.8 ± 0.5	1.9 ± 0.8

FA, Fatty acids; ARA, arachidonic; DHA, docosahexaenoic; SFA, Saturated FA; MUFA, mono-unsaturated FA; MCFA, medium-chain FA; PUFA, polyunsaturated FA. * Values are presented as median ± standard deviation (SD). Values within a row with a symbol indicate statistically significant differences. † $p < 0.05$ versus colostrum. ‡ $p < 0.05$ versus transitional milk.

3.3. Phospholipids

PL classes were determined by LC-ELSD, as previously described by Giuffrida et al. [28] and the results are listed in Table 3.

We did not measure minor constituents, such as lysophosphatidylcholine, which may contribute only to small amounts of the infant's diet.

From the total population, total PL content in HM decreased along the lactation period from 33.0 in colostrum to 24.2 mg/100 mL in mature milk, being significant lower ($p < 0.05$) in mature milk (Table 3). PtdCho was the most abundant PL in HM (from 12.0 mg/100 mL in colostrum to 8.2 mg/100 mL in mature milk) followed by CerPCho (from 9.1 mg/100 mL in colostrum to 7.2 mg/100 mL in mature milk), PtdEtn (from 8.5 mg/100 mL in colostrum to 6.4 mg/100 mL in mature milk), PtdIns (from 1.8 mg/100 mL in colostrum to 1.5 mg/100 mL in mature milk), and PtdSer (from 1.5 mg/100 mL to 1.0 mg/100 mL in mature milk). The PL class distribution was similar in colostrum, transitional, and mature milk (Figure 2).

Among the cities, PtdCho content did not show significant difference ($p > 0.05$) (Table 3); however, when considering the mature milk data at different lactation stages (Figure 3), PtdCho content was significant higher at 2–4 months in Suzhou (9.0 mg/100 mL) when compared to Beijing (7.1 mg/100 mL) and Guangzhou (6.4 mg/100 mL). CerPCho content was significant higher ($p < 0.05$) in colostrum (10.9 mg/100 mL) of lactating mothers from Beijing and in transitional milk (8.5 mg/100 mL) of lactating mothers from Suzhou (Table 3); when considering the different lactation stages of mature milk (Figure 3), Beijing showed significantly higher content (12.9 mg/100 mL) at 12–30 days and Suzhou at 1–2 months (10.9 mg/100 mL). PtdEtn content was significant lower ($p < 0.05$) in colostrum (7.6 mg/100 mL) and mature milk (5.3 mg/100 mL) of lactating mother from Beijing and significant higher ($p < 0.05$) in colostrum (12.6 mg/100 mL) and transitional milk (10.8 mg/100 mL) of lactating mothers from Suzhou (Table 3); when considering the mature of the milk data at different lactation stages (Figure 3) Suzhou showed the highest contents of PtdEtn at 1–2 months (8.6 mg/100 mL). PtdIns content was significant low ($p < 0.05$) in mature milk (1.2 mg/100 mL) of lactating mothers from Beijing and significant higher ($p < 0.05$) in colostrum (2.3 mg/100 mL), transitional (2.4 mg/100 mL), and mature milk (1.7 mg/100 mL) of lactating mothers from Suzhou (Table 3); within mature milk (Figure 3) Suzhou showed the highest content of PtdIns (2.0 mg/100 mL) at 1–2 months. PtdSer content was significant higher ($p < 0.05$) in colostrum (1.8 mg/100 mL) of lactating mothers from Beijing and significantly different ($p < 0.05$) in transitional (1.3 mg/100mL) and mature milk (1.2 mg/100 mL) of lactating mothers from Suzhou (Table 3). Within mature milk (Figure 3) Beijing showed the highest PtdSer content (1.7 mg/100 mL) at 12–30 days and Suzhou at 1–2 months (1.5 mg/100 mL, respectively). Finally, Suzhou showed significant higher ($p < 0.05$) PL content in colostrum (38.9 mg/100 mL), transitional milk (34.9 mg/100 mL), and mature milk (26.0 mg/100 mL), and Beijing showed the lowest content in mature milk (22.3 mg/100 mL) (Table 3).

3.4. Gangliosides

Gangliosides were determined by LC-MS/MS as described by Giuffrida et al. [29] and the results are listed in Table 4.

From the total population, the amount of GD changed during the lactation period (Table 4), with GM3 significantly increasing ($p < 0.05$) from 3.8 mg/mL in colostrum to 10.1 mg/L in mature milk and GD3 significantly decreasing ($p < 0.05$) from 4.1 mg/mL in colostrum to 1.0 mg/mL in mature milk. Total gangliosides increased significantly ($p < 0.05$) from 8.0 mg/L in colostrum to 11.0 mg/L in mature milk (Table 4). However, variability was high and total ganglioside content ranged from 1.66–28.44 mg/L in colostrum, 2.77–22.04 mg/L in transitional milk, and between 0.90–36.88 mg/L in mature milk; GM3 contents ranged between 0.63–13.03 mg/L in colostrum, 1.01–17.71 mg/L in transitional milk, 3.45–25.97 mg/L at 1–2 months, 3.45–25.97 mg/L at 2–4 months, and between 5.17–34.41 mg/L at 4–8 months; GD3 contents ranged between 0.55–18.04 mg/L in colostrum, 0.06–15.52 mg/L in transitional milk, 0.15–4.93 mg/L at 1–2 months, 0.06–5.0 mg/L at 2–4 months, and between 0.05 and 6.77 mg/L at 4–8 months. The GM3/GD3 ratio also increased over the lactation period, to 0.9 in colostrum and 10.1 in mature milk, consistent with the variation of GM3 and GD3 described above.

Table 3. Median phospholipids composition of HM expressed as mg/100 mL.

mg/100 mL	Total Population			Guangzhou			Beijing			Suzhou		
	Colostrum (0–5 Days) $n = 113$	Transitional (6–15 Days) $n = 81$	Mature (16 Days–8 Months) $n = 345$	Colostrum (0–5 Days) $n = 38$	Transitional (6–15 Days) $n = 22$	Mature (16 Days–8 Months) $n = 120$	Colostrum (0–5 Days) $n = 45$	Transitional (6–15 Days) $n = 21$	Mature (16 Days–8 Months) $n = 113$	Colostrum (0–5 Days) $n = 30$	Transitional (6–15 Days) $n = 38$	Mature (16 Days–8 Months) $n = 112$
PtdCho	12.0 ± 5.8	10.1 ± 5.5 [†]	8.2 ± 5.0 [†‡]	12.5 ± 4.6 [a]	11.3 ± 5.6 [b]	8.6 ± 5.1 [c]	10.9 ± 4.8 [a]	8.3 ± 3.7 [b]	7.6 ± 4.5 [c]	12.6 ± 7.7 [a]	11.9 ± 6.1 [b]	8.5 ± 5.3 [c]
CerPCho	9.1 ± 4.0	7.3 ± 4.1 [†]	7.2 ± 4.0 [†]	7.7 ± 1.6 [a]	6.8 ± 2.7 [b]	7.1 ± 4.0 [c]	10.9 ± 4.9 [d]	6.2 ± 3.8 [b]	7.3 ± 3.9 [c]	9.7 ± 3.1 [a]	8.5 ± 4.7 [e]	7.4 ± 4.2 [c]
PtdEtn	8.5 ± 5.2	8.2 ± 5.3	6.4 ± 3.4 [†‡]	9.9 ± 2.6 [a]	5.6 ± 3.7 [b]	7.1 ± 3.9 [c]	7.6 ± 3.1 [d]	7.3 ± 2.4 [b]	5.3 ± 2.6 [e]	12.6 ± 7.4 [f]	10.8 ± 5.8 [g]	7.3 ± 3.2 [c]
PtdIns	1.8 ± 0.7	1.8 ± 1.0	1.5 ± 0.7 [†‡]	1.8 ± 0.5 [a]	1.2 ± 0.7 [b]	1.5 ± 0.8 [c]	1.6 ± 0.5 [a]	1.5 ± 0.4 [b]	1.2 ± 0.5 [d]	2.3 ± 1.0 [e]	2.4 ± 1.1 [f]	1.7 ± 0.8 [g]
PtdSer	1.5 ± 1.6	1.1 ± 0.8 [†]	1.0 ± 1.0 [†]	1.3 ± 0.4 [a]	0.8 ± 0.4 [b]	1.0 ± 0.6 [c]	1.8 ± 2.3 [d]	1.0 ± 1.4 [b]	0.9 ± 1.2 [c]	1.7 ± 0.5 [a]	1.3 ± 0.5 [e]	1.2 ± 1.4 [f]
Total PL (mg/100 mL)	33.0 ± 13.2	28.5 ± 14.4 [†]	24.2 ± 11.4 [†‡]	33.2 ± 8.1 [a]	25.6 ± 11.1 [b]	25.3 ± 12.5 [c]	33.0 ± 11.2 [a]	24.4 ± 8.1 [b]	22.3 ± 9.9 [d]	38.9 ± 18.8 [e]	34.9 ± 16.6 [f]	26.02 ± 11.3 [c]

PL, phospholipids. * Values are presented as median ± standard deviation. Values within a row with a symbol indicate statistically significant differences. [†] $p < 0.05$ versus colostrum. [‡] $p < 0.05$ versus transitional milk. [a,b,c,d,e,f,g] $p < 0.05$ among cities.

Table 4. Average GD composition of HM expressed as mg/L.

GD mg/L	Total Population			Guangzhou			Beijing			Suzhou		
	Colostrum (0–5 Days) $n = 113$	Transitional (6–15 Days) $n = 81$	Mature (16 Days–8 Months) $n = 345$	Colostrum (0–5 Days) $n = 38$	Transitional (6–15 Days) $n = 22$	Mature (16 Days–8 Months) $n = 120$	Colostrum (0–5 Days) $n = 45$	Transitional (6–15 Days) $n = 21$	Mature (16 Days–8 Months) $n = 113$	Colostrum (0–5 Days) $n = 30$	Transitional (6–15 Days) $n = 38$	Mature (16 Days–8 Months) $n = 112$
GM3	3.8 ± 2.5	5.5 ± 3.2 [†]	10.1 ± 4.6 [†‡]	4.0 ± 2.7 [a]	7.7 ± 4.5 [b]	10.5 ± 4.6 [c]	3.7 ± 2.3 [a]	3.3 ± 1.6 [d]	9.0 ± 3.8 [c]	4.0 ± 2.6 [a]	5.4 ± 2.0 [e]	10.8 ± 5.2 [c]
GD3	4.1 ± 4.5	3.0 ± 3.4 [†]	1.0 ± 1.7 [†‡]	2.8 ± 2.5 [a]	3.0 ± 3.5 [b]	1.0 ± 2.3 [c]	2.2 ± 2.0 [a]	3.0 ± 2.8 [b]	0.7 ± 0.9 [c]	8.6 ± 5.9 [d]	2.9 ± 3.7 [b]	1.1 ± 1.5 [c]
GM3 + GD3	8.0 ± 5.3	8.5 ± 4.5 [†]	11.0 ± 5.0 [†‡]	6.6 ± 3.2 [a]	10.7 ± 4.7 [b]	11.5 ± 5.1 [c]	5.9 ± 2.7 [a]	6.3 ± 3.4 [d]	9.7 ± 4.0 [c]	12.6 ± 7.0 [e]	8.3 ± 4.3 [f]	11.9 ± 5.6 [c]
GM3/GD3	0.9	1.8 [†]	10.1 [†‡]	1.4	2.6	10.4	1.7	1.1	12.5	0.5	1.8	9.4

* Values are presented as average ± standard deviation. Values within a row with a symbol indicate statistically significant differences. [†] $p < 0.05$ versus colostrum. [‡] $p < 0.05$ versus transitional milk. [a,b,c,d,e,f] $p < 0.05$ among cities.

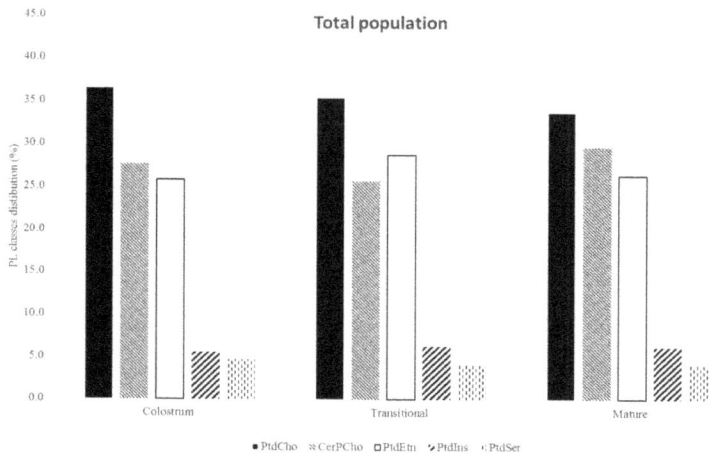

Figure 2. Change in phospholipid (PL) classes distribution in colostrum, transitional and mature milk.

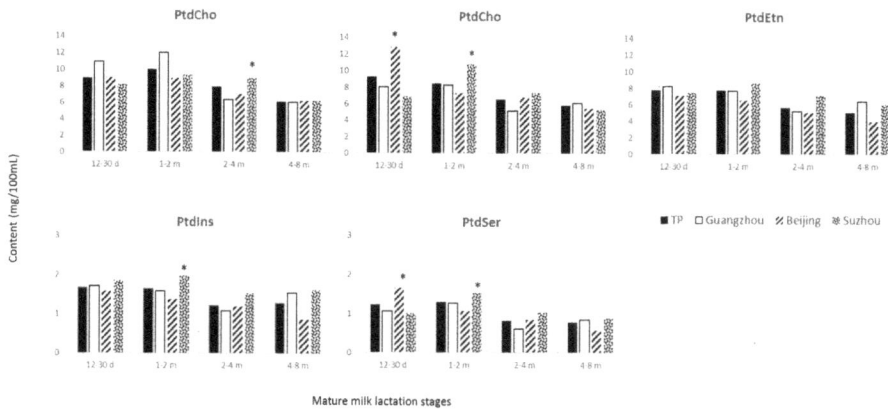

Figure 3. PL contents at different lactation stages, i.e., 12–30 days, 1–2 months, 2–4 months, and 4–8 months postpartum are shown in the total population and cities. TP stands for total population. * indicates significant difference ($p < 0.05$) among cities within the lactation stage.

Among the different cities, GM3 content was comparable ($p > 0.05$) in colostrum; GM3 highest content ($p < 0.05$) in transitional milk (7.7 mg/L) was observed in HM of lactating mothers from Guangzhou and in mature milk in lactating mothers from Guangzhou and Suzhou, at 10.5 and 10.8 mg/L, respectively (Table 4). Within mature milk (Figure 4) Beijing, Guangzhou, and Suzhou showed the highest GM3 content at 4–8 months (11.0 ± 3.9, 12.3 ± 5.5, and 15.6 ± 6.1 mg/L, respectively). The highest content ($p < 0.05$) of GD3 was observed in colostrum of lactating mothers from Suzhou (8.6 mg/L); GD3 content was comparable ($p > 0.05$) in transitional milk among the different cities and between Guangzhou and Suzhou in mature HM (Table 4). However, when considering mature milk at different lactation stages (Figure 4), Beijing, Guangzhou, and Suzhou showed the highest GD3 content at 12–30 days (0.9 ± 1.3, 1.1 ± 1.1, and 1.5 ± 2.2 mg/L, respectively). Suzhou showed the highest content ($p < 0.05$) of total GD in colostrum and mature milk (12.6 and 11.9 mg/L, respectively), the highest content ($p < 0.05$) of total GD in transitional milk was observed in Guangzhou (10.7 mg/L) (Table 4).

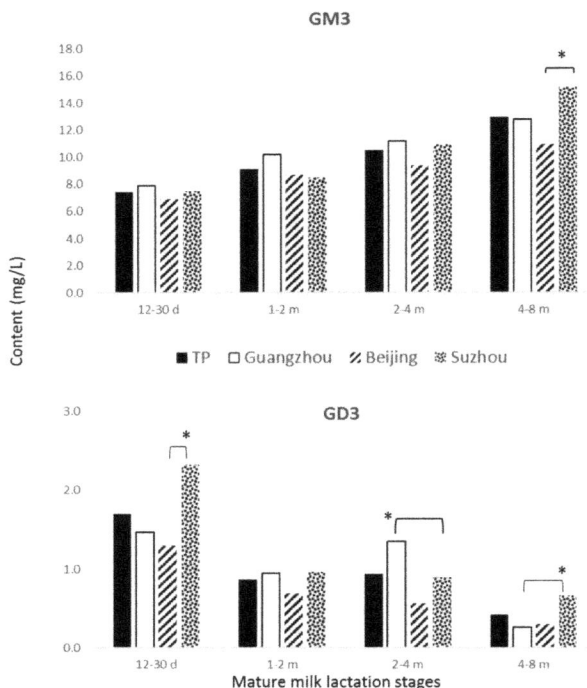

Figure 4. GM3 and GD3 contents at different mature milk lactation stages, i.e., 12–30 days, 1–2 months, 2–4 months, and 4–8 months postpartum are shown in total population (TP) and cities. * stands for significant difference ($p < 0.05$) at 4–8 months between Beijing and Suzhou for GM3, at 12–30 days between Beijing and Suzhou, and at 2–4 months and at 4–8 months between Guangzhou and Suzhou for GD3.

4. Discussion

This study measured the FA, PL, and GD content and the profile of 539 HM samples from Beijing, Guangzhou, and Suzhou.

4.1. FA

Results from the total population (Table 2) showed a total SFA content of 35.7% ± 3.9% in colostrum, of 38.9% ± 4.1% in transitional milk, and of 36.2% ± 4.7% in mature milk. Chinese studies have reported SFA level in colostrum ranging from 36.8% to 41.3% [30,31], in transitional milk from 35.2% to 42.6% [31,32] and in mature milk from 35.1% to 41.1% [30–34], in agreement with our results. When considering other populations (e.g., Caucasian, American) the SFA level in colostrum was 42.3%–43.7% [35–37], in transitional milk it ranged from 43.1% to 45.2% [36,37] and, in mature milk, from 37.4% to 57.1% [34–38], therefore, Chinese populations seem to show lower amount of total SFA in colostrum, transitional and mature milk when compared to other populations.

In this study, main SFA, lauric (12:0), myristic (14:0), palmitic (16:0), and stearic (18:0) acid contents were 2.6% ± 1.6%, 3.8% ± 1.7%, 23.2% ± 1.9%, and 5.2% ± 1.0% of total FA, respectively, in colostrum (Table 2); 6.1% ± 2.3%, 5.5% ± 2.2%, 20.5% ± 2.3%, and 5.0% ± 0.8% of total FA in transitional milk (Table 2); and 5.2% ± 1.9%, 4.2% ± 1.7%, 19.8% ± 2.6%, and 5.1% ± 1.1% of total FA, respectively, in mature milk (Table 2). Among the Chinese population, lauric, myristic, palmitic, and stearic acids ranged between 3.0%–4.9%, 5.2%–5.3%, 20.1%–23.3%, and 6.0%–7.0% of total

FA, respectively, in colostrum [30,31]; between 4.2%–6.5%, 3.8%–6.4%, 19.7%–23.3%, and 5.4%–8.1% of total FA, respectively, in transitional milk [31,32]; and finally between 3.8%–6.3%, 3.4%–6.5%, 17.3%–22.3%, and 5.0%–8.0% of total FA, respectively, in mature milk [30–34]. When considering other populations, lauric, myristic, palmitic, and stearic acids ranged between 1.2%–4.5%, 4.8%–7.3%, 24.0%–27.3%, and 5.5%–7.1% of total FA, respectively, in colostrum [35–37]; between 5.2%–6.5%, 6.5%–7.7%, 22.2%–22.6%, and 5.7%–7.4% of total FA, respectively, in transitional milk [36,37]; and finally between 3.7%–6.1%, 4.9%–7.0%, 18.7%–23.0%, and 4.8%–7.6% of total FA, respectively, in mature milk [34–38]. Philippian population showed high lauric (13.82%) and myristic (12.12%) FA contents [34] and it was reported [20,21] that 10:0, 12:0, and 14:0 FA content increases when lactating women consumed high-carbohydrate diets, whereas the secretion of the 18-carbon chain unsaturated FA, which are derived from the diet, decreased. High contents of lauric (10.2%) and myristic FA (9.1%) have been also reported in the milk of women from Nigeria [4] as a typical response to a high-carbohydrate diet.

Results from the total population (Table 2) showed total MUFA content of 40.7% ± 3.8% in colostrum, of 37.7% ± 4.3% in transitional milk, and of 36.9% ± 4.1% in mature milk. Chinese studies have reported MUFA levels in colostrum ranging from 34.7% [30] to 43.1% [31], in transitional milk from 30.8% to 42.9% [31,32], and in mature milk from 28.5% to 45.6% [30–34], in agreement with our results.

When considering other population, MUFA levels in colostrum ranged between 32.1%–44.4% of total FA [35–37], in transitional milk it was 35.1% of total FA [37], and in mature milk ranged from 30.3%–44.4% of total FA [34,35,37,38], therefore, Chinese populations seem to show comparable MUFA content in colostrum, transitional and mature milk to other populations.

Among MUFA, oleic acid was the most abundant FA and its content ranged from 34.4% in colostrum to 31.9% in transitional and mature milk. In the Chinese population oleic acid ranged from 28.4%–36.3% of total FA in colostrum [30,31]; from 25.9%–36.5% of total FA in transitional milk [31,32], and from 24.9%–38.1% in mature milk [30–34], and in other populations from 28.4%–40.1%, from 27.7%–32.1%, and from 21.9%–40.5% of total FA in colostrum [35–37], transitional [36,37], and mature milk [34–38], respectively.

Results from the total population (Table 2) showed total *n*-6 and *n*-3 PUFA content of 21.7 ± 3.6 and 1.4% ± 0.5% in colostrum, respectively, of 21.6 ± 3.8 and 1.9% ± 0.7% in transitional milk, and of 24.1 ± 5.0 and 1.9% ± 0.9% of total FA in mature milk. Chinese studies have reported PUFA levels in colostrum ranging from 14.8%–22.5% for *n*-6PUFA and from 2.9%–3.9% for *n*-3PUFA [30,31], in transitional milk from 13.7%–27.6% for *n*-6PUFA and from 2.5%–5.1% for *n*-3PUFA [31,32], and in mature milk from 14.1%–27.8% for *n*-6PUFA and from 2.6%–6.8% for *n*-3PUFA [30–34], therefore, the values are in agreement with the *n*-6PUFA results of this study, but higher for *n*-3PUFA.

When considering other populations, PUFA levels in colostrum ranged between 11.2%–14.0% for *n*-6PUFA and from 1.9%–3.5% of total FA for *n*-3PUFA [35–37], in transitional milk from 12.3%–14.1% for *n*-6PUFA and from 1.5%–3.3% of total FA for *n*-3PUFA [36,37], and in mature milk from 9.5%–20.3% for *n*-6PUFA and from 1.3%–3.2% of total FA for *n*-3PUFA [34–38]. Therefore, the Chinese populations seem to show higher contents of total *n*-6 PUFA when compared to other populations.

Among PUFA, LA (18:2*n*-6), and ALA (18:3*n*-3), considered essential FA because humans lack the enzymes required for their biosynthesis, were the most abundant FA we observed in colostrum, mature and transitional milk (18.9% ± 3.6%, 19.7% ± 3.8%, and 22.8% ± 4.9% of total FA for LA, respectively and for 0.9% ± 0.4%, 1.4% ± 0.6%, and 1.5% ± 0.9% of total FA for ALA, respectively).

In the Chinese population, LA and ALA ranged from 10.3%–19.2% and from 0.9%–1.3% of total FA, respectively, in colostrum [30–32]; from 9.8%–23.3% and from 0.9%–2.2% of total FA, respectively, in transitional milk [31,32]; and from 10.9%–23.7% and from 0.9%–3.0% of total FA, respectively, in mature milk [30–34], in agreement with our findings.

In other populations, LA and ALA ranged from 8.6%–11.9% and from 0.7%–1.1% of total FA, respectively, in colostrum [35–37]; from 10.3%–12.5% and from 0.8%–1.3% of total FA, respectively, in transitional milk [36,37]; and from 7.9%–17.8% and from 0.4%–1.4% of total FA, respectively, in mature milk [34–38].

Finally, in our study, DHA contents for the total population ranged from 0.3%, in mature milk, to 0.5% in colostrum and transitional milk, therefore, lower than the DHA content reported for Chinese marine populations in colostrum (1.5%) [30], transitional (0.6%) [31], and mature milk (0.5%–2.8%) [30,33]. The ratio ARA/DHA (1.8–2.2) was comparable to average worldwide ratio of about 1.5 [22].

Among different cities, over lactation time, HM from Beijing showed slightly higher SFA content (Table 2), Guangzhou the highest MUFA content (Table 2), and Suzhou the highest *n*-3PUFA content (Table 2).

It is known that the type of fat/oil in the maternal diet influences the FA composition of breast milk. Francois et al. [22] showed that the consumption of six different dietary fats, each providing a specific FA, caused an acute response in HM FA composition, especially within 24 h, and that the response remained significantly elevated for 1–3 days after consumption of dietary fat. Therefore, difference observed in HM FA composition may reflect variation in maternal diet [33].

However, a careful analyses of dietary habits of Guangzhou, Beijing, and Suzhou needs to be performed for correlating to HM composition.

4.2. Phospholipids

Several studies have recognized the importance of PL for infant growth [39–41]. At the same time, PL are involved in immunity and inflammatory responses [42], and in neuronal signaling [43].

PL content in HM significantly ($p < 0.005$) decreased along the lactation period from 33.0 in colostrum to 24.2 mg/100 mL in mature milk, in agreement with previous studies performed elsewhere [12,44]. The PL class distribution was similar in colostrum, transitional and mature milk (Figure 2).

PL as emulsifiers are essential for the solubilization of dietary fats and as a consequence for their digestion and absorption. In this regard, the higher content of PL in colostrum and transitional HM compared to mature milk might explain the good fat absorption from HM by the newborn, despite poor pancreatic secretion, as suggested by Harzer et al. [11]. A decrease in PL content in HM along the lactation stage might occur because the diameter of the milk fat globule membrane increases [11,45], decreasing the PL/TAG ratio [7,8].

Our study showed that PtdCho was the most abundant PL in HM (Figure 2), followed by CerPCho and PtdEtn, and PtdIns and PtdSer, in agreement with previous studies [3,11,12,44,46]. PtdCho and CerPCho are important sources of choline considered as an essential nutrient for infants. Choline is a precursory amino alcohol of the neurotransmitter acetylcholine, it acts by regulating the transduction signal, and serves as a source of methyl groups in intermediate metabolism, being considered essential for optimum development of the brain [7,8]. In addition, CerPCho can reduce cholesterol absorption between 20.4%–85.5%, depending on the ingested dose (0.1% and 5.0%, respectively) [47], being possibly involved in cholesterol regulation programming.

The amount of total PL in colostrum (33.0 ± 13.2 mg/100 mL), transitional (28.5 ± 14.4 mg/100 mL), and mature milk (24.2 ± 11.4 mg/100 mL), was comparable to the values reported by Bitman et al. [44] (35, 31, and 27 mg/100 mL, respectively), Thakkar et al. [48] (20.8–24.2 mg/100 mL in mature milk), and Garcia et al. [49] (15.3–47.4 mg/100 mL in mature milk); higher than the values reported by Sala-Vila et al. [12] (13.5, 14.0, and 9.8 mg/100 mL, respectively), Lopez et al. [50] (13.5 mg/100 mL in mature milk) and Zou et al. [51] (16.8, 22.3, and 19.2 mg/100 mL, respectively).

In the total population PtdCho contents in colostrum, transitional, and mature milk were 12.0 ± 5.8, 10.1 ± 5.5, and 8.2 ± 5.0 mg/100 mL, respectively, comparable to values reported in literature, 4.3–11.2, 5.7–9.4, and 2.0–11.2 mg/100 mL, respectively [44,48–56].

CerPCho contents in colostrum, transitional, and mature milk were 9.1 ± 4.0, 7.3 ± 4.1, and 7.2 ± 4.0 mg/100 mL, respectively, comparable to values reported in the literature of 5.3–11.0, 9.0–11.6, and 3.1–13.5 mg/100 mL, respectively [44,48–57].

PtdEtn contents in colostrum, transitional, and mature milk were 8.5 ± 5.2, 8.2 ± 5.3, and 6.4 ± 3.4 mg/100 mL, respectively, higher than values reported in the literature for colostrum and transitional milk 1.4–6.4 and 1.5–5.6 mg/100 mL, respectively [44,51], and comparable to values reported for mature milk of 0.2–8.1 mg/100 mL [3,11,12,44,48,49,51,52].

PtdIns and PtdSer contents in colostrum (1.8 ± 0.7 and 1.5 ± 1.6 mg/100 mL, respectively), transitional (1.8 ± 1.0 and 1.1 ± 0.8 mg/100mL, respectively), and mature milk (1.5 ± 0.7 and 1.0 ± 1.1 mg/100 mL, respectively) were comparable to values reported in previous studies for PtdIns, 1.4–3.3, 1.5–2.2, and 0.2–2.2 mg/100 mL, respectively, and for PtdSer, 2.1–3.6, 1.5–2.2, and 0.8–4.5 mg/100 mL [44,48–51,53].

Among the different cities, Suzhou showed the highest total PL and PtdEtn levels in colostrum, transitional, and mature milk (Table 3). Dietary sources of PtdEtn may be lecithin from rapeseed oil, whose consumption may explain also the higher content of ALA in HM from Suzhou. However, a careful analyses of dietary habits of this region needs to be performed for correlating to HM composition.

It is well known [58] that lipid and liposoluble nutrients content increases towards the latter part of a feeding session, a phenomenon that has been corroborated by biochemical analyses of total milk fat in fore-milk, and hind-milk [59,60]. Therefore, in order to assure sample homogeneity in our study all efforts have been made to collect fully-expressed milk. Among the cited studies, only Bitman et al., Thakkar et al., Holmes et al., and Fischer et al. [44,48,54,56] refer to full breast milk samples, Sala-Vila et al. [12] to fore-milk, and no detailed sampling procedure is described in the other studies. Analysis performed in fore-milk and hind-milk rather than fully-expressed milk could explain the discrepancy among results.

4.3. Gangliosides

GD are widely distributed in almost all human tissues, with the highest amount found in neural tissue and extra-neural organs, such the lung, spleen, and gut. It has been reported that during the first stages of life, dietary GD may have an important role in preventing infections [61] and in cognitive development functions [10,62].

Our data confirmed, as previously reported [14,16,17,29,63,64], that the amount of GD changes during the lactation period, with GD3 decreasing and GM3 increasing over the lactation period. Rueda et al. [15] postulated that a high concentration of GD3 in early milk may reflect its biological role in the development of organs, such as the intestine, as was observed in our study in all cities. The increase in GM3 in mature milk has been associated with signal transduction, cell adhesion, and growth factor receptors, leading to the development of the immune and central nervous systems [14,17,61]. In the studied population, the sum of GM3 and GD3 increased from 8.0 mg/L in colostrum to 11.0 mg/L in mature milk, as previously published [29]. It has been reported [64] that the sum of GM3 and GD3 can range from as low as 2 mg/L to as high as 25 mg/L, depending on breast milk sampling, population demographics, diet, and analytical methodologies. In this study, total ganglioside content ranged from 1.66–28.44 mg/L in colostrum, 2.77–22.04 mg/L in transitional milk, and between 0.90–36.88 mg/L in mature milk, covering total GD contents previous reported, i.e., 2.8–59.7 mg/L in colostrum [14,15,17,18,29,63,65], 0.9–30.7 mg/L in transitional [14,15,17,18,63,65], and 1.6–68.6 mg/L in mature milk [14,15,17,18,29,48,63,65,66]. When considering average values, in colostrum and transitional milk, GM3 content (3.8 and 5.5 mg/L, respectively) was lower than the one reported by Ma et al. [63] (6.5–7.1 and 8.3–9.6 mg/L, respectively). Within mature milk, at 1–2 months GM3 content (9.08 mg/L) was comparable to the one reported by Ma et al. [63,64] (8.3–11.3 mg/L) and higher than the content reported by Thakkar et al. [48] (2.3–2.9 mg/L); after 3–8 months GM3 content (10.46–12.92 mg/L) was lower than what reported by Ma et al. [63,64] (17.4–21.4 mg/L) and higher than the content reported by Thakkar et al. [48] (3.9 mg/L). However, when considering minimum and maximum values, GM3 contents (0.63–13.03, 1.01–17.71, and 0.8–34.41 mg/L, in colostrum, transitional, and mature milk, respectively) were comparable with GM3 contents previously reported [48,63,64].

As for GM3, when considering average values, in colostrum and transitional milk, GD3 content (4.1 and 3.0 mg/L, respectively) was lower than the one reported by Ma et al. [63] (20 and 10 mg/L, respectively). Within mature milk, at 1–2 months GD3 content (0.87 mg/L) was lower than the one reported by Ma et al. [63,64] (4.6–7.0 mg/L) and by Thakkar et al. [48] (1.9–2.3 mg/L); after 3–8 months GD3 content (0.25–0.50 mg/L) was lower than that reported by Ma et al. [63,64] (1.5–2.7 mg/L) and by Thakkar et al. [48] (1.7 mg/L). However, when considering minimum and maximum values, GD3 contents (0.6–18.0, 0.1–15.5, and 0.1–9.3 mg/L, in colostrum, transitional, and mature milk, respectively) were comparable with GD3 contents previously reported [48,63,64]. Among the cities Suzhou showed the highest GM3 and GD3 contents (Table 4) in colostrum and mature milk.

Ma et al. [64] suggested that the ganglioside concentrations in HM at any time point may be influenced by the mother's dietary intake of gangliosides or their precursors. It was demonstrated [67] that GD3 and GM3 are transferred across the human placenta using an ex vivo model of dually-perfused isolated human placental lobules, suggesting that they are available to the developing fetus. Therefore, a careful analysis of dietary habits in this region needs to be performed for correlating to HM GD composition.

5. Conclusions

In this study, FA, PL, and GD contents and compositions of HM from lactating women living in Suzhou, Guangzhou, and Beijing were evaluated.

HM was collected over a period of eight months, allowing the observation of lipid compositional changes during lactation.

SFA, MUFA, and PL content decreased during lactation, PUFA and GD content increased. Among different cities, over lactation time, HM from Beijing showed the highest SFA content, HM from Guangzhou showed the highest MUFA content, and HM from Suzhou showed the highest *n*-3PUFA content. The highest total PL and GD contents were observed in HM from Suzhou. In order to investigate the influence of the diet on maternal milk composition, a careful analysis of dietary habits of these population needs to be performed in future work.

Acknowledgments: The authors would like to thank the participants who volunteered for this study, Lawrence Li for project support and guidance, Celia Ning for project management, Qiaoji Li for clinical project management, Emilie Ba for data management and local project staff at Peking University School of Public Health, Guangzhou University School of Public Health and Soochow University School of Public Health for recruitment and data collection.

Author Contributions: S.K.T., G.V.-P., Y.Z. and P.W. conceived and designed the experiments; F.G., C.C.-H., E.B., P.F., I.M.E., I.T., C.M., B.S.-B. developed, validated and performed the experiments; F.G., C.C.-H., S.K.T. and C.A.D.-C. analyzed the data; F.G. wrote the paper.

Conflicts of Interest: This study was funded by Nestlé Nutrition Institute, China, and Nestlé Research Centre, Beijing, China. F.G., C.C.-H., E.B., P.F., I.M.E., I.T., C.M., B.S.-B., S.K.T., C.A.D.-C and G.V.-P. were all employees of Nestec Ltd. when this work was done. The opinions expressed in the article are those of the authors alone and do not necessarily reflect the views or recommendations of their respective affiliations.

Abbreviations

FA (FA), phospholipids (PL), gangliosides (GD), gas chromatography (GC), evaporative light scattering detector (ELSD), with time of flight (TOF), triacylglycerols (TAG), saturated FA (SFA), mono-unsaturated (MUFA), polyunsaturated (PUFA), long chain polyunsaturated FA (LCPUFA), linoleic (LA), linolenic acids (ALA), arachidonic (ARA), docosahexaenoic (DHA), phosphatydilinositol (PtdIns), phosphatydylethanolamine (PtdEtn), phosphatydylserine (PtdSer), phosphatidylcholine (PtdCho), sphingomyelin (CerPCho), methyl esters of FA (FAMEs).

References

1. Kramer, M.; Ritsuko, S.K. *The Optimal Duration of Exclusive Breastfeeding: A Systematic Review*; World Health Organization: Geneva, Switzerland, 2002.

2. Giovannini, M.; Riva, E.; Agostoni, C. FA in pediatric nutrition (Review). *Pediatr. Clin. North. Am.* **1995**, *42*, 861. [CrossRef]

3. Bitman, J.; Wood, L.; Metha, N.R.; Hamosh, P.; Hamosh, M. Comparison of phospholipid composition of breast milk from mothers of term and preterm infants during lactation. *Am. J. Clin. Nutr.* **1984**, *40*, 1103–1119. [PubMed]

4. Jensen, R.G. Lipids in HM. *Lipids* **1999**, *12*, 1243–1271. [CrossRef]

5. Innis, S.M. Essential FA in growth and development. *Prog. Lipid Res.* **1991**, *30*, 39–103. [CrossRef]

6. Pruett, S.T.; Bushnev, A.; Hagedorn, K.; Adiga, M.; Haynes, C.A.; Sullards, M.C.; Liotta, D.C.; Merrill, A.H., Jr. Biodiversity of sphingoid bases ("sphingosines") and related amino alcohols. *J. Lipid Res.* **2008**, *49*, 1621–1639. [CrossRef] [PubMed]

7. Zeisel, S.H.; Blusztajn, J.K. Choline and human nutrition. *Ann. Rev. Nutr.* **1994**, *14*, 269–296. [CrossRef] [PubMed]

8. Zeisel, S.H. The fetal origins of memory: The role of dietary choline in optimal brain development. *J. Pediatr.* **2006**, *149*, 131s–136s. [CrossRef] [PubMed]

9. Schauer, R. Achievements and challenges of sialic acid research. *Glycoconj. J.* **2000**, *17*, 485–499. [CrossRef] [PubMed]

10. Gurnida, D.A.; Rowan, A.M.; Idjradinata, P.; Muchtadi, D.; Sekarwana, N. Association of complex lipids containing gangliosides with cognitive development of 6-month-old infants. *Early Hum. Dev.* **2012**, *88*, 595–601. [CrossRef] [PubMed]

11. Harzer, G.; Haug, M.; Bindels, J.G. Biochemistry of human milk in early lactation. *Z. Ernahrungswissenschaft* **1986**, *25*, 77–90. [CrossRef]

12. Sala Vila, A.; Castellote, A.I.; Rodriguez-Palmero-Seuma, M.; Campoy, C.; Lopez-Sabater, M.C. Lipid composition in human breast milk from Granada (Spain): Changes during lactation. *Nutrition* **2005**, *21*, 467–473. [CrossRef] [PubMed]

13. Cilla, A.; Diego-Quintaes, K.; Barbera, R.; Alegria, A. Phospholipids in HM and infant formula: Benefits and needs for correct infant nutrition. *Crit. Rev. Food Sc. Nutr.* **2016**, *56*, 1880–1892. [CrossRef] [PubMed]

14. Takamizawa, K.; Iwamori, K.; Mutai, M.; Nagai, Y. Selective changes in gangliosides of HM during lactation: A molecular indicator for the period of lactation. *Biochim. Biophys. Acta* **1986**, *879*, 73–77. [PubMed]

15. Rueda, R.; Puente, R.; Hueso, P.; Maldonado, J.; Gil, A. New data on content and distribution of gangliosides in HM. *Biol. Chem. Hoppe-Seyler* **1995**, *376*, 723–727. [CrossRef] [PubMed]

16. Rueda, R.; Maldonado, J.; Gil, A. Comparison of content and distribution of HM gangliosides from Spanish and Panamanian mothers. *Ann. Nutr. Metab.* **1996**, *40*, 194–201. [CrossRef] [PubMed]

17. Pan, X.L.; Izumi, T. Variation of the ganglioside compositions of HM, cow's milk and infant formulas. *Early Hum. Dev.* **2000**, *57*, 25–31. [CrossRef]

18. Martin-Sosa, S.; Martin, M.-J.; Garcia-Pardo, L.A.; Hueso, P. Distribution of sialic acids in the milk of Spanish mothers of full term infants during lactation. *J. Pediatr. Gastr. Nutr.* **2004**, *39*, 111–116.

19. Uchiyama, S.-I.; Sekiguchi, K.; Akaishi, M.; Anan, A.; Maeda, T.; Izumi, T. Characterization and chronological changes of preterm HM gangliosides. *Nutrition* **2011**, *27*, 998–1001. [CrossRef] [PubMed]

20. Read, W.W.C.; Lutz, P.G.; Tashjian, A. HM lipids. II the influence of dietary carbohydrates and fat on the FA of mature milk. A study in four ethnic groups. *Am. J. Clin. Nutr.* **1965**, *17*, 180–183. [PubMed]

21. Van Beusekom, C.M.; Martini, I.A.; Rutgers, H.M.; Boersma, E.R.; Muskiet, F.A. A carbohydrate-rich diets not only leads to incorporation of medium-chain FA (6:0–14:0) in triglycerides but also in each milk-phospholipid subclass. *Am. J. Clin. Nut.* **1990**, *52*, 326–334.

22. Francois, C.A.; Connor, S.L.; Wander, R.C.; Connor, W.E. Acute effects of dietary FA on the FA of HM. *Am. J. Clin. Nutr.* **1998**, *67*, 301–308. [PubMed]

23. Samur, G.; Topcu, A.; Turan, S. *Trans* FA and fatty acid composition of mature breast milk in Turkish women and their association with maternal diets. *Lipids* **2009**, *44*, 405. [CrossRef] [PubMed]

24. Lauritzen, L.; Jørgensen, M.H.; Hansen, H.S.; Michaelsen, K.F. Fluctuations in HM long-chain PUFA levels in relation to dietary fish intake. *Lipids* **2002**, *37*, 237. [CrossRef] [PubMed]

25. Ryan, J.M.; Rice, E.G.; Mitchell, M.D. The role of gangliosides in brain development and the potential benefits of perinatal supplementation. *Nutr. Res.* **2013**, *33*, 877–887. [CrossRef] [PubMed]

26. Yang, T.; Zhang, Y.; Ning, Y.; You, L.; Ma, D.; Zheng, Y.; Yang, X.; Li, W.; Wang, J.; Wang, P. Breast milk macronutrient composition and the associated factors in urban Chinese mothers. *Chin. Med. J. Assoc.* **2014**, *9*, 127.

27. Cruz-Hernandez, C.; Goeuriot, S.; Giuffrida, F.; Thakkar, S.K.; Destaillats, F. Direct quantification of FA in HM by gas chromatography. *J. Chrom. A* **2013**, *9*, 174. [CrossRef] [PubMed]

28. Giuffrida, F.; Cruz-Hernandez, C.; Fluck, B.; Tavazzi, I.; Thakkar, K.S.; Destaillats, F.; Braun, M. Quantification of Phospholipids Classes in HM. *Lipids* **2013**, *48*, 1051–1058. [CrossRef] [PubMed]

29. Giuffrida, F.; Masserey-Elmelegy, I.; Thakkar, S.K.; Marmet, C.; Destaillats, F. Longitudinal Evolution of the Concentration of Gangliosides GM3 and GD3 in HM. *Lipids* **2014**, *49*, 997–1004. [CrossRef] [PubMed]

30. Wu, T.-C.; Lau, B.-H.; Chen, P.-H.; Wu, L.-T.; Tang, R.-B. Fatty acid composition of Taiwanese HM. *J. Chin. Med. Assoc.* **2012**, *73*, 581–588. [CrossRef]

31. Chen, Z.Y.; Kwan, K.Y.; Tong, K.K.; Ratnayake, W.M.N.; Li, H.Q.; Leung, S.S.F. Breast milk fatty acid composition: A comparative study between Hong Kong and Chongqing Chinese. *Lipids* **1997**, *32*, 1061–1067. [CrossRef] [PubMed]

32. Li, J.; Fan, Y.; Zhang, Z.; Yu, H.; An, Y.; Kramer, J.K.G.; Deng, Z. Evaluating the trans fatty acid, CLA, PUFA and erucic acid diversity in HM from five region in China. *Lipids* **2009**, *44*, 257–271. [CrossRef] [PubMed]

33. Ruan, C.-L.; Liu, X.-F.; Man, H.-S.; Ma, X.-L.; Lu, G.-Z.; Duan, G.-H.; DeFrancesco, C.A.; Connor, W.E. Milk composition in women from five different regions of China: The great diversity of milk FA. *Hum. Clin. Nutr.* **1995**, 2993–2998.

34. Yuhas, R.; Pramuk, K.; Lien, E.L. HM fatty acid composition from nine countries varies most in DHA. *Lipids* **2006**, *41*, 851–858. [CrossRef] [PubMed]

35. Xiang, M.; Alfvén, G.; Blennow, M.; Trygg, M.; Zetterstrom, R. Long-Chain polyunsaturated FA in HM and brain growth during early infancy. *Acta Pediatr.* **2000**, *89*, 142–147. [CrossRef]

36. Genzel-Boroviczény, O.; Wahle, J.; Koletzko, B. Fatty acid composition of HM during the 1st month after term and preterm delivery. *Eur. J. Pediatr.* **1997**, *156*, 142–147. [CrossRef] [PubMed]

37. Idota, T.; Sakurai, M.; Sugawara, Y.; Ishiyama, Y.; Murakami, Y.; Moriguchi, H.; Takeuchi, M.; Shimoda, K.; Asai, Y. The latest survey for the composition of milk obtained from Japanese mothers. Part II. Changes of fatty acid composition, phospholipids and cholesterol contents during lactation. *Jpn. J. Pediatr. Gastroenterol. Nutr.* **1991**, *5*, 159–173.

38. Chardigny, J.-M.; Wolff, R.L.; Sébédio, J.-L.; Martine, L.; Juaneda, P. Trans mono- and polyunsaturated FA in HM. *Eur. J. Clin. Nutr.* **1995**, *49*, 523–531. [PubMed]

39. Tanaka, K.; Hosozawa, M.; Kudo, N.; Yoshikawa, N.; Hisata, K.; Shoji, H.; Shinohara, K.; Shimizu, T. The pilot study: Sphingomyelin-Fortified milk has a positive association with the neurobehavioural development of very low birth weight infants during infancy, randomized control trial. *Brain Dev.* **2013**, *35*, 45–52. [CrossRef] [PubMed]

40. Küllenberg, D.; Taylor, L.A.; Schneider, M.; Massing, U. Health effects of dietary phospholipids. *Lipids Health Dis.* **2012**, *11*, 1–16. [CrossRef] [PubMed]

41. German, J.B. Dietary lipids from an evolutionary perspective: Sources, structures and functions. *Mater. Child. Nutr.* **2011**, *7*, 2–16. [CrossRef] [PubMed]

42. Nixon, G.F. Sphingolipids in inflammation: Pathological implications and potential therapeutic targets. *Br. J. Pharmacol.* **2009**, *158*, 982–993. [CrossRef] [PubMed]

43. McDaniel, M.A.; Maier, S.F.; Einstein, G.O. "Brain-specific" nutrients: A memory cure? *Nutrition* **2003**, *19*, 957–975. [CrossRef]

44. Bitman, J.; Freed, L.M.; Neville, M.C.; Wood, D.L.; Hamosh, P.; Hamosh, M. Lipid composition of prepartum human mammary secretion and postpartum milk. *J. Ped. Gastr. Nutr.* **1986**, *5*, 608–615. [CrossRef]

45. Harzer, G.; Haug, M.; Dieterich, I.; Gentner, P.G. Changing patterns of HM lipids in the course of the lactation and during the day. *Am. J. Clin. Nutr.* **1983**, *37*, 612–621. [PubMed]

46. Morrison, W.R.; Smith, L.M. Fatty Acid Composition of Milk Phospholipids. II. Sheep, Indian Buffalo and HMs. *Lipids* **1967**, *2*, 178–182. [CrossRef] [PubMed]

47. Rombaut, R.; Dewettinck, K. Properties, analysis and purification of milk polar lipids. *Int. Dairy J.* **2006**, *16*, 1362–1373. [CrossRef]

48. Thakkar, S.K.; Giuffrida, F.; Cruz-Hernandez, C.; De Castro, A.C.; Mukherjee, R.; Tran, L.-A.; Steenhout, P.; Lee, L.Y.; Destaillats, F. Dynamic composition of HM nutrient composition of women from Singapore with special focus on lipids. *Am. J. Nutr. Biol.* **2013**, *25*, 770–779.

49. Garcia, C.; Millet, V.; Coste, T.C.; Mimoun, M.; Ridet, A.; Antona, C.; Simeoni, U.; Armand, M. French Mothers' Milk Deficient in DHA Contains Phospholipid Species of Potential Interest for Infant Development. *J. Pediatr. Gastroenterol. Nutr.* **2011**, *53*, 206–212. [CrossRef] [PubMed]

50. Lopez, C.; Briard-Bion, V.; Menard, O.; Rousseau, F.; Pradel, P.; Besle, J.-M. Phospholipid, sphingolipid, and fatty acid compositions of the milk fat globule membrane are modified by diet. *J. Agric. Food Chem.* **2008**, *56*, 5226–5236. [CrossRef] [PubMed]

51. Zou, X.-Q.; Guo, Z.; Huang, J.-H.; Jin, Q.-Z.; Cheong, L.-Z.; Wang, X.-G.; Xu, X.-B. HM fat globules from different stages of lactation: A lipid composition analysis and microstructure characterization. *J. Agric. Food Chem.* **2012**, *60*, 7158–7167. [CrossRef] [PubMed]

52. Zeisel, S.H.; Char, D.; Sheard, N.F. Choline, phosphatidylcholine and sphingomyelin in human and bovine milk and infant formulas. *J. Nutr.* **1986**, *116*, 50–58. [PubMed]

53. Kynast, G.; Schmitz, C. Determination of the phospholipid content of HM, cow's milk and various infant formulas. *Z. Ernährungswiss* **1988**, *27*, 252–265. [CrossRef] [PubMed]

54. Holmes-McNary, M.Q.; Cheng, W.-L.; Mar, M.-H.; Fussell, S.; Zeisel, S.H. Choline and choline esters in human and rat milk and in infant formulas. *Am. J. Clin. Nutr.* **1996**, *64*, 572–576. [PubMed]

55. Ilcol, Y.O.; Ozbek, R.; Hamurtkin, E.; Ulus, I.H. Choline status in newborns, infants, children, breast-feeding women, breast-fed infants and human breast milk. *J. Nutr. Biochem.* **2005**, *16*, 489–499. [CrossRef] [PubMed]

56. Fischer, L.M.; Costa, K.A.; Galanko, J.; Sha, W.; Stephenson, B.; Vick, J.; Zeisel, S.H. Choline intake and genetic polymorphisms influence choline metabolite concentrations in human breast milk and plasma. *Am. J. Clin. Nutr.* **2010**, *92*, 336–346. [CrossRef] [PubMed]

57. Blaas, N.; Schüürmann, C.; Bartke, N.; Stahl, B.; Humpf, H.-U. Structural profiling and quantification of sphingomyelin in human breast milk by HPLC-MS/MS. *J. Agric. Food Chem.* **2011**, *59*, 6018–6024. [CrossRef] [PubMed]

58. Neville, M.C.; Picciano, M.F. Regulation of milk lipid secretion and composition. *Ann. Rev. Nutr.* **1997**, *17*, 159–184. [CrossRef] [PubMed]

59. Hytten, F.E. Clinical and chemical studies in human lactation. *Br. Med. J.* **1954**, *1*, 249–255. [CrossRef] [PubMed]

60. Saarela, T.; Kokkonen, J.; Koivisto, M. Macronutrient and energy contents of HM fractions during the first six months of lactation. *Acta Paediatr.* **2005**, *94*, 1176–1181. [CrossRef] [PubMed]

61. Rueda, R. The role of dietary gangliosides on immunity and the prevention of infection. *Brit. J. Nutr.* **2007**, *98*, 68–73. [CrossRef] [PubMed]

62. Wang, B.; McVeagh, P.; Petocz, P.; Brand-Miller, J. Brain gangliosides and glycoprotein sialic acid in breastfed compared with formula-fed infants. *Am. J. Clin. Nutr.* **2003**, *78*, 1024–1029. [PubMed]

63. Ma, L.; MacGibbon, A.K.H.; Mohamed, H.J.B.J.; Loy, S.L.; Rowan, A.; McJarrow, P.; Fong, B.Y. Determination of ganglioside concentrations in breast milk and serum from Malaysian mothers using a high performance liquid chromatography-mass spectrometry-multiple reaction monitoring method. *Intern. Dairy J.* **2015**, *49*, 62–71. [CrossRef]

64. Ma, L.; Liu, X.; MacGibbon, A.K.H.; Loy, S.L.; Rowan, A.; McJarrow, P.; Fong, B.Y. Lactational changes in concentration and distribution of ganglioside molecular species in human breast milk from Chinese mothers. *Lipids* **2015**, *50*, 1145–1154. [CrossRef] [PubMed]

65. Nakano, T.; Sugawara, M.; Kawakami, H. Sialic acid in HM: Composition and functions. *Acta Paediatr. Taiwan* **2001**, *42*, 11–17. [PubMed]

66. Laegreid, A.; Otnaess, A.B.K.; Fuglesang, J. Human and bovine-milk: Comparison of ganglioside composition and enterotoxin-inhibitory activity. *Pediatr. Res.* **1986**, *20*, 416–421. [CrossRef] [PubMed]

67. Mitchell, M.D.; Henare, K.; Balakrishnan, B.; Lowe, E. Transfer of gangliosides across the human placenta. *Placenta* **2012**, *33*, 312–316. [CrossRef] [PubMed]

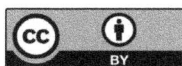

nutrients

MDPI

Article

A Comparison of Nutritional Antioxidant Content in Breast Milk, Donor Milk, and Infant Formulas

Corrine Hanson [1],*, Elizabeth Lyden [2], Jeremy Furtado [3], Matthew Van Ormer [4] and Ann Anderson-Berry [4]

[1]   College of Allied Health Professions, University of Nebraska Medical Center, Medical Nutrition Education, 984045 Nebraska Medical Center, Omaha, NE 68198-4045, USA
[2]   College of Public Health, University of Nebraska Medical Center, 984375 Nebraska Medical Center, Omaha, NE 68198-4375, USA; elyden@unmc.edu
[3]   Department of Nutrition, Harvard School of Public Health, 655 Huntington Avenue, Boston, MA 02215, USA; jfurtado@hsph.harvard.edu
[4]   Pediatrics, University of Nebraska Medical Center, 981205 Nebraska Medical Center, Omaha, NE 68198-1205, USA; Matthew.vanormer@unmc.edu (M.V.O.); alanders@unmc.edu (A.A.-B.)
*   Correspondence: ckhanson@unmc.edu; Tel.: +1-402-559-3658; Fax: +1-402-559-7565

Received: 23 August 2016; Accepted: 24 October 2016; Published: 28 October 2016

Abstract: Human milk is the optimal food for human infants, including infants born prematurely. In the event that a mother of a hospitalized infant cannot provide breast milk, donor milk is considered an acceptable alternative. It is known that the macronutrient composition of donor milk is different than human milk, with variable fat content and protein content. However, much less is known about the micronutrient content of donor milk, including nutritional antioxidants. Samples of breast milk from 12 mothers of infants hospitalized in the Newborn Intensive Care Unit until were collected and analyzed for concentrations of nutritional antioxidants, including α-carotene, β-carotene, β-cryptoxanthin, lycopene, lutein + zeaxanthin, retinol, and α-tocopherol. Additionally, a homogenized sample of donor milk available from a commercial milk bank and samples of infant formulas were also analyzed. Concentrations of nutritional antioxidants were measured using high-performance liquid chromatography. Compared to breast milk collected from mothers of hospitalized infants, commercially available donor milk had 18%–53% of the nutritional antioxidant content of maternal breast milk. As donor milk is becoming a common nutritional intervention for the high risk preterm infant, the nutritional antioxidant status of donor milk–fed premature infants and outcomes related to oxidative stress may merit further investigation.

Keywords: antioxidants; breast milk; infant feeding; infant formula; breast milk substitutes; human milk

1. Introduction

Human milk is the optimal food for infants, including infants born prematurely. In the event that a mother of a hospitalized infant cannot provide breast milk, donor milk is often considered an acceptable or even ideal alternative to the mother's own milk. It is known that the macronutrient composition of donor milk is different from human milk, with variable fat content and protein content lower than that of mature milk [1–4]. However, much less is known about the micronutrient content of donor milk, including nutritional antioxidants.

There is increasing evidence that links early exposure to oxidative stress with potentially lifelong consequences. The premature infant is especially susceptible to damage from oxidative stress for two reasons: (1) adequate concentrations of antioxidants may be absent at birth; (2) the ability to increase synthesis of antioxidants is impaired. This can lead to an increased risk for the development of oxidative stress–induced diseases such as bronchopulmonary dysplasia (BPD), retinopathy of prematurity (ROP), necrotizing enterocolitis (NEC), and periventricular leukomalacia (PVL) [5,6]. Therefore, it is critical in premature infants to ensure an adequate supply of dietary antioxidants. The objective of this analysis was to compare the nutritional antioxidant profile of different types of feedings for premature infants, including samples of maternal breast milk collected during neonatal hospitalization and pasteurized pooled donor milk.

2. Materials and Methods

A total of 12 breast milk samples from women with singleton infants who were admitted to the Neonatal Intensive Care Unit were collected for analysis. These samples were obtained as a subset of subjects ($n = 30$) who were enrolled in a study of nutritional antioxidant status of Newborn Intensive Care Unit (NICU) hospitalized infants who had excess breast milk available after clinical use. Institutional Review Board approval was obtained prior to collection of any samples. The median gestational age was 37.1 weeks, with a range 30.3–42.0 weeks. A 2.0 mL sample was collected from each participant in a sterile plastic tube, protected from heat and light, and stored at $-80\,^\circ$F freezers until they were analyzed. In addition, a single 2 mL aliquot of the commercially available, pooled donor milk sample was collected for analysis, and single 2 mL samples of the commercially available preterm infant formula, transitional infant formula, and term infant formula used in the study unit were collected. All formulas were from a single manufacturer (Abbott Nutrition®). Analysis of samples was performed at the Biomarker Research Institute at the Harvard School of Public Health. Measurements of lutein + zeaxanthin, β-cryptoxanthin, *trans*-lycopene, *cis*-lycopene, total lycopene, α-carotene, *trans*-β-carotene, *cis*-β-carotene, total-β-carotene, retinol, α-tocopherol and γ-tocopherol were obtained. Concentrations in plasma samples were measured as described by El-Sohemy et al [7]. Plasma samples (250 μL) were mixed with 250 mL ethanol containing 10 μg *rac*-tocopherol/mL (Tocol) as an internal standard, extracted with 4 mL hexane, evaporated to dryness under nitrogen, and reconstituted in 100 mL ethanol-dioxane (1:1, by vol) and 150 mL acetonitrile. Samples are quantitated by high-performance liquid chromatography (HPLC) on a Restek Ultra C_{18} 150 mm × 4.6 mm column with a 3 μm particle size encased in a column oven (Hitachi L-2350, Hitachi, San Jose, CA, USA) to prevent temperature fluctuations, and equipped with a trident guard cartridge system (Restek, Corp., Bellefonte, PA, USA). A mixture of acetonitrile, tetrahydrofuran, methanol, and a 1% ammonium acetate solution (68:22:7:3) was used as the mobile phase at a flow rate of 1.1 mL/min, with a Hitachi L-2130 pump in isocratic mode, a Hitachi L-2455 diode array detector (300 nm and 445 nm), and a Hitachi L-2200 auto-sampler with water-chilled tray. The Hitachi System Manager software (D-2000 Elite, Version 3.0) was used for peak integration and data acquisition. Because lutein and zeaxanthin co-elute on the chromatogram, the two are grouped and provided as lutein + zeaxanthin. Internal quality control was monitored with four control samples analyzed within each run. These samples consisted of two identical high-level plasmas and two identical low-level plasmas. Comparison of data from these samples allowed for within-run and between-run variation estimates. In addition, external quality control was monitored by participation in the standardization program for carotenoid analysis from the National Institute of Standards and Technology U.S.A. Descriptive statistics included means and standard deviations. A one sample *t*-test was used to compare the mean value from the 12 maternal breast milk (MBM) to the known value of the donor or infant formulas values $p < 0.05$ was considered statistically significant.

3. Results

The results for the concentrations of α-carotene, total β-carotenes, β-cryptoxanthin, total lycopenes, lutein + zeaxanthin, retinol, α-tocopherol, and γ-tocopherol for each of the feeding types are shown in Table 1.

When the concentrations of carotenoids between the 12 breast milk samples and the pooled donor milk sample were compared, the donor milk sample was descriptively lower in all carotenoids.

A statistically significant difference was found between concentrations of total lycopene ($p = 0.006$). A comparison of levels of carotenoids breast milk vs. donor milk is shown in Figure 1.

Table 1. Nutrition antioxidant content of infant feedings.

Nutritional Antioxidant (µg/L)	Premature Formula	Transitional Formula	Term Standard Formula	Breast Milk Mean (SD) N = 12	Donor Milk
α-carotene	0.51	1.40	0.5	7.7 (14.5)	3.6
β-carotene	71.1	63.9	25.0	49.1 (75.5)	13.7
β-cryptoxanthin	0.9	0.9	0.48	21.7 (40.0)	3.8
Lycopene	1.5	5.8	79.8	66.1 (55.9)	11.9
Lutein + zeaxanthin	65.5	56.9	58.4	40.1 (42.5)	21.4
Retinol	3086.2	911.8	571.2	401.6 (516.3)	185.8
α-tocopherol	20,109.1	13,360.2	8520.0	5880.8 (4971.7)	1381.9
γ-tocopherol	6787.1	6561.6	4204.0	1207.1 (668.4)	622.8

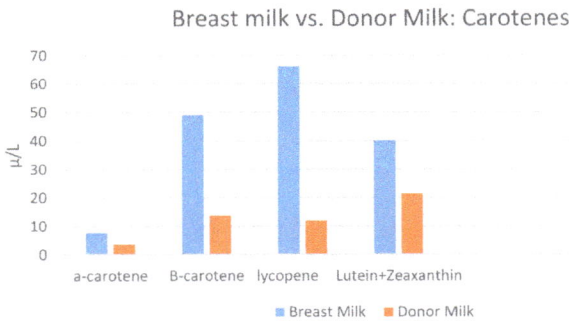

Figure 1. The concentrations of α-carotene, β-carotene, lycopene, and lutein + zeaxanthin in maternal breast milk vs. donor milk samples. Lycopene was statistically significant ($p = 0.006$).

Samples of the transitional formula and premature formula were also significantly lower in lycopene when compared to breast milk ($p = 0.003$ and 0.002, respectively) (see Table 1).

When concentrations of tocopherols between the 12 breast milk samples and the pooled donor milk sample were compared, a statistically significant difference was found between concentrations of both α- and γ-tocopherols ($p = 0.009$ and 0.01, respectively). A comparison of concentrations of tocopherols in breast milk vs. donor milk is shown in Figure 2.

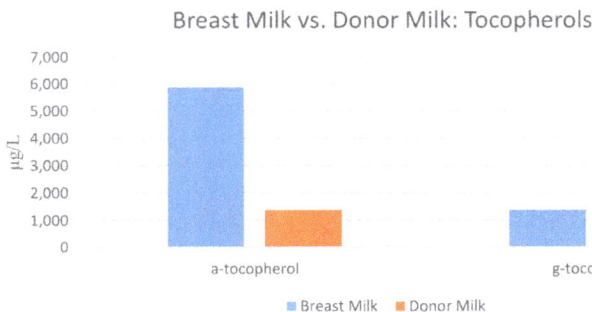

Figure 2. The concentrations of α-tocopherol and γ-tocopherol in maternal breast milk vs. donor milk samples. All values were significantly different ($p = 0.009$ and 0.01 for α-tocopherol and γ-tocopherol, respectively).

Samples of the transitional formula and premature formula were significantly higher in α-tocopherol when compared to breast milk ($p = 0.003$ and 0.002) and all infant formulas were significantly higher in γ-tocopherol when compared to breast milk ($p < 0.0001$ for term, transitional, and premature formulas) (see Table 1).

4. Discussion

Donor milk is considered to be an effective alternative source of nutrition when the mother's own milk is not available, and preterm infants are the primary recipients. Donor milk is obtained from healthy, lactating mothers who consent to donate their surplus which is collected, processed, and stored by specialized centers such as human milk banks. Donor milk is pasteurized to reduce microbial growth and ensure its safety for consumption. The most common pasteurization procedure is Holder pasteurization, in which milk is exposed to a temperature of approximately 62.5 °C (144.5 °F) for at least 30 min [8]. Pasteurization is necessary to inactivate most viral and bacterial compounds, but can affect the nutrition and immunological properties of breast milk. While it has been shown that pasteurized mother's milk retains some of the beneficial and protective effects [1,4,9] there does appear to be an impact on the antioxidant capacity of donor milk [10,11]. Significant decreases in the anti-oxidant compounds malondialdehye and glutathione have been found after pasteurization [12]. The pasteurization of human milk has also been shown to result in significant losses of vitamin D, with reductions of 10%–20% [13].

Preterm infants are born relatively deficient in antioxidant defenses, with increased oxidant stress [5]. Many events, such as infection, mechanical ventilation, intravenous nutrition, and blood transfusions result in oxidative stress. Oxidative stress is associated with serious conditions in the newborn, such as bronchopulmonary dysplasia (BPD), respiratory distress, retinopathy of prematurity (ROP), and necrotizing enterocolitis (NEC), as well as an increased risk of infection [6]. Ensuring adequate nutritional antioxidant status may provide protective benefits to infants at an increased risk of developing these conditions or may positively impact an infant's recovery from these complications.

Studies have shown that there are significant differences in the antioxidant capacity of different types of infant feeding. One study has shown that the total antioxidant capacity in the breast milk of mothers who deliver prematurely is higher than the breast milk of mothers who deliver at term [14], while another study has found them to be equal [15]. However, both have superior antioxidant capacity when compared to formula [15,16]. Breast-fed and formula-fed infants show significant differences in plasma antioxidant nutrient concentrations [17]. The mother's diet also affects the antioxidant capacity of human milk. An increased consumption of dairy products, fruits and vegetables, cereals and nuts has been shown to increase the total antioxidant capacity of the breastmilk [16].

Major nutritional antioxidants include α- and β-carotenes, lutein + zeaxanthin, lycopene, and α-tocopherol. Humans cannot synthesize these compounds and thus they must be provided exogenously through dietary intake. Carotene levels in colostrum have been shown to be five times higher than in mature breast milk [17]. Similarly, breast-fed premature infants have been shown to have higher serum carotenoids than formula-fed premature infants [18]. In one study, carotenoid supplementation was associated with a blunted increase in C-reactive protein (CRP) concentrations from one to 40 weeks post-menstrual age, whereas CRP levels rose in controls [19]. The association of a lower CRP with higher carotenoid consumption likely reflects carotenoid antioxidant and immunomodulatory properties. In populations of children with acute infections, a significant inverse correlation was shown between serum CRP and carotene concentrations [20]. Plasma β-carotene concentrations have indeed been found to be lower in infants with bronchopulmonary dysplasia [21], which may result in a reduction of their antioxidant protection. Our study does report that β-carotene concentrations in donor milk were less than one-third of those in fresh breast milk, and our *p*-value of 0.13, which approaches statistical significance, may be more likely due to the limited power of our study. This may indicate that further investigation into carotenoid anti-inflammatory effects in sick, preterm infants is warranted.

It is thought that lutein + zeaxanthin influence the maturation of cells in the macular region of the retina [22] and protect against stress and oxidation in the retinal pigment epithelium [23]. Vishwanathan et al. determined that the mean concentration of lutein was significantly greater than the other carotenoids in brain tissue samples of infants who died within the first 18 months of life [22]. Preterm infants also had significantly lower concentrations of lutein + zeaxanthin compared to term infants in most of the brain regions [22]. These findings, in addition to previous research, help support the role lutein + zeaxanthin plays in visual and cognitive development. Breast-fed infants have been shown to have higher serum lutein levels than formula-fed infants, possibly due to increased bioavailability of the compound in breast milk, and a dose-dependent relationship exists between lutein in the diet and lutein in the serum [24]. It was calculated that four times more lutein is needed in infant formula than in human milk to achieve similar serum lutein concentrations among breast-fed and formula-fed infants [24]. In a recent pilot randomized controlled trial in healthy newborns, lutein administration proved effective in increasing the levels of biological antioxidant potential by decreasing the total hydroperoxides as markers of oxidative stress [25]. In another study by Mazoni et al., the effect of lutein + zeaxanthin on prevention of BPD appears relevant, although not statistically significant ($p = 0.07$) [26]. Lutein supplementation also has been shown to result in greater rod photoreceptor sensitivity responses when compared to controls [19]. A pilot study showed a potential antioxidant effect of lutein in the neonatal period [25]; however, another study showed that lutein supplementation did not enhance the biological antioxidant capacity [27], although this second study did not achieve a statistically significant difference in the serum lutein concentrations between the placebo and intervention group. A positive association was seen between plasma lutein levels and total antioxidant status ($r = 0.13$, $p = 0.02$) [27]. Our study finds that concentrations of lutein + zeaxanthin were approximately half of the concentrations found in maternal breast milk. Both donor milk and maternal breast milk had lower lutein + zeaxanthin concentrations when compared to the infant formulas tested; however, given the study that demonstrated possible improved bioavailability from breast milk [24], it cannot be assumed that the formula-fed infants would have higher serum concentrations. Additionally, it is important to note that not all formula manufacturers provide supplemental lutein in preterm formula, and therefore infant intake may vary widely based on formula selection.

Vitamin E is an antioxidant that protects cell membranes against free radicals [28]. Although vitamin E deficiency is thought to be rare in healthy adults, it is much more common in premature infants [29]. Vitamin E occurs naturally in several different isoforms, including α- and γ-tocopherol. These isoforms differ by one methyl group and are not interconvertible in human metabolism [30]. As a result, increased intakes of α- or γ-tocopherol will cause a rise in serum concentrations of that specific tocopherol [31,32]. Importantly, serum and tissue levels of vitamin E isoforms correlate [33], meaning the dietary intake of tocopherols has the potential to influence biological mechanisms.

One change in infant nutrition that has occurred in the last several decades is the increase in the γ-tocopherol isoform in the diet of infants. This is primarily due to in the use of soy oils, which are extremely high in γ-tocopherol, as the primary lipid component in infant formulas [34]. While human breast milk has been shown to contain some γ-tocopherol, previous studies have shown the content of γ-tocopherol in infant formula to be up to seven times higher than that in human milk [35]. Our findings concur with this report, demonstrating γ-tocopherol levels in our formula samples to be 3.5–5.6 times higher than in maternal breast milk samples. This level of γ-tocopherol in infant formula does not appear to provide similar protection from lipid peroxidation as human milk [36]. Serum levels of γ-tocopherol in infants have been shown to increase during the first week of life [37], presumably from dietary sources [35]. Recently, our understanding of these tocopherols isoforms has expanded as new evidence indicates that vitamin E isoforms have different roles in influencing inflammation. In contrast to the anti-inflammatory properties of the α-tocopherol isoform, the γ-tocopherol isoform has been shown to increase cytokine production (i.e., IL-2) and demonstrate pro-inflammatory properties [38–42].

Importantly, serum γ-tocopherol isoforms at as little as 10% of the concentration of α-tocopherol have been shown to ablate the anti-inflammatory benefit of alpha-tocopherol [41]. With regard to α-tocopherol, long-term supplementation (six months minimum and up to 24 months) has been shown to positively impact mental development, particularly intelligence quocient (IQ), in school-age children who were extremely low-birth-weight infants (ELBW) [43], raising the possibility that α-tocopherol might be a functional molecule in a developing brain. Although some NICU infants receive donor milk for only a limited amount of time, other institutions use donor milk as a primary source of nutrition throughout NICU hospitalization; our finding that α-tocopherol levels in donor milk samples were significantly decreased when compared to breast milk may make consideration of vitamin E status important in these infants.

Donor milk still has unique advantages compared to formula and continues to represent an important alternative if maternal milk is not available, specifically with regard to necrotizing enterocolitis [44]. In a Cochrane systematic review and meta-analysis, Quigley et al. demonstrated both benefits and risks associated with the use of donor milk. Importantly, there was a higher incidence of NEC among infants with birth weights <2500 g and in those fed formula versus those fed donor milk (relative risk of 2.5 (95% CI, 1.2, 5.1) [44]. Because NEC is the most common gastrointestinal emergency among very-low-birth-weight (VLBW) infants, its prevention is a powerful argument in favor of donor milk as an alternative supplement to formula when the mother's own milk is not available. The Quigley et al. review and meta-analysis, however, concluded that infants fed donor milk experienced slower weight ($p < 0.0001$), length ($p < 0.0003$) and head circumference ($p < 0.0001$) gains than those fed formula [44]. These risks associated with donor milk are of significant concern because VLBW infants are born with impoverished nutrient reserves, and are subject to metabolic stresses that further elevate nutritional requirements [45]. Nutrient deficits and sub-optimal growth have significant long-term neurodevelopmental consequences [46,47]. Quigley et al. point out that all but one of the randomized controlled trials examined in their meta-analysis were >25 years old, when smaller VLBW infants did not survive, and these studies also may not be reflective of current practice [44]. In a more recent study conducted in 2012–2014, The Early Nutrition Study Randomized Clinical Trial found no difference in infections, necrotizing enterocolitis, or mortality during the first 60 days of life in 373 infants fed pasteurized donor milk or preterm formula for supplemental feedings [48]. Another study 2014 of 201 ELBW infants found no difference in NEC or infection rates between infants receiving human milk (including donor milk) and infants receiving formula; however, the duration of mechanical ventilation was significantly higher among formula-fed infants (24 vs. 60 h, $p = 0.016$) in the group exposed to formula [48].

Our analysis has several limitations. First, the antioxidant capacity of breast milk includes many other compounds than the ones highlighted in this study, including uric acid, enzymes, and lipids. However, the antioxidants targeted in this study are modifiable by maternal diet, which may allow for interventions targeted at increasing the antioxidant potential of human milk. Additionally, we did not have the serum levels of donor milk–fed infants to compare to infants receiving maternal breast milk to compare the impact of decreased intake. Additionally, our statistical power was limited by low numbers of analyzed breast milk, a precious commodity to a premature neonate. The median gestational age of 37 weeks in our cohort includes preterm breast milk samples, and the donor milk samples are from a commercial pooled supply. Future studies evaluating the serum nutritional antioxidant status of infants receiving the mother's own milk, donor milk, and infant formulas will expand our knowledge in this area.

5. Conclusions

As donor milk is becoming a common nutritional intervention for the high risk preterm infant, the nutritional antioxidant status of donor milk–fed premature infants and outcomes related to oxidative stress may merit further investigation.

Acknowledgments: This research and publication was supported by a grant from the Department of Pediatrics, University of Nebraska Medical Center.

Author Contributions: C.H., E.L., J.F., M.O. and A.A.B. conceived and designed the experiments, performed the experiments, analyzed the data, and wrote the paper.

Conflicts of Interest: C.H., E.L. and J.F. declare no conflicts of interest. A.A.B. has provided educational lectures on neonatal nutrition for Abbott Nutrition.

References

1. ESPGHAN Committee on Nutrition; Arslanoglu, S.; Corpeleijn, W.; Moro, G.; Braegger, C.; Campoy, C.; Colomb, V.; Decsi, T.; Domellöf, M.; Fewtrell, M.; et al. Donor human milk for preterm infants: Current evidence and research directions. *J. Pediatr. Gastroenterol. Nutr.* **2013**, *57*, 535–542. [CrossRef] [PubMed]

2. Bertino, E.; Giuliani, F.; Baricco, M.; Di Nicola, P.; Peila, C.; Vassia, C.; Chiale, F.; Pirra, A.; Cresi, F.; Martano, C.; et al. Benefits of donor milk in the feeding of preterm infants. *Early Hum. Dev.* **2013**, *89* (Suppl. 2), S3–S6. [CrossRef] [PubMed]

3. Vieira, A.A.; Soares, F.V.; Pimenta, H.P.; Abranches, A.D.; Moreira, M.E. Analysis of the influence of pasteurization, freezing/thawing, and offer processes on human milk's macronutrient concentrations. *Early Hum. Dev.* **2011**, *87*, 577–580. [CrossRef] [PubMed]

4. Bertino, E.; Arslanoglu, S.; Martano, C.; Di Nicola, P.; Giuliani, F.; Peila, C.; Cester, E.; Pirra, A.; Coscia, A.; Moro, G. Biological, nutritional and clinical aspects of feeding preterm infants with human milk. *J. Biol. Regul. Homeost. Agents* **2012**, *26* (Suppl. 3), 9–13. [PubMed]

5. Sandal, G.; Uras, N.; Gokmen, T.; Oguz, S.S.; Erdeve, O.; Dilmen, U. Assessment of oxidant/antioxidant system in newborns and their breast milks. *J. Matern. Fetal Neonatal Med.* **2013**, *26*, 540–543. [CrossRef] [PubMed]

6. Weber, D.; Stuetz, W.; Bernhard, W.; Franz, A.; Raith, M.; Grune, T.; Breusing, N. Oxidative stress markers and micronutrients in maternal and cord blood in relation to neonatal outcome. *Eur. J. Clin. Nutr.* **2014**, *68*, 215–222. [CrossRef] [PubMed]

7. El-Sohemy, A.; Baylin, A.; Kabagambe, E.; Ascherio, A.; Spiegelman, D.; Campos, H. Individual carotenoid concentrations in adipose tissue and plasma as biomarkers of dietary intake. *Am. J. Clin. Nutr.* **2002**, *76*, 172–179. [PubMed]

8. O'Connor, D.L.; Ewaschuk, J.B.; Unger, S. Human milk pasteurization: Benefits and risks. *Curr. Opin. Clin. Nutr. Metab. Care* **2015**, *18*, 269–275. [CrossRef] [PubMed]

9. Peila, C.; Coscia, A.; Bertino, E.; Cavaletto, M.; Spertino, S.; Icardi, S.; Tortone, C.; Visser, G.H.A.; Gazzolo, D. Effects of holder pasteurization on the protein profile of human milk. *Ital. J. Pediatr.* **2016**, *42*. [CrossRef] [PubMed]

10. Ewaschuk, J.B.; Unger, S.; Harvey, S.; O'Connor, D.L.; Field, C.J. Effect of pasteurization on immune components of milk: Implications for feeding preterm infants. *Appl. Physiol. Nutr. Metab.* **2011**, *36*, 175–182. [CrossRef] [PubMed]

11. Ewaschuk, J.B.; Unger, S.; O'Connor, D.L.; Stone, D.; Harvey, S.; Clandinin, M.T.; Field, C.J. Effect of pasteurization on selected immune components of donated human breast milk. *J. Perinatol.* **2011**, *31*, 593–598. [CrossRef] [PubMed]

12. Silvestre, D.; Miranda, M.; Muriach, M.; Almansa, I.; Jareno, E.; Romero, F.J. Antioxidant capacity of human milk: Effect of thermal conditions for the pasteurization. *Acta Paediatr.* **2008**, *97*, 1070–1074. [CrossRef] [PubMed]

13. Gomes, F.P.; Shaw, P.N.; Whitfield, K.; Koorts, P.; McConachy, H.; Hewavitharana, A.K. Effect of pasteurisation on the concentrations of vitamin D compounds in donor breastmilk. *Int. J. Food Sci. Nutr.* **2016**, *67*, 16–19. [CrossRef] [PubMed]

14. Turhan, A.H.; Atici, A.; Muslu, N. Antioxidant capacity of breast milk of mothers who delivered prematurely is higher than that of mothers who delivered at term. *Int. J. Vitam. Nutr. Res.* **2011**, *81*, 368–371. [CrossRef] [PubMed]

15. Friel, J.K.; Martin, S.M.; Langdon, M.; Herzberg, G.R.; Buettner, G.R. Milk from mothers of both premature and full-term infants provides better antioxidant protection than does infant formula. *Pediatr. Res.* **2002**, *51*, 612–618. [CrossRef] [PubMed]

16. Oveisi, M.R.; Sadeghi, N.; Jannat, B.; Hajimahmoodi, M.; Behfar, A.O.; Jannat, F.; MokhtariNasab, F. Human breast milk provides better antioxidant capacity than infant formula. *Iran. J. Pharm. Res.* **2010**, *9*, 445–449. [PubMed]

17. Sommerburg, O.; Meissner, K.; Nelle, M.; Lenhartz, H.; Leichsenring, M. Carotenoid supply in breast-fed and formula-fed neonates. *Eur. J. Pediatr.* **2000**, *159*, 86–90. [CrossRef] [PubMed]

18. Chan, G.M.; Chan, M.M.; Gellermann, W.; Ermakov, I.; Ermakova, M.; Bhosale, P.; Bernstein, P.; Rau, C. Resonance Raman spectroscopy and the preterm infant carotenoid status. *J. Pediatr. Gastroenterol. Nutr.* **2013**, *56*, 556–559. [CrossRef] [PubMed]

19. Rubin, L.P.; Chan, G.M.; Barrett-Reis, B.M.; Fulton, A.B.; Hansen, R.M.; Ashmeade, T.L.; Oliver, J.S.; Mackey, A.D.; Dimmit, R.A.; Hartmann, E.E. Effect of carotenoid supplementation on plasma carotenoids, inflammation and visual development in preterm infants. *J. Perinatol.* **2012**, *32*, 418–424. [CrossRef] [PubMed]

20. Cser, M.A.; Majchrzak, D.; Rust, P.; Rust, P.; Sziklai-Laszlo, I.; Kovacs, I.; Bocskai, E.; Elmadfa, I. Serum carotenoid and retinol levels during childhood infections. *Ann. Nutr. Metab.* **2004**, *48*, 156–162. [CrossRef] [PubMed]

21. Vogelsang, A.; van Lingen, R.A.; Slootstra, J.; Dikkeschei, B.D.; Kollen, B.J.; Schaafsma, A.; van Zoeren-Grobben, D. Antioxidant role of plasma carotenoids in bronchopulmonary dysplasia in preterm infants. *Int. J. Vitam. Nutr. Res.* **2009**, *79*, 288–296. [CrossRef] [PubMed]

22. Vishwanathan, R.; Kuchan, M.J.; Sen, S.; Johnson, E.J. Lutein and preterm infants with decreased concentrations of brain carotenoids. *J. Pediatr. Gastroenterol. Nutr.* **2014**, *59*, 659–665. [CrossRef] [PubMed]

23. Lipkie, T.E.; Morrow, A.L.; Jouni, Z.E.; McMahon, R.J.; Ferruzzi, M.G. Longitudinal survey of carotenoids in human milk from urban cohorts in China, Mexico, and the USA. *PLoS ONE* **2015**, *10*, e0127729. [CrossRef] [PubMed]

24. Bettler, J.; Zimmer, J.P.; Neuringer, M.; DeRusso, P.A. Serum lutein concentrations in healthy term infants fed human milk or infant formula with lutein. *Eur. J. Nutr.* **2010**, *49*, 45–51. [CrossRef] [PubMed]

25. Perrone, S.; Longini, M.; Marzocchi, B.; Picardi, A.; Bellieni, C.V.; Proietti, F.; Rodriguez, A.; Turrisi, G.; Buonocore, G. Effects of lutein on oxidative stress in the term newborn: A pilot study. *Neonatology* **2010**, *97*, 36–40. [CrossRef] [PubMed]

26. Manzoni, P.; Guardione, R.; Bonetti, P.; Priolo, C.; Maestri, A.; Mansoldo, C.; Mostert, M.; Anselmetti, G.; Sardei, D.; Bellettato, M.; et al. Lutein and zeaxanthin supplementation in preterm very-low-birth-weight neonates in neonatal intensive care units: A multicenter randomized controlled trial. *Am. J. Perinatol.* **2013**, *30*, 25–32. [CrossRef] [PubMed]

27. Costa, S.; Giannantonio, C.; Romagnoli, C.; Barone, G.; Gervasoni, J.; Perri, A.; Zecca, E. Lutein and zeaxanthin concentrations in formula and human milk samples from Italian mothers. *Eur. J. Clin. Nutr.* **2015**, *69*, 531–532. [CrossRef] [PubMed]

28. Food and Nutrition Board, Institute of Medicine. *Dietary Reference Intakes for Vitamin C, Vitamin E, Selenium, and Carotenoids*; National Academy Press: Washington, WA, USA, 2000.

29. Tanaka, H.; Mino, M.; Takeuchi, T. A nutritional evaluation of vitamin E status in very low birth weight infants with respect to changes in plasma and red blood cell tocopherol levels. *J. Nutr. Sci. Vitaminol. (Tokyo)* **1988**, *34*, 293–307. [CrossRef] [PubMed]

30. Cook-Mills, J.M. Isoforms of vitamin E differentially regulate PKC and inflammation: A review. *J. Clin. Cell Immunol.* **2013**, *4*. [CrossRef] [PubMed]

31. Wu, D.; Han, S.N.; Meydani, M.; Meydani, S.N. Effect of concomitant consumption of fish oil and vitamin E on T cell mediated function in the elderly: A randomized double-blind trial. *J. Am. Coll. Nutr.* **2006**, *25*, 300–306. [CrossRef] [PubMed]

32. Meydani, M.; Cohn, J.S.; Macauley, J.B.; McNamara, J.R.; Blumberg, J.B.; Schaefer, E.J. Postprandial changes in the plasma concentration of α- and γ-tocopherol in human subjects fed a fat-rich meal supplemented with fat-soluble vitamins. *J. Nutr.* **1989**, *119*, 1252–1258. [PubMed]

33. Redlich, C.A.; Grauer, J.N.; van Bennekum, A.M.; Clever, S.L.; Ponn, R.B.; Blaner, W.S. Characterization of carotenoid, vitamin A, and α-tocopheral levels in human lung tissue and pulmonary macrophages. *Am. J. Respir. Crit. Care Med.* **1996**, *154*, 1436–1443. [CrossRef] [PubMed]

34. Uauy, R.; Hoffman, D.R.; Birch, E.E.; Birch, D.G.; Jameson, D.M.; Tyson, J. Safety and efficacy of omega-3 fatty acids in the nutrition of very low birth weight infants: Soy oil and marine oil supplementation of formula. *J. Pediatr.* **1994**, *124*, 612–620. [CrossRef]

35. Martysiak-Zurowska, D.; Szlagatys-Sidorkiewicz, A.; Zagierski, M. Concentrations of α- and γ-tocopherols in human breast milk during the first months of lactation and in infant formulas. *Matern. Child. Nutr.* **2013**, *9*, 473–482. [CrossRef] [PubMed]

36. Elisia, I.; Kitts, D.D. Differences in vitamin E and C profile between infant formula and human milk and relative susceptibility to lipid oxidation. *Int. J. Vitam. Nutr. Res.* **2013**, *83*, 311–319. [CrossRef] [PubMed]

37. Bell, E.F.; Hansen, N.I.; Brion, L.P.; Ehrenkranz, R.A.; Kennedy, K.A.; Walsh, M.C.; Shankaran, S.; Acarregui, M.J.; Johnson, K.J.; Hale, E.C.; et al. Serum tocopherol levels in very preterm infants after a single dose of vitamin E at birth. *Pediatrics* **2013**, *132*, e1626–e1633. [CrossRef] [PubMed]

38. Cook-Mills, J.M.; Abdala-Valencia, H.; Hartert, T. Two faces of vitamin E in the lung. *Am. J. Respir. Crit. Care Med.* **2013**, *188*, 279–284. [CrossRef] [PubMed]

39. McCary, C.A.; Yoon, Y.; Panagabko, C.; Cho, W.; Atkinson, J.; Cook-Mills, J.M. Vitamin E isoforms directly bind PKCα and differentially regulate activation of PKCα. *Biochem. J.* **2012**, *441*, 189–198. [CrossRef] [PubMed]

40. McCary, C.A.; Abdala-Valencia, H.; Berdnikovs, S.; Cook-Mills, J.M. Supplemental and highly elevated tocopherol doses differentially regulate allergic inflammation: Reversibility of α-tocopherol and γ-tocopherol's effects. *J. Immunol.* **2011**, *186*, 3674–3685. [CrossRef] [PubMed]

41. Berdnikovs, S.; Abdala-Valencia, H.; McCary, C.; McCary, C.; Somand, M.; Cole, R.; Garcia, A.; Bryce, P.; Cook-Mills, J.M. Isoforms of vitamin E have opposing immunoregulatory functions during inflammation by regulating leukocyte recruitment. *J. Immunol.* **2009**, *182*, 4395–4405. [CrossRef] [PubMed]

42. Abdala-Valencia, H.; Berdnikovs, S.; Cook-Mills, J.M. Vitamin E isoforms as modulators of lung inflammation. *Nutrients.* **2013**, *5*, 4347–4363. [CrossRef] [PubMed]

43. Kitajima, H.; Kanazawa, T.; Mori, R.; Hirano, S.; Ogihara, T.; Fujimura, M. Long-term α-tocopherol supplements may improve mental development in extremely low birthweight infants. *Acta Paediatr.* **2015**, *104*, e82–e89. [CrossRef] [PubMed]

44. Quigley, M.; McGuire, W. Formula versus donor breast milk for feeding preterm or low birth weight infants. *Cochrane Database Syst. Rev.* **2014**. [CrossRef]

45. Stoll, B.J.; Hansen, N.I.; Bell, E.F.; Shankaran, S.; Laptook, A.R.; Walsh, M.C.; Hale, E.C.; Newman, N.S.; Schibler, K.; Carlo, W.A.; et al. Neonatal outcomes of extremely preterm infants from the NICHD neonatal research network. *Pediatrics* **2010**, *126*, 443–456. [CrossRef] [PubMed]

46. Ehrenkranz, R.A.; Dusick, A.M.; Vohr, B.R.; Wright, L.L.; Wrage, L.A.; Poole, W.K. Growth in the neonatal intensive care unit influences neurodevelopmental and growth outcomes of extremely low birth weight infants. *Pediatrics* **2006**, *117*, 1253–1261. [CrossRef] [PubMed]

47. Corpeleijn, W.E.; de Waard, M.; Christmann, V.; van Goudoever, J.B.; der Jansen-van Weide, M.C.; Kooi, E.M.; Koper, J.F.; Kouwenhoven, S.M.; Lafeber, H.N.; Mank, E.; et al. Effect of donor milk on severe infections and mortality in very low-birth-weight infants: The Early Nutrition Study randomized clinical trial. *JAMA Pediatr.* **2016**, *170*, 654–661. [CrossRef] [PubMed]

48. Verd, S.; Porta, R.; Botet, F.; Gutierrez, A.; Ginovart, G.; Barbero, A.H.; Ciurana, A.; Plata, I.I. Hospital outcomes of extremely low birth weight infants after introduction of donor milk to supplement mother's milk. *Breastfeed Med.* **2015**, *10*, 150–155. [CrossRef] [PubMed]

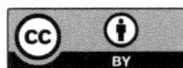

nutrients

MDPI

Article

Assessment of Breast Milk Iodine Concentrations in Lactating Women in Western Australia

Anita Jorgensen [1,*], Peter O'Leary [2], Ian James [3], Sheila Skeaff [4] and Jillian Sherriff [1]

1   School of Public Health, Curtin University, Perth 6102, Australia; j.sherriff@curtin.edu.au
2   Faculty of Health Sciences, Curtin University, Perth 6102, Australia; peter.oleary@curtin.edu.au
3   Institute for Immunology & Infectious Diseases, Murdoch University, Murdoch 6150, Australia; i.james@murdoch.edu.au
4   Department of Human Nutrition, University of Otago, Dunedin 9054, New Zealand; sheila.skeaff@otago.ac.nz
*   Correspondence: a.jorgensen@curtin.edu.au; Tel.: +61-8-9266-1083

Received: 30 September 2016; Accepted: 1 November 2016; Published: 4 November 2016

Abstract: Breast-fed infants may depend solely on an adequate supply of iodine in breast milk for the synthesis of thyroid hormones which are essential for optimal growth and cognitive development. This is the first study to measure breast milk iodine concentration (BMIC) among lactating women in Western Australian ($n = 55$). Breast milk samples were collected between 2014 and 2015 at a mean ($\pm$SD) of 38.5 ($\pm$5.5) days post-partum. The samples were analysed to determine median BMIC and the percentage of samples with a BMIC < 100 µg/L, a level considered adequate for breast-fed infants. The influence of (a) iodine-containing supplements and iodised salt use and (b) consumption of key iodine-containing foods on BMIC was also examined. The median (p25, p75) BMIC was 167 (99, 248) µg/L and 26% of samples had a BMIC < 100 µg/L. Overall, BMIC tended to be higher with iodine-containing supplement usage (ratio 1.33, 95% confidence interval (CI) (1.04, 1.70), $p = 0.030$), cow's milk consumption (ratio 1.66, 95% CI (1.23, 2.23), $p = 0.002$) and lower for Caucasians (ratio 0.61, 95% CI (0.45, 0.83), $p = 0.002$), and those with secondary school only education (ratio 0.66, 95% CI (0.46, 0.96), $p = 0.030$). For most women, BMIC was adequate to meet the iodine requirements of their breast-fed infants. However, some women may require the use of iodine-containing supplements or iodised salt to increase BMIC to adequate levels for optimal infant nutrition.

Keywords: iodine; breast milk; supplementation; iodine status

1. Introduction

Iodine, an essential nutrient, is required by humans for the synthesis of thyroid hormones which are vital for normal growth and development [1,2]. A regular and adequate supply of iodine is particularly important during the critical period for brain and central nervous system development, namely, from the second trimester of pregnancy to 3 years of age [1]. Iodine deficiency during this time results in a spectrum of adverse effects known as iodine deficiency disorders, with the most severe outcomes, irreversible mental impairment and cretinism, resulting from severe iodine deficiency during pregnancy. In infants, iodine deficiency leading to inadequate thyroid activity results in delayed growth and physical development, and impaired cognitive function [1,2].

During intrauterine life, iodine is transferred from the mother to the fetus [3]. This results in a pool of iodine stored in the fetal thyroid gland, with the size of the pool strongly reflecting maternal dietary iodine intake. However, even under conditions of maternal iodine sufficiency, this fetal iodine pool is small and turns over rapidly after birth to partly support the iodine demand of newborns [4]. Infants, however, rely solely on dietary sources to meet their iodine needs. Breast-fed infants are particularly vulnerable to iodine deficiency as they may be completely dependent on the iodine concentration of breast milk for their intake of iodine [5]. Consequently, maternal iodine requirements are increased during breastfeeding to provide sufficient amounts for the mother and to also meet the iodine demands of the developing infant, via breast milk. Given that 40%–45% of the iodine ingested by the mother appears in breast milk [6], a maternal iodine intake during breastfeeding of 190 µg/day (Australian Estimated Average Requirement (EAR)) would provide just under the Australian Adequate Intake (AI) of 90 µg/day for infants aged 0–6 months [7]. This is achieved by a physiological response during breastfeeding whereby iodine is strongly concentrated by the lactating mammary gland due to the increased expression of the sodium iodide symporter, the main iodine transporter in lactating breast cells [8]. This results in human milk having an iodine concentration 20–50 times higher than that of plasma [4].

Breast milk iodine concentration (BMIC) is influenced by, and may be an indicator of, maternal iodine status during breastfeeding [4,5,8–11]. BMIC is also influenced by other factors including recent maternal iodine intake [12] and duration of lactation [5]. While no reference ranges for the adequate iodine concentration of breast milk have been specified, values above 75 µg/L have been suggested to indicate sufficient maternal iodine intake [4]. An iodine balance study of full-term infants found that a positive iodine balance is only achieved when iodine intake is 15 µg/kg per day, which equates to a BMIC of 100–200 µg/L [8].

A wide range of median or mean BMIC values has been reported in several reviews conducted in areas of varying iodine sufficiency [4,8,10]. BMIC typically ranges from <50 µg/L in iodine-deficient areas [5] to 100–150 µg/L in areas of iodine sufficiency [4] and as high as 150–180 µg/L in areas of good iodine supply [8,10]. A BMIC < 100 µg/L has been identified in studies from France, Germany, Belgium, Sweden, Spain, Italy, Denmark, Thailand and Zaire while studies from Iran, China, USA and some parts of Europe have identified above this level [4]. A recent study in Nepal identified a median BMIC of 250 µg/L, and the estimated iodine intake of the infants involved (0–6 months) was 200 µg/day [13]. WHO's recommended maximum iodine intake for infants <2 years old is 180 µg/day [14], therefore some infants in this area may be consuming excessive iodine intakes through breast milk [13]. This can result in subclinical hypothyroidism and permanently affect their neurodevelopment [15].

In recent decades, Australia has been regarded as a country with mild iodine deficiency. Two initiatives introduced in response to the re-emergence of this public health issue are the mandatory fortification of all bread (except organic) with iodised salt in 2009 [16] and the 2010 National Health and Medical Research Council recommendation that all pregnant and breastfeeding women take a daily supplement containing 150 µg of iodine [17]. Despite this recommendation, only two studies have examined the iodine content of breast milk in Australia to assess either iodine provision to breastfed infants or maternal iodine status. The first was a small (*n* = 50) cross-sectional study of breastfeeding women in Sydney, conducted more than a decade ago and prior to mandatory iodine fortification. This study identified a median BMIC of 84 µg/L [18], indicating inadequate maternal iodine intake based on the adequate cut-off of 100 µg/L. The second larger and more recent study compared the BMIC of lactating women in South Australia pre- (*n* = 291) and post- (*n* = 653) mandatory fortification. The median BMIC of samples from both periods were indicative of adequate breast milk iodine levels, however, BMIC was significantly higher in the post-fortification samples compared with the pre-fortification samples (187 vs. 103 µg/L; *p* < 0.05) [19].

To date, there is no information regarding BMIC for lactating mothers in Western Australia (WA), nor for iodine status of WA breastfeeding women. WA has long been considered an iodine-sufficient area of Australia, based on measures of iodine status in studies involving school-children and adults [20,21]. However, this outcome may not reflect the iodine status in breastfeeding women, who have substantially greater requirements for iodine [1]. In the present study we examined BMIC in breastfeeding women in a local cohort to determine adequacy of iodine provision to breastfed infants. We also investigated the influence of iodine-containing supplements and iodised salt use, as well as the consumption of key iodine-containing foods, on this biomarker of iodine status.

2. Materials and Methods

2.1. Subjects and Design

Participants were recruited in 2013–2014 as part of the Perth Iodine and Pregnancy Study II (PIPS II) via advertising (flyer in private women's ultrasound practices $n = 15$ and newspaper, radio and websites $n = 7$), in-person by study coordinator (public maternity hospital antenatal clinics $n = 21$ and pathology centre $n = 3$) and word of mouth ($n = 8$). At the time of recruitment, women were aged 18 years and over and were in the first or second trimester of pregnancy (gestation range 5–22 weeks). Other inclusion criteria were no history of thyroid disease, not currently taking thyroid medication, having a singleton birth and not currently breastfeeding but with the intention to breastfeed their baby. Women were excluded from the study if English was not the main language spoken at home. The study was approved by the Curtin University (Approval No. HR 47/2013; 15 April 2013) and Women and Newborn Health Service Human Research Ethics Committees (Approval No. 2014075EW; 4 August 2014) and informed written consent was obtained from each participant.

Breast milk samples were collected between February 2014 and August 2015. Participants were mailed vials for sampling together with instructions to provide (duplicate) 5 mL nonfasted breast milk samples at home at the start of a single morning feed (preferably between 0900 and 1200 h) when their baby was aged 4–6 weeks. Women were asked to record baby's age and time of day of sampling. Participants were also asked to provide information on current medication use, daily use of dietary supplements, daily intake (yes/no) of any amount of six key iodine-containing foods (cow's milk, cheese, ice cream, yoghurt, bread/bread products, eggs), use of iodised salt (yes/no) and whether or not they smoke cigarettes. Sociodemographic characteristics of the women, namely parity, age, postcode, ethnicity, household income and education, had been collected previously.

2.2. Laboratory Procedures

Breast milk samples were stored at -20 °C from time of sampling until collection and then at -80 °C until analysis. After thawing, milk samples were homogenized before analysis by inductively coupled plasma mass spectrometry (ICPMS) in an accredited commercial laboratory (PathWest Laboratory Medicine WA, Nedlands, Australia). ICPMS is considered the gold standard to determine iodine concentration in complex sample matrices such as breast milk [9,22]. An optimised ICPMS method for breast milk has been published recently [22] and was adapted for this study. In brief, sonicated breast milk samples were diluted in mild alkali solution, ionized with inductively coupled plasma and the ions separated and quantified in a Perkin Elmer NexION 300 ICP-MS mass spectrometer (PerkinElmer Inc., Waltham, MA, USA).

2.3. Statistical Analysis

Distributions of BMIC were skewed and descriptive statistics reported as medians and 25th, 75th percentile. The proportion of women with BMIC < 100 µg/L, the suggested cut-off for providing an adequate iodine supply to breast-fed infants, was also determined. Statistical analyses of BMIC were carried out on the log base 10 scale to better approximate normality. Multiple regression analyses were used to assess associations of BMIC with: (a) use of iodine supplements and iodised salt; (b) daily consumption of six key iodine-containing foods (yes/no); and (c) all studied factors simultaneously. Associations of cohort characteristics with use of iodised salt or iodine supplements were assessed via logistic regressions. Data were analysed using IBM SPSS version 20 (IBM Corporation, Tokyo, Japan) and TIBCO Spotfire S+ version 8.2 (TIBCO Software Inc., Boston, MA, USA). A 5% level of significance was chosen.

3. Results

Sociodemographic characteristics of the 55 study participants are shown in Table 1. The mean age (±standard deviation (SD)) of the study women was 31.4 (±4.7) years. This is consistent with the average age of women who gave birth in WA in 2013 of 29.8 years [23]. The majority of women were pregnant for the first time (52.7%), were tertiary educated (72.3%), had a total household income of >$AUS100K (67.3%) and were Caucasian (80.0%). Compared with available Western Australian data from the Australian Bureau of Statistics Census 2011, our cohort included an over representation of women with a higher reported education level and higher household incomes [24]. All women provided breast milk samples, however one woman was excluded as she reported being a smoker, thus leaving 54 women for breast milk analysis. Breast milk samples were collected at 28–56 days postpartum with a mean (±SD) of 38.5 (±5.5) days. All samples were provided in the morning between 0600 h and 1200 h. The median (p25, p75) BMIC was 167 (99, 248) μg/L indicating adequate maternal iodine intake for the group. However, 26% of women had BMIC less than the suggested cut-off level for adequacy of 100 μg/L (see Figure 1).

Table 1. Sociodemographic characteristics of study participants (*n* = 55).

	n	%
First pregnancy		
Yes	29	52.7
No	26	47.3
Highest education [1]		
Secondary school	7	12.7
Trade or technical	3	5.5
Diploma	5	9.1
Professional	2	3.6
Bachelor degree	22	40.0
Postgraduate university	16	29.1
Total household income		
<$AUS50K	8	14.5
$AUS50–100K	8	14.5
>$AUS100K	37	67.3
Don't wish to answer	2	3.6
Ethnicity		
Caucasian	44	80.0
Non-Caucasian	11	20.0

[1] Tertiary educated includes Professional, Bachelor degree and Postgraduate university.

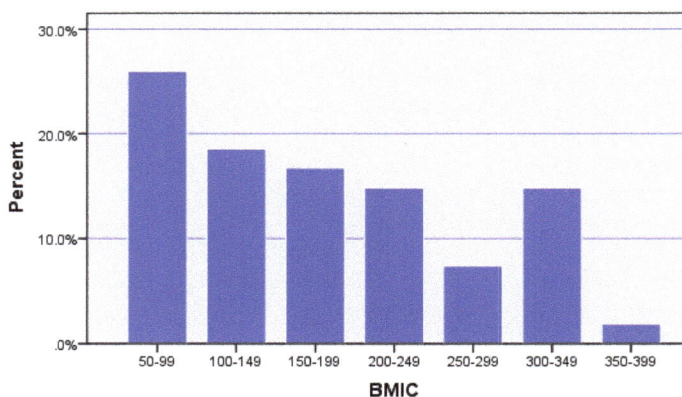

Figure 1. Percentage distribution of breast milk iodine concentration (BMIC) (μg/L).

Thirty-one women (57.4%) reported the daily use of an iodine-containing supplement, some of which contained less than the amount recommended (i.e., 150 µg). Use of iodised salt and iodine-containing supplements were independently associated with increases of similar magnitudes in BMIC (ratio 1.37, 95% CI (1.05, 1.80), p = 0.025 and ratio 1.37, 95% CI (1.04, 1.79), p = 0.029, respectively—see Table 2). There was no significant difference (p = 0.96) between the median BMIC values for the use of either iodised salt or iodine-containing supplements without the other. Among all cohort characteristics jointly considered only low household income (<$AUS50K) remained significantly (negatively) associated with iodine supplement usage (1/8 vs. 30/46, p = 0.010 Fisher test). Exactly half of the women reported using iodised salt, with usage higher among non-Caucasians (10/11 vs. 17/43, p = 0.005).

Table 2. Effect of iodine supplement and iodised salt use on BMIC.

	n	Median BMIC (µg/L)
Yes supplement + Yes salt	15	272 **
Yes supplement + No salt	16	151 *
No supplement + Yes salt	12	156 *
No supplement + No salt	11	98 **

Overall p = 0.028; * There was no difference between the 'Yes supplement + No salt' and 'No Supplement + Yes salt' groups (p = 0.960); ** There was a significant difference between the 'Yes supplement + Yes salt' and 'No supplement + No salt' groups (p = 0.003).

For the six key iodine-containing foods, the majority of women reported daily consumption of bread/bread products (79.6%) and cow's milk (77.8%) and with just less than half of women (46.3%) reporting daily intake of cheese. Furthermore, about a third of women (37.0%) reported daily consumption of yoghurt, around a quarter (27.8%) ate eggs daily and 5.6% of women said they ate ice cream each day. However, only daily cow's milk intake was significantly associated with higher BMIC values after adjusting for the other foods or on its own (ratio 1.44, 95% CI (1.01, 2.06), p = 0.49 and ratio 1.44, 95% CI (1.03, 2.01), p = 0.040, respectively). None of the other foods were significant, jointly or marginally, in influencing BMIC values. Furthermore, cow's milk remained the only food positively associated with BMIC after adjustment for iodine-containing supplements and iodised salt use (ratio 1.50, 95% CI (1.10, 2.04), p = 0.013). Overall in the joint model, BMIC tended to be higher with iodine-containing supplement usage and cow's milk consumption and lower for Caucasians and those with secondary school only education (see Table 3).

Table 3. Significant joint explanatory variables for BMIC *.

Variable	Ratio ** (95% CI)	p-Value
Caucasian ethnicity	0.61 (0.45, 0.83)	0.002
School only education	0.66 (0.46, 0.96)	0.030
Iodine supplement use	1.33 (1.04, 1.70)	0.030
Cow's milk consumption	1.66 (1.23, 2.23)	0.002

* Analyses carried out on the log BMIC scale with non-significant terms (sociodemographic and dietary factors) removed by backwards elimination; ** Exponentiated coefficient from the joint model for log (BMIC) predicts the ratio of BMIC for the listed category relative to those not in the category, given fixed values of the other variables.

4. Discussion

This is the first study to report BMIC values for breastfeeding women in Western Australia. The median BMIC value of women would provide an adequate iodine supply for breastfed infants. However, BMIC levels were below the suggested adequate cut-off (100 µg/L) for 26% of women, indicating some infants may be at risk for iodine deficiency, especially if exclusively breast-fed as is recommended. These findings are consistent with results for the post-fortification cohort of the recent South Australian study. However, compared to our study, the proportion of women with BMIC below the adequate cut-off level was considerably lower in the study by Huynh et al. (26% vs. 13%) [19]. The one participant who reported being a smoker in the present study was excluded from breast milk analysis as the chemical thiocyanate found in cigarettes competitively inhibits the sodium iodide transporter in the lactating breast and impairs iodine transport into breast milk [25], thereby distorting BMIC values.

Despite the NHMRC recommendation for all breastfeeding women to use a daily 150 µg iodine supplement, only about half of the women (54%) in the present study reported behaviour consistent with this (an additional two women reported use of a daily iodine supplement containing less than the recommended iodine amount). In a recent study of breastfeeding women conducted in regional New South Wales (n = 60), iodine-containing supplements were being taken by 45% of women, although frequency of use and iodine content were not documented [26]. These results suggest a low level of awareness and/or compliance amongst Australian breastfeeding women regarding the national iodine supplement recommendations. In contrast, 90% of South Australian women in the post-fortification cohort reported use of supplements containing any iodine [19], although again details of frequency of use and iodine content were not documented. Furthermore, given the low use of iodine-containing supplements in low income cases compared to higher income participants (12.5% vs. 65.2%, respectively) in the present study, perhaps the availability of government subsidized iodine supplements is warranted in Australia, as is the case in New Zealand. Interestingly, in the Perth Infant Feeding Study Mark II conducted in 2002–2003 prior to the supplement recommendation, no breastfeeding women reported taking iodine supplements [27].

In addition, 50% of women in the present study reported using iodised salt. This is similar to the 45% of lactating women using iodised salt in the regional New South Wales study by Charlton et al. [26]. In the present study, use of iodised salt was significantly higher among non-Caucasians (p = 0.013), possibly explaining why BMIC tended to be higher in non-Caucasian mothers compared with Caucasian mothers (p = 0.002). This later finding is consistent with the results of the South Australian study by Huynh et al. [19].

As shown in Table 2, use of both iodine-containing supplements and iodised salt together resulted in the highest median BMIC value (272 µg/L). The use of either iodine-containing supplements or iodised salt had similar positive effects on median BMIC values, suggesting both methods are equally effective in improving the iodine content of breast milk. Our results are consistent with other recent studies that have examined the effect of supplementation and/or iodised salt use on breast milk iodine content [28,29]. The lowest median BMIC was recorded for those women using neither iodine-containing supplements nor iodised salt. This median BMIC value of 98 µg/L is borderline for inadequate BMIC using the cut-off of 100 µg/L. This suggests that for women in our study, food sources alone may not provide the amounts of iodine required during breastfeeding to meet maternal and infant needs. Furthermore, given breast milk samples in the present study were provided in the early post-partum period and BMIC of iodine-deficient lactating women has been shown to decrease in the first 6 months postpartum [5], the use of some form of iodine supplementation by these women is important.

Of the six key iodine-containing foods examined in the study, only daily cow's milk consumption was significantly associated with higher BMIC values, independent of other foods and supplement and iodised salt use. Some cow's milk was consumed daily by more than three-quarters of women in the study. Despite quantity not being examined in the present study, this suggests the importance of cow's milk consumption in terms of iodine intake for breastfeeding women. Interestingly, milk and dairy foods were the highest contributors to iodine intake in the study by Charlton et al. which used a self-administered validated iodine-specific food frequency questionnaire to assess dietary iodine intake of Australian breastfeeding women [26]. Conversely, daily consumption of bread/bread products was not associated with higher BMIC values, despite the fact that a very high proportion of women reported consumption of these foods daily and their known fortification with iodine. This finding therefore questions the impact of the bread fortification initiative for lactating women in relation to BMIC.

There are some limitations to the interpretation of our study findings. Firstly, the impact of time of supplement intake, iodised salt use and consumption of key iodine-containing foods relative to breast milk sampling were not examined. Leung et al. [12] reported a rise in BMIC following acute oral ingestion of 600 µg potassium iodide, with peak levels at 6 h post-ingestion, and concluded that recent maternal iodine intake would influence the interpretation of BMIC values. Furthermore, as BMIC values fluctuate throughout the day, single breast milk samples provide an imprecise measurement of daily iodine output or maternal iodine sufficiency [30]. In addition, actual compliance with reported supplement use, use of iodised salt or intake of foods examined in the 24-h prior to breast milk sampling could not be confirmed with participants. Finally, while the study included a cross-section of breastfeeding women from both public and private health care systems, the sample size is relatively small and all women who participated (bar one) lived in the Perth metropolitan area, so generalisability of results to the wider breastfeeding population is made with qualifications.

5. Conclusions

Despite these limitations, for the majority of women in the present study, BMIC was adequate to meet the iodine requirement of their breast-fed infants. However, the study also indicates that some breast-fed infants may be at risk of iodine deficiency, which could potentially be reduced by the maternal use of iodine-containing supplements and/or iodised salt. Further studies of women representing the social and regional diversity of the population will be needed to confirm our findings.

Acknowledgments: The authors sincerely thank the women who participated in the study, staff at recruitment sites for their cooperation and staff at PathWest Laboratory Medicine WA for their assistance with sample analysis.

Author Contributions: J.S., S.S. and P.O.L. conceived, designed and supervised the study; A.J. performed the data collection; I.J. and A.J. analysed and interpreted the data; A.J. wrote the first draft of the manuscript; J.S., S.S. and P.O.L. edited the manuscript. All authors reviewed and approved the manuscript submitted.

Conflicts of Interest: The authors declare no conflict of interest.

References

1. World Health Organisation; United Nations International Children's Emergency Fund; International Council for Control of Iodine Deficiency Disorders. *Assessment of Iodine Deficiency Disorders and Monitoring Their Elimination, a Guide for Programme Managers*; World Health Organisation Press: Geneva, Swizerland, 2007.
2. Zimmermann, M.B.; Jooste, P.L.; Pandav, C.S. Iodine-deficiency disorders. *Lancet* **2008**, *372*, 1251–1262. [CrossRef]
3. Delange, F. Optimal iodine nutrition during pregnancy, lactation and the neonatal period. *Int. J. Endocrinol. Metab.* **2004**, *2*, 1–12.
4. Azizi, F.; Smyth, P. Breastfeeding and maternal and infant iodine nutrition. *Clin. Endocrinol.* **2009**, *70*, 803–809. [CrossRef] [PubMed]
5. Mulrine, H.M.; Skeaff, S.A.; Ferguson, E.L.; Gray, A.R.; Valeix, P. Breast-milk iodine concentration declines over the first 6 mo postpartum in iodine-deficient women. *Am. J. Clin. Nutr.* **2010**, *92*, 849–856. [CrossRef] [PubMed]
6. Laurberg, P.; Andersen, S.L. Nutrition: Breast milk—A gateway to iodine-dependent brain development. *Nat. Rev. Endocrinol.* **2014**, *10*, 134–135. [CrossRef] [PubMed]
7. National Health and Medical Research Council (NHMRC); New Zealand Ministry of Health. *Nutrient Reference Values for Australia and New Zealand Including Recommended Dietary Intakes*; Commonwealth of Australia: Canberra, Australia, 2006.
8. Semba, R.D.; Delange, F. Iodine in human milk: Perspectives for infant health. *Nutr. Rev.* **2001**, *59*, 269–278. [CrossRef] [PubMed]

9. Dold, S.; Baumgartner, J.; Zeder, C.; Krzystek, A.; Osei, J.; Haldimann, M.; Zimmermann, M.B.; Andersson, M. Optimization of a new mass spectrometry method for measurement of breast milk iodine concentrations and an assessment of the effect of analytic method and timing of within-feed sample collection on breast milk iodine concentrations. *Thyroid* **2016**, *26*, 287–295. [CrossRef] [PubMed]

10. Dorea, J.G. Iodine nutrition and breast feeding. *J. Trace Elem. Med. Biol.* **2002**, *16*, 207–220. [CrossRef]

11. Zimmermann, M. Iodine deficiency. *Endocr. Rev.* **2009**, *30*, 376–408. [CrossRef] [PubMed]

12. Leung, A.M.; Braverman, L.E.; He, X.; Heeren, T.; Pearce, E.N. Breastmilk iodine concentrations following acute dietary iodine intake. *Thyroid* **2012**, *22*, 1176–1180. [CrossRef] [PubMed]

13. Henjum, S.; Kjellevold, M.; Ulak, M.; Chandyo, R.; Shrestha, P.; Frøyland, L.; Strydom, E.; Dhansay, M.; Strand, T. Iodine concentration in breastmilk and urine among lactating women of Bhaktapur, Nepal. *Nutrients* **2016**, *8*, 255. [CrossRef] [PubMed]

14. Andersson, M.; de Benoist, B.; Delange, F.; Zupan, J. Prevention and control of iodine deficiency in pregnant and lactating women and in children less than 2-years-old: Conclusions and recommendations of the technical consultation. *Public Health Nutr.* **2007**, *10*, 1606–1611. [PubMed]

15. Zimmermann, M.B. The role of iodine in human growth and development. *Semin. Cell Dev. Biol.* **2011**, *22*, 645–652. [CrossRef] [PubMed]

16. Food Standards Australia New Zealand. *Proposal p1003—Mandatory Iodine Fortification for Australia—Approval Report*; Food Standards Australia New Zealand (FSANZ): Canberra, Australia, 2008.

17. National Health and Medical Research Council. *NHMRC Public Statement: Iodine Supplementation for Pregnant and Breastfeeding Women*; National Health and Medical Research Council: Canberra, Australia, 2010.

18. Chan, S.S.Y.; Hams, G.; Wiley, V.; Wilcken, B.; McElduff, A. Postpartum maternal iodine status and the relationship to neonatal thyroid function. *Thyroid* **2003**, *13*, 873–876. [CrossRef] [PubMed]

19. Huynh, D.; Condo, D.; Gibson, R.; Makrides, M.; Muhlhausler, B.; Zhou, S.J. Comparison of breast-milk iodine concentration of lactating women in Australia pre and post mandatory iodine fortification. *Public Health Nutr.* **2016**. [CrossRef] [PubMed]

20. Li, M.; Ma, G.; Boyages, S.C.; Eastman, C.J. Re-emergence of iodine deficiency in australia. *Asia Pac. J. Clin. Nutr.* **2001**, *10*, 200–203. [CrossRef] [PubMed]

21. Australian Bureau of Statistics. *Australian Health Survey: Biomedical Results for Nutrients, 2011–2012. Feature Article: Iodine*; Australian Bureau of Statistics: Canberra, Australia, 2013.

22. Huynh, D.; Zhou, S.J.; Gibson, R.; Palmer, L.; Muhlhausler, B. Validation of an optimized method for the determination of iodine in human breast milk by inductively coupled plasma mass spectrometry (ICPMS) after tetramethylammonium hydroxide extraction. *J. Trace Elem. Med. Biol.* **2015**, *29*, 75–82. [CrossRef] [PubMed]

23. Hutchinson, M.; Joyce, A. *Western Australia's Mother's and Babies, 2013: 31st Annual Report of the Western Australian Midwives' Notification System*; Department of Health, Western Australia: Perth, Australia, 2016.

24. Australian Bureau of Statistics. *Census of Population and Housing: Community Profile Western Australia*; Australian Bureau of Statistics: Canberra, Australia, 2011.

25. Laurberg, P.; Nøhr, S.B.; Pedersen, K.M.; Fuglsang, E. Iodine nutrition in breast-fed infants is impaired by maternal smoking. *J. Clin. Endocrinol. Metab.* **2004**, *89*, 181–187. [CrossRef] [PubMed]

26. Charlton, K.; Yeatman, H.; Lucas, C.; Axford, S.; Gemming, L.; Houweling, F.; Goodfellow, A.; Ma, G. Poor knowledge and practices related to iodine nutrition during pregnancy and lactation in Australian women: Pre- and post-iodine fortification. *Nutrients* **2012**, *4*, 1317–1327. [CrossRef] [PubMed]

27. Kyung Lee, M.; Binns, C.; Zhao, Y.; Scott, J.; Oddy, W. Nutritional supplements during breastfeeding. *Curr. Pediatr. Rev.* **2012**, *8*, 292–298. [CrossRef]

28. Andersen, S.L.; Møller, M.; Laurberg, P. Iodine concentrations in milk and in urine during breastfeeding are differently affected by maternal fluid intake. *Thyroid* **2013**, *24*, 764–772. [CrossRef] [PubMed]

29. Brough, L.; Jin, Y.; Shukri, N.H.; Wharemate, Z.R.; Weber, J.L.; Coad, J. Iodine intake and status during pregnancy and lactation before and after government initiatives to improve iodine status, in Palmerston North, New Zealand: A pilot study. *Matern. Child Nutr.* **2013**, *11*, 646–655. [CrossRef] [PubMed]

30. Kirk, A.B.; Kroll, M.; Dyke, J.V.; Ohira, S.I.; Dias, R.A.; Dasgupta, P.K. Perchlorate, iodine supplements, iodized salt and breast milk iodine content. *Sci. Total Environ.* **2012**, *420*, 73–78. [CrossRef] [PubMed]

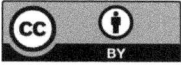

nutrients

MDPI

Article

Colostrum and Mature Human Milk of Women from London, Moscow, and Verona: Determinants of Immune Composition

Daniel Munblit [1,2,3,*], Marina Treneva [2,4], Diego G. Peroni [2,5], Silvia Colicino [6], LiYan Chow [1], Shobana Dissanayeke [7], Priya Abrol [1], Shreya Sheth [1], Alexander Pampura [2,4], Attilio L. Boner [8], Donna T. Geddes [2,9], Robert J. Boyle [1,2,†] and John O. Warner [1,2,†]

[1] Department of Paediatrics, Imperial College London, London W2 1NY, UK; lychow8@gmail.com (L.C.); p.abrol@doctors.org.uk (P.A.); shreya.sheth10@imperial.ac.uk (S.S.); r.boyle@nhs.net (R.J.B.); j.o.warner@imperial.ac.uk (J.O.W.)

[2] International Inflammation (in-FLAME) Network of the World Universities Network, Sydney 2006, NSW, Australia; trenevamarina@mail.ru (M.T.); diego.peroni@unipi.it (D.G.P.); apampura1@mail.ru (A.P.); donna.geddes@uwa.edu.au (D.T.G.)

[3] Faculty of Pediatrics, I. M. Sechenov First Moscow State Medical University, Moscow 119991, Russia

[4] Allergy Department, Veltischev Clinical Pediatric Research Institute of Pirogov Russian National Research Medical University, Moscow 125412, Russia

[5] Department of Clinical and Experimental Medicine, Section of Paediatrics, University of Pisa, 56126 Pisa, Italy

[6] National Heart and Lung Institute, Imperial College London, London SW3 6NP, UK; s.colicino@imperial.ac.uk

[7] Royal Holloway University of London School of Biological Sciences, Biomedical Sciences, London TW20 0EX, UK; shobanadis@hotmail.com

[8] Department of Life and Reproduction Sciences, Section of Paediatrics, University of Verona, 37124 Verona, Italy; attilio.boner@univr.it

[9] School of Chemistry and Biochemistry, The University of Western Australia, Perth 6009, WA, Australia

[*] Correspondence: daniel.munblit08@imperial.ac.uk; Tel.: +44-07-898-257-151

[†] These authors contributed equally to this work.

Received: 30 August 2016; Accepted: 28 October 2016; Published: 3 November 2016

Abstract: Cytokines and growth factors in colostrum and mature milk may play an important role in infant immune maturation, and may vary significantly between populations. We aimed to examine associations between environmental and maternal factors, and human milk (HM) cytokine and growth factor levels. We recruited 398 pregnant/lactating women in the United Kingdom, Russia, and Italy. Participants underwent skin prick testing, questionnaire interview, and colostrum and mature milk sampling. HM cytokine and growth factor levels were quantified by electro-chemiluminescence. We found significant geographical variation in growth factor levels, but no evidence of variation between sites in cytokine detectability. There was an inverse correlation between time of milk sampling and growth factor levels in colostrum for Hepatocyte Growth Factor (HGF) and TGFβ1 and TGFβ3, but not TGFβ2, and levels were significantly higher in colostrum than mature milk for all growth factors. The kinetics of decline were different for each growth factor. Cytokines were present at much lower levels than growth factors, and the decline over time was less consistent. HM growth factors and cytokine levels vary between populations for unknown reasons. Levels of HM mediators decline at different rates postpartum, and these findings suggest specific biological roles for HM growth factors and cytokines in early postnatal development.

Keywords: colostrum; human milk; immune modulators; immunologically active molecules; cytokines; growth factors; environmental influence

1. Introduction

Human milk (HM) is usually the first source of nutrition for a newborn, and an important factor assisting infants in the first months of life, not only as a nutrition source but also as a manner of adapting infants to their extra-uterine environment. Breastfeeding is known to have positive short- and long-term effects on child health, although its influence on allergy development is still debatable [1]. There have been few attempts to investigate relationships between maternal and environmental factors and immune active profiles of HM. Data from a variety of studies suggest that factors such as country of maternal origin, diet, exercise, and exposure to smoke or farming environment in early life may influence colostrum and HM constituents [2–22].

It has been shown that Hepatocyte Growth Factor (HGF) is known to regulate vascular endothelial growth factor (VEGF) production from endothelial cells [23] and complements VEGF biological activity in the infant gut [24]. HGF levels in maternal serum change throughout pregnancy, peaking at 30 to 40 weeks of gestation and then decreasing upon delivery [25]. As levels of HGF are 20 to 30 times higher in colostrum than in maternal serum [26] it is reasonable to propose that HGF is actively excreted into HM in order to support infant's gut immunity maturation and growth.

Inverse relationships between the risk of atopic diseases, associated with T-helper lymphocyte type 2 (TH2) immune response, and indicators of early-life exposure to infections, such as high birth order or sibship size, early attendance at day care, and early exposure to pets or other animals are well described [27]. The "hygiene hypothesis" remains one of the most popular current hypotheses on early-life exposures and allergy risk [28]. It has been suggested that farming environment [6], higher bacterial exposure [7], or maternal country of origin [5] may have significant impacts on HM immune composition, and such effects on HM composition may be an important pathway through which early variations in microbial exposures influence risk of allergy development.

Our study aimed to prospectively investigate the relationship between maternal and environmental factors and levels of HGF, Transforming Growth Factor beta (TGFβ)1,2,3 and detectability of TH1 and TH2 cytokines using colostrum and HM samples collected from birth cohorts in three regions; the UK, eastern Europe, and continental Europe.

2. Materials and Methods

2.1. Study Setting, Eligibility Criteria, and Ethics

The investigations and sample collection have been conducted following ethical approval by Ethics committee in three countries participating in the study: West London Rec 3 (UK) (Ref. number 10/H0706/32) and all paperwork has been completed according to the hospital R&D Joint Research Office (UK) (JROSM0072) policy; Ethical Committee of the Azienda Ospedaliera di Verona (Italy) (approval No. 1288), and Moscow Institute of Paediatrics and Child Health of Ministry of Health of Russian Federation (Russia) (approval No. 1-MS/11). All women provided written informed consent.

Women were enrolled at antenatal and postnatal units of three participating centres—St. Mary's Hospital, London, UK; Maternity Hospital No. 1, Moscow, Russia; G.B. Rossi Hospital, Verona, Italy. Inclusion criteria for the study were: healthy term infants and their mothers intending to breastfeed and willing to comply with the study procedures.

Exclusion criteria were: maternal immunosuppressive treatment during lactation, or severe illness; infants with a major birth defect, admitted to neonatal intensive care, other severe illness, born prematurely (<37 weeks gestation), or with low birth weight (<2nd centile).

2.2. Medical Records and Interview

Following enrolment, participants underwent allergy skin prick testing (SPT) and answered a 10 min interview-based questionnaire regarding their medical history. Exposure variables recorded were selected based on a detailed review of known determinants of HM composition [29].

Information collected from the recruited women included parity; age; mode of delivery; details of residence environment, such as mould presence at home, regular contact with animals and/or pets at home; exposure to tobacco smoke (smoker or living in household with smoker or self-reported passive smoker); any reports of infections during pregnancy. We also obtained information on maternal dietary preferences—fish, fresh fruit, and probiotic intake. Participant medical records were reviewed by study personnel to extract relevant health information which was not available from questionnaires, prior to breast milk analysis. SPT was undertaken using the following solutions: Histamine 1% Positive Control, Glycerol Negative Control, House Dust Mite (*Dermatophagoides pteronyssinus*), Cat (*Felix domesticus*), Grass Pollen, Birch pollen, Peanut, Hazelnut, Egg (all from Stallergenes, SA 92160 Anthony, France), and Cow's milk (ALK-Abello, Hørsholm, Denmark). SPT was performed by standard technique using 1 mm lancets (ALK-Abello, Hørsholm, Denmark), and were read at 15 min. Allergic sensitization was defined as a wheal $\geq$3 mm to at least one allergen, in the context of a wheal $\geq$3 mm to histamine and no wheal to the negative control.

2.3. Human Milk Sampling

Participants were given sterile tubes to collect their own colostrum (once in the first 6 days of life) and mature HM (once at 4–6 weeks postpartum). Local site investigators and participating mothers were asked to collect colostrum or milk at the first morning breastfeed, by manual expression (colostrum) or collecting the drip (mature milk) from the contra-lateral breast during feeding [15]. Colostrum samples were frozen at -50 °C to -80 °C within 12 h of collection. HM samples were collected at home, stored in the fridge for not longer than 4 h, and transported to participating units by study staff, and frozen at 50 °C to -80 °C within 12 h of collection. It has been previously demonstrated that storage for 6 months at either -20 °C or -80 °C did not influence the concentration of immune active factors in human milk [30]. After thawing, samples were centrifuged at $1500\times g$ for 15 min at 4 °C. The lipid layer was removed with a pipette and aqueous fraction was analysed for immune modulators [31]. All milk samples were transported to London at -70 °C where the samples were stored at -80 °C until analysis.

2.4. Electro-Chemiluminescence

We used electro-chemiluminescence to measure immune mediators in colostrum and breast milk samples for Th1 and Th2 cytokines, HGF, and TGFβ1-3 (MesoScale Discovery, Rockville, MD, USA). Laboratory experiments were run according to manufacturer's protocol, using an eight-point standard curve. No dilution was used for Th1 and Th2 cytokines and HGF, and 1:2 dilution for TGFβ assays, following pilot experiments which showed that TGFβ2 levels in undiluted milk samples were often greater than the upper limit of detection. Assays were run in duplicate, and mediator levels were excluded where the CV was >25%—Median (IQR) levels and assay detection limits for each immune mediator studied are shown in Table A1.

2.5. Protein Analysis

We used turbidimetry to assess total protein concentration in colostrum samples (Abbott Architect Analyser C8000, Abbott, Abbott Park, IL, USA). For turbidimetry colostrum, proteins were denatured by benzethonium chloride, then measured at 404 nm. Pilot experiments determined that a 1:30 onboard dilution was needed to bring the colostrum protein concentration to within the linear measurement range of the Architect Analyser (3–60 g/L). Prior to protein analysis samples were thawed and centrifuged at $3000\times g$ for 15 min at 4 °C. Next, 300 μL of supernatant were carefully transferred to the tubes and loaded into the Architect device for the analysis.

2.6. Statistical Analysis

Maternal factors and levels/detection of cytokines and growth factors were summarized using standard descriptive statistics. As outcome variables were not normally distributed, non-parametric tests such as the Mann–Whitney *U*-test, were used to compare independent observations of different populations for unadjusted analyses. All growth factors have been presented as a continuous variable (pg/mL), whilst data on cytokines were transformed into a binary variable (detectable versus undetectable). Since concentration of growth factors and cytokines were assayed twice (in both colostrum and breast milk) for many participants, we used a mixed-effect regression model to account for the absence of independence between those two measures and to evaluate a broad range of variables. Continuous data with non-parametric distribution were log-transformed for inclusion in regression models.

Model selection was based on major approaches such as Akaike and Bayesian information criteria. Difference between groups effects (maternal and environmental factors) as well as within subject effects were evaluated using multilevel mixed-effect regression model. Factors and covariates included in the models were: parity, maternal sensitisation, maternal age, site of collection, mode of delivery—vaginal birth/caesarean section, mould presence at home, pets at home or regular contact; exposure to tobacco smoke (i.e., maternal active smoking or living in household with smoker or self-reported passive smoker) at recruitment; at least one self-reported maternal infection during pregnancy; maternal diet—fish intake at least once per week versus less often; daily fresh fruit versus less often; daily probiotic versus none/less often.

As models were used for the statistical analysis, the sample size reduced slightly, due to incomplete data for one or more variables included in the multivariate model in 56 individuals. This explains discrepancy in colostrum numbers. Reduced numbers were included in analysis of human milk samples, due to missing samples. Milk samples were missing due to cessation of breastfeeding before this time, due to mother's not supplying a sample within the four to six week time window for sampling, and due to loss to follow up/not contactable women.

Outcomes assessed were levels of HGF, TGFβ1, TGFβ2, TGFβ3, and cytokine detectability. Relationship between corrected growth factor levels and time (measured as HGF/Protein, TGFβ1/Protein, TGFβ2/Protein, and TGFβ3/Protein in pg/g) was assessed using the Spearman rank correlation coefficient. Results were considered significant when p-values were reported at a level less than 0.05. Bonferroni correction was used in mixed models analyses to control for false discovery.

3. Results

3.1. Study Population

Total of 481 mothers were recruited into the study from June 2011 to March 2012 from the birth centres and antenatal and postnatal units of secondary and tertiary hospitals from three countries, located in Northern Europe, Eastern Europe, and the Mediterranean area. Of 481 women, 398 (UK $n = 101$, Russia $n = 221$, Italy $n = 76$) provided samples and were included in this study. The 83 mothers unwilling or unable to provide colostrum samples postnatally were not evaluated further.

Demographic data of the participants is presented in Table 1. Significant differences between groups were seen for most variables recorded. Maternal age (highest in Italy), maternal allergic sensitization (highest in UK), rate of Caesarean section (highest in UK), tobacco smoke exposure (highest in Russia), antenatal infections (highest in Italy), and time of colostrum collection (earlier in Russia than other sites) all differed significantly. There was also weak evidence for differences in parity and birth weight across centres). Infant sex did not significantly differ across sites.

3.2. Association between Collection Time and Colostrum/Breast Milk Composition

Among the environmental and maternal factors analysed we found time of milk sample collection postpartum to have the most significant influence on growth factor levels, and a mixed effect on cytokine detectability. A significant decline over time in colostrum was seen for HGF, TGFβ1 and TGFβ3, IL2, IL5, IL10, and IFNγ. No significant influence but similar trends were seen for most of the other mediators (Table 2 and Figure 1). Differences between colostrum and mature milk showed similar findings for growth factors, which were all statistically significant. For cytokine detectability in breast milk versus colostrum, findings were mixed and not entirely consistent with the changes seen over time in colostrum. IL10 was more commonly detected in colostrum than in HM, but IL4 and IFNγ were more commonly detected in HM, despite no change or a decline in detectability over time in colostrum samples. Other cytokines showed no significant difference between colostrum and HM (Table 2).

Table 1. Characteristics of study participants.

	UK	Russia	Italy	*p*-Value (Three Countries)
Maternal allergic sensitisation *	35/94 (37)	22/156 (14)	9/40 (23)	<0.01 [a]
Maternal Age (years)	32.8 (4.78)	29.8 (4.45)	37.4 (5.38)	<0.01 [b]
Vaginal Delivery	70/101 (69)	188/219 (86)	62/76 (82)	<0.01 [a]
Male sex	54/101 (53)	118/216 (55)	41/76 (54)	0.98 [a]
Birth Weight (grams)	3527 (535.37)	3526 (438.97)	3328 (476.95)	0.05 [b]
Primiparous women	55/100 (55)	93/216 (43)	29/75 (39)	0.06 [a]
Household tobacco smoke exposure	30/99 (30)	135/218 (62)	25/76 (33)	<0.01 [a]
Antenatal Infections [†]	16/100 (16)	61/211 (29)	29/76 (38)	<0.01 [a]
Time of colostrum collection (hours)	58.61 (33.2)	50.03 (14.34)	57.84 (26.52)	<0.01 [b]

[a] Pearson χ^2 test has been used; [b] ANOVA test has been used. Data shown are (*n*/(%)) for binary variables, and (mean (S.D.)) for continuous variables; * Defined as skin prick test wheal ≥3 mm to at least one of a panel of common allergens; [†] Antenatal infection is defined as at least one self-reported maternal infection during pregnancy.

Table 2. Relationship between time of sample collection and milk composition.

Immune Modulator	Colostrum Composition			Paired Differences between HM and Colostrum of Colostrum and Breast Milk Composition		
	Change over Time	β	*p*-Value	Difference between Colostrum and HM over Time	β	*p*-Value
HGF	Lower	−0.01	<0.001 **	Higher in colostrum	−1.35	<0.001 **
TGFβ1	Lower	−0.003	0.01 *	Higher in colostrum	−0.93	<0.001 **
TGFβ2	No change	−0.003	0.12	Higher in colostrum	−1.12	<0.001 **
TGFβ3	Lower	−0.01	<0.001 **	Higher in colostrum	−2.03	<0.001 **
IL2	Lower	−0.02	0.02 *	No difference	0.32	0.30
IL4	No change	−0.01	0.22	Higher in HM	0.72	0.04 *
IL5	Lower	−0.03	<0.001 **	No difference	−0.54	0.09
IL10	Lower	−0.02	<0.001 **	Higher in colostrum	−1.66	<0.001 **
IFNγ	Lower	−0.01	0.04 *	Higher in HM	1.20	<0.001 **
IL12	No change	−0.01	0.12	No difference	−0.11	0.73
IL13	No change	−0.01	0.09	No difference	0.09	0.72

Data shown are concentration (pg/mL) for growth factors, and detectable versus not detectable for cytokines. A multilevel mixed-effect regression model was used for all analyses, which were adjusted to the following factors: Parity, Maternal Atopy, Maternal age, Site of collection, Mode of delivery, Mould presence at home, Pets at home or regular contact; Exposure to tobacco smoke; At least one self-reported maternal infection during pregnancy; Maternal diet. HM, human milk; HGF, Hepatocyte Growth Factor. * *p* value < 0.05; ** *p* value < 0.01.

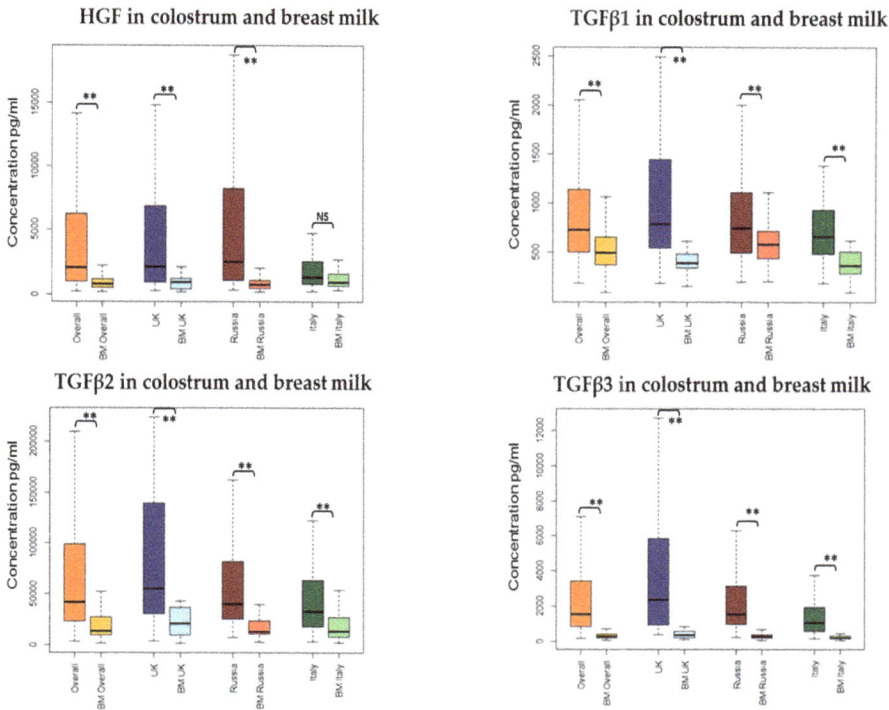

Figure 1. Unadjusted growth factors concentration (pg/mL) in colostrum and breast milk across all sites (overall) and at each site of collection (London, Moscow, and Verona). ** *p* value < 0.01.

3.3. Association between Collection Site and Colostrum/Breast Milk Composition

3.3.1. Growth Factors

We found a significant influence of country of residence on some growth factor concentrations (Table 3 and Figure 2). TGFβ2 and TGFβ3 showed consistent findings in colostrum and HM samples—levels of both factors were higher in UK and lower in Italy, with intermediate levels in Russian women. HGF was lowest in the colostrum, but not HM, of mothers in Italy (mean log HGF 7.38, SE 0.12 in Italy; 7.98 (0.11) UK; 7.99 (0.10) Russia). TGFβ1 did not show consistent differences between sites in colostrum and HM analyses, with higher levels in UK colostrum samples compared with Italy (mean log TGFβ1 6.80 (0.07) in the UK; 6.53 (0.08) Italy); and high levels in Russian HM samples (6.36 (0.08)) compared with Italy (5.86 (0.11)) or the UK (5.96 (0.11)). We evaluated a number of other maternal factors for association with growth factor concentrations, and found weak evidence of an association between fish consumption less than once a week and higher levels of TGFβ1 (mean log TGFβ1 6.72 (0.06) for less than once a week; 6.57 (0.05) for more than once a week); and primiparity with higher levels of HGF in colostrum (7.87 (0.08) for primiparous; 7.69 (0.08) for multiparous) and HM (6.92 (0.11) for primiparous; 6.75 (0.11) for multiparous).

Table 3. Concentration (pg/mL) of growth factors in colostrum and breast milk and exposures associated with the levels.

	Median (IQR) pg/mL	Important Growth Factor Level Difference between the Groups	
		Colostrum	
HGF	2055.31 (964–6239)	UK and Russia higher than in Italy	$p < 0.001$
		Primipara higher than Multipara	$p = 0.05$
TGFβ1	731.534 (505–1142)	UK higher than Italy	$p = 0.01$
		Fish consumption Less than once a week higher than At least once a week	$p = 0.04$
TGFβ2	42,209.88 (23,847–98,597)	UK higher than Russia and Italy	$p < 0.05$
TGFβ3	1535.081 (847–3395)	UK higher than Russia higher than Italy	$p < 0.05$
		Breast Milk	
HGF	784.041 (508–1189)	Primiparous higher than Multigravida	$p = 0.05$
TGFβ1	493.514 (375–653)	Russia higher than UK and Italy	$p < 0.05$
TGFβ2	14,040.62 (10,080–27,262)	UK higher than Russia and Italy	$p < 0.05$
TGFβ3	279.41 (183–395)	UK higher than Russia higher than Italy	$p < 0.05$

A multilevel mixed-effect regression model was used for all analyses, which was adjusted using Bonferroni correction, to the following factors: Parity, Maternal Atopy, Maternal age, Site (Country) of collection, Mode of delivery—labour versus no labour, Mould presence at home, Pets at home or regular contact; Exposure to tobacco smoke (i.e., smoker or living in household with smoker or self-reported passive smoker) at recruitment; At least one self-reported maternal infection during pregnancy; Maternal diet—fish intake at least once per week versus less often; daily fresh fruit versus less often; daily probiotic versus none/less often.

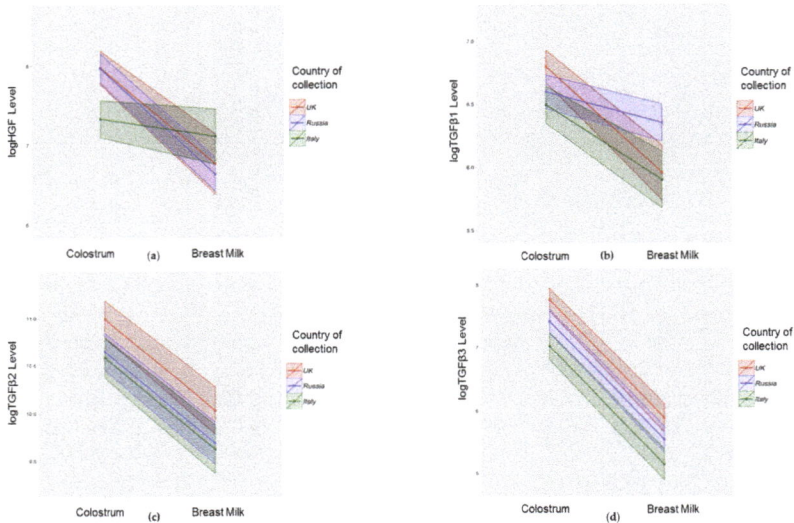

Figure 2. Association between site of collection and growth factor concentrations in colostrum and breast milk. Data shown are mean (bold line) and 95% CI (shaded area) for log transformed concentrations of HGF (**a**); TGFβ1 (**b**); TGFβ2 (**c**); and TGFβ3 (**d**) in the UK (**red**), Russia (**blue**), and Italy (**green**). A multilevel mixed-effect regression model was used for all analyses which were adjusted to the following factors: Parity, Maternal Atopy, Maternal age, Site (Country) of collection, Mode of delivery, Mould presence at home, Pets at home or regular contact; Exposure to tobacco smoke, at recruitment; At least one self-reported maternal infection during pregnancy; Maternal diet.

3.3.2. Cytokines

Women reporting infections during pregnancy had detectable levels of IL5 less often in comparison to mothers reporting no antenatal infections (Table 4). Smoking, type of delivery, and antenatal infections were not related to detection of cytokines in HM or colostrum.

Table 4. Detectability of Th1 and Th2 Cytokines in Colostrum and Human Milk.

	Colostrum Detectable	Human Milk Detectable	Factors Associated with Cytokines Detectability
IL2	49/342 (14%)	38/190 (20%)	NA
IL4	35/342 (10%)	30/190 (16%)	NA
IL5	77/342 (23%)	27/190 (14%)	Antenatal infections OR 0.49 (95% CI 0.25–0.98)
IL10	225/342 (66%)	69/190 (36%)	NA
IFNγ	66/342 (19%)	92/190 (48%)	NA
IL12	63/342 (18%)	31/190 (16%)	NA
IL13	86/342 (25%)	58/190 (31%)	NA

NA—no association. A multilevel mixed-effect regression model was used for all analyses which were adjusted to the following factors: Parity, Maternal Atopy, Maternal age, Site (Country) of collection, Mode of delivery, Mould presence at home, Pets at home or regular contact; Exposure to tobacco smoke, at recruitment; At least one self-reported maternal infection during pregnancy; Maternal diet.

3.3.3. Protein and Sodium in Colostrum

Protein in human colostrum declines over time ($r = -0.42$; $p < 0.001$) with all growth factor levels demonstrating a significant and marked decline over time, although the slope of decline varied between growth factors. When corrected for protein, the correlation between growth factor levels and time of collection was inconsistent between factors, with a significant decline seen for HGF/Protein, an increase over time seen for TGFβ1/Protein and TGFβ2/Protein, and no change over time seen for TGFβ3/Protein. The relationship between time of colostrum collection and growth factor or growth factor/Protein level for the four growth factors measured is shown in Table A2 and Figure 3.

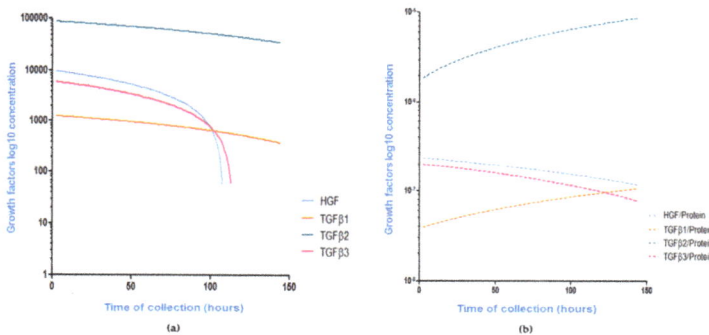

Figure 3. Effect of correcting growth factor concentrations for total protein level on the relationship between concentration and time. Data show nonlinear curves for unadjusted concentrations (pg/mL) of HGF (**blue**), TGFβ1 (**orange**), TGFβ2 (**green**), and TGFβ3 (**pink**) in colostrum in relation to time of sampling. Correlations were explored using raw data (**a**); and the ratio of growth factor concentration to protein concentration in the same sample (**b**). Trends in absolute and relative growth factors concentration in colostrum change over time. All correlation coefficients were statistically significant apart from the TGFβ3/Protein ratio in Figure 3b.

4. Discussion

In this large prospective cohort study, we have confirmed earlier findings of significant differences in milk composition between sites, but were not able to explain these differences through maternal or environmental factors. We identified important differences between mediators in kinetics of decline postpartum and these data suggest specific mechanisms controlling HM immune composition, and support important biological roles for HM immune factors in the developing infant.

Data from a variety of studies suggest that colostrum and HM constituents may be influenced by the country of origin and a number of environmental conditions which may differ significantly from one location to another [3–7,32], but the cause of this difference is still unclear. Our data suggest that HGF levels were lower in the colostrum/milk of Italian mothers and TGFβ2 and TGFβ3 were higher in colostrum/milk of UK mothers with the same significant difference for colostral TGFβ1 (Figure 2). Amoudruz showed that Mali women have higher levels of TGF-β1 in comparison with women born in Sweden [5]. Peroni reported higher HM TGF-β1 in a farming compared with urban environment [6]. Tomicic found Estonian mothers have lower HM TGFβ2 than Swedish mothers [7] which the authors suggested may be due to differences in microbial exposure. Orivuori et al. assessed HM samples collected in four countries of continental Europe and Finland and showed TGFβ1 levels to be highest in Finland and sIgA lowest in Germany [32]. We explored a number of maternal and demographic variables including markers of microbial load such as maternal report of probiotic, pet, and mould exposure, but we were not able to confirm these previous findings.

At present, we do not possess strong evidence of maternal allergic status influences on qualitative and quantitative immunological constituents in HM. We did not find any relationship between the levels of growth factors and/or detectability of cytokines and maternal allergy; this is in agreement with data from other studies which found no obvious trend in HM composition of allergic mothers compared to non-allergic [32–34].

Our data show some evidence for higher levels of HGF and TGFβ3 in the colostrum of primiparous women. Data from some studies suggest that parity does not influence HM composition. This borderline trend can be seen in some (but not all [3,35]) other studies [4,36,37], suggesting that higher levels of certain immune active markers can be found in the HM of primiparous mothers, which may be an additional mechanism to explain decreased allergy risk with an increase of birth order.

We found some evidence that fish intake during pregnancy can influence HM composition [3]—we found higher colostrum TGFβ1 in women eating fish less than once a week. This adds to a confusing picture, with Urwin reporting TGF-β1 levels to be highest in the colostrum of women residing in the river and lake region of China [3], well known for high fish consumption and Hawkes not finding any relationship between fish oil intervention and TGFβ1 levels [38]. Thus, the reasons behind differences in the HM immunological profile between countries remain unclear. Further work should consider genetic and gene/environment influences, as well as detailed dietary assessments, in addition to the factors evaluated in this study. Data from So-Yeon Lee and co-authors show that breastfeeding was found to be associated with a reduced risk of allergic sensitisation in children with CT/CC geno-type, suggesting gene-environment interaction between the CD14C-159T polymorphism and breastfeeding in relation to aeroallergen sensitisation [39].

It is well established that colostrum is particularly rich in immunologically active molecules and that levels of immunological factors are lower in mature HM [6,12,40,41]. Although our study did not involve HM collection in the same individuals over multiple timepoints, the sample size was large enough to identify a strong relationship between time of sampling postpartum and growth factor levels. We observed a strong relationship between growth factor levels and time postpartum both within colostrum, and between colostrum and mature milk samples, which was independent of geographical location. Although the difference between colostrum and mature milk composition is well established in the literature [6,12,40,41], our finding of a rapid decline in growth factor levels (HGF, TGFβ1, TGFβ3) and evidence for reduced detectability of cytokines (IL2, IL5, IL10, IFNγ) in colostrum with time postpartum has not been consistently demonstrated by others. Soto-Ramirez et al.

found none of the immune markers to correlate with the time of milk collection in a study conducted in the USA [42]; this may be partially explained by a wide range in collection times (week one to eight) and absence of colostral samples. In a study done in China with a narrower range of collection times, levels of TGF-β1 and TGF-β2 decreased significantly over time [3]. Studies which do not adequately account for variations in sampling time may explain some of the inconsistency of HM composition and its determinants in the literature [29].

Dilution could be a potential explanation of the growth factor decline over time. During the first week of life the infant's volume requirements are low. Later levels of the immune active molecules decrease as the volume and nutritional requirements of the infant increase. Immune active constituents of colostrum and breast milk represent a minor component but one of the most biologically active parts of HM total protein. In this study, we attempted to adjust for dilutional effects by correcting growth factor colostrum levels for total protein level in the same sample. Correction for colostrum total protein failed to consistently remove the relationship between factor level and time postpartum, and highlighted significant variation between factors in the kinetics of decline. This implies active transport of these growth factors using varied mechanisms specific to each factor. If we assume biological relevance, then these results suggest that infants need relatively higher amounts of TGFβ1 and TGFβ2 for longer than that of TGFβ3 or HGF. TGFβ3 is significantly different from TGFβ1 and TGFβ2 in its detailed tertiary structure of the active domain despite homology in amino acid sequence [43]. There is some evidence [43] that TGFβ3 may also have distinct functions to other TGFβ isoforms. TGFβ3 is up-regulated by milk stasis, and induces apoptosis in mammary gland epithelium during involution, in contrast to TGFβ1 and TGFβ2 [44]. The biological relevance of HM TGFβ is illustrated by the observed direct correlation between the levels of TGFβ in human milk and infant serum IgA [45]. As the infant's immune response matures there is likely to be less need for an extrinsic supply of immune stimulants.

The main limitations of our study are first that we did not assess maternal diet using a food frequency questionnaire, did not collect detailed information on the strain of probiotics and/or fish oil supplements used, and did not evaluate maternal genotype as a potentially important determinant or modulator of HM composition. This means that while we were able to explore our primary focus of maternal and demographic factors influence on HM composition, we were not able to reliably identify reasons for the difference in HM composition identified between sites. Second, we sampled single colostrum and HM specimens from each subject. Our findings regarding the kinetics of growth factor decline in colostrum and HM need to be explored further in prospective studies with longitudinal sampling at multiple timepoints within the same participants. Third, we only made preliminary attempts to adjust for the effect of time or milk maturity on compositional analysis. Since time postpartum may be a surrogate for milk/breast maturity, we aimed to identify a 'correction factor' that might reflect milk maturity. We did not find evidence that any growth factor concentration was related to HM protein concentration, but further work is needed to identify markers of HM maturity in order to control for this in compositional analysis of colostrum. Maternal body mass index (BMI) data has not been assessed due to a difficulty in one of the participating countries. Finally, due to logistical, funding, and sample size constraints our analysis covers only a small number of growth factors and cytokines, so may not be generalisable to all immune factors in HM.

5. Conclusions

In this large international cohort study of HM composition, we have found an important influence of time after birth on colostrum composition, which must be adjusted for in any further research. Despite adjusting for this and other factors, we identified unexplained and significant variation in HM immune composition between geographically distant populations. Overall, our data suggest that levels of human milk mediators decline at different rates post-partum, and this may suggest that these factors are likely to have specific biological roles in early postnatal development. An important aim of future research should be to optimize the analysis of HM composition, accounting for maturity of milk, and aim to better understand the biological roles and consequences for the developing infant of variations in HM immune composition.

Acknowledgments: We are grateful to the staff of birth centres and postnatal units involved and all the women and their babies, participating in our study. Robert Boyle and John Warner are supported by a National Institute for Health Research Biomedical Research Centre (BRC). Both JW and RB have received research grant income from Danone in relation to studies of the value of prebiotics in allergy prevention and Airsonette to evaluate Temperature controlled laminar airflow for asthma. JW is on a Danone, UCB and Airsonette scientific advisory board and both JW and RB have given paid lectures for the companies. DM has received travel funding from Nutricia. DG receives an unrestricted research grant from Medela AG and has received travel funding and support for lectures.

Author Contributions: J.O.W., R.J.B. and D.M. conceived and designed the experiments; D.M., S.D., L.Y.C., P.A. and S.S. performed the experiments; D.M., L.Y.C. collected data in London; D.G.P. and A.L.B. collected data in Verona; M.T. and A.P. collected data in Moscow; S.C. analysed the data; D.M., D.T.G., R.J.B. and J.O.W. wrote the paper. For research articles with several authors, a short paragraph specifying their individual contributions must be provided. The following statements should be used "X.X. and Y.Y. conceived and designed the experiments; X.X. performed the experiments; X.X. and Y.Y. analysed the data; W.W. contributed reagents/materials/analysis tools; Y.Y. wrote the paper". Authorship must be limited to those who have contributed substantially to the work reported.

Conflicts of Interest: The authors declare no conflict of interest.

Appendix A

Table A1. Lower limit of detection values (pg/mL) for cytokines and growth factors analysis and overall locations median concentrations for all immune active molecules (values below LLOD for all cytokines have been transformed into $1/2$ of LLOD).

Immune Active Molecule	Median Lower Limit of Detection	Median (IQR) Colostrum	Median (IQR) HM
IFN-γ	3.49	1.23 (0.51–3.49)	3.49 (1.54–7.8)
IL2	2.06	0.6 (0.29–1.47)	0.98 (0.23–2.06)
IL4	1.83	1.83 (0.24–1.83)	1.83 (0.50–1.83)
IL5	2.89	1.44 (0.57–2.85)	1.57 (0.33–2.89)
IL10	1.50	2.67 (1.01–9.04)	1.5 (0.74–2.66)
IL12	3.50	1.85 (0.34–3.5)	2.13 (0.32–3.5)
IL13	4.60	4.6 (1.85–4.69)	4.6 (3.52–6.76)
HGF	73.00	2055.31 (964–6239)	784.041 (508–1189)
TGFβ1	8.73	731.534 (505–1142)	493.514 (375–653)
TGFβ2	265.00	42,209.88 (23,847–98,597)	14,040.62 (10,080–27,262)
TGFβ3	8.37	1535.081 (847–3395)	279.41 (183–395)

Standard curve ranges: IFN-γ, IL2, IL4, IL5, IL10, IL12, IL13 0—2500 pg/mL; HGF, TGFβ1, TGFβ2 0—100.000; TGFβ3 0—50.000. All values presented in pg/mL.

Table A2. Absolute and relative decline of growth factors over time.

Growth Factor Concentration (pg/mL)/Time of Collection	Raw Concentration (pg/mL)	Growth Factor/Protein Ratio
HGF	$r = -0.39, p < 0.001 \downarrow$	$r = -0.19, p = 0.003 \downarrow$
TGFβ1	$r = -0.21, p < 0.001 \downarrow$	$r = 0.25, p < 0.001 \uparrow$
TGFβ2	$r = -0.16, p = 0.01 \downarrow$	$r = 0.20, p = 0.004 \uparrow$
TGFβ3	$r = -0.35, p < 0.001 \downarrow$	$r = -0.06, p = 0.34 \downarrow$

↑—Positive correlation with time of collection; ↓—Negative correlation with time of collection.

References

1. Matheson, M.C.; Allen, K.J.; Tang, M.L. Understanding the evidence for and against the role of breastfeeding in allergy prevention. *Clin. Exp. Allergy* **2012**, *42*, 827–851. [CrossRef] [PubMed]
2. Hoppu, U.; Isolauri, E.; Laakso, P.; Matomaki, J.; Laitinen, K. Probiotics and dietary counselling targeting maternal dietary fat intake modifies breast milk fatty acids and cytokines. *Eur. J. Nutr.* **2012**, *51*, 211–219. [CrossRef] [PubMed]

3. Urwin, H.J.; Miles, E.A.; Noakes, P.S.; Kremmyda, L.S.; Vlachava, M.; Diaper, N.D.; Perez-Cano, F.J.; Godfrey, K.M.; Calder, P.C.; Yaqoob, P. Salmon consumption during pregnancy alters fatty acid composition and secretory IgA concentration in human breast milk. *J. Nutr.* **2012**, *142*, 1603–1610. [CrossRef] [PubMed]

4. Amoudruz, P.; Holmlund, U.; Schollin, J.; Sverremark-Ekstrom, E.; Montgomery, S.M. Maternal country of birth and previous pregnancies are associated with breast milk characteristics. *Pediatr. Allergy Immunol.* **2009**, *20*, 19–29. [CrossRef] [PubMed]

5. Holmlund, U.; Amoudruz, P.; Johansson, M.A.; Haileselassie, Y.; Ongoiba, A.; Kayentao, K.; Traore, B.; Doumbo, S.; Schollin, J.; Doumbo, O.; et al. Maternal country of origin, breast milk characteristics and potential influences on immunity in offspring. *Clin. Exp. Immunol.* **2010**, *162*, 500–509. [CrossRef] [PubMed]

6. Peroni, D.G.; Pescollderungg, L.; Piacentini, G.L.; Rigotti, E.; Maselli, M.; Watschinger, K.; Piazza, M.; Pigozzi, R.; Boner, A.L. Immune regulatory cytokines in the milk of lactating women from farming and urban environments. *Pediatr. Allergy Immunol.* **2010**, *21*, 977–982. [CrossRef] [PubMed]

7. Tomicic, S.; Johansson, G.; Voor, T.; Bjorksten, B.; Bottcher, M.F.; Jenmalm, M.C. Breast milk cytokine and IgA composition differ in Estonian and Swedish mothers-relationship to microbial pressure and infant allergy. *Pediatr. Res.* **2010**, *68*, 330–334. [CrossRef] [PubMed]

8. Striker, G.A.; Casanova, L.D.; Nagao, A.T. Influence of type of delivery on A, G and M immunoglobulin concentration in maternal colostrum. *J. Pediatr.* **2004**, *80*, 123–128. [CrossRef]

9. Bottcher, M.F.; Jenmalm, M.C.; Garofalo, R.P.; Bjorksten, B. Cytokines in breast milk from allergic and nonallergic mothers. *Pediatr. Res.* **2000**, *47*, 157–162. [CrossRef] [PubMed]

10. Laiho, K.; Lampi, A.M.; Hamalainen, M.; Moilanen, E.; Piironen, V.; Arvola, T.; Syrjanen, S.; Isolauri, E. Breast milk fatty acids, eicosanoids, and cytokines in mothers with and without allergic disease. *Pediatr. Res.* **2003**, *53*, 642–647. [CrossRef] [PubMed]

11. Prokesova, L.; Lodinova-Zadnikova, R.; Zizka, J.; Kocourkova, I.; Novotna, O.; Petraskova, P.; Sterzl, I. Cytokine levels in healthy and allergic mothers and their children during the first year of life. *Pediatr. Allergy Immunol.* **2006**, *17*, 175–183. [CrossRef] [PubMed]

12. Rigotti, E.; Piacentini, G.L.; Ress, M.; Pigozzi, R.; Boner, A.L.; Peroni, D.G. Transforming growth factor-beta and interleukin-10 in breast milk and development of atopic diseases in infants. *Clin. Exp. Allergy* **2006**, *36*, 614–618. [CrossRef] [PubMed]

13. Marek, A.; Zagierski, M.; Liberek, A.; Aleksandrowicz, E.; Korzon, M.; Krzykowski, G.; Kaminska, B.; Szlagatys-Sidorkiewicz, A. TGF-beta(1), IL-10 and IL-4 in colostrum of allergic and nonallergic mothers. *Acta Biochim. Pol.* **2009**, *56*, 411–414. [PubMed]

14. Sidor, K.; Jarmolowska, B.; Kaczmarski, M.; Kostyra, E.; Iwan, M.; Kostyra, H. Content of beta-casomorphins in milk of women with a history of allergy. *Pediatr. Allergy Immunol.* **2008**, *19*, 587–591. [CrossRef] [PubMed]

15. Snijders, B.E.; Damoiseaux, J.G.; Penders, J.; Kummeling, I.; Stelma, F.F.; van Ree, R.; van den Brandt, P.A.; Thijs, C. Cytokines and soluble CD14 in breast milk in relation with atopic manifestations in mother and infant (KOALA study). *Clin. Exp. Allergy* **2006**, *36*, 1609–1615. [CrossRef] [PubMed]

16. Bottcher, M.F.; Abrahamsson, T.R.; Fredriksson, M.; Jakobsson, T.; Bjorksten, B. Low breast milk tgf-beta2 is induced by lactobacillus reuteri supplementation and associates with reduced risk of sensitization during infancy. *Pediatr. Allergy Immunol.* **2008**, *19*, 497–504. [CrossRef] [PubMed]

17. Boyle, R.J.; Ismail, I.H.; Kivivuori, S.; Licciardi, P.V.; Robins-Browne, R.M.; Mah, L.J.; Axelrad, C.; Moore, S.; Donath, S.; Carlin, J.B.; et al. Lactobacillus GG treatment during pregnancy for the prevention of eczema: A randomized controlled trial. *Allergy* **2011**, *66*, 509–516. [CrossRef] [PubMed]

18. Prescott, S.L.; Wickens, K.; Westcott, L.; Jung, W.; Currie, H.; Black, P.N.; Stanley, T.V.; Mitchell, E.A.; Fitzharris, P.; Siebers, R.; et al. Supplementation with *Lactobacillus Rhamnosus* or *Bifidobacterium Lactis* probiotics in pregnancy increases cord blood interferon-gamma and breast milk transforming growth factor-beta and immunoglobin a detection. *Clin. Exp. Allergy* **2008**, *38*, 1606–1614. [CrossRef] [PubMed]

19. Rautava, S.; Kalliomaki, M.; Isolauri, E. Probiotics during pregnancy and breast-feeding might confer immunomodulatory protection against atopic disease in the infant. *J. Allergy Clin. Immunol.* **2002**, *109*, 119–121. [CrossRef] [PubMed]

20. Kuitunen, M.; Kukkonen, A.K.; Savilahti, E. Impact of maternal allergy and use of probiotics during pregnancy on breast milk cytokines and food antibodies and development of allergy in children until 5 years. *Int. Arch. Allergy Immunol.* **2012**, *159*, 162–170. [CrossRef] [PubMed]

21. Zanardo, V.; Nicolussi, S.; Cavallin, S.; Trevisanuto, D.; Barbato, A.; Faggian, D.; Favaro, F.; Plebani, M. Effect of maternal smoking on breast milk interleukin-1alpha, beta-endorphin, and leptin concentrations and leptin concentrations. *Environ. Health Perspect.* **2005**, *113*, 1410–1413. [CrossRef] [PubMed]

22. Burch, J.; Karmaus, W.; Gangur, V.; Soto-Ramirez, N.; Yousefi, M.; Goetzl, L.M. Pre- and perinatal characteristics and breast milk immune markers. *Pediatr. Res.* **2013**, *74*, 615–621. [CrossRef] [PubMed]

23. Min, J.K.; Lee, Y.M.; Kim, J.H.; Kim, Y.M.; Kim, S.W.; Lee, S.Y.; Gho, Y.S.; Oh, G.T.; Kwon, Y.G. Hepatocyte growth factor suppresses vascular endothelial growth factor-induced expression of endothelial ICAM-1 and VCAM-1 by inhibiting the nuclear factor-kappaB pathway. *Circ. Res.* **2005**, *96*, 300–307. [CrossRef] [PubMed]

24. Kobata, R.; Tsukahara, H.; Ohshima, Y.; Ohta, N.; Tokuriki, S.; Tamura, S.; Mayumi, M. High levels of growth factors in human breast milk. *Early Hum. Dev.* **2008**, *84*, 67–69. [CrossRef] [PubMed]

25. Horibe, N.; Okamoto, T.; Itakura, A.; Nakanishi, T.; Suzuki, T.; Kazeto, S.; Tomoda, Y. Levels of hepatocyte growth factor in maternal serum and amniotic fluid. *Am. J. Obstet. Gynecol.* **1995**, *173*, 937–942. [CrossRef]

26. Yamada, Y.; Saito, S.; Morikawa, H. Hepatocyte growth factor in human breast milk. *Am. J. Reprod. Immunol.* **1998**, *40*, 112–120. [CrossRef] [PubMed]

27. Strachan, D.P. Family size, infection and atopy: The first decade of the "hygiene hypothesis". *Thorax* **2000**, *55* (Suppl. 1), S2–S10. [CrossRef] [PubMed]

28. Strachan, D.P. Hay fever, hygiene, and household size. *BMJ* **1989**, *299*, 1259–1260. [CrossRef] [PubMed]

29. Munblit, D.; Boyle, R.J.; Warner, J.O. Factors affecting breast milk composition and potential consequences for development of the allergic phenotype. *Clin. Exp. Allergy* **2015**, *45*, 583–601. [CrossRef] [PubMed]

30. Ramirez-Santana, C.; Perez-Cano, F.J.; Audi, C.; Castell, M.; Moretones, M.G.; Lopez-Sabater, M.C.; Castellote, C.; Franch, A. Effects of cooling and freezing storage on the stability of bioactive factors in human colostrum. *J. Dairy Sci.* **2012**, *95*, 2319–2325. [CrossRef] [PubMed]

31. Jones, C.A.; Holloway, J.A.; Popplewell, E.J.; Diaper, N.D.; Holloway, J.W.; Vance, G.H.; Warner, J.A.; Warner, J.O. Reduced soluble CD14 levels in amniotic fluid and breast milk are associated with the subsequent development of atopy, eczema, or both. *J. Allergy Clin. Immunol.* **2002**, *109*, 858–866. [CrossRef] [PubMed]

32. Orivuori, L.; Loss, G.; Roduit, C.; Dalphin, J.C.; Depner, M.; Genuneit, J.; Lauener, R.; Pekkanen, J.; Pfefferle, P.; Riedler, J.; et al. Soluble immunoglobulin A in breast milk is inversely associated with atopic dermatitis at early age: The PASTURE cohort study. *Clin. Exp. Allergy* **2014**, *44*, 102–112. [CrossRef] [PubMed]

33. Savilahti, E.; Siltanen, M.; Kajosaari, M.; Vaarala, O.; Saarinen, K.M. IgA antibodies, TGF-beta1 and -beta2, and soluble CD14 in the colostrum and development of atopy by age 4. *Pediatr. Res.* **2005**, *58*, 1300–1305. [CrossRef] [PubMed]

34. Kondo, N.; Suda, Y.; Nakao, A.; Oh-Oka, K.; Suzuki, K.; Ishimaru, K.; Sato, M.; Tanaka, T.; Nagai, A.; Yamagata, Z. Maternal psychosocial factors determining the concentrations of transforming growth factor-beta in breast milk. *Pediatr. Allergy Immunol.* **2011**, *22*, 853–861. [CrossRef] [PubMed]

35. Ismail, I.H.; Licciardi, P.V.; Oppedisano, F.; Boyle, R.J.; Tang, M.L. Relationship between breast milk sCD14, Tgf-beta1 and total IgA in the first month and development of eczema during infancy. *Pediatr. Allergy Immunol.* **2013**, *24*, 352–360. [CrossRef] [PubMed]

36. Groer, M.W.; Shelton, M.M. Exercise is associated with elevated proinflammatory cytokines in human milk. *J. Obstet. Gynecol. Neonatal Nurs.* **2009**, *38*, 35–41. [CrossRef] [PubMed]

37. Walter, J.; Kuhn, L.; Ghosh, M.K.; Kankasa, C.; Semrau, K.; Sinkala, M.; Mwiya, M.; Thea, D.M.; Aldrovandi, G.M. Low and undetectable breast milk interleukin-7 concentrations are associated with reduced risk of postnatal HIV transmission. *J. Acquir. Immune Defic. Syndr.* **2007**, *46*, 200–207. [CrossRef] [PubMed]

38. Hawkes, J.S.; Bryan, D.L.; Neumann, M.A.; Makrides, M.; Gibson, R.A. Transforming growth factor beta in human milk does not change in response to modest intakes of docosahexaenoic acid. *Lipids* **2001**, *36*, 1179–1181. [CrossRef] [PubMed]

39. Lee, S.Y.; Kang, M.J.; Kwon, J.W.; Park, K.S.; Hong, S.J. Breastfeeding might have protective effects on atopy in children with the CD14C-159T CT/CC genotype. *Allergy Asthma Immunol. Res.* **2013**, *5*, 239–241. [CrossRef] [PubMed]

40. Takahata, Y.; Takada, H.; Nomura, A.; Ohshima, K.; Nakayama, H.; Tsuda, T.; Nakano, H.; Hara, T. Interleukin-18 in human milk. *Pediatr. Res.* **2001**, *50*, 268–272. [CrossRef] [PubMed]

41. Ustundag, B.; Yilmaz, E.; Dogan, Y.; Akarsu, S.; Canatan, H.; Halifeoglu, I.; Cikim, G.; Aygun, A.D. Levels of cytokines (IL-1beta, IL-2, IL-6, IL-8, TNF-alpha) and trace elements (Zn, Cu) in breast milk from mothers of preterm and term infants. *Mediat. Inflamm.* **2005**, *2005*, 331–336. [CrossRef] [PubMed]

42. Soto-Ramirez, N.; Karmaus, W.; Yousefi, M.; Zhang, H.; Liu, J.; Gangur, V. Maternal immune markers in serum during gestation and in breast milk and the risk of asthma-like symptoms at ages 6 and 12 months: A longitudinal study. *Allergy Asthma Clin. Immunol.* **2012**, *8*, 11. [CrossRef] [PubMed]

43. Laverty, H.G.; Wakefield, L.M.; Occleston, N.L.; O'Kane, S.; Ferguson, M.W. TGF-β3 and cancer: A review. *Cytokine Growth Factor Rev.* **2009**, *20*, 305–317. [CrossRef] [PubMed]

44. Nguyen, A.V.; Pollard, J.W. Transforming growth factor beta3 induces cell death during the first stage of mammary gland involution. *Development* **2000**, *127*, 3107–3118. [PubMed]

45. Ogawa, J.; Sasahara, A.; Yoshida, T.; Sira, M.M.; Futatani, T.; Kanegane, H.; Miyawaki, T. Role of transforming growth factor-beta in breast milk for initiation of IgA production in newborn infants. *Early Hum. Dev.* **2004**, *77*, 67–75. [CrossRef] [PubMed]

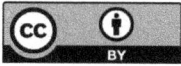

nutrients

MDPI

Article

Leptin Levels Are Higher in Whole Compared to Skim Human Milk, Supporting a Cellular Contribution

Sambavi Kugananthan [1,2], Ching Tat Lai [2], Zoya Gridneva [2], Peter J. Mark [1], Donna T. Geddes [2,*] and Foteini Kakulas [2]

[1] School of Anatomy, Physiology and Human Biology, The University of Western Australia, Perth 6009, Australia; 21141062@student.uwa.edu.au (S.K.); peter.mark@uwa.edu.au (P.J.M.)
[2] School of Chemistry and Biochemistry, The University of Western Australia, Perth 6009, Australia; ching-tat.lai@uwa.edu.au (C.T.L.); zgridneva@gmail.com (Z.G.); foteini.kakulas@bigpond.com (F.K.)
* Correspondence: donna.geddes@uwa.edu.au; Tel.: +61-8-6488-4467

Received: 27 September 2016; Accepted: 2 November 2016; Published: 8 November 2016

Abstract: Human milk (HM) contains a plethora of metabolic hormones, including leptin, which is thought to participate in the regulation of the appetite of the developing infant. Leptin in HM is derived from a combination of de novo mammary synthesis and transfer from the maternal serum. Moreover, leptin is partially lipophilic and is also present in HM cells. However, leptin has predominately been measured in skim HM, which contains neither fat nor cells. We optimised an enzyme-linked immunosorbent assay for leptin measurement in both whole and skim HM and compared leptin levels between both HM preparations collected from 61 lactating mothers. Whole HM leptin ranged from 0.2 to 1.47 ng/mL, whilst skim HM leptin ranged from 0.19 to 0.9 ng/mL. Whole HM contained, on average, 0.24 ± 0.01 ng/mL more leptin than skim HM ($p < 0.0001$, $n = 287$). No association was found between whole HM leptin and fat content ($p = 0.17$, $n = 287$), supporting a cellular contribution to HM leptin. No difference was found between pre- and post-feed samples (whole HM: $p = 0.29$, skim HM: $p = 0.89$). These findings highlight the importance of optimising HM leptin measurement and assaying it in whole HM to accurately examine the amount of leptin received by the infant during breastfeeding.

Keywords: leptin; human milk; whole human milk; skim human milk; appetite; obesity

1. Introduction

Human milk (HM) is a heterogeneous fluid composed of a combination of macro- and micro-nutrients, cells, and a plethora of biomolecules that provide the necessary elements to sustain infant growth, protection and development [1–3]. The developmental effects of breastfeeding extend to the programming of various organs and systems of the newborn, including that of appetite regulation [4]. This early developmental programming results in a reduction in obesity and other metabolic diseases not only in the short-term, but also in adulthood [5–9]. The complex system of breastfeeding-mediated appetite regulation is attributable to various factors associated with the practice of breastfeeding, such as feeding on demand, but also potentially to a host of appetite regulatory molecules present in HM [4]. These include whey and casein proteins, HM oligosaccharides, and recently discovered in HM appetite regulatory hormones, including the well-documented adipokine leptin, adiponectin, and many others [10–14].

Amongst these appetite molecules, leptin is the most widely studied, being primarily known for promoting satiety and energy expenditure in adults through binding to the full length leptin receptor (ObRb) expressed on the arcuate nucleus of the hypothalamus [15]. In addition, leptin stimulates cell proliferation, regulates blood pressure, and is also involved in the T-cell immune response, thus displaying pleiotropic roles [16,17]. White adipose tissue is one of the main sources of serum leptin, secreting leptin proportionally to the number of white adipocytes present in the body [18]. Further, gastric chief cells, the placenta, and the mammary epithelium also synthesise and secrete leptin in adults [19–22].

In infants, HM is believed to be a major source of leptin early in life, with the endogenous leptin-synthesising mechanisms being still immature [23]. Leptin in HM has been hypothesised to be involved both in the short-term control of appetite and in developmental programming of appetite and energy-signalling pathways, promoting efficient energy control and storage throughout life [9,24]. Leptin administered during the first 14 days of life has been shown to act as a neurotrophic agent, promoting neural growth from the arcuate nucleus of the hypothalamus to additional appetite control centres located in the central nervous system [25]. HM leptin may provide short-term appetite control in the infant also by up-regulating circulating melanocortins, potent anorexigenic agents that promote satiety [26]. Leptin in HM is sourced both endogenously from the mammary gland and from the maternal serum, following secretion from white adipocytes and gastric chief cells into the bloodstream [9]. In the lactating mammary gland, serum-derived leptin combines with locally-synthesised leptin by the mammary epithelium to yield the total leptin content of HM [22].

Leptin in HM has been predominately measured in skim HM, which does not contain the cellular and fat components of HM [26–28]. Considering that the leptin peptide is capable of lipophilic interactions [29,30], it is plausible it may associate with the fat globule in whole HM. Moreover, HM cells, which are predominantly of epithelial origin in mature HM of healthy mother/infant dyads [1,31], are also thought to contribute to the leptin concentration of whole HM [22]. Few previous studies have measured leptin in whole HM using a radioimmuno-assay (RIA) [21,32]. However, RIA is not considered appropriate for measuring leptin in a lipid-rich medium such as whole HM due to interference of triglycerides with the binding of radioactive-labelled antigens to antibodies, which compromises the sensitivity of the assay [33,34]. Given the lack of an optimised assay to detect leptin in whole HM and the absence of reliable comparisons of leptin levels between whole and skim HM, we developed an enzyme-linked immunosorbent assay (ELISA) as a more appropriate means of measuring leptin in HM, with two antibodies assisting in immobilising the leptin antigen, and compared the leptin concentration between pre- and post-feed samples, as well as whole and skim HM.

2. Materials and Methods

2.1. Study Participants

All procedures involving the recruitment of lactating mothers and HM sample collection and analyses were approved by, and conducted in accordance with, the guidelines of the Human Research Ethics Committee of The University of Western Australia (ethics approval number RA/4/1/4253). All mothers provided informed written consent in the form of a secure online questionnaire that was administered and securely stored by The University of Western Australia. A single sample of whole HM expressed by a mother in her first month of lactation was used for optimisation of the leptin assay. Following assay optimisation, 61 lactating mothers (38 Caucasian, 23 non-Caucasian) with a mean maternal age of 33.6 ± 4.39 years, of full-term healthy infants were recruited to assess leptin differences between whole and skim HM (Table 1). HM samples (~5 mL) were obtained at approximately 1100 h aseptically, as previously described by Hassiotou et al. [35], from each breast before and after the infant fed from a single breast session either by using a Medela Symphony (Medela AG, Baar, Zug, Switzerland) breast pump or by hand expression. Samples were stored at -20 °C prior to analysis. Samples were collected at the second, fifth, ninth, and 12th months of lactation (Table 1).

Table 1. Maternal and infant anthropometric and demographic characteristics (*n* = 61). Values are mean ± SD (range). Table includes mothers who provided samples for multiple months.

Stage of Lactation (Month)	2	5	9	12
Maternal age (years)	32.9 ± 4.21 (28–40)	33.4 ± 4.27 (24–40)	34.0 ± 4.57 (25–43)	34.1 ± 4.35 (26–44)
Maternal BMI	27.1 ± 7.15 (20.1–38.5)	23.5 ± 4.46 (18.0–35.2)	24.0 ± 5.15 (18.7–37.2)	24.8 ± 5.6 (18.2–34.6)
Parity	2.10 ± 0.75 (1–4)	2.13 ± 0.85 (1–4)	1.96 ± 0.94 (1–4)	2.05 ± 0.98 (1–4)
Infant sex (Male/Female)	12/9	16/16	17/13	12/12
Infant birth weight (kg)	3.58 ± 0.64 (2.66–4.23)	3.49 ± 0.45 (2.66–4.46)	3.49 ± 0.46 (2.82–4.46)	3.59 ± 0.46 (2.80–4.46)
Infant body length (cm)	57.6 ± 2.17 (54.2–61.3)	64.5 ± 2.09 (61.5–69.5)	70.9 ± 2.11 (68.0–74.5)	73.9 ± 2.38 (71.5–78.5)

BMI: body mass index.

2.2. Measurement of Leptin in Whole and Skim Human Milk by an Enzyme-Linked Immunosorbent Assay (ELISA)

Whole HM samples were thawed at room temperature, vortexed for 10 s and aliquoted (2 × 750 µL) into 1.5 mL microfuge tubes (Sarstedt, Numbrecht, Germany). One whole HM aliquot was centrifuged (05PR-22 Refrigerated Centrifuge, Hitachi, Tokyo, Japan) at 1500× *g* for 10 min at 4 °C and the resultant skim HM portion was aspirated. Both skim and whole HM aliquots were sonicated on ice at 100 Hz for three cycles of 5 s pulses, with a 20 s rest interval using an ultrasonic processor VCX130 (Sonics and Material, Newton, CT, USA). Eleven dilutions ranging from 1 to 50-fold were prepared from both milk preparations using 1% bovine serum albumin (BSA; Sigma-Aldrich, Castle Hill, NSW, Australia) in phosphate-buffered saline (PBS; Gibco Life Technologies, Paisley, Scotland).

Leptin concentration for each dilution was measured using the Human Leptin ELISA DuoSet (R&D Systems, Minneapolis, MN, USA). Capture antibody (4 ng/mL, diluted with PBS, pH 7.4) was pipetted (100 µL per well) to coat the bottom of the wells of flat bottom 96-well microtiter plates (Flow Laboratories, McLean, VA, USA). Plates were sealed and incubated overnight at room temperature. Wells were washed three times with PBS/Tween wash buffer (0.05% Tween 20; (Bio-Rad Laboratories, Gladesville, NSW, Australia) in PBS, pH 7.4), dispensed at 400 µL per well, using a plate washer (Immunowash 1575, Bio-Rad Laboratories, Hercules, CA, USA). Washed plates were inverted and blotted against absorbent paper to ensure no remaining solution was present inside the wells. Blocking buffer (1% *w/v* BSA in PBS, pH 7.4) was added (300 µL per well) to block non-specific binding sites. Plates were sealed and incubated for one hour at room temperature. Blocking buffer was washed according to the wash procedure described earlier. Diluted samples and standards (0–0.9 ng/mL) were added (100 µL per well) in duplicates and plates were sealed and incubated for 2 h at room temperature. Unbound components from samples and standards were washed, and biotinylated detection antibody (4 ng/mL, diluted in 1% *w/v* BSA in PBS, pH 7.4) was added (100 µL per well). Plates were sealed and incubated for 2 h at room temperature. Unbound detection antibody was washed, and streptavidin-horseradish peroxidase (HRP; R&D Systems, Minneapolis, MN, USA) (50 ng/mL in PBS, pH 7.4) was added (100 µL per well), and plates were sealed, wrapped in aluminium foil to avoid exposure to direct light, and incubated for 20 min at room temperature. Streptavidin-HRP was washed and substrate colour reagent (1:1 mixture of 12 mL/vial hydrogen peroxide and 4 mL/vial enhanced luminol, R&D Systems, Minneapolis, MN, USA) was added (100 µL per well). Plates were sealed and wrapped in aluminium foil and were incubated for 20 min at room temperature. Sulphuric acid (1 M, R&D Systems, Minneapolis, MN, USA) stop solution was added (50 µL per well) and absorbance was read at 450 nm by a plate spectrophotometer (Enspire Multimode Plate Reader, Waltham, MA, USA). Standard curves and leptin concentrations were calculated using linear regression (Figures 1 and 2).

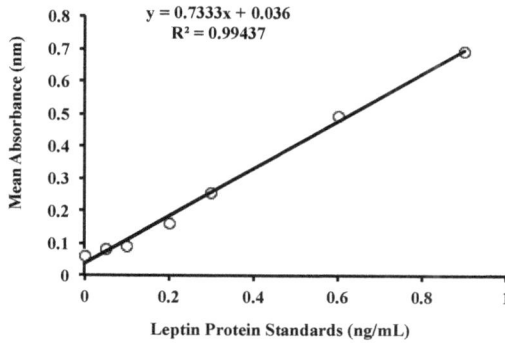

Figure 1. Standard curve for the leptin enzyme-linked immunoassay (ELISA) for whole and skim human milk. Standards were selected according to previous literature investigating levels of leptin in skim human milk, as well as recommendations provided by the leptin kit manufacturer [36].

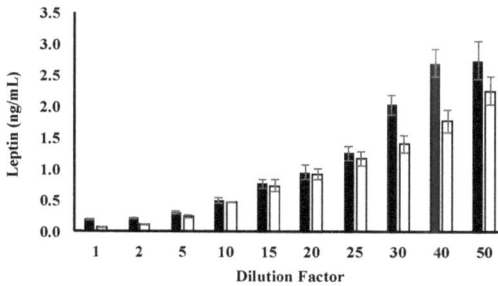

Figure 2. Leptin concentration for whole and skim human milk for each dilution tested. Values are mean $\pm$ SEM (n = 100 diluted human milk preparations). Leptin levels in whole and skim human milk are shown by black and white bars, respectively.

Recovery assays to discern the optimal dilution factor for leptin detection were conducted on dilutions reporting leptin concentrations within the range of the protein standards used (Table 2). Following optimisation of the dilution factor, leptin concentration in matched whole and skim HM samples from the study population was measured. All whole and skim HM samples were prepared according to the same centrifugation and sonication protocol used in the assay optimisation. Recovery of a known amount of the leptin protein when added to samples was 97.7% $\pm$ 9.7% (n = 10) (Table 2), with the leptin kit reporting an intra-assay variability of <5% and an inter-assay variability of <7.2%.

Table 2. Recovery percentages for each dilution factor for skim and whole human milk leptin measurement.

Dilution Factor	Skim Human Milk Leptin (%)	Whole Human Milk Leptin (%)
1	61.5 $\pm$ 2.09	17.1 $\pm$ 2.9
2	179.0 $\pm$ 0.82	14.0 $\pm$ 2.7
5	96.3 $\pm$ 1.2	14.0 $\pm$ 1.4
10	71.3 $\pm$ 1.6	97.1 $\pm$ 9.1

2.3. Measurement of Fat Content in Human Milk

The total fat content of HM samples was measured using the creamatocrit method [37,38]. Samples were placed in micro-haematocrit tubes, plugged with sealant and centrifuged at $12,000 \times g$ for ten min in a micro-haematocrit centrifuge (Hermle Z230H Labortechnik, Wehingen, Germany). The resultant milk column was placed on the creamatocrit analyser (Creamatocrit Plus, Medela Inc., McHenry, IL, USA) and the length of the fat layer and the total milk column was measured, from which the total fat content was calculated. It has been shown that Creamatocrit measurements strongly correlate with the biochemical spectroscopic esterified fatty acid assay [38–40].

2.4. Statistical Analyses

Statistical analyses were performed using Microsoft Excel 2013 (Microsoft Corporation, Redmond, WA, USA) and R 2.9.10 (R Core Team, Vienna, Austria) [41] for Windows 10, with the additional R package "nlme" (R Core Team, Vienna, Austria) used for linear mixed effects modelling [42]. Student's paired *t*-tests were conducted to assess leptin differences between matched skim and whole HM samples in the entire study population. Differences between whole and skim HM leptin concentrations were subsequently analysed within each month of breastfeeding, also using matched Student's *t*-test.

Linear mixed effects modelling was used to examine any associations between HM fat content and whole HM leptin concentration. Responses were modelled with and without controlling for the volume of milk that had been removed from the breast during the collection of the HM sample. To discern the significant random effects to use for each statistical model analysing the association between HM fat content and whole HM leptin concentration, three separate models were devised; one linear model with no random effects and two linear mixed effects models with the following random effects: the effect of general inter-individual variation present in the study population, and the effect of the stage of lactation in addition to inter-individual variation. Analysis of variance (ANOVA) tests were then used to compare each model with the same fixed effects, namely fat content and fat content when controlled for volume of milk removed from the breast. The final model for the association between whole HM leptin concentration and fat content accounted for inter-individual variation and the stage of lactation as random effects when volume removed was not controlled for in the model. Similarly, when volume of milk removed from the breast was controlled for in the linear mixed effects models, inter-individual variation and stage of lactation were also considered as significant random variables to include in the analysis of associations between fat content and whole HM leptin concentration.

Similarly, the association between leptin concentration in whole HM samples and the corresponding fat content was also analysed within each month of lactation. Given that the volume of HM removed during feeding was only collected for 74 samples out of the entire study population, the liner mixed effects models used for intra-month analysis did not control for volume of milk removed from the breast. As with the analysis between the association of leptin levels in whole HM samples and fat content for the entire population, for each month, three statistical models were devised; one linear model with no random effects, and two linear mixed effects models with the following random variables included: the effect of inter-individual variation present in the study population and the effect of the stage of lactation in addition to inter-individual variation. Analysis of variance (ANOVA) was then used to compare each model within each month. For each month of breastfeeding, the only significant random effect found was general inter-individual variation. $p < 0.05$ was considered statistically significant. All values presented are mean $\pm$ standard deviation (SD), unless stated otherwise. All R^2 values were generated from the linear regression line of best fit equations.

3. Results

3.1. Participants

The demographic characteristics of mothers and infants in the study population are shown in Table 2. All infants ($n = 61$) were born at term, healthy, and were growing appropriately for their age according to the World Health Organisation's (WHO) growth charts for exclusively-breastfed infants [43,44]. Mean maternal body mass index (BMI) was highest at 27.1 ± 7.15 kg/m^2 during the second month of lactation and lowest during the fifth month of lactation at 23.5 ± 4.46 kg/m^2 (Table 1). Compared to the second month of lactation, maternal BMI decreased by 2.30 ± 1.55 kg/m^2 over the first 12 months of breastfeeding ($p < 0.01$).

3.2. Leptin Optimisation

Measurement of leptin in whole and skim HM was optimised using an ELISA-based assay. One- to 20-fold dilutions for both skim and whole HM yielded leptin concentrations within the standard range of the assay (0–0.9 ng/mL), whilst dilutions above 20-fold reported values Redmond outside of the upper protein standard used (Figure 2). Mean leptin concentrations for 15-fold (whole HM: 0.8 ± 0.07 ng/mL, skim HM: 0.75 ± 0.09 ng/mL) and 20-fold (whole HM: 0.9 ± 0.11 ng/mL, skim HM: 0.9 ± 0.09 ng/mL) dilutions were close to the highest protein standard, thus further consideration was not given to these dilution factors (Figure 2). Ten-fold dilution of whole HM yielded the best recovery rates ($97.7\% \pm 9.7\%$) (Table 2). Five-fold-diluted skim HM recovered $96.3\% \pm 1.2\%$ of leptin (Table 2). Therefore, subsequent samples were diluted by 10-fold and five-fold with the diluent reagent for whole and skim HM samples, respectively, given these dilution factors recovered the highest percentage of leptin protein when the assay was performed for whole and skim HM.

3.3. Whole and Skim Human Milk Leptin

Leptin levels measured using the optimised assay were compared between whole and skim HM obtained during different stages of lactation from 61 lactating mothers. Whole HM leptin levels ranged from 0.2–1.47 ng/mL, whilst a 0.19–0.9 ng/mL range was obtained for skim HM leptin (Figure 3). Whole HM leptin was 0.24 ± 0.01 ng/mL higher than skim HM leptin across all samples ($p < 0.0001$, $n = 287$) (Figure 3). Leptin levels were also higher in whole HM compared to skim HM within each month of lactation (Table 3). Matched pre-feed whole HM samples contained 0.24 ± 0.07 ng/mL more leptin than pre-feed skim preparations ($p < 0.01$, $n = 157$), with 0.25 ng/mL $\pm$ 0.05 ng/mL more leptin measured in post-feed whole HM samples compared to paired skim post-feed aliquots ($p < 0.01$, $n = 137$).

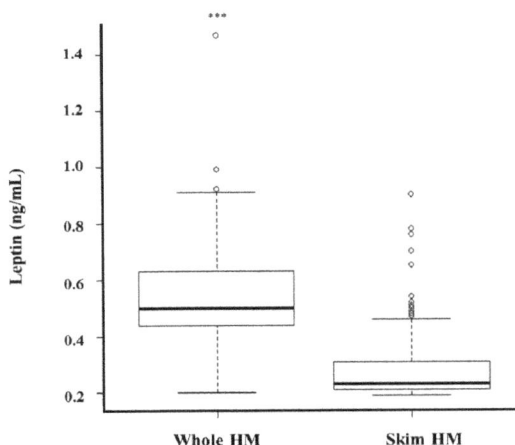

Figure 3. Comparison between whole and skim human milk (HM) leptin concentration (n = 287). *** Indicates significant difference between matched whole and skim human milk leptin values (p < 0.001).

No association was observed between whole and skim HM leptin (p = 0.55, n = 287) (Figure 4a). HM fat content was not related to leptin concentration in whole HM when the volume of milk removed from the breast during sample collection was not accounted for (p = 0.52, n = 283) (Figure 4b) or accounted for (p = 0.24, n = 74) in the analysis. Further, no association between leptin levels in whole HM samples and fat content were found within each stage of lactation (Table 4).

Table 3. Leptin concentrations for whole and skim human milk at each month of lactation. Values are mean ± SD.

Month of Lactation	Whole Human Milk Leptin (ng/mL)	Skim Human Milk Leptin (ng/mL)	p-Value *
2	0.50 ± 0.16	0.32 ± 0.16	p < 0.0001
5	0.48 ± 0.16	0.26 ± 0.07	p < 0.0001
9	0.56 ± 0.11	0.22 ± 0.03	p < 0.0001
12	0.54 ± 0.14	0.21 ± 0.02	p < 0.0001

* p-values indicate significant differences between whole and skim human milk leptin concentrations at given time points.

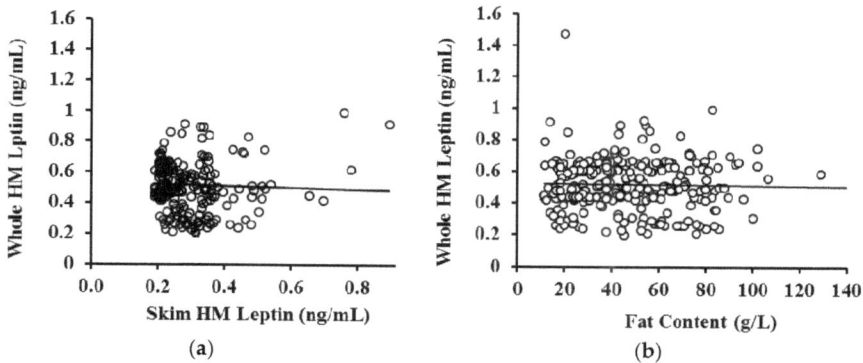

Figure 4. (a) Association between skim and whole human milk (HM) leptin ($n = 287$). No association was detected between skim and whole HM leptin levels in matched samples ($R^2 = 0.001$, $p = 0.552$); (b) no association was detected between fat content and leptin concentration in whole HM ($R^2 = 0.0004$, $p = 0.17$, $n = 284$). The solid black line is the line of best fit.

Table 4. Association between leptin levels in whole human milk and fat content at each stage of lactation.

Month of Lactation	N (Samples)	R^2	p-Value *
2	66	0.0013	0.782
5	72	0.018	0.686
9	83	0.069	0.577
12	66	0.153	0.889

* p-values indicate absence of associations between whole human milk leptin concentrations and fat concentrations at given time points.

No differences between pre- and post-feed whole ($p = 0.29$, $n = 74$) and skim ($p = 0.89$, $n = 74$) leptin levels were detected after accounting for the volume of milk consumed by the infant during the session (Figure 5). Post-feed samples contained 36.2 ± 2.82 g/L more fat compared to matched pre-feed samples ($p < 0.01$, $n = 74$).

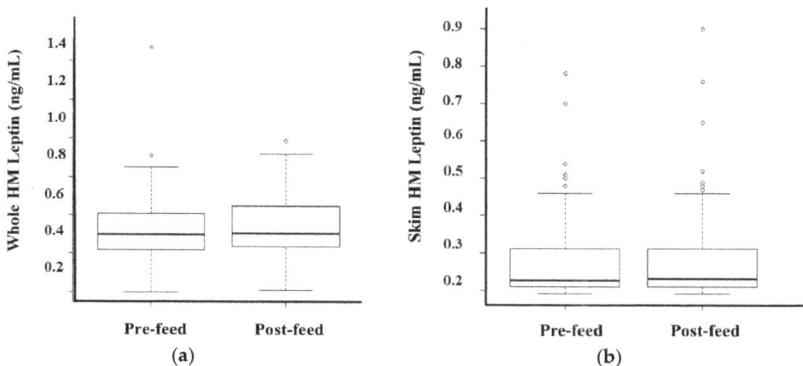

Figure 5. After accounting for the volume of milk consumed by the infant during the session, no differences in pre- and post-feed (a) whole and (b) skim human milk (HM) leptin values were detected in the study population.

4. Discussion

This study has shown that whole HM contains significantly higher levels of leptin compared to skim HM and that sampling either before or after a breastfeed does not influence this level.

Leptin has been previously shown to be present in HM and has been hypothesised to participate in the short- and long-term regulation of appetite in the breastfed infant [9,45]. In addition, HM leptin may be involved in other functions in the breastfed infant given its known pleiotropic properties, and in mammary development [46,47]. Although many studies have previously measured leptin in HM, optimisation of the methodology has not been well documented and most studies have focused on the levels of leptin in skim HM. However, leptin has been proposed to have lipophilic properties [29] and is also synthesised by mammary epithelial cells [22], which comprise the majority of cells in mature HM from healthy mother/infant dyads [1,48,49]. It is, therefore, conceivable that leptin in HM is associated with the fat and/or cells, which are not present in its skim fraction, suggesting that previous measurements of skim HM leptin have underestimated the concentration of leptin in HM. In this study, we performed a comparison of leptin levels between whole and skim HM and optimised an ELISA assay to accurately measure it in both HM preparations.

Leptin levels were found to be, on average, two-fold higher in whole HM compared to skim HM (Figure 3, Table 3). There are limited studies that have compared whole and skim HM leptin levels and they utilized RIA based methodologies. While results of our study are in agreement with two previous studies that found higher levels of leptin in whole than skim HM, the actual values are different. Houseknecht et al. [32] reported whole HM leptin levels (10.1 ± 2.6 ng/mL, $n = 23$) that were approximately seven times higher than in skim HM (1.5 ± 0.87 ng/mL, $n = 23$) and, on average, 20 times higher than levels found in this study (Figure 3). Moreover, Smith-Kirwin et al. [21] reported 56-fold higher leptin levels in whole HM (73.2 ± 39.0 ng/mL, $n = 8$) compared to skim HM (approximately 1.3 ng/mL), and a 130-fold higher mean whole HM leptin concentration compared to the present study. For skim HM both studies observed leptin levels 1.5–2.5 times greater than those found here [21]. The higher absolute leptin levels measured in these studies may be attributable to the analysis. Both studies used the RIA technique, which is not as reliable as ELISA in measuring leptin levels in whole HM due to its known inaccuracies of immune-reactive antibodies binding to the epitopes of antigens suspended in a lipid-rich medium, such as whole HM, or of interference of iron and emulsifiers with the assay [33,34]. In addition, differences in the technique optimisation between the two previous studies are apparent, as the whole HM leptin level in one study is seven times greater than the other. Both commercially available RIA and ELISA kits are originally designed to measure leptin in serum, not in HM; therefore, optimisation is critical. On the other hand, our results are comparable to leptin levels in many other studies that measured it in skim HM using ELISA, or whole and skim HM using RIA. ELISA in skim HM detected similar leptin levels (from 0.30 ± 0.04 ng/mL at 1 month to 0.10 ± 0.02 ng/mL at 12 months, $n = 72$) in a study by Bronsky et al. [50], (0.28 ± 0.38 ng/mL, $n = 651$) in a study by Weyermann et al. [27], and (0.16 ± 0.04 ng/mL, $n = 28$) in a study by Miralles et al. [26]. RIA in skim HM also detected close leptin levels: (0.18 ± 0.15 ng/mL, $n = 23$) in a study by Schuster et al. [28] and (1.00 ± 0.80 ng/mL, $n = 13$) in a study by Schueler et al. [51]. RIA results in whole HM (1.34 ± 0.14, $n = 24$) in a study by Bielicki et al. [52] were also comparable to our whole HM leptin levels.

Whilst it has been hypothesised that leptin may be associated with fat globules present in whole HM due to its lipophilic nature [21,29] this was not borne out in this study (Figure 4b, tab:nutrients-08-00711-t004) despite analysing pre- and post-feeding milk samples with a wide range of fat content of 11.0–128.8 g/L. The lack of an association between HM fat content and whole HM leptin levels suggests that fat may not have a strong contribution to HM leptin levels compared to the cellular fraction of HM. Lactocytes, myoepithelial cells, and stem cells present in HM have been previously shown to express the leptin gene [22]. Additionally, flow cytometric analysis of HM cells has revealed that the majority of lactocytes and stem cells contain the leptin protein [22]. Given that lactocytes are the dominant cell type in mature whole HM when both the mother and infant are healthy [1,48,49,53,54], it is likely that lactocytes contribute significantly to HM leptin levels. Indeed, the cellular fraction of HM can constitute a significant portion of milk, comparable to its skim and fat fractions [1,31]. This warrants investigation to further discern the cellular contribution to leptin levels in whole HM, and emphasises the need to assay whole HM for leptin and, potentially, for other appetite hormones, to obtain accurate measurements of the levels of these hormones in HM. Importantly, the procedures of whole HM preparation for such measurements must enable complete lysis of the milk cells for accurate results. This is also very important during sample preparation for whole HM ELISA, achieved in the present study by sonication.

Higher leptin levels in whole HM compared to the skim fraction indicate that infants ingest a larger dose of leptin than that calculated from skim HM. Whilst HM cells likely contribute to the increased leptin level in whole HM the bioavailability of this source is unknown. However, we speculate that the process of digestion would release leptin proteins from HM cells. It is also possible that these cells are absorbed through the stomach mucosa after ingestion and enter the circulation, as has been confirmed with HM leukocytes and stem cells [35,55].

The lack of an association between whole HM leptin and milk fat content may be also attributable to the biochemical properties of the leptin peptide. Although paradoxical to the notion that leptin is synthesised by white adipocytes which exhibit a lipophilic nature, leptin may also consist of hydrophilic regions, enabling it to primarily interact with aqueous fluids. The specific hydrophilic regions exhibited on the leptin peptide are hypothesised to be conserved cysteine residues tethered to disulphide bridges [29,56], which may form polar bonds with water molecules, given sulphide's strong electronegativity properties [57]. Leptin crystallization studies could further confirm its hydrophilic properties [56], providing insight into the lack of an association between the leptin protein and the fat component of whole HM.

Upon analysis, we also found no difference between the concentration of whole HM leptin in pre- and post-feed samples, indicating the small samples taken either pre- or post-feed provide the same levels of leptin despite differences in fat content. To measure the cellular contribution of leptin in HM, it may be possible to acquire larger pre- and post-feed sample volumes and examine the number of cells in the sample. Hassiotou et al. [1] has shown that cell content increases post-feed, as does fat, when larger sample volumes were attained or the breast was well drained of milk.

5. Conclusions

We describe the first standardised and optimised ELISA assay for the measurement of leptin in both skim and whole HM, demonstrating higher concentrations of leptin in whole HM preparations compared to skim HM samples. Further, we provide evidence supporting the lack of an association between the fat component of HM and its leptin content, suggesting a contribution of HM cells, which merits further investigation. Accurate analysis of whole HM leptin will assist in clarifying the biological role of this milk component for the breastfed infant, improving our understanding of early developmental programming of appetite and its implications for obesity prevention later in life.

Acknowledgments: This study was supported by an unrestricted research grant from Medela AG (Switzerland). Sambavi Kugananthan received a Margaret Lomann-Hall Scholarship from the School of Anatomy, Physiology and Human Biology, The University of Western Australia. Zoya Gridneva received an Australian Postgraduate Award from The University of Western Australia (Australia). Many thanks are extended to all mothers who participated in this study, and to the Australian Breastfeeding Association for assistance in recruitment of participants.

Author Contributions: Sambavi Kugananthan designed the study, conducted experiments and data analyses, interpreted results, and wrote the manuscript; Ching Tat Lai conducted experiments and data analyses, and critically reviewed the manuscript; Zoya Gridneva conducted experiments, collected the data, and critically reviewed the manuscript; Peter J. Mark designed the study, interpreted results, and critically reviewed the manuscript; Donna T. Geddes designed the study, interpreted results, and critically reviewed the manuscript; Foteini Kakulas designed the study, interpreted results and critically reviewed the manuscript.

Conflicts of Interest: The authors declare that Medela AG provides an unrestricted research grant to Donna T. Geddes from which salaries to Foteini Kakulas, Donna T. Geddes and Ching Tat Lai are paid. Medela AG provided a Top-up Scholarship for Zoya Gridneva, and has provided speaker's fees to Donna T. Geddes for educational lectures. The funding sponsors had no role in the design of the study; in the collection, analyses, or interpretation of data; in the writing of the manuscript, or in the decision to publish the results.

Abbreviations

The following abbreviations are used in this manuscript:

HM	Human milk
ELISA	Enzyme linked immunosorbent assay
RIA	Radioimmunoassay
PBS	Phosphate-buffered solution
BMI	Body mass index
SD	Standard deviation
SEM	Standard error of the mean

References

1. Hassiotou, F.; Geddes, D.T.; Hartmann, P.E. Cells in Human Milk: State of the Science. *J. Hum. Lact.* **2013**, *29*, 171–182. [CrossRef] [PubMed]
2. Ballard, O.; Morrow, A.L. Human Milk Composition: Nutrients and Bioactive Factors. *Pediatr. Clin. N. Am.* **2013**, *60*, 49–74. [CrossRef] [PubMed]
3. Hamosh, M. Bioactive Factors in Human Milk. *Pediatr. Clin. N. Am.* **2001**, *48*, 69–86. [CrossRef]
4. Hassiotou, F.; Geddes, D.T. Programming of Appetite Control during Breastfeeding as a Preventative Strategy against the Obesity Epidemic. *J. Hum. Lact.* **2014**, *30*, 136–142. [CrossRef] [PubMed]
5. Von Kries, R.; Koletzko, B.; Sauerwald, T.; von Mutius, E.; Barnert, D.; Grunert, V.; von Voss, H. Breast feeding and obesity: cross sectional study. *BMJ* **1999**, *319*, 147–150. [CrossRef] [PubMed]
6. Gillman, M.W.; Rifas-Shiman, S.L.; Camargo, C.A., Jr.; Berkey, C.S.; Frazier, A.L.; Rockett, H.R.; Field, A.E.; Colditz, G.A. Risk of overweight among adolescents who were breastfed as infants. *JAMA* **2001**, *285*, 2461–2467. [CrossRef] [PubMed]
7. Armstrong, J.; Reilly, J.J. Breastfeeding and lowering the risk of childhood obesity. *Lancet* **2002**, *359*, 2003–4. [CrossRef]
8. Bouret, S.G.; Bates, S.H.; Chen, S.; Myers, M.G.; Simerly, R.B. Distinct Roles for Specific Leptin Receptor Signals in the Development of Hypothalamic Feeding Circuits. *J. Neurosci.* **2012**, *32*, 1244–1252. [CrossRef] [PubMed]
9. Pico, C.; Oliver, P.; Sanchez, J.; Miralles, O.; Caimari, A.; Priego, T.; Palou, A. The intake of physiological doses of leptin during lactation in rats prevents obesity in later life. *Int. J. Obes.* **2007**, *31*, 1199–1209. [CrossRef] [PubMed]
10. Savino, F.; Liguori, S.A.; Petrucci, E.; Lupica, M.M.; Fissore, M.F.; Oggero, R.; Silvestro, L. Evaluation of leptin in breast milk, lactating mothers and their infants. *Eur. J. Clin. Nutr.* **2010**, *64*, 972–977. [CrossRef] [PubMed]
11. Savino, F.; Lupica, M.M.; Benetti, S.; Petrucci, E.; Liguori, S.A.; Cordero Di Montezemolo, L. Adiponectin in breast milk: Relation to serum adiponectin concentration in lactating mothers and their infants. *Acta Paediatr.* **2012**, *101*, 1058–1062. [CrossRef] [PubMed]
12. Savino, F.; Sorrenti, M.; Benetti, S.; Lupica, M.M.; Liguori, S.A.; Oggero, R. Resistin and leptin in breast milk and infants in early life. *Early Hum. Dev.* **2012**, *88*, 779–782. [CrossRef] [PubMed]
13. Alderete, T.L.; Autran, C.; Brekke, B.E.; Knight, R.; Bode, L.; Goran, M.I.; Fields, D.A. Associations between human milk oligosaccharides and infant body composition in the first 6 mo of life. *Am. J. Clin. Nutr.* **2015**, *102*, 1381–1388. [CrossRef] [PubMed]
14. Alvarez, M. Proteins in human milk. *Breastfeed. Rev.* **2007**, *15*, 5–16.
15. Tartaglia, L.A.; Dembski, M.; Weng, X.; Deng, N.; Culpepper, J.; Devos, R.; Richards, G.J.; Campfield, L.A.; Clark, F.T.; Deeds, J.; et al. Identification and expression cloning of a leptin receptor, OB-R. *Cell* **1995**, *83*, 1263–1271. [CrossRef]
16. Bassi, M.; Furuya, W.I.; Zoccal, D.B.; Menani, J.V.; Colombari, E.; Hall, J.E.; do Carmo, J.M.; Colombari, D.S. Control of respiratory and cardiovascular functions by leptin. *Life Sci.* **2015**, *125*, 25–31. [CrossRef] [PubMed]
17. Magariños, M.P.; Sánchez-Margalet, V.; Kotler, M.; Calvo, J.C.; Varone, C.L. Leptin Promotes Cell Proliferation and Survival of Trophoblastic Cells. *Biol. Reprod.* **2007**, *76*, 203–210. [CrossRef] [PubMed]
18. Klein, S.; Coppack, S.W.; Mohamed-Ali, V.; Landt, M. Adipose Tissue Leptin Production and Plasma Leptin Kinetics in Humans. *Diabetes* **1996**, *45*, 984–987. [CrossRef] [PubMed]

19. Myers, M.G., Jr. Leptin receptor signaling and the regulation of mammalian physiology. *Recent Prog. Horm. Res.* **2004**, *59*, 287–304. [CrossRef] [PubMed]

20. Mix, H.; Widjaja, A.; Jandl, O.; Cornberg, M.; Kaul, A.; Goke, M.; Beil, W.; Kuske, M.; Brabant, G.; Manns, M.P.; et al. Expression of leptin and leptin receptor isoforms in the human stomach. *Gut* **2000**, *47*, 481–486. [CrossRef] [PubMed]

21. Smith-Kirwin, S.M.; O'Connor, D.M.; De Johnston, J.; Lancey, E.D.; Hassink, S.G.; Funanage, V.L. Leptin expression in human mammary epithelial cells and breast milk. *J. Clin. Endocrinol. Metab.* **1998**, *83*, 1810–1813. [CrossRef] [PubMed]

22. Hassiotou, F.; Savigni, D.; Hartmann, P.; Geddes, D. Mammary cells synthesize appetite hormones that may contribute to breastmilk. In Proceedings of the Bi-annual Conference of International Society for Research in Human Milk and Lactation, Charleston, SC, USA, 27 October 2014.

23. Oliver, P.; Pico, C.; De Matteis, R.; Cinti, S.; Palou, A. Perinatal expression of leptin in rat stomach. *Dev. Dyn. Off. Publ. Am. Assoc. Anat.* **2002**, *223*, 148–154. [CrossRef] [PubMed]

24. Bouret, S.G.; Draper, S.J.; Simerly, R.B. Formation of projection pathways from the arcuate nucleus of the hypothalamus to hypothalamic regions implicated in the neural control of feeding behavior in mice. *J. Neurosci. Off. J. Soc. Neurosci.* **2004**, *24*, 2797–2805. [CrossRef] [PubMed]

25. Proulx, K.; Richard, D.; Walker, C.D. Leptin regulates appetite-related neuropeptides in the hypothalamus of developing rats without affecting food intake. *Endocrinology* **2002**, *143*, 4683–4692. [CrossRef] [PubMed]

26. Miralles, O.; Sanchez, J.; Palou, A.; Pico, C. A physiological role of breast milk leptin in body weight control in developing infants. *Obesity (Silver Spring, MD)* **2006**, *14*, 1371–1377. [CrossRef] [PubMed]

27. Weyermann, M.; Beermann, C.; Brenner, H.; Dietrich, R. Adiponectin and Leptin in Maternal Serum, Cord Blood, and Breast Milk. *Clin. Chem.* **2006**, *52*, 2095–2102. [CrossRef] [PubMed]

28. Schuster, S.; Hechler, C.; Gebauer, C.; Kiess, W.; Kratzsch, J. Leptin in maternal serum and breast milk: association with infants' body weight gain in a longitudinal study over 6 months of lactation. *Pediatr. Res.* **2011**, *70*, 633–637. [CrossRef] [PubMed]

29. Kline, A.D.; Becker, G.W.; Churgay, L.M.; Landen, B.E.; Martin, D.K.; Muth, W.L.; Rathnachalam, R.; Richardson, J.M.; Schoner, B.; Ulmer, M.; et al. Leptin is a four-helix bundle: Secondary structure by NMR. *FEBS Lett.* **1997**, *407*, 239–242. [CrossRef]

30. Xie, X.; Steiner, S.H.; Bickel, M.H. Kinetics of distribution and adipose tissue storage as a function of lipophilicity and chemical structure. II. Benzodiazepines. *Drug Metab. Dispos.* **1991**, *19*, 15–19. [PubMed]

31. Hassiotou, F.; Hartmann, P.E. At the Dawn of a New Discovery: The Potential of Breast Milk Stem Cells. *Adv. Nutr. Int. Rev. J.* **2014**, *5*, 770–778. [CrossRef] [PubMed]

32. Houseknecht, K.L.; McGuire, M.K.; Portocarrero, C.P.; McGuire, M.A.; Beerman, K. Leptin Is Present in Human Milk and Is Related to Maternal Plasma Leptin Concentration and Adiposity. *Biochem. Biophys. Res. Commun.* **1997**, *240*, 742–747. [CrossRef] [PubMed]

33. Resto, M.; O'Connor, D.; Leef, K.; Funanage, V.; Spear, M.; Locke, R. Leptin Levels in Preterm Human Breast Milk and Infant Formula. *Pediatrics* **2001**, *108*, e15. [CrossRef] [PubMed]

34. Grundy, S.M.; Mok, H.Y.I.; Zech, L.; Steinberg, D.; Berman, M. Transport of Very Low Density Lipoprotein Triglycerides in Varying Degrees of Obesity and Hypertriglyceridemia. *J. Clin. Investig.* **1979**, *63*, 1274–1283. [CrossRef] [PubMed]

35. Hassiotou, F.; Beltran, A.; Chetwynd, E.; Stuebe, A.M.; Twigger, A.J.; Metzger, P.; Trengove, N.; Lai, C.T.; Filgueira, L.; Blancafort, P.; et al. Breastmilk is a novel source of stem cells with multilineage differentiation potential. *Stem Cells* **2012**, *30*, 2164–2174. [CrossRef] [PubMed]

36. Cannon, A.; Kakulas, F.; Hepworth, A.; Lai, C.; Hartmann, P.; Geddes, D. The Effects of Leptin on Breastfeeding Behaviour. *Int. J. Environ. Res. Public Health* **2015**, *12*, 12340. [CrossRef] [PubMed]

37. Khan, S.; Hepworth, A.R.; Prime, D.K.; Lai, C.T.; Trengove, N.J.; Hartmann, P.E. Variation in Fat, Lactose, and Protein Composition in Breast Milk over 24 Hours: Associations with Infant Feeding Patterns. *J. Hum. Lact.* **2013**, *29*, 81–89. [CrossRef] [PubMed]

38. Mitoulas, L.R.; Kent, J.C.; Cox, D.B.; Owens, R.A.; Sherriff, J.L.; Hartmann, P.E. Variation in fat, lactose and protein in human milk over 24 h and throughout the first year of lactation. *Br. J. Nutr.* **2002**, *88*, 29–37. [CrossRef] [PubMed]

39. Czank, C.; Simmer, K.; Hartmann, P.E. A method for standardizing the fat content of human milk for use in the neonatal intensive care unit. *Int. Breastfeed. J.* **2009**, *4*, 3. [CrossRef] [PubMed]

40. Hassiotou, F.; Hepworth, A.R.; Williams, T.M.; Twigger, A.-J.; Perrella, S.; Lai, C.T.; Filgueira, L.; Geddes, D.T.; Hartmann, P.E. Breastmilk Cell and Fat Contents Respond Similarly to Removal of Breastmilk by the Infant. *PLoS ONE* **2013**, *8*, 1–11. [CrossRef] [PubMed]

41. R Core Team. *A Language and Environment for Statistical Computing*; R Foundation for Statistical Computing: Vienna, Austria, 2014.

42. Pinheiro, J.; Bates, D.; DebRoy, S.; Sarkar, D. *Linear and Nonlinear Mixed Effects Models*; Foundation for Statistical Computing: Vienna, Austria, 2008.

43. World Health Organization. *Birth to 24 Months: Boys Head Circumference-for-Age and Weight-for-Length Percentiles*; Centres for Disease Control and Prevention: Atlanta, GA, USA, 2009.

44. World Health Organization. *Birth to 24 Months: Girls Head Circumference-for-Age and Weight-for-Length Percentiles*; Centres for Disease Control and Prevention: Atlanta, GA, USA, 2009.

45. Bouret, S.G.; Simerly, R.B. Developmental programming of hypothalamic feeding circuits. *Clin. Genet.* **2006**, *70*, 295–301. [CrossRef] [PubMed]

46. Lord, G.M.; Matarese, G.; Howard, J.K.; Baker, R.J.; Bloom, S.R.; Lechler, R.I. Leptin modulates the T-cell immune response and reverses starvation-induced immunosuppression. *Nature* **1998**, *394*, 897–901. [PubMed]

47. Lord, G.M.; Matarese, G.; Howard, J.K.; Bloom, S.R.; Lechler, R.I. Leptin inhibits the anti-CD3-driven proliferation of peripheral blood T cells but enhances the production of proinflammatory cytokines. *J. Leukoc. Biol.* **2002**, *72*, 330–338. [PubMed]

48. Ho, F.C.; Wong, R.L.; Lawton, J.W. Human colostral and breast milk cells. A light and electron microscopic study. *Acta Paediatr. Scand.* **1979**, *68*, 389–396. [CrossRef] [PubMed]

49. Boutinaud, M.; Jammes, H. Potential uses of milk epithelial cells: A review. *Reprod. Nutr. Dev.* **2002**, *42*, 133–147. [CrossRef] [PubMed]

50. Bronsky, J.; Mitrova, K.; Karpisek, M.; Mazoch, J.; Durilova, M.; Fisarkova, B.; Stechova, K.; Prusa, R.; Nevoral, J. Adiponectin, AFABP, and leptin in human breast milk during 12 months of lactation. *J. Pediatr. Gastroenterol. Nutr.* **2011**, *52*, 474–477. [CrossRef] [PubMed]

51. Schueler, J.; Alexander, B.; Hart, A.M.; Austin, K.; Larson-Meyer, D.E. Presence and dynamics of leptin, GLP-1, and PYY in human breast milk at early postpartum. *Obesity (Silver Spring, MD)* **2013**, *21*, 1451–1458. [CrossRef] [PubMed]

52. Bielicki, J.; Huch, R.; von Mandach, U. Time-Course of leptin levels in term and preterm human milk. *Eur. J. Endocrinol./Eur. Fed. Endocr. Soc.* **2004**, *151*, 271–276. [CrossRef]

53. King, B.L.; Crisi, G.M.; Tsai, S.C.; Haffty, B.G.; Phillips, R.F.; Rimm, D.L. Immunocytochemical analysis of breast cells obtained by ductal lavage. *Cancer Cytopathol.* **2002**, *96*, 244–249. [CrossRef] [PubMed]

54. Hassiotou, F.; Geddes, D.T. Immune cell-mediated protection of the mammary gland and the infant during breastfeeding. *Adv. Nutr. (Bethesda, MD)* **2015**, *6*, 267–275. [CrossRef] [PubMed]

55. Weiler, I.J.; Hickler, W.; Sprenger, R. Demonstration That Milk Cells Invade the Suckling Neonatal Mouse. *Am. J. Reprod. Immunol.* **1983**, *4*, 95–98. [CrossRef] [PubMed]

56. Imagawa, K.; Numata, Y.; Katsuura, G.; Sakaguchi, I.; Morita, A.; Kikuoka, S.; Matumoto, Y.; Tsuji, T.; Tamaki, M.; Sasakura, K.; et al. Structure-Function Studies of Human Leptin. *J. Biol. Chem.* **1998**, *273*, 35245–35249. [CrossRef] [PubMed]

57. Bergstrom, F.W. Solutions of the electronegative elements in liquid ammonia; the actions of selenium, tellurium, arsenic acid and a solution of sulfur in liquid ammonia upon cyanides. *J. Am. Chem. Soc.* **1926**, *48*, 2319–2327. [CrossRef]

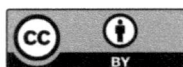

nutrients

MDPI

Article

The Effect of Gestational and Lactational Age on the Human Milk Metabolome

Ulrik K. Sundekilde [1,*], Eimear Downey [2], James A. O'Mahony [2], Carol-Anne O'Shea [3], C. Anthony Ryan [3], Alan L. Kelly [2] and Hanne C. Bertram [1]

[1]   Department of Food Science, Aarhus University, Årslev 5792, Denmark; hannec.bertram@food.au.dk
[2]   School of Food and Nutritional Sciences, University College Cork, Cork T12 YN60, Ireland;
      eimeardowney@gmail.com (E.D.); sa.omahony@ucc.ie (J.A.M.); a.kelly@ucc.ie (A.L.K.)
[3]   Department of Paediatrics and Child Health, University College Cork, Cork T12 YN60, Ireland;
      Ca.OShea@ucc.ie (C.A.S.); tony.ryan@ucc.ie (C.A.R.)
*   Correspondence: uksundekilde@food.au.dk; Tel.: +45-87154882

Received: 1 April 2016; Accepted: 16 May 2016; Published: 19 May 2016

Abstract: Human milk is the ideal nutrition source for healthy infants during the first six months of life and a detailed characterisation of the composition of milk from mothers that deliver prematurely (<37 weeks gestation), and of how human milk changes during lactation, would benefit our understanding of the nutritional requirements of premature infants. Individual milk samples from mothers delivering prematurely and at term were collected. The human milk metabolome, established by nuclear magnetic resonance (NMR) spectroscopy, was influenced by gestational and lactation age. Metabolite profiling identified that levels of valine, leucine, betaine, and creatinine were increased in colostrum from term mothers compared with mature milk, while those of glutamate, caprylate, and caprate were increased in mature term milk compared with colostrum. Levels of oligosaccharides, citrate, and creatinine were increased in pre-term colostrum, while those of caprylate, caprate, valine, leucine, glutamate, and pantothenate increased with time postpartum. There were differences between pre-term and full-term milk in the levels of carnitine, caprylate, caprate, pantothenate, urea, lactose, oligosaccharides, citrate, phosphocholine, choline, and formate. These findings suggest that the metabolome of pre-term milk changes within 5–7 weeks postpartum to resemble that of term milk, independent of time of gestation at pre-mature delivery.

Keywords: pre-term; infant; nutrition; human milk; metabolites; NMR; metabolomics

1. Introduction

Human milk (HM) is the recognised gold standard for feeding new-born full-term healthy infants. HM is a unique food source that contains all the exacting amounts of required nutrients to support the growth and development of term infants during the first six months of life. The health benefits of HM have been well documented [1]. Current data suggest that the quantity of HM consumed by healthy term infants is on average 0.778 kg human milk/day, with males consuming 0.056 kg/day more than females. Human milk consumption rises rapidly during the first month postpartum to ~0.6 kg/day and increases to ~0.82 kg/day in 3–4 month old infants [2].

Human milk is also regarded as particularly important for feeding pre-mature infants. There are many health benefits related to providing a pre-term infant with HM, including improvements in digestion, nutrient absorption, gastrointestinal function, and neurodevelopment of the infant [3,4]. In addition, an exclusive HM diet has been associated with lower rates of necrotizing enterocolitis, a potentially fatal gastrointestinal complication, in premature infants [5]. Human milk oligosaccharides (HMO) are known to affect the gut microbiota and it has been speculated that HMOs could account for the lower observed incidences of necrotizing enterocolitis [6].

Mother's milk is inadequate for rapidly growing pre-term neonates, which can be ascribed to a higher protein and energy requirement of pre-term neonates, particularly those of low birth weight and <28 weeks gestation, leading to insufficient weight gain and nutrition deficits [7,8]. For extremely pre-term and very low birth weight infants, the fortification of HM using commercial fortifiers is often recommended in order to supply the neonate with the nutrients required to support its rapid rate of growth. Studies have shown that the addition of HM fortifier can improve weight, length, and head circumference growth, in addition to bone mineralization and neurological outcomes [9–13].

It is known that the composition of pre-term milk differs from that of milk of full-term mothers, with higher reported levels of total protein, fat, carbohydrate and energy in pre-term milk [14]. Differences in the proteome of the two types of milk have also been reported [15]. Generally, studies have focused on the macronutrient content of pre-term and term HM without consideration of micronutrients such as biologically significant metabolites [14].

Previous work on milk metabolomes has predominantly considered bovine milk [16–20] and human milk [21–28]. Recently, a multi-analytical platform study identified 710 metabolites in human milk by using a combination of MS- and NMR-based analytical techniques [21]. Moreover, a recent study identified subtle differences between some milk metabolites during the first month of lactation [27]. However, the changes in pre-term and full-term human milk metabolomes over a full lactation time course have not yet been reported in detail.

In this study, we report how gestational age affects the low-molecular-weight metabolome of HM from mothers of pre-term and term infants over range of stages of lactation. The milk metabolomes were compared using proton nuclear magnetic resonance spectroscopy (^{1}H NMR)-based metabolomics from milk samples from mothers at different gestational ages. Longitudinal samples were also examined to analyse how pre-term milk develops with time postpartum compared with term milk.

2. Materials and Methods

2.1. Ethical Approval

Ethical approval for this study was granted by The Clinical Research Ethics Committee of the Cork Teaching Hospitals, Cork, Ireland (clinical number reference ECM 4(s) 06/08/13).

2.2. Samples and Sample Collection

2.2.1. Pre-term Samples

Multiple frozen (−20 °C) longitudinal pre-term HM samples were collected from 15 individual mothers of pre-term infants (Table 1). The HM samples were collected from the freezers of the neonatal intensive care unit of Cork University Maternity Hospital (Wilton, Co. Cork, Ireland). Each bottle of HM was dated allowing for an accurate calculation of the gestational age of the infant when the milk was expressed. The HM samples from each individual mother were pooled according to 'day postpartum' up to 14 days and according to 'week postpartum' after this, creating $n = 62$ pre-term HM samples. For one donor (Pre-1), information on number of days postpartum was unavailable and accordingly samples from this donor were removed from multivariate models using gestational age or days postpartum for modelling or visualization purposes.

2.2.2. Full-term Samples

Frozen (−20 °C) HM samples ($n = 30$) were obtained from The Western Trust Milk Bank, Irvinestown, Co. Fermanagh, Ireland (Table 2). The HM samples were from 30 individual mothers of healthy full-term infants who donated milk with consent for use for research purposes. The mothers expressed milk in a domestic setting and stored milk at −20 °C before shipping to The Western Trust Milk Bank, Ireland. HM was pasteurised and microbiologically screened before being frozen and shipped to University College Cork where it was stored at −20 °C. Milk samples were categorized according to the length of time postpartum; colostrum (<5 days postpartum; $n = 5$), transitional (6 days–2 weeks postpartum; $n = 4$), mature (>2 weeks, $n = 21$).

Table 1. Sample information from mothers of pre-term infants.

Sample Id	Secretor Status	Gestation	Infant Weight, Grams	Age of Mother, Years	Gravida [1]	Para [2]	Number of Samples	Postpartum Span [3]
Pre 01	Se⁺	–	–	–	–	–	4	–
Pre 02	Se⁺	38 weeks	3210	35	2	2	4	7–11 weeks
Pre 03	Se⁺	28 weeks	1190	33	1	1	9	4–12 days
Pre 04	Se⁺	31 weeks	1830	36	3	3	5	1–5 weeks
Pre 05	Se⁺	30 weeks	1340	29	1	1	7	4 days–7 weeks
Pre 06	Se⁺	32 weeks + 2 days	2340	42	2	2	1	8 days
Pre 07	Se⁻	24 weeks + 4 days	540	33	1	1	4	1–4 days
Pre 08	Se⁻	31 weeks	1680	35	2	2	2	5–14 weeks
Pre 09	Se⁺	35 weeks + 6 days	2410	33	1	1	3	2–5 weeks
Pre 10	Se⁺	35 weeks + 2 days	3100	26	1	1	2	4–5 days
Pre 11	Se⁺	33 weeks + 4 days	1800	29	6	5	2	4–6 days
Pre 12	Se⁺	35 weeks + 4 days	3260	45	4	3 + 2 [4]	2	9–10 days
Pre 13	Se⁺	26 weeks	650	40	–	–	15	6 days–8 weeks
Pre 14	Se⁻	28 weeks + 3 days	–	–	–	–	1	13 weeks
Pre 15	Se⁺	32 weeks	–	–	–	–	1	9 weeks

[1] Number of pregnancies, including the current pregnancy; [2] number of times the mother has given birth; [3] time range indicates days postpartum of first and last samples from that donor; [4] indicates twin pregnancy.

2.3. NMR Spectroscopy

NMR spectroscopy was essentially performed as described earlier [29]. Briefly, the samples skimmed by centrifugation at 4000 *g* for 15 min and removal of the top fat layer before filtering to remove residual lipids and protein using Amicon Ultra 0.5 mL 10 kDa (Millipore, Billerica, MA, USA) spin filters at 10,000 *g* for 30 min at 4 °C. A filtered sample (500 μL) was mixed with 100 μL D_2O containing 0.025% 3-(trimethylsilyl) propionic-2,2,3,3-d_4 acid, sodium salt (TSP; Sigma-Aldrich, St. Louis, MO, USA) as an internal chemical shift reference. ^1H NMR spectroscopy was performed at 298 K on a Bruker Avance III 600 spectrometer, operating at a ^1H frequency of 600.13 MHz, and equipped with a 5-mm ^1H TXI probe (Bruker BioSpin, Rheinstetten, Germany). The sample sequence was randomized prior to acquisition and standard one-dimensional spectra were acquired using a single 90° pulse experiment with a relaxation delay of 5 s. Water suppression was achieved by irradiating the water peak during the relaxation delay, and a total of 64 scans were collected into 32,768 data points spanning a spectral width of 12.15 ppm. All ^1H spectra were initially referenced to the TSP signal at 0 ppm. Prior to Fourier transformation, the data were multiplied by a 0.3 Hz line-broadening function. The proton NMR spectra were phase and baseline corrected manually using Topspin 3.2 (Bruker Biospin, Rheinstetten, Germany). NMR signals were assigned in accordance with existing literature [20,21,25,29], 2D NMR spectroscopy, Chenomx NMR Suite 8.1.2 (Chenomx Inc, Edmonton, AB, Canada) and the Human Metabolome Database [30].

Table 2. Sample information from mothers of term infants.

Sample ID	Secretor status	Time postpartum	Group
Term 01	Se$^+$	<5 days	Colostrum
Term 02	Se$^+$	<5 days	Colostrum
Term 03	Se$^+$	<5 days	Colostrum
Term 04	Se$^+$	<5 days	Colostrum
Term 05	Se$^+$	<5 days	Colostrum
Term 06	Se$^+$	2 weeks	Transitional
Term 07	Se$^+$	2 weeks	Transitional
Term 08	Se$^-$	6 days	Transitional
Term 09	Se$^-$	2 weeks	Transitional
Term 10	Se$^-$	15 weeks	Mature
Term 11	Se$^-$	9 weeks	Mature
Term 12	Se$^+$	15 weeks	Mature
Term 13	Se$^-$	11 weeks	Mature
Term 14	Se$^-$	15 weeks	Mature
Term 15	Se$^-$	11 weeks	Mature
Term 16	Se$^+$	16 weeks	Mature
Term 17	Se$^-$	9 weeks	Mature
Term 18	Se$^+$	19 weeks	Mature
Term 19	Se$^+$	24 weeks	Mature
Term 20	Se$^+$	11 weeks	Mature
Term 21	Se$^+$	7–10 weeks	Mature
Term 22	Se$^+$	13 weeks	Mature
Term 23	Se$^+$	13 weeks	Mature
Term 24	Se$^+$	14 weeks	Mature
Term 25	Se$^+$	5 weeks	Mature
Term 26	Se$^+$	27 weeks	Mature
Term 27	Se$^-$	33 weeks	Mature
Term 28	Se$^-$	27 weeks	Mature
Term 29	Se$^+$	29 weeks	Mature
Term 30	Se$^+$	33 weeks	Mature

2.4. Secretor Status

Maternal secretor status was determined as previously described [25]. In brief the absence or presence of 2-FL was used to determine secretor status quantified by NMR spectroscopy (2-FL corresponds to NMR signal at δ 5.32 ppm). Milk from mothers classified as non-secretors did not have any detectable levels of 2-FL, whereas milk from mothers classified as secretors did contain 2-FL.

2.5. Multivariate Data and Statistical Analyses

NMR spectra of milk samples were aligned using Icoshift by co-shifting of the whole spectra according to the anomeric lactose proton at 5.23 ppm [31]. The proton NMR spectra were subdivided into 0.01 ppm bins, reducing each spectrum into 957 separate variables in the regions 10.00–5.00 and 4.72–0.5 ppm. Principal component analysis (PCA) and orthogonal partial least squares discriminant analysis (OPLS-DA) were performed in order to identify differences in the metabolite profiles. The data was mean-centred and Pareto-scaled prior to analysis. The OPLS-DA model was cross-validated using segmentation with seven splits. Covariance was investigated by analysis of OPLS-DA regression coefficients back-transformed to original data and colour coded by the loading weights [32]. The multivariate data analysis was performed using SIMCA-P + 13 (Umetrics AB, Umeå, Sweden). Alignment by Icoshift, binning, and analysis of OPLS-DA plots were performed in MATLAB 7.13 using in-house developed scripts (MathWorks Inc., Natick, MA, USA). Univariate statistical significance was evaluated by Student's *t*-test using the Statistics Toolbox in MATLAB 7.13 (MathWorks Inc., Natick, MA, USA).

3. Results

HM samples (*n* = 92) were collected from 45 individual mothers with different gestational ages at delivery, ranging from 24.6–35.8 weeks in the case of pre-term samples and more than 37 weeks for full-term samples (Tables 1 and 2). For pre-mature deliveries, infant birth weight ranged from 540 g to 3260 g. Age of the mothers of pre-term infants ranged from 26–45 years, and all had at least one previous pregnancy longer than 24 weeks gestation (Table 1).

The median spectrum of all 92 milk samples is shown in Figure 1. Each signal corresponds to proton resonances in milk metabolites according to assignments in Table 3. Differences in fucosylated human milk oligosaccharides (HMO) have previously been described to depend on maternal secretor status [33]. Accordingly, secretor status of the mothers was determined by examining the specific patterns of fucosylated oligosaccharides (Figure 1B) [25]. Thirteen mothers were found to be non-secretors, accounting for 28.9% of the mothers included in the study (Tables 1 and 2).

The collected milk samples were analysed for changes during lactation following both full-term (Figure 2) and pre-term (Figure 3) delivery. Figure 2 shows a scores plot of principal component (PC) 2 and PC3 from a principal component analysis (PCA) model of full-term milk samples. The samples are grouped into colostrum, transitional, and mature groups and coloured according to days postpartum. The scores plot shows the distinct groupings of the milk samples, and indicates a gradual change in the milk metabolome as the milk develops from colostrum towards mature milk (Figure 2). In addition, no detectable differences were observed between mature milk samples in the intervals before 26 weeks and after 26 weeks (Figure 2). There was an apparent difference in milk metabolites depending on secretor status in term milk samples, as the milk samples were separated into secretor or non-secretor groups along PC2 (Figure 2).

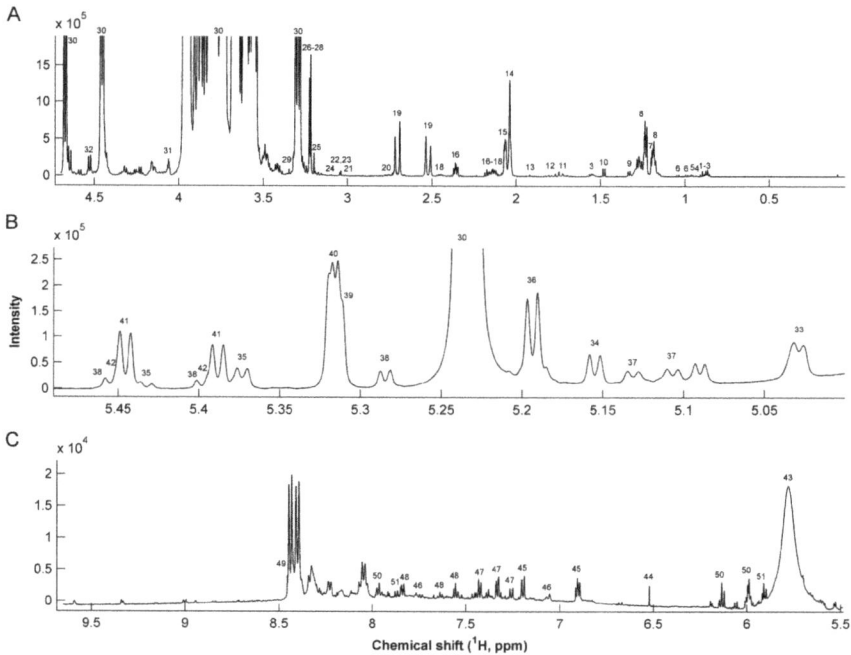

Figure 1. Median ^{1}H NMR spectrum of 92 human milk samples. (**A**) Aliphatic region 4.6–0 ppm (**B**) Human milk oligosaccharides in 5.45–5.00 ppm region; and (**C**) aromatic region 9.7–5.5 ppm region. For peak assignments refer to Table 3.

Table 3. List of metabolites in human milk with chemical shifts in ppm from internal TSP standard and assignment of resonances.

#	Metabolite	¹H Chemical shift (ppm)	Assignment	#	Metabolite	¹H Chemical shift (ppm)	Assignment
1	Caprylate	0.85	CH₃	29	Methanol	3.37	CH₃
		1.53	CH₂	30	Lactose	3.23, 3.5–4.0	Multiple
2	Caprate	0.85	CH₃	31	Gluconate	4.05	CH
		1.53	CH₂	32	Galactose	4.57	CH
3	Butyrate	0.88	CH₃	33	Fuc α1,4 GlcNAc	5.03	CH-1
		1.55	β-CH₂	34	Fuc α1,3 GlcNAc	5.19	CH-1
		2.16	α-CH₂			5.03	Fuc (α1-4) CH-1
4	Pantothenate	0.91	CH₃	35	LNDFH II	5.38	Fuc (α1-3) αGlc CH-1
5	Leucine	0.94	CH₃			5.43	Fuc (α1-3) βGlc CH-1
6	Valine	0.98	γ-CH₃	36	LNDFH I	5.16	Fuc (α1-2) CH-1
		1.03	γ'-CH₃			5.03	Fuc (α1-4) CH-1
7	3-BHBA	1.18	CH₃	37	LNFP III	5.11	Fuc (α1-3) GlcNAc CH-1
		2.39	CH₂			5.13	Fuc (α1-3) GlcNAc CH-1
8	Fucosyl moieties	1.19	CH₃-6	38	LDFT	5.29	Fuc (α1-2) CH-1
		1.23–1.29	CH₃-6			5.4	Fuc (α1-3) αGlc CH-1
9	Lactate	1.32	CH₃			5.46	Fuc (α1-3) βGlc CH-1
10	Alanine	1.47	CH₃	39	LNFP I	5.32	Fuc (α1-2) CH-1
11	6'-SL	1.73	CH₃	40	2'FL	5.32	Fuc (α1-2) CH-1
12	3'-SL	1.78	CH₃	41	3'FL	5.39	Fuc (α1-3) αGlc CH-1
13	Acetate	1.91	CH₃			5.44	Fuc (α1-3) βGlc CH-1
14	GlcNAc	2.04	CH₃	42	LNFP V	5.39	Fuc(α1-3)αGlc CH-1
15	Sialic acid	2.06	CH₃			5.44	Fuc (α1-3) βGlc CH-1
16	Glutamate	2.12	β-CH₂	43	Urea	5.76	NH₂
		2.33	γ-CH₂	44	Fumarate	6.51	CH = CH
17	Methionine	2.13	CH₃	45	Tyrosine	6.9	CH-3,5
18	Glutamine	2.11	β-CH₂			7.2	CH-2,6
		2.46	γ-CH₂	46	Methylhistidine	7.06	CH-4
19	Citrate	2.51	α-CH₂			7.8	CH-2
		2.69	α'-CH₂	47	Phenylalanine	7.32	CH-2,6
20	Dimethylamine	2.72	2 CH₃			7.37	CH-4
21	2-oxogluturate	2.99	CH₂			7.42	CH-3,5
22	Creatinine	3.02	CH₃			7.54	CH-2,6
23	Creatine	3.03	CH₃	48	Hippurate	7.63	CH-4
24	Malonate	3.12	CH₂			7.82	CH-3,5
25	Choline	3.19	3 CH₃	49	Formate	8.44	CH
26	O-Phosphocholine	3.21	3 CH₃	50	Cytidine triphosphate	5.99	CH-2
		4.16	CH₂			6.13	CH-10
27	Carnitine	2.42	CH₂			7.97	CH-11
		3.21	3 CH₃	51	Uridine	5.89	CH-2
28	Betaine	3.24	3 CH₃			5.91	CH-10
						7.87	CH-11

Abbreviations: 3-BHBA, 3-betahydroxybutyrate; FL, fucosyllactose; Fuc, Fucose; GlcNAc, N-acetylglucosamine; LDFT, lactodifucotetraose; LNDFH, lacto-N-difucohexaose, LNFP, lacto-N-fucopentaose; SL, sialyllactose.

Several milk metabolites were found to be present in significantly different concentration in colostrum, transitional, and mature milk. Fucosylated oligosaccharides, and also components of oligosaccharides (Fucose, N-acetylneuraminic acid, N-acetylglucosamine), were found at the highest levels in colostrum, and levels decreased in mature milk samples (Figure 2B). Moreover, levels of valine, leucine, pantothenate, citric acid, lactic acid, betaine, and creatinine were higher in colostrum and transitional milk compared with mature HM, and levels of glutamate, butyrate, caprylate, and caprate were higher in mature HM compared with colostrum and transitional milk. The level of β-hydroxybutyrate was found to be independent of milk maturity in full-term HM (Figure 2B). Milk from non-secretor mothers did not contain oligosaccharides with α1-2 fucosylated structures (Figure 2B); however, the level of 3' fucosyllactose (3'-FL) was increased in non-secretor mothers compared with secretor mothers.

Similarly, the pre-term milk samples were also examined for an effect of stage of lactation on the milk metabolome. The scores plot of a two component PCA model of milk samples from pre-term mothers is shown in Figure 3, in which samples are coloured according to number of days postpartum. The scores and loadings plots clearly show the changes in milk metabolome occurring over time in pre-term milk. Levels of fucosyl moieties, N-acetylneuraminic acid, N-acetylglucosamine, 3'-sialyllactose, 6'-sialyllactose, 2'-fucosyllactose, citric acid, choline, and creatinine decreased with time postpartum (Figure 3B), while levels of 3-FL, lacto-N-difucohexaose I (LNDFH I), butyrate, caprylate, caprate, lactic acid, valine, leucine, alanine, glutamate, and pantothenate increased with time postpartum (Figure 3B). Only two mothers, who donated seven milk samples in total, were identified as non-secretors (Table 1). Thus, it was not possible to identify differences in the PCA model for pre-term samples on the basis of secretor status.

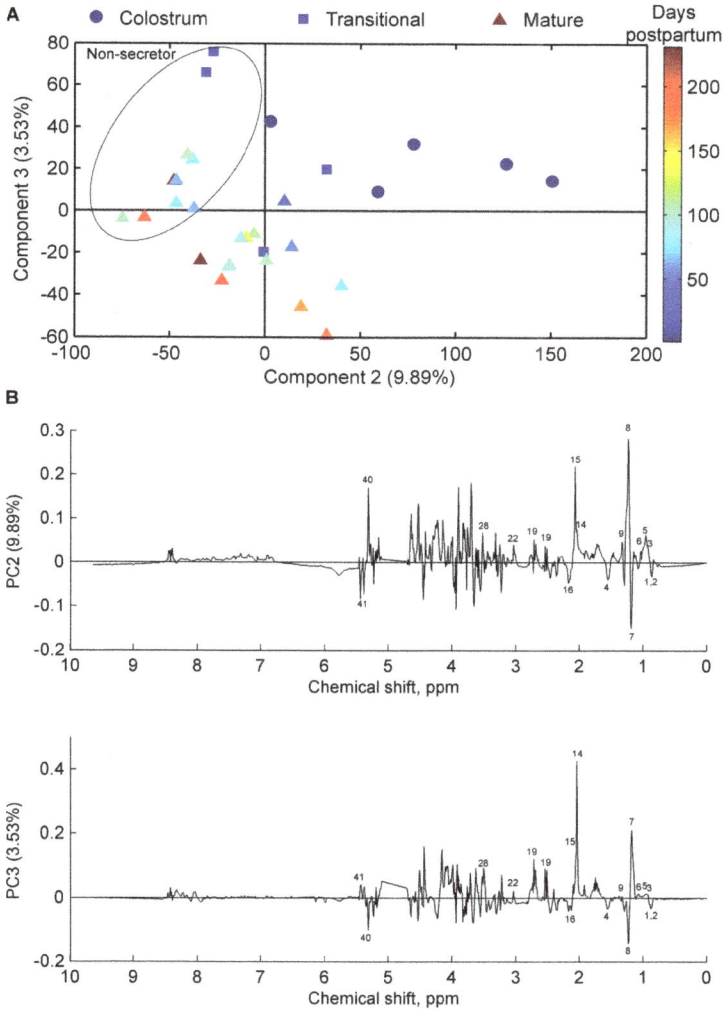

Figure 2. (A) Principal component analysis scores plot of full-term milk samples from 30 mothers ($n = 30$)); samples are coloured according to days postpartum; Colostrum (dots), transitional (squares), and mature (triangles); the circle denotes samples from non-secretor mothers, while remaining samples are from secretor mothers; and **(B)** corresponding loading line plots. For peak assignments refer to Table 3.

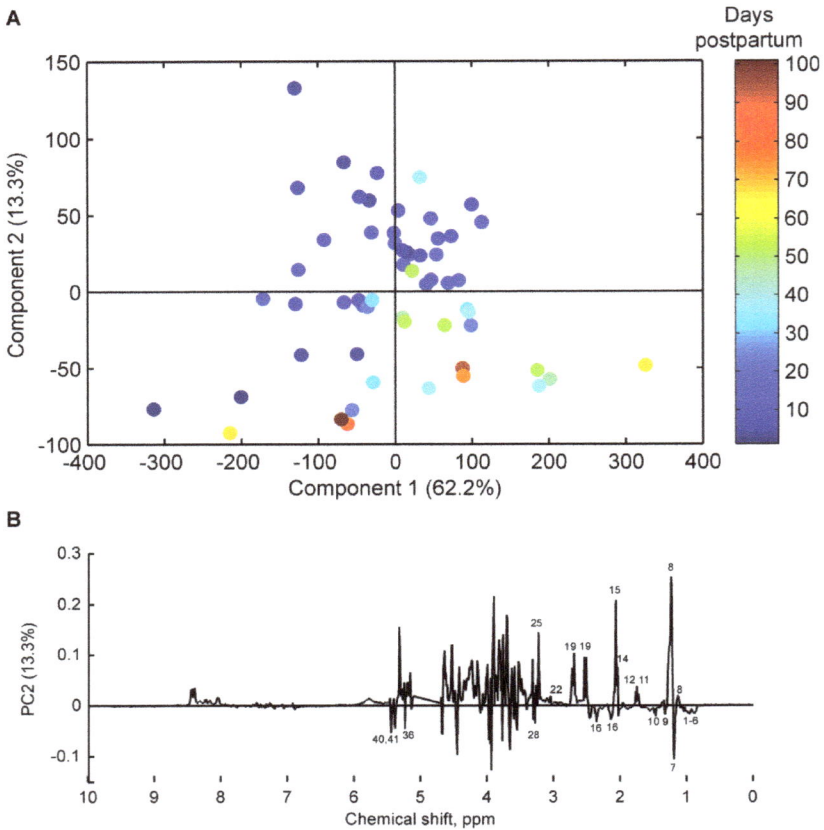

Figure 3. (**A**) Principal component analysis scores plot of pre-term milk samples from 15 mothers (*n* = 58), coloured according to number of days postpartum; and (**B**) corresponding loading line plot. For peak assignments refer to Table 3.

As some of the same time-related changes were apparent in both pre-term and full-term milk samples, the difference between the pre-term and full-term milk metabolomes of similar days postpartum was investigated. Citrate (*P* = 0.00057), lactose (*P* = 0.0039), and phosphocholine (*P* = 0.049) were found to be present in significantly higher levels in pre-term milk samples compared with full-term milk samples (Figure 4). Citrate level is known to decrease with time postpartum [28], while lactose is the major milk metabolite identified by NMR spectroscopy [20].

Thus, in the following analysis, NMR resonances originating from lactose were removed in order to increase the weight of other metabolites in the multivariate models. A PCA of pre-term and full-term milk samples (*n* = 88) was generated using two principal components which, together, explained 80.8% of the total variance described by the PCA model (Figure 5). From the PCA model, it is apparent that the milk metabolite profile from mothers of pre-term infants older than 5–7 weeks resembles that of full-term milk, as they are positioned in close proximity to the full-term milk samples, independent of time of gestation at delivery (Figure 5).

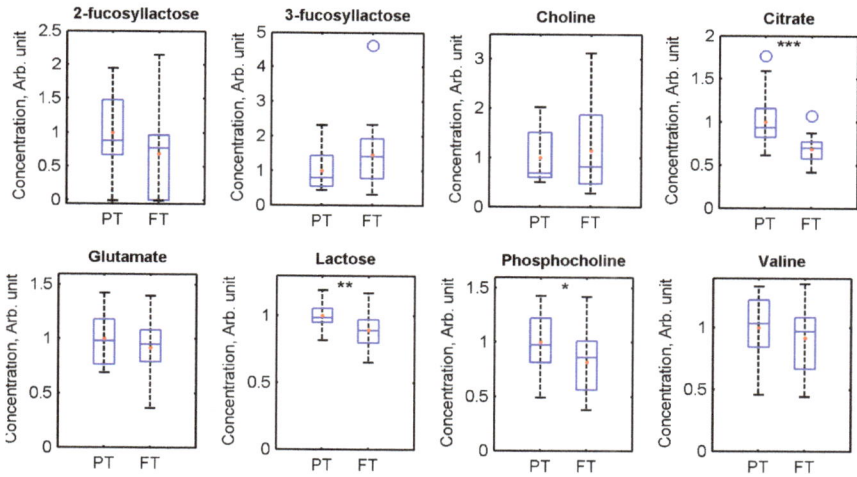

Figure 4. Box plots showing the distributions of 2-fucosyllactose, 3-fucosyllactose, choline, citrate, glutamate, lactose, phosphocholine, and valine concentrations in pre-term (PT) and full-term (FT) milk. Pre-term milk samples <14 days postpartum and full-term colostrum, transitional, and mature >26 weeks were excluded from the analysis in order to compare milk with a similar range of days postpartum. Horizontal lines indicate medians; coloured boxes specify interquartile ranges and dashed lines the ranges without outliers. The open circles indicate outliers (falls in-between 1.5× and 3× the interquartile range). *** = $P < 0.001$, ** = $P < 0.01$, * = $P < 0.05$; the comparisons were made using two-tailed Student's *t*-test.

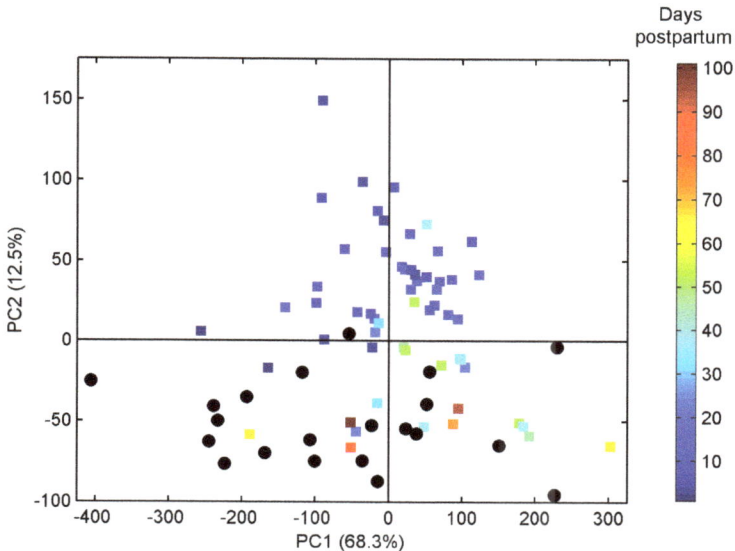

Figure 5. Principal component analysis scores plot of mature milk samples from pre-term (squares, $n = 58$) and full-term (circles, $n = 30$) mothers. Pre-term milk samples are coloured according to days postpartum.

OPLS-DA was also performed on the pre-term and full-term milk samples (Figure 6). Full-term and pre-term colostrum and transitional milk were excluded from the analysis, due to there being too few samples of these, and to be able to compare milk samples with similar days postpartum. The OPLS-DA model shows that significant differences exist between the metabolite profiles of pre-term and full-term milk (Figure 6B). In full-term milk, carnitine, caprylate, caprate, pantothenate, beta-hydroxybutyrate, and urea were found to be present in higher levels compared with pre-term milk, while lactose (Figure 4), Fucosyl moieties, *N*-acetylneuraminic acid, *N*-acetylglucosamine, 3′-sialyllactose, 6′-sialyllactose, lacto-*N*-difucohexaose I (LNDFH I), glutamate, citric acid, phosphocholine, choline, and formic acid were found in higher levels in pre-term milk (Figure 6).

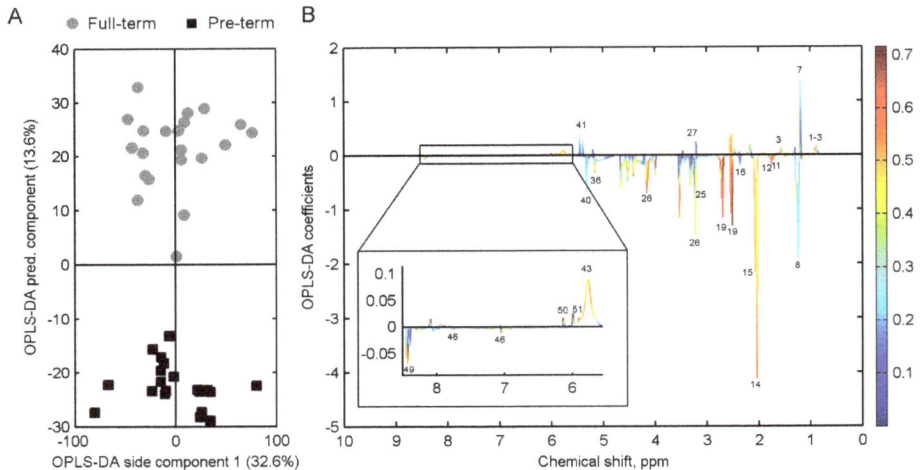

Figure 6. (**A**) Orthogonal partial least squares discriminant analysis of pre-term (*n* = 20, days postpartum range 3–14 weeks) and full-term (*n* = 21, days postpartum range 3–26 weeks) milk. Full-term colostrum, transitional, and pre-term milk <2 weeks postpartum have been excluded. Cross-validation, Q2: 0.70; (**B**) corresponding OPLS-DA coefficients plot. Each variable has been coloured according to the OPLS-DA loadings (correlation between NMR variables and pre-term/full-term classes); for peak assignments refer to Table 3.

4. Discussion

Pre-mature birth is considered to have long-lasting adverse effects on health, and it has been proposed that the introduction of metabolomics technologies may facilitate better understanding of these effects [34]. The exact causes of preterm delivery are not clear, but often associated with inflammation [35]. In the present study, causes of the preterm delivery were not known. In this study, differences in metabolomic profiles of HM were associated with gestational age. Previous studies have shown many health benefits of breast-feeding pre-term infants. However, mother's milk may not always be adequate for pre-term infants with high nutrition density requirements, which can lead to insufficient weight gain and nutrition deficits. To date, only a few metabolomics studies have been performed on pre-term human milk in the first few weeks of lactation [27]. To our knowledge, this is the first study to comprehensively characterize and compare the pre-term and full-term human milk metabolome over a lactation time-course (up to 14 weeks postpartum). Milk metabolomics may be used in a clinical setting [23], in order to establish the milk metabolome for infant nutrition in cases where the optimal nutrition is a key advantage as in pre-term infants. Milk metabolomics studies in cows' milk have previously shown an ability to yield information about the health status of the cow [29,36]. It can likewise be hypothesized that the milk metabolome of lactating mothers can give information that can be used in a clinical setting.

Previous studies have shown that several factors influence the variability in the milk metabolome. The epithelial cells in the mammary gland are accountable for the milk production, and these cells are ultimately responsible for converting most precursors into milk components, but many other cell types are also involved in milk production [37]. Development of the mammary epithelial cells during pregnancy has been shown to influence transport pathways in the mammary gland responsible for different protein profiles of milk [38]. Moreover, insulin has been shown to be actively transported into milk and maternal diabetes affect milk insulin levels [39]. Maternal factors such as diet, lifestyle and phenotype have been shown to influence the milk composition [26]. Moreover, secretor status is also important for the biosynthesis of milk oligosaccharides [26]. The presence of α1,2 fucosyltransferase gene (FUT2) is important for the milk oligosaccharides since non-secretors, which lack the FUT2 gene, are unable to biosynthesize HMOs with a fucose bound to a N-acetylglucosamine via a glycosidic α1,2 linkage. Non-secretor status occurs in approximately 20% of most human populations [40,41]. In the present study, non-secretor status, identified by increased level of 3-FL, was found in 28.9 % of milk donors. Gestational age and the stage of lactation are also known to influence the milk proteins [14], lipids [42], and lactose [43]. Preliminary HM metabolomic studies have shown a difference between the metabolite profiles of pre-term and full-term HM [22,24]. Additionally, the metabolite extraction procedure in sample preparation prior to NMR spectroscopy has shown to influence the milk metabolite levels. In a recent paper, a sample preparation method using ultrafiltration as employed in the present study, was found to be superior compared with methanol/chloroform extraction in terms of separating small molecules from proteins and lipids [28]. Levels of HMO and its components are known to decrease with time [44]. A specific HMO, lacto-N-tetraose, has also been shown to be elevated in pre-term milk [45]. Interestingly, specific HMOs, LNDFH I, 3'-sialyllactose, and 6'-sialyllactose, and common components of HMO, including fucose, N-acetylglucosamine, and N-acetylneuraminic acid were identified to be present in higher concentrations in pre-term milk. HMOs have previously been shown to prevent necrotizing enterocolitis in neonatal rats [6], which may be linked to alterations in the microbiota of the infant's gut [46]. Thus, the elevated amounts of HMOs in pre-term milk may be a factor in the observed association of lower rates of necrotizing enterocolitis in premature infants fed HM [5].

Most of the free amino acids in HM steadily decrease in level as the milk matures [42]. However, the pre-term milk amino acid composition has not been well characterized throughout the course of lactation [47–49]. Glutamate is known to increase with lactation time [47] and this was also found in both pre-term and full-term milk in the present study. Valine and leucine, two essential amino acids, were found at the highest concentration in full-term colostrum and decreased with time postpartum, in agreement with other human milk metabolomics studies [27]. In contrast, increases in valine and leucine levels were observed in pre-term milk with time post-partum, which is in contrast to the pattern observed in full-term milk and that previously reported for pre-term milk [48,49].

Short- and medium-chain fatty acids (SMCFA; butyrate, caprylate, and caprate) were found in higher concentrations in full-term milk compared with pre-term milk. Moreover, the levels of SMCFA increased with time postpartum, as previously reported [50]. Choline is of high nutritional value, as it is abundant in cell membranes and acts as a precursor for the important messenger acetylcholine, and infants require high amounts of choline in order to sustain their rapid growth. Phosphocholine was found in higher levels in pre-term milk than in full-term milk, which is in agreement with previous reports on phosphocholine [51]. In contrast, pre-term milk has previously been shown to contain lesser amounts of choline [51], which is contradictory to findings in the present study.

In this study, it was shown that, after 5–7 weeks the metabolite profiles of pre-term milk resembled that of full-term milk, independently of gestational age. For extremely early pre-term infants born at a gestational age of, e.g., 24 weeks, these findings suggest that mother's milk becomes equivalent to mature milk for term infants by the time the infant reaches ~29 weeks post-menstrual age. This is a significant finding concerning a period in which the infant still requires advanced nutritional support to maintain its growth and long-term developmental requirements. Clinical metabolomics could potentially be advantageous to determine when milk metabolites levels become inadequate due to maturation of milk, if causal relationships between milk metabolites and infant growth parameters can be established. Previous studies have shown that protein concentration remains at higher levels in pre-term human milk even after 8 weeks of lactation [13]; however, we believe this to be the first study to document the changes in the metabolomics profile of pre-term human milk as it evolves to resemble that of full-term milk, and to show that this occurs independent of gestational age at delivery.

In conclusion, specific differences in milk metabolites exist between milk from mothers delivering pre-maturely and at term. Moreover, milk metabolite composition is associated with gestational age and the metabolome of pre-term milk changes within 5–7 weeks postpartum to resemble that of full-term milk, independent of time of gestation at delivery. However, as this study did not systematically collect samples from a cohort of mothers in a longitudinal design, further studies of this kind are recommended to more fully understand the significance of the changes reported herein.

Acknowledgments: The authors would like to acknowledge the Western Trust Milk Bank, Irvinestown, Co. Fermanagh, Ireland, the staff of the neonatal intensive care unit of Cork University Maternity Hospital and all of the mother and infants that kindly donated their milk. The authors are grateful for financial support from the Danish Research Council FTP through the project "Advances in Food quality and Nutrition Research through implementation of metabolomic strategies".

Author Contributions: All authors participated in the conception, design and writing of the manuscript. All authors read and approved the final manuscript.

Conflicts of Interest: The authors declare no conflict of interest.

Abbreviations

The following abbreviations are used in this manuscript:

HM   Human milk
HMO   Human milk oligosaccharide
NMR   Nuclear magnetic resonance

1.   Wu, T.C.; Chen, P.H. Health consequences of nutrition in childhood and early infancy. *Pediatr. Neonatol.* **2009**, *50*, 135–142. [CrossRef]
2.   Da Costa, T.H.M.; Haisma, H.; Wells, J.C.K.; Mander, A.P.; Whitehead, R.G.; Bluck, L.J.C. How much human milk do infants consume? Data from 12 countries using a standardized stable isotope methodology. *J. Nutr.* **2010**, *140*, 2227–2232. [PubMed]
3.   Isaacs, E.B.; Morley, R.; Lucas, A. Early diet and general cognitive outcome at adolescence in children born at or below 30 weeks gestation. *J. Pediatr.* **2009**, *155*, 229–234. [CrossRef] [PubMed]
4.   Lawrence, R.M. Breastfeeding, Host-resistance factors and immunologic significance of human milk. In *Breastfeeding. A guide for the medical profession*; Lawrence, R.A., Lawrence, R.M., Eds.; Elsevier: Philadelphia, PA, USA, 2006; pp. 171–214.
5.   Sullivan, S.; Schanler, R.J.; Kim, J.H.; Patel, A.L.; Trawöger, R.; Kiechl-Kohlendorfer, U.; Chan, G.M.; Blanco, C.L.; Abrams, S.; Cotten, C.M.; *et al.* An exclusively human milk-based diet is associated with a lower rate of necrotizing enterocolitis than a diet of human milk and bovine milk-based products. *J. Pediatr.* **2010**, *156*, 562–567. [CrossRef] [PubMed]
6.   Jantscher-Krenn, E.; Zherebtsov, M.; Nissan, C.; Goth, K.; Guner, Y.S.; Naidu, N.; Choudhury, B.; Grishin, A.V.; Ford, H.R.; Bode, L. The human milk oligosaccharide disialyllacto-*N*-tetraose prevents necrotising enterocolitis in neonatal rats. *Gut* **2012**, *61*, 1417–1425. [CrossRef] [PubMed]
7.   Mikkola, K.; Ritari, N.; Tommiska, V.; Salokorpi, T.; Lehtonen, L.; Tammela, O.; Pääkkönen, L.; Olsen, P.; Korkman, M.; Fellman, V. Neurodevelopmental outcome at 5 years of age of a national cohort of extremely low birth weight infants who were born in 1996–1997. *Pediatrics* **2005**, *116*, 1391–1400. [CrossRef] [PubMed]

8. Sauer, P.J. Can extrauterine growth approximate intrauterine growth? Should it? *Am. J. Clin. Nutr.* **2007**, *85*, 608S–613S. [PubMed]

9. Faerk, J.; Petersen, S.; Peitersen, B.; Michaelsen, K.F. Diet and bone mineral content at term in premature infants. *Pediatr. Res.* **2000**, *47*, 148–156. [CrossRef] [PubMed]

10. Gross, S.J. Bone mineralization in preterm infants fed human milk with and without mineral supplementation. *J. Pediatr.* **1987**, *111*, 450–458. [CrossRef]

11. Martins, E.C.; Krebs, V.L.J. Effects of the use of fortified raw maternal milk on very low birth weight infants. *J. Pediatr.* **2009**, *85*, 157–162. [CrossRef]

12. Nicholl, R.M.; Gamsu, H.R. Changes in growth and metabolism in very low birthweight infants fed with fortified breast milk. *Acta. Paediatr.* **1999**, *88*, 1056–1061. [CrossRef] [PubMed]

13. Pettifor, J.M.; Rajah, R.; Venter, A.; Moodley, G.P.; Opperman, L.; Cavaleros, M.; Ross, F.P. Bone mineralization and mineral homeostasis in very low-birth-weight infants fed either human milk or fortified human milk. *J. Pediatr. Gastroenterol. Nutr.* **1989**, *8*, 217–224. [CrossRef] [PubMed]

14. Bauer, J.; Gerss, J. Longitudinal analysis of macronutrients and minerals in human milk produced by mothers of preterm infants. *Clin. Nutr.* **2011**, *30*, 215–220. [CrossRef] [PubMed]

15. Armaforte, E.; Curran, E.; Huppertz, T.; Ryan, C.A.; Caboni, M.F.; O'Connor, P.M.; Ross, R.P.; Hirtz, C.; Sommerer, N.; Chevalier, F.; *et al.* Proteins and proteolysis in pre-term and term human milk and possible implications for infant formulae. *Int. Dairy J.* **2010**, *20*, 715–723. [CrossRef]

16. Boudonck, K.J.; Mitchell, M.W.; Wulff, J.; Ryals, J.A. Characterization of the biochemical variability of bovine milk using metabolomics. *Metabolomics* **2009**, *5*, 375–386. [CrossRef]

17. Buitenhuis, A.J.; Sundekilde, U.K.; Poulsen, N.A.; Bertram, H.C.; Larsen, L.B.; Sørensen, P. Estimation of genetic parameters and detection of quantitative trait loci for metabolites in Danish Holstein milk. *J. Dairy Sci.* **2013**, *96*, 3285–3295. [CrossRef] [PubMed]

18. Klein, M.S.; Almstetter, M.F.; Schlamberger, G.; Nurnberger, N.; Dettmer, K.; Oefner, P.J.; Meyer, H.H.D.; Wiedemann, S.; Gronwald, W. Nuclear magnetic resonance and mass spectrometry-based milk metabolomics in dairy cows during early and late lactation. *J. Dairy Sci.* **2010**, *93*, 1539–1550. [CrossRef] [PubMed]

19. Maher, A.D.; Hayes, B.; Cocks, B.; Marett, L.; Wales, W.J.; Rochfort, S. Latent biochemical relationships in the blood-milk metabolic axis of dairy cows revealed by statistical integration of ^{1}H NMR spectroscopic data. *J. Proteome Res.* **2013**, *12*, 1428–1435. [CrossRef] [PubMed]

20. Sundekilde, U.K.; Larsen, L.B.; Bertram, H.C. NMR-Based Milk Metabolomics. *Metabolites* **2013**, *3*, 204–222. [PubMed]

21. Andreas, N.J.; Hyde, M.J.; Gomez-Romero, M.; Lopez-Gonzalvez, M.A.; Villaseñor, A.; Wijeyesekera, A.; Barbas, C.; Modi, N.; Holmes, E.; Garcia-Perez, I. Multiplatform characterization of dynamic changes in breast milk during lactation. *Electrophoresis* **2015**, *36*, 2269–2285. [CrossRef] [PubMed]

22. Longini, M.; Tataranno, M.L.; Proietti, F.; Tortoriello, M.; Belvisi, E.; Vivi, A.; Tassini, M.; Perrone, S.; Buonocore, G. A metabolomic study of preterm and term human and formula milk by proton MRS analysis: Preliminary results. *J. Matern. Neonatal Med.* **2014**, *27*, 27–33. [CrossRef] [PubMed]

23. Marincola, F.C.; Dessì, A.; Corbu, S.; Reali, A.; Fanos, V. Clinical impact of human breast milk metabolomics. *Clin. Chim. Acta.* **2015**, *451*, 103–106. [CrossRef] [PubMed]

24. Marincola, F.C.; Noto, A.; Caboni, P.; Reali, A.; Barberini, L.; Lussu, M.; Murgia, F.; Santoru, M.L.; Atzori, L.; Fanos, V. A metabolomic study of preterm human and formula milk by high resolution NMR and GC/MS analysis: Preliminary results. *J. Matern. Neonatal Med.* **2012**, *25*, 62–67. [CrossRef] [PubMed]

25. Praticò, G.; Capuani, G.; Tomassini, A.; Baldassarre, M.E.; Delfini, M.; Miccheli, A. Exploring human breast milk composition by NMR-based metabolomics. *Nat. Prod. Res.* **2014**, *28*, 95–101. [CrossRef] [PubMed]

26. Smilowitz, J.T.; O'Sullivan, A.; Barile, D.; German, J.B.; Lönnerdal, B.; Slupsky, C.M. The human milk metabolome reveals diverse oligosaccharide profiles. *J. Nutr.* **2013**, *143*, 1709–1718. [CrossRef] [PubMed]

27. Spevacek, A.R.; Smilowitz, J.T.; Chin, E.L.; Underwood, M.A.; German, J.B.; Slupsky, C.M. Infant maturity at birth reveals minor differences in the maternal milk metabolome in the first month of lactation. *J. Nutr.* **2015**, *145*, 1698–1708. [CrossRef] [PubMed]

28. Wu, J.; Domellöf, M.; Zivkovic, A.M.; Larsson, G.; Öhman, A.; Nording, M.L. NMR-based metabolite profiling of human milk: A pilot study of methods for investigating compositional changes during lactation. *Biochem. Biophys. Res. Commun.* **2015**, *469*, 626–632. [CrossRef] [PubMed]

29. Sundekilde, U.K.; Poulsen, N.A.; Larsen, L.B.; Bertram, H.C. Nuclear magnetic resonance metabonomics reveals strong association between milk metabolites and somatic cell count in bovine milk. *J. Dairy Sci.* **2013**, *96*, 290–299. [CrossRef] [PubMed]

30. Wishart, D.S.; Knox, C.; Guo, A.C.; Eisner, R.; Young, N.; Gautam, B.; Hau, D.D.; Psychogios, N.; Dong, E.; Bouatra, S.; *et al.* HMDB: A knowledgebase for the human metabolome. *Nucleic Acids Res.* **2009**, *37*, D603–D610. [CrossRef] [PubMed]

31. Savorani, F.; Tomasi, G.; Engelsen, S.B. icoshift: A versatile tool for the rapid alignment of 1D NMR spectra. *J. Magn. Reson.* **2010**, *202*, 190–202. [CrossRef] [PubMed]

32. Cloarec, O.; Dumas, M.E.; Trygg, J.; Craig, A.; Barton, R.H.; Lindon, J.C.; Nicholson, J.K.; Holmes, E. Evaluation of the orthogonal projection on latent structure model limitations caused by chemical shift variability and improved visualization of biomarker changes in ^{1}H NMR spectroscopic metabonomic studies. *Anal. Chem.* **2005**, *77*, 517–526. [CrossRef] [PubMed]

33. Thurl, S.; Munzert, M.; Henker, J.; Boehm, G.; Müller-Werner, B.; Jelinek, J.; Stahl, B. Variation of human milk oligosaccharides in relation to milk groups and lactational periods. *Br. J. Nutr.* **2010**, *104*, 1261–1271. [CrossRef] [PubMed]

34. Dessì, A.; Ottonello, G.; Fanos, V. Physiopathology of intrauterine growth retardation: From classic data to metabolomics. *J. Matern. Neonatal Med.* **2012**, *25* (Suppl. 5), 13–18. [CrossRef] [PubMed]

35. Palmas, F.; Fattuoni, C.; Noto, A.; Barberini, L.; Dessì, A.; Fanos, V. The choice of amniotic fluid in metabolomics for the monitoring of fetus health. *Expert Rev. Mol. Diagn.* **2016**, *7159*, 1–14. [CrossRef] [PubMed]

36. Klein, M.S.; Buttchereit, N.; Miemczyk, S.P.; Immervoll, A.K.; Louis, C.; Wiedemann, S.; Junge, W.; Thaller, G.; Oefner, P.J.; Gronwald, W. NMR metabolomic analysis of dairy cows reveals milk glycerophosphocholine to phosphocholine ratio as prognostic biomarker for risk of ketosis. *J. Proteome Res.* **2012**, *11*, 1373–1381. [CrossRef] [PubMed]

37. McManaman, J.L.; Neville, M.C. Mammary physiology and milk secretion. *Adv. Drug Deliv. Rev.* **2003**, *55*, 629–641. [CrossRef]

38. Molinari, C.E.; Casadio, Y.S.; Hartmann, B.T.; Livk, A.; Bringans, S.; Arthur, P.G.; Hartmann, P.E. Proteome mapping of human skim milk proteins in term and preterm milk. *J. Proteome Res.* **2012**, *11*, 1696–1714. [CrossRef] [PubMed]

39. Whitmore, T.J.; Trengove, N.J.; Graham, D.F.; Hartmann, P.E. Analysis of insulin in human breast milk in mothers with type 1 and type 2 diabetes mellitus. *Int. J. Endocrinol.* **2012**, *2012*, 296368. [CrossRef] [PubMed]

40. Kelly, R.J.; Rouquier, S.; Giorgi, D.; Lennon, G.G.; Lowe, J.B. Sequence and Expression of a Candidate for the Human Secretor Blood Group (1,2) Fucosyltransferase Gene (FUT2): Homozygosity for an enzyme-inactivating nonsense mutation commonly correlates with the non-secretor phenotype. *J. Biol. Chem.* **1995**, *270*, 4640–4649. [CrossRef] [PubMed]

41. Totten, S.M.; Zivkovic, A.M.; Wu, S.; Ngyuen, U.; Freeman, S.L.; Ruhaak, L.R.; Darboe, M.K.; German, J.B.; Prentice, A.M.; Lebrilla, C.B. Comprehensive profiles of human milk oligosaccharides yield highly sensitive and specific markers for determining secretor status in lactating mothers. *J. Proteome Res.* **2012**, *11*, 6124–6133. [CrossRef] [PubMed]

42. Beijers, R.J.W.; Schaafsma, A. Long-chain polyunsaturated fatty acid content in Dutch preterm breast milk; differences in the concentrations of docosahexaenoic acid and arachidonic acid due to length of gestation. *Early Hum. Dev.* **1996**, *44*, 215–223. [CrossRef]

43. Coppa, G.V.; Gabrielli, O.; Pierani, P.; Catassi, C.; Carlucci, A.; Giorgi, P.L. Changes in carbohydrate composition in human milk over 4 months of lactation. *Pediatrics* **1993**, *91*, 637–641. [PubMed]

44. Villaseñor, A.; Garcia-Perez, I.; Garcia, A.; Posma, J.M.; Fernández-López, M.; Nicholas, A.J.; Modi, N.; Holmes, E.; Barbas, C. Breast milk metabolome characterization in a single-phase extraction, multiplatform analytical approach. *Anal. Chem.* **2014**, *86*, 8245–8252. [CrossRef] [PubMed]

45. De Leoz, M.L.A.; Gaerlan, S.C.; Strum, J.S.; Dimapasoc, L.M.; Mirmiran, M.; Tancredi, D.J.; Smilowitz, J.T.; Kalanetra, K.M.; Mills, D.A.; German, J.B.; *et al.* Lacto-N-tetraose, fucosylation, and secretor status are highly variable in human milk oligosaccharides from women delivering preterm. *J. Proteome Res.* **2012**, *11*, 4662–4672. [CrossRef] [PubMed]

46. Torrazza, R.M.; Neu, J. The altered gut microbiome and necrotizing enterocolitis. *Clin. Perinatol.* **2013**, *40*, 93–108. [CrossRef] [PubMed]

47. Zhang, Z.; Adelman, A.S.; Rai, D.; Boettcher, J.; Lönnerdal, B. Amino acid profiles in term and preterm human milk through lactation: A systematic review. *Nutr.* **2013**, *5*, 4800–4821. [CrossRef] [PubMed]

48. Atkinson, S.; Anderson, G.; Bryan, M. Human milk: Comparison of the nitrogen composition in milk from mothers of premature and full-term infants. *Am. J. Clin. Nutr.* **1980**, *33*, 811–815. [PubMed]

49. Chuang, C.K.; Lin, S.P.; Lee, H.C.; Wang, T.J.; Shih, Y.S.; Huang, F.Y.; Yeung, C.Y. Free amino acids in full-term and pre-term human milk and infant formula. *J. Pediatr. Gastroenterol. Nutr.* **2005**, *40*, 496–500. [CrossRef] [PubMed]

50. Moltó-Puigmartí, C.; Castellote, A.I.; Carbonell-Estrany, X.; López-Sabater, M.C. Differences in fat content and fatty acid proportions among colostrum, transitional, and mature milk from women delivering very preterm, preterm, and term infants. *Clin. Nutr.* **2011**, *30*, 116–123. [CrossRef] [PubMed]

51. Holmes-McNary, M.Q.; Cheng, W.L.; Mar, M.H.; Fussell, S.; Zeisel, S.H. Choline and choline esters in human and rat milk and in infant formulas. *Am. J. Clin. Nutr.* **1996**, *64*, 572–576. [PubMed]

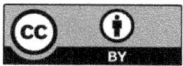

nutrients

MDPI

Article

Retinol and α-Tocopherol in the Breast Milk of Women after a High-Risk Pregnancy

Reyna Sámano [1], Hugo Martínez-Rojano [2,3,*], Rosa M. Hernández [1], Cristina Ramírez [1], María E. Flores Quijano [1], José M. Espíndola-Polis [4] and Daniela Veruete [5]

[1] Departamento de Nutrición y Bioprogramación, Instituto Nacional de Perinatología, Secretaría de Salud Montes Urales 800, Miguel Hidalgo, Lomas Virreyes, Ciudad de México CP. 11000, Mexico; ssmr0119@yahoo.com.mx (R.S.); rmh080868@yahoo.com (R.M.H.); crisra07@yahoo.com.mx (C.R.); maru_fq@yahoo.com (M.E.F.Q.)

[2] Departamento de Posgrado e Investigación, Escuela Superior de Medicina del Instituto Politécnico Nacional, Plan de San Luis y Díaz Mirón s/n, Colonia Casco de Santo Tomas, Delegación Miguel Hidalgo, Ciudad de México CP. 11340, Mexico

[3] Coordinación de Medicina Laboral, Instituto de Diagnóstico y Referencia Epidemiológicos (InDRE) "Dr. Manuel Martínez Báez", Secretaría de Salud Francisco de P. Miranda 177, Lomas de Plateros, Ciudad de México CP. 01480, Mexico

[4] Departamento de Nutrición Humana, Universidad del Altiplano, Mirasol 1, Tlacomulco, Tlaxcala de Xicohténcatl CP. 90102, Mexico; jjmartinezr@yahoo.com

[5] Universidad del Valle de México, campus Chapultepec Av. Constituyentes No. 151, Miguel Hidalgo, San Miguel Chapultepec I Secc, Ciudad de México CP. 11850, Mexico; analilia_000@hotmail.com

[*] Correspondence: hmartinez_59@yahoo.com.mx or hugo.martinezr@salud.gob.mx; Tel.: +52-555-062-1600 (ext. 59343)

Received: 18 September 2016; Accepted: 21 December 2016; Published: 1 January 2017

Abstract: Background: There is scant information about whether, after a high-risk pregnancy, breast milk provides enough vitamins for assuring satisfactory bodily reserves in newborns. Objective: To comparatively evaluate, in women with high-risk and normal pregnancy, the concentration of retinol and α-tocopherol in breast milk. Methods: This cross-sectional, analytical study was evaluated with reverse-phase high-performance liquid chromatography (HPLC). Informed consent was signed by 95 mothers with a high-risk pregnancy and 32 mothers with a normal pregnancy. From the mothers with a high-risk pregnancy were obtained: 23 samples of colostrum, 24 of transitional milk, and 48 of mature milk. From the normal pregnancy group, 32 mature milk samples were collected. Pregestational Body Mass Index (BMI) and the gestational weight gain were noted. Models of logistic regression were constructed to identify the variables related to a low concentration of either retinol or α-tocopherol in breast milk. Results: The concentration of retinol and α-tocopherol in mature milk was 60 (interquartile range (IQR), 41–90) and 276 (103–450) μg/dL, respectively, for the high-risk pregnancy group, and 76 (65–91) and 673 (454–866) μg/dL, respectively, for the normal pregnancy group ($p = 0.001$). The concentration of retinol and α-tocopherol was similar in the subgroups of mothers with different disorders during gestation. A clear correlation was found between a greater pregestational weight and a lower concentration of retinol ($Rho = -0.280$, $p = 0.006$), and between α-tocopherol and retinol in all cases ($Rho = 0.463$, $p = 0.001$). Among women having a high-risk pregnancy, those delivering prematurely rather than carrying their pregnancy to term had a reduced concentration of retinol (54 (37–78) vs. 70 (49–106) μg/dL; $p = 0.002$) and a tendency to a lower concentration of α-tocopherol in breast milk (185 (75–410) vs. 339 (160–500) μg/dL; $p = 0.053$). Compared to mothers with a normal pregnancy, those with a high-risk pregnancy (whether carried to term or ending in preterm delivery) exhibited a reduced concentration of retinol in mature milk ($p = 0.003$), as well as a tendency to a lower concentration of α-tocopherol ($p = 0.054$). Conclusion: Even though the women in the high-risk pregnancy group showed a deficiency of vitamins A and E in their breast milk, the unique biological benefits of this milk justify the promotion of breast feeding as the optimal method of nourishing neonates and infants. In these cases, it should be recommended that the woman increase her consumption of certain nutrients during pregnancy. Additionally, after childbirth mothers should consider the use of supplements to produce milk of adequate quality and thus meet the needs of the baby and prevent any deficiency in micronutrients.

Keywords: breast milk; liposoluble vitamins; high-performance liquid chromatography; pregestational obesity

1. Introduction

Approximately 22% of all pregnancies are high-risk in Mexico each year [1]. One of the risk factors for complications during pregnancy is being overweight, leading to a higher prevalence of gestational diabetes, hypertension, pre-eclampsia, asthma, and thromboembolic disease [2]. Around 60% of Mexican women in reproductive age are overweight [3]. Additionally, excessive weight gain during pregnancy also increases the risk of adverse outcomes for both mother and child [4], and a high percentage of Mexican women gain more weight than recommended [5].

Similarly, gestational diabetes is a risk factor for the increased incidence today of teratogenicity, which has been observed more frequently in fetuses of diabetic versus healthy mothers. These malformations are the result of tissue injury caused by the activity of free radicals [6]. Natural antioxidants reduce the adverse effects of these radicals, since they can capture and neutralize reactive oxygen species, thus preventing lipid peroxidation. This neutralization is essential, especially in situations where oxidative stress is elevated, such as gestational diabetes and preeclampsia [7]. One of the essential natural antioxidants is vitamin E, which comprises a group of eight fat-soluble compounds that are classified as α-, β-, γ-, and δ-tocopherol or tocotrienol. Of these, α-tocopherol is the most active compound [8].

The variation of glycaemia during pregnancy leads to serious complications for the mother-child binomial [7,8]. Although there is currently little evidence of the association between the concentration of retinol and diabetes in pregnant women [9], this disease makes such women more prone to a marginal or poor biochemical status of vitamin A [9]. In addition to potentiating the complications caused by diabetes in pregnant women, low levels of vitamin A leave their children vulnerable to developing a deficiency of the same [10,11].

An adequate nutritional status during the first 2–3 years of life is necessary for subsequent health and well-being. Deficient development cannot be reversed after passing this critical window [12]. In this sense, a study in Egypt stressed that vitamin E is a key micronutrient for development, with its deficiency leading to a delay in growth [13]. The authors also noted that 78.2% of children showing a delay in their growth were deficient in vitamin E, having plasma concentrations of α-tocopherol at 7.7 mmol/L versus 14.1 mmol/L for the group of control children [13]. Fares et al. [14] revealed that deficiencies of vitamins A, E, and D were very common among infants with very low birth weight in Tunisia, and were associated with preeclampsia. However, the risk of preeclampsia did not diminish after the administration of vitamin C and E in a series of studies in Western countries [15,16].

The results of administering vitamin E supplements have been variable. One reason is that the appropriate status of α-tocopherol during pregnancy has not yet been defined. Moreover, in the various global reports on the usefulness of vitamin E supplements during pregnancy, the plasma concentration of α-tocopherol is often not even determined. In situations where a low concentration of α-tocopherol was documented, the administration of supplements of vitamin E has proven beneficial. In a Hungarian population, for instance, supplementation of vitamin E in women was associated with a decreased incidence of premature babies [17]. The establishment of a clear criteria for adequate levels of vitamin E deserves further investigation.

It is also known that placental transfer of vitamins A and E during pregnancy is limited and that the reserve of these micronutrients in the newborn is low, especially in the case of premature babies. Consequently, exclusive breastfeeding is the only way to meet their nutritional needs [8]. Since exposure to hyperoxia at birth increases the risk of free radical formation [18], it is essential that the mother provide the infant a sufficient supply of vitamin E through breastfeeding.

Due to the importance of vitamins A and E for the mother and child, the aim of the present study was to determine the concentration of retinol and α-tocopherol in the breast milk of mothers after undergoing a high-risk versus normal pregnancy, as well as after giving birth preterm versus carrying their pregnancy to term. Associations were examined between low levels of vitamins A and E in breast milk and maternal characteristics.

2. Material and Methods

2.1. Study Design and Population

A cross-sectional and analytical study was conducted to determine the presence of retinol and α-tocopherol in the breast milk of 95 mothers with a high-risk pregnancy (and whose newborns were confined in the neonatal intensive care unit during the first and second month after birth) and 32 mothers with a normal pregnancy and healthy newborns. The study took place from January 2013 to October 2016. It was conducted at the Instituto Nacional de Perinatología (National Institute of Perinatology) and the School of Medicine, National Polytechnic Institute, in Mexico City.

The sample size was calculated with a 95% confidence interval, utilizing information from previous reports that estimated the mean content of vitamin A in breast milk [19]. After the mothers had agreed to participate and signed informed consent, they were asked to fill out a survey to provide data about their obstetrical background.

The manner of sampling mothers was not probabilistic or based on consecutive cases. Inclusion criteria were that the women lived in the metropolitan area of Mexico City, agreed to provide all data requested through a survey (maternal age, sociodemographic characteristics, medical and obstetrical history, course of current pregnancy and term, mode of delivery, pregnancy-related complications, weight, and complications of the neonates), were breastfeeding their newborns/infants and secreting breast milk in adequate quantities, were 18–45 years old, and were not taking medications or vitamin/multivitamin supplements. All participating mothers had been eating customary Mexican food during pregnancy and none had adopted special diets.

The 127 mothers that participated in the study were recruited by the nutrition team of the National Perinatology Institute (all women in this unit who consented were included). In the high-risk pregnancy group, all the newborns and some of the women were hospitalized. Contrarily, in the normal pregnancy group, none of the infants were hospitalized. Among the 95 mothers with a high-risk pregnancy, 48 delivered preterm and 47 carried their pregnancy to term. All 32 mothers with a history of normal pregnancy carried their pregnancy to term.

Preterm childbirth was defined as a gestation lasting less than 37 weeks. A normal pregnancy was defined as the lack of complications or disorders before and/or during gestation. When there were pregnancy-related complications, illnesses, or events that represented a health risk, the situation was considered high risk. Especially important was any appearance of the woman or an increase in complications that could have caused maternal/perinatal morbidity/mortality. The following conditions were examined for any possible association with low levels of retinol or α-tocopherol: (i) multiple gestation (involving twins, triplets, etc.), which increases the risk of infants being born prematurely (before 37 weeks of pregnancy); (ii) pregnancy with triplets or quadruplets, which implies a greater the probability of delivery by cesarean section; (iii) pregnancy after age 30 and/or after taking fertility drugs (both related to multiple births); and (iv) gestational diabetes, preeclampsia or eclampsia.

Preeclampsia, a syndrome marked by a sudden rise in the blood pressure of a pregnant woman after the 20th week of pregnancy, can affect the kidneys, liver, and brain. When left untreated, the condition may result in long term health problems or be fatal for the mother and/or the fetus. Eclampsia is a more severe form of preeclampsia, marked by anemia, seizures, and coma in the mother (implying an increased risk for a first-time pregnancy in women over 35 years of age). Preeclampsia and gestational diabetes were based on the criteria of the American College of Obstetricians and Gynecologists [20,21].

2.2. Milk Sampling

Samples of breast milk were aseptically obtained from the mothers, either at home or in the hospital, during the morning (08:00–10:00) and after 8–10 h of fasting. The first sample of breast milk from mothers with a history of high-risk pregnancy was obtained in the hospital during the 48 h immediately after birth. These samples were considered as colostrum. Transitional milk was obtained from these same mothers at eight days postpartum. Mature milk samples were obtained from both groups of women between the first and second month postpartum. Breast milk was delivered by mothers to the hospital milk bank with the high-risk pregnancy group, because the newborns were in the Neonatal Intensive Care. This milk was deposited in sterile polypropylene bottles and stored at 4 °C or colder. The women with a history of normal pregnancy delivered their sample of breast milk to the nutritionist when they brought their healthy child to the hospital. From each recipient, an aliquot of 15 mL was filled without leaving any air pockets (to avoid oxygenation). This aliquot was taken from a full breast sample, previously homogenized. Each aliquot was protected from ultraviolet light with aluminum foil and placed in refrigeration at –20 °C.

2.3. Type of Milk

From the high-risk pregnancy group, 23 of the breast milk samples obtained were considered as colostrum, 24 transitional milk, and 48 mature milk. From the normal pregnancy group, 32 mature milk samples were obtained. Colostrum is considered as the breast milk from delivery to approximately five days postpartum, transitional milk from day 6–15 postpartum, and mature milk from day 15 onwards.

2.4. Laboratory Methods

The procedure for determining the concentration of vitamins A and E (as retinol and α-tocopherol) was based on high-performance liquid chromatography (HPLC) in the reverse phase. The internal standard was all-trans-retinyl-acetate (800-Across-01. Software Total Chrome, version 6.3.2.0646, Whippany, NJ, USA). This determination was carried out on all of the breast milk samples from the 127 participating mothers.

Retinol and α-tocopherol levels were determined in breast milk by using a binary HPLC pump (Flexar model, Perkin-Elmer, Naperville, IL, USA) with an injector (loop size 100 µL, Flexar model), a sensitive UV7 detector (Flexar model, Norwalk, CT, USA), a three-column microbondapak rp-18 Pecosphere C-18 of 3 µm and 33.46 mm (Perkin-Elmer), and an acrodisc CR-13 mm syringe filter with a 0.2 µm PTFE (polytetrafluoroethylene) membrane (Teflon).

After the extraction, vitamins A and E were isolated from the samples of breast milk. First the matrix was saponified, followed by extraction of the analytes of interest. The esters of retinal were hydrolyzed to retinol by saponification. To 15 mL of breast milk was added 24 mL of potassium hydroxide in a solution of 16% methanol (weight per volume). This alkaline mixture was heated to 75 °C and maintained at that temperature for 30 min, then cooled for 5 min. For the extraction of the vitamins, 16 mL of petroleum ether was added in a separatory funnel, and then the solution was stirred and left to stand for 30 min. The aqueous phase was drained and disposed of three times. The etheric dissolution was washed with deionized water to eliminate the alkaline excess, reaching pH 7 (measured with pH paper). The solvent was recovered in Falcon tubes of 50 mL, to be evaporated in a steam bath at 70 °C. The residue was dissolved with 2 mL of ethanol, then filtered with acrodisk CR 13 mm syringe filters with a 0.2 µm PTFE membrane. An injection volume was taken from this solution for the chromatography with 50 µL, which was run for 10 min. To obtain the target of the reactives, a process of saponification and extraction was carried out in the absence of breast milk. All samples were processed in duplicate and each replicate was injected twice [22].

Microbondapak columns with a UV/visible detector were utilized to establish the conditions for the chromatographic system, with methanol/water (96:4) for the mobile phase and a wavelength of 325 nm for retinol and 290 nm for α-tocopherol. The analytic parameters for linearity were $R^2 = 0.9955$ for retinol and $R^2 = 0.9808$ for α-tocopherol, while the detection and quantification limits were 1.1 µg/dL and 2.7 µg/dL for retinol and 0.9 µg/dL and 2.3 µg/dL for α-tocopherol. Regarding accuracy, relative standard deviation (RSD) was 4.5% for the same day and RSD 4.8% between days for retinol, and 4.9% for the same day and 4.1% between days for α-tocopherol. The recovery was 85.8 ± 7.8% µg/dL for retinol and 98 ± 1.9% µg/dL for α-tocopherol. Once validated, the method was applied to the quantification of retinol and α-tocopherol in samples of breast milk [23].

2.5. Evaluating Maternal Body Mass Index (BMI) and Morbidity in Mothers and Newborns/Infants

The pregestational weight and height of the mother was obtained from the clinical history. The BMI was calculated considering ≤18.49 kg/m^2 as underweight, 18.50–24.99 kg/m^2 as normal, 25–29.9 kg/m^2 as overweight and ≥30 kg/m^2 as obese. The evaluation of the gestational weight was based on both the pregestational BMI and the tables of the Institute of Medicine (IOM, Washington, DC, USA). The increase in gestational weight was calculated by subtracting the pregestational weight from the maximum gestational weight, and the result was classified as adequate or below/above the recommended level, according to the guidelines of the IOM [24]. The absence or presence of morbidity in mothers and newborns/infants was determined by reviewing the corresponding clinical history.

3. Statistical Analysis

For clinical data, anthropometric and sociodemographic characteristics of the mothers and newborns were reported as the mean ± Standard Deviation (SD) and the median with an interquartile range (IQR) of p25–p75. Due to the nature of the variables, a parametric analysis was performed with the Student's *t*-test and a non-parametric analysis with the Mann-Whitney *U* test and the Kruskal-Wallis test. Additionally, frequency and percentages for categorical variables were analyzed with the Pearson's X^2 test. For qualitative variables, such as marital status, occupation, level of education, and pregnancy outcome, frequency measurements were calculated. For numerical variables, including the age of the mother and pregestational weight and height, measurements of central tendency and dispersion were utilized. With the Kruskal-Wallis test, analysis was made of the difference between the concentration of retinol and α-tocopherol between groups and in relation to the pregestational BMI of the mother. For the concentration of the vitamins and the outcome of the pregnancy, the Mann-Whitney *U* test was employed. We used the median value for women with high-risk or normal pregnancy as a comparison group. The two values used in the logistic regression model were considered risk variables when they were below these medians. A statistical significance was considered at $p < 0.05$. Data entry and analysis were performed with the statistical program SPSS version 20 for Windows (SPSS Inc., Chicago, IL, USA).

4. Ethical Aspects

Data gathering and analysis was confidential, taking such ethical questions as autonomy and security into account. The guidelines of the Helsinki Declaration were followed. The project protocol was approved by the Scientific and Ethics Committee of our institution. All women participating in this study were given medical attention at the highest level of medical specialties in a health center in Mexico City (with ethical approval code number 212250-49501).

5. Results

Of the 95 mothers with a high-risk pregnancy and 32 with a normal pregnancy, the median age was 28 years (IQR = 20–34 years), cohabitation was the most common marital status, and homemaker was the most common occupation. Regarding educational level, nearly 90% had finished middle school. Concerning obstetric background, 44% of the participants were primigravida, 98% of the births took place by caesarean section, and the average weight of the neonates was 1686 g (Table 1).

Table 1. Clinical, anthropometric and sociodemographic characteristics of the mothers and newborns (*n* = 127).

Clinical and Anthropometric Characteristics			
	High-risk pregnancy *n* = 95	Normal pregnancy *n* = 32	*p*
	Mean ± SD		
Age (years) [a]	28 ± 5	27 ± 8	0.456
Pregestational weight (kg) [a]	62.2 ± 10	59.9 ± 10	0.253
Maximum gestational weight (kg) [a]	70.4 ± 13	67 ± 13	0.239
Height (cm) [a]	156 ± 6	156 ± 5	0.632
Pregestational BMI [a]	25.5 ± 4	24.5 ± 3	0.176
Number of prenatal check-ups [a]	4 ± 2	4 ± 0.5	0.211
Gynecological age (years) [a]	15 ± 8	16.5 ± 5	0.890
Menarche (age in years) [a]	12 ± 2	12 ± 1	0.878
Weight of the newborn (g) [a]	1686 ± 843	2167 ± 689	0.004
Length of the newborn (cm) [a]	40 ± 5	48.2 ± 5	0.006
Sociodemographic characteristics [b]	Frequency (%)		
Marital status			
Single	23 (24)	4 (13)	
Married	35 (37)	11 (34)	0.556
Cohabitation	37 (39)	17 (53)	
Occupation			
Homemaker	73 (77)	24 (75)	0.883
Working outside the home	22 (23)	8 (25)	
Level of education			
Primary or less	10 (11)	2 (6)	
Middle school	40 (42)	14 (44)	0.823
High school	33 (35)	13 (41)	
Professional	12 (12)	3 (9)	
Socioeconomic level			
Lower to lower-middle class	95 (100)	31 (96)	0.983

Data expressed as the [a] mean ± standard deviation—Student's *t*; [b] frequency (%)—Pearson's X^2.

There were differences between the two groups of mothers (normal versus high-risk pregnancy) in relation to the concentration of retinol and α-tocopherol in mature breast milk (Figures 1 and 2), as well as in neonate weight and length. Concerning anthropometric characteristics, women with a high-risk pregnancy had an average pregestational BMI of 25.5 kg/m² and those with a normal pregnancy 24.5 kg/km², while the average gestational weight gain was 8.2 kg for both groups (Table 1).

For the women with a high-risk pregnancy, the most common disorder or condition related to risk was preeclampsia (40/95), followed by anemia (29/95), advanced maternal age (14/95), and gestational diabetes (12/95). The complications of the neonates born of these women were preterm birth or low birth weight (62/95), infant respiratory distress syndrome or gastroschisis (18/95), and lesions related to the birth canal (6/95). The rest showed no complications (9/95).

When comparing the distinct subgroups of women with different disorders during gestation, there were similar concentrations of retinol and α-tocopherol in breast milk (Table 2). However, the concentration of retinol and α-tocopherol in breast milk was lower in women that gave preterm birth compared to those who carried their pregnancy to term. Considering the women with a high-risk pregnancy, the concentration of retinol was higher in the mature milk of women with normal pregestational weight, while no significant difference was found in the concentration of α-tocopherol among those having adequate gestational weight gain.

266

Table 2. Concentrations of retinol and α-tocopherol in breast milk, in relation to some perinatal data of the women with a high-risk pregnancy (*n* = 95).

		Retinol				α-Tocopherol		
		n	Colostrum µg/dL Median (IQR)	Transition Milk µg/dL Median (IQR)	Mature Milk µg/dL Median (IQR)	Colostrum µg/dL Median (IQR)	Transition Milk µg/dL Median (IQR)	Mature Milk µg/dL Median (IQR)
Maternal age (years)	≤19	21	73 (37–93)	57 (52–70)	67 (49–70)	500 (103–654)	276 (55–445)	207 (48–270)
	20–29	29	67 (35–128)	84 (64–103)	60 (49–82)	298 (127–492)	204 (103–321)	321 (68–436)
	30–34	23	42 (33–50)	93 (64–120)	42 (35–56)	500 (405–597)	654 (348–727)	103 (46–255)
	≥35	22	79 (52–106)	62 (39–81)	67 (49–70)	275 (192–570)	201 (167–475)	339 (180–423)
p [a]			0.225	0.340	0.173	0.632	0.407	0.330
Pregestational BMI	Normal weight	41	60 (47–96)	80 (66–97)	60 (42–80)	575 (154–654)	180 (131–410)	321 (55–448)
	Overweight	40	60 (38–94)	64 (41–93)	45 (34–64)	321 (130–540)	249 (90–450)	190 (54–340)
	Obesity	14	33 (33–33)	42 (32–52)	49 (38–55)	455 (410–500)	295 (146–445)	146 (103–423)
p [a]			0.209	0.095	0.003	0.575	0.945	0.620
Gestational weight increase	Adequate	19	31 (29–33)	72(44–120)	50 (34–60)	270 (130–410)	549 (323–727)	340 (61–423)
	Low	35	60 (42–93)	73 (70–110)	62 (49–90)	470 (120–654)	180 (107–433)	218 (63–339)
	Excessive	41	61 (45–94)	64 (53–89)	55 (40–79)	400 (253–602)	249 (103–372)	180 (103–423)
p [a]			0.090	0.136	0.337	0.802	0.911	0.951
Gestational age	To term	47	60 (46–102)	103 (73–120)	59 (49–91)	470 (275–654)	445 (160–676)	330 (63–441)
	Preterm	48	41 (33–89)	62 (47–77)	48 (38–70)	400 (125–525)	132 (233–371)	135 (61–276)
p [b]			0.069	0.005	0.058	0.260	0.290	0.118
Complication during pregnancy	Gestational diabetes	12	49 (44–93)	94 (70–119)	47 (35–99)	400 (321–500)	433 (189–676)	38 (18–431)
	Preeclampsia	40	60 (41–92)	62 (40–76)	59 (46–76)	343 (230–654)	233 (115–445)	218 (104–450)
	Anemia, myomas	29	49 (32–83)	93 (70–103)	47 (35–67)	545 (125–654)	321 (160–450)	205 (59–416)
	Advanced maternal age	14	90 (62–96)	76 (52–100)	68 (49–85)	360 (183–500)	274 (103–445)	180 (103–321)
p [a]			0.690	0.260	0.378	0.905	0.906	0.661

[a] Kruskal-Wallis; [b] Mann–Whitney *U*; IQR, interquartile ranges.

Women with normal pregestational BMI had a higher concentration of retinol compared to those who were overweight or obese (see Table 2). The Spearman correlation revealed that the greater the pregestational weight (relative to normal), the lower the concentration of retinol (*Rho* = −0.280, *p* = 0.006). Moreover, there was a correlation between α-tocopherol and retinol (*Rho* = 0.463, *p* = 0.001).

Compared to women with a normal pregnancy, the mature breast milk of those with a high-risk pregnancy who delivered at full term showed a similar concentration of retinol but a lower concentration of α-tocopherol. Compared to the mature milk of women with a normal pregnancy, in contrast, the breast milk of those with a high-risk pregnancy who delivered preterm had a reduced concentration of retinol and α-tocopherol in the diverse types of milk (colostrum, transition milk, and mature milk) (Figures 1 and 2).

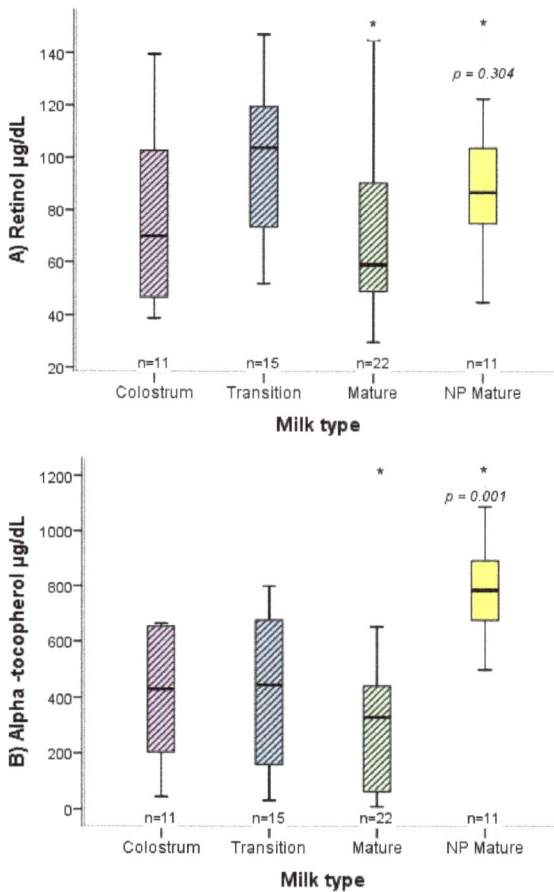

Figure 1. Box plot distribution of the concentration of retinol (**A**) and α-tocopherol (**B**) in breast milk, comparing the women with a full-term, high-risk pregnancy to those with a normal pregnancy. For the high-risk pregnancy, the distinct types of breast milk are shown (colostrum, transition milk, and mature milk). * *p*; Mann-Whitney *U*. The bottom and top of the box represent the first and third quartiles (IQR), and the band inside the box the median. The ends of the whiskers denote the lowest and highest values still within 1.5 IQR. Outlier values are not displayed. NP, normal pregnancy.

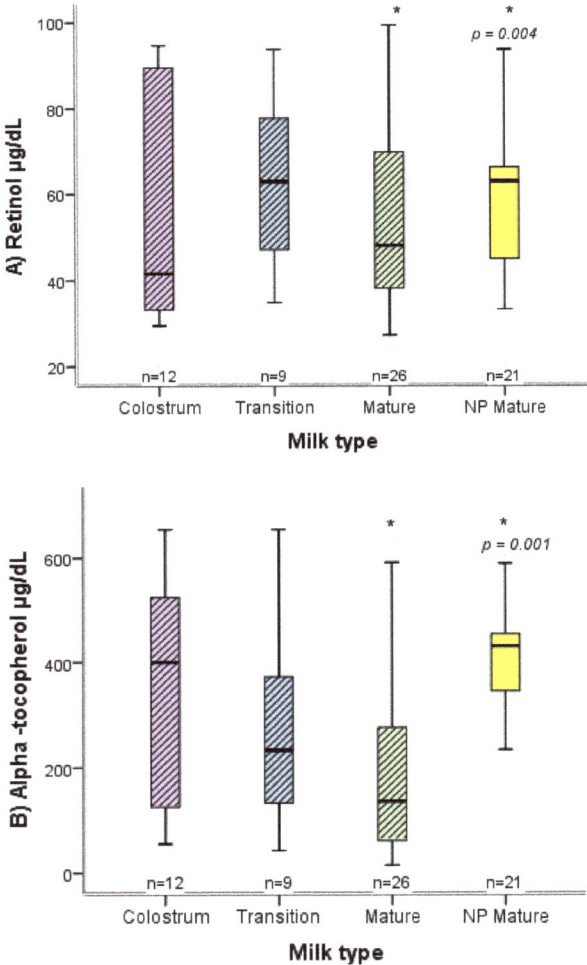

Figure 2. Box plot distribution of the concentration of retinol (**A**) and α-tocopherol (**B**) in breast milk, comparing women with a preterm, high-risk pregnancy to those with a normal pregnancy. For the high-risk pregnancy, the distinct types of breast milk (colostrum, transition milk and mature milk) are shown. * *p*; Mann-Whitney *U*. The bottom and top of the box represent the first and third quartiles (IQR), and the band inside the box the median. The ends of the whiskers denote the lowest and highest values still within 1.5 IQR. Outlier values are not displayed. NP, normal pregnancy.

When the logistic regression model included variables that corresponded to a high-risk pregnancy, it was observed that in all cases the concentration of both vitamin precursors was lower with high-risk versus normal pregnancy. However, no particular risk factors were associated with these lower concentrations. Hence, the following model was performed.

For the regression model, we utilized the median values for concentrations of retinol below 60 µg/dL and for α-tocopherol below 276 µg/dL in the group high-risk pregnancy, while using these values below 76 and 673 µg/dL for retinol and α-tocopherol, respectively, in the group with a history of normal pregnancy. For the high-risk pregnancy group, the variables associated with a low concentration of retinol in breast milk were preterm childbirth and pregestational overweight or obesity. For the normal pregnancy group, only pregestational overweight or obesity was significant. Meanwhile, for all the women (whether having a high-risk pregnancy or a history of normal pregnancy), a significant risk of a low concentration of α-tocopherol was correlated with preterm childbirth and a tendency was associated with preeclampsia (Table 3).

Table 3. Variables associated with low concentrations of retinol and α-tocopherol in mothers that underwent a high-risk pregnancy ($n = 95$).

Maternal variables	The Median Concentration in Mature Milk of Mothers Who Underwent a High-Risk Pregnancy			The Median Concentration in Mature Milk of Mothers Who Experienced a Normal Pregnancy		
	OR	CI 95%	p *	OR	CI 95%	p *
	Retinol concentration ($\leq$60 µg/dL)			($\leq$76 µg/dL)		
Preterm childbirth	2.618	1.111–6.169	0.028	2.112	0.858–5.856	0.112
Preeclampsia	1.512	0.429–5.450	0.512	0.992	0.992–1.138	0.102
Gestational diabetes	0.879	0.277–3.122	0.575	0.272	0.023–3.249	0.273
Anemia	0.877	0.281–3.629	0.258	0.955	0.906–1.006	0.331
Maternal age: under 19 or over 29 years	0.818	0.364–1.838	0.390	2.189	0.858–5.586	0.101
Pregestational overweight or obesity	1.179	1.822–2692	0.039	3.563	1.422–8.927	0.007
	α-tocopherol concentration ($\leq$276 µg/dL) [a]			($\leq$673 µg/dL) [b]		
Preterm childbirth	2.243	0.985–5.111	0.039	2.091	1.689–2.588	0.038
Preeclampsia	1.304	0.567–3.001	0.532	1.063	0.992–1.138	0.051
Gestational diabetes	0.892	0.228–3.483	0.869	0.289	0.023–2.951	0.336
Anemia	0.914	0.252–3.319	0.892	0.955	0.906–1.006	0.331
Maternal age: under 19 or over 29 years	1.879	0.459–2.484	0.879	0.402	0.035–4.591	0.441
Pregestational overweight or obesity	1.056	0.447–2.494	0.870	0.772	0.064–9.302	0.838

CI 95%: 95% confidence interval. OR: odds ratio. Low concentrations of retinol and α-tocopherol: value below the median in mothers after a high-risk pregnancy and those with a history of a normal pregnancy. * p Value in logistic regression model.

Regarding the different types of breast milk (Table 4), the concentration of both α-tocopherol and retinol were lower among women who gave preterm childbirth. A positive correlation existed in all cases between the concentration of retinol and that of α-tocopherol in the different types of milk, with *Rho* values of 0.325 for colostrum, 0.375 for transition milk, and 0.300 for mature milk ($p \leq 0.001$).

Table 4. Concentration of retinol and α-tocopherol in relation to the type of breast milk.

Pregnancy Length	Colostrum	Transition	Mature
	Retinol, median (IQR), µg/dL		
Preterm ($n = 48$)	36 (32–63)	60 (39–81)	43 (36–66)
Full term ($n = 47$)	49 (39–86)	73 (49–115)	52 (37–72)
p [a]	0.010	0.020	0.032
	α-tocopherol, median (IQR), µg/dL		
Preterm ($n = 48$)	405 (109–676)	233 (90–372)	175 (59–465)
Full term ($n = 47$)	654 (205–2313)	676 (174–1884)	285 (55–477)
p [a]	0.004	0.001	0.012

Data expressed as the median (IQR). [a] *Mann Whitney U*; IQR, interquartile range.

There was a reduced level of retinol and α-tocopherol in mothers giving preterm birth or having low birth-weight neonates compared to those that carried their pregnancy to term. However, the concentration of retinol ($p = 0.244$) and α-tocopherol ($p = 0.090$) did not show a significant difference in relation to complications of the newborn. Likewise, no significant difference existed for the concentration of retinol ($p = 0.243$) or α-tocopherol ($p = 0.897$) in regard to the history of pregnancies.

When comparing women with preterm delivery to those who carried their pregnancy to term, the concentration of retinol was 54 (IQR; 37–78) vs. 70 (IQR; 49–106) µg/dL ($p = 0.002$), while that of α-tocopherol was 155 (IQR; 74–410) vs. 445 (IQR; 160–500) µg/dL ($p = 0.053$). On the other hand, compared to women with a high-risk pregnancy, those with a normal pregnancy had a higher level of both vitamin precursors in mature milk.

6. Discussion

There was an association between a lower concentration of retinol and α-tocopherol in mature breast milk and two risk factors: pregestational overweight or obesity and preterm delivery. This significance was established with the original statistical analysis and confirmed by the logistic regression model. No significant difference in the concentration of retinol or α-tocopherol was found in relation to either of the morbidities existing among women in the high-risk pregnancy group. Although no direct association was detected between preeclampsia and lower levels of these vitamin precursors, this morbidity is related to overweight and obesity, a condition that, in turn, may cause preterm delivery.

6.1. Concentration of Retinol and α-Tocopherol

Considering that breast milk is the only source of nutrition for newborns, it is important to determine whether the content of vitamins A and E are adequate, especially when the neonate is premature or of very low weight [25,26]. In the majority of reports, the concentration of α-tocopherol in the colostrum of women is two to three times higher than that detected presently in Mexican women after a high-risk pregnancy. For the women with a normal evolutive pregnancy, some of the current results are similar to those described for women from Bangladesh and Poland [27,28].

Concerning retinol, for the group of mothers in this study with a history of normal pregnancy and having a normal delivery, the average concentration of this vitamin precursor is close to that commonly reported. In contrast, the women in the present study with a high-risk pregnancy had, on the average, about half the concentration of retinol previously found for women with a normal pregnancy, and a third of this concentration in the cases of preterm childbirth. These values are close to those observed in a group of women in Bangladesh [27,29,30].

The similarities in the concentration of these two vitamins between Mexico and Bangladesh [27] may be due to the characteristics of the particular populations under study. That is, the women in both studies had a low socioeconomic status and poor health indicators, which makes them more prone to the development of nutritional deficiencies. Although the nutrient concentrations found in the women are low, Ahmed et al. demonstrated that this amount is sufficient to satisfy the nutritional needs of infants.

In relation to transitional milk, the concentration of retinol and α-tocopherol described in diverse populations [31–35] is higher than that evidenced in the present study after a high-risk pregnancy. Kodentsova and Vrzhesinskaya reported a mean concentration for each of these vitamin precursors in Russian women that was very similar to the present high-risk pregnancy group. This similarity is likely due to the fact that approximately 50% of Russian women who participated in the study experienced a preterm pregnancy [36].

Regarding mature milk in the current contribution, the mean concentration of α-tocopherol and retinol for both groups of women (with a normal pregnancy and high-risk pregnancy) is very similar to most reports on these micronutrients. However, for women who, herein, had a high-risk pregnancy, the median concentration of α-tocopherol was higher than that detected in Polish women [37–43] and in a group of adolescent mothers in Brazil [44]. In another study by Tokusoglu et al. [45], the concentration of α-tocopherol in the mature milk of Turkish women was similar to that commonly observed in colostrum. Quiles et al. [26] found higher than average values for mature milk in Spain, but this was based on only 15 women. The small sample size likely influenced the results.

The level of α-tocopherol and retinol in breast milk is normally greater in colostrum and thereafter exhibits a downward trend during the different stages of lactation. In this study, the women with a high-risk pregnancy showed this downward trend. We compared the average concentration of α-tocopherol previously reported for different groups of women, mostly with a normal evolutive pregnancy, to that found presently for women with a high-risk pregnancy. This concentration was herein found to be 2–3 times lower in colostrum, approximately two times lower in transitional milk, and very similar in mature milk [31,32,46–48].

Although an inverse correlation has been reported between the concentration of retinol and α-tocopherol in colostrum [49], the current results evidence a positive correlation between these two vitamins, which implies the existence of suboptimal concentrations. This manifests the need for supplementation [50] to prevent deficiencies in any given population.

6.2. Preterm Childbirth

For women in the present study with preterm birth, the median concentration of 405 (IQR; 109–676) µg/dL of α-tocopherol in colostrum was lower than that detected in the colostrum of some other groups of women having the same gestational age. For example, there were 1450 µg/dL in a group of German women [51], 1292.1–1722.8 µg/dL in Spanish women [26], and 1222 ± 772 µg/dL in Tunisian women [14]. Nevertheless, the current findings coincide with the concentration of α-tocopherol in the colostrum of women in other studies that gave preterm birth, such as the 250 µg/dL detected in Canadian women [52] and the 260.0 ± 30.0 µg/dL for Russian women [31]. In the case of retinol in the colostrum of women having given preterm birth, the median value of 36 (32–63) µg/dL observed herein is lower than the 57.5 ± 50.1 µg/dL described by Fares et al. [14]. This suggests the need to focus on reinforcing vitamin levels in women with preterm births and their neonates.

The hypothesis that the concentration of vitamin E depends on gestational age is still very controversial [49,53]. Nonetheless, this idea is supported by the current findings. Similar results were reported for a group of Spanish women by Quiles et al. [26], who found significantly higher concentrations of vitamin E at all stages of lactation in women who had carried their pregnancy to term compared to those giving preterm birth.

Compared to the women that carried their pregnancy to term in the present study, those that gave preterm birth had lower concentrations of retinol and α-tocopherol. The greatest deficiency was detected for the latter vitamin precursor. These results coincide with the findings of Souza et al. [54]. To compensate for this deficiency, supplementation of these vitamins should be provided during pregnancy (especially when involving high-risk) and breastfeeding. Unlike the current results, a Brazilian study reported variable concentrations of α-tocopherol, without any difference between women giving premature birth and those carrying their pregnancy to term. It has been postulated that the concentration of this vitamin is associated with birth weight more than prematurity [53]. However, this idea was not corroborated presently, evidencing multifactorial causes for the deficiency of this vitamin.

The current findings emphasize the fact that the neonate of a preterm birth requires special care, such as optimal nutrition. Not only does the prematurity of birth imply low reserves of vitamins A and E, but also the poor nutritional status of the mother indicates a limited transfer of the same through the placenta. For these reasons, liposoluble vitamins (e.g., retinol and α-tocopherol) should be assimilated by women with high-risk pregnancies [55] to avoid complications such as a delay in intrauterine growth or in neurodevelopment. A deficiency of these vitamins can even induce miscarriage [29].

Furthermore, it is recommended that preterm neonates immediately begin enteral feeding with breast milk and, if possible, vitamin supplementation [55]. Indeed, clinical assays have been conducted in which pregnant women were given a supplement of RRR α-tocopherol acetate, resulting in a significantly elevated concentration of this vitamin in transition milk and mature milk, as well as in the mothers themselves who gave preterm birth [50].

6.3. Does the BMI Affect the Concentrations of Retinol and α-Tocopherol?

The current results reveal that the higher the pregestational BMI (relative to normal) and the greater the gap between the real and recommended gestational weight gain, the lower the concentration of retinol tends to be. In this sense, the simple fact of having a high BMI is a risk factor for increased production of proinflammatory cytokines, a problem that can be counteracted if women are protected by adequate concentrations of two antioxidant substances, retinol and α-tocopherol. Perhaps it was the deficiency of retinol and α-tocopherol that, in large part, caused the relatively high frequency of preeclampsia among the women presently studied, considering that this deficiency (as well as others) can lead to greater oxidative stress [37] which, in turn, when coupled with other factors, tends to trigger this disorder [56,57].

A negative correlation was observed herein between pregestational BMI and the concentration of retinol and α-tocopherol. Like any population with overweight and obesity, pregnant women lack antioxidants and are exposed to cytokines that can harm their health and that of their offspring, thus affecting fetal programming and the first 1000 days of life [58–60].

The results suggest that the present participants showed no association between gestational diabetes (or other morbidities correlated with pregnancy) and low concentrations of retinol and α-tocopherol in breast milk, in agreement with another report that found no such association [11]. Since breast milk is the only source of these vitamins, however, there may be a greater risk, especially in the case that the newborn is premature or suffers from complications that increase oxidative stress.

The current results, like the vast majority of studies on liposoluble vitamins in breast milk [61–63], evidence a wide range in the concentration of vitamins A and E (especially vitamin E) among participants. This variation could be related to differences in lifestyle, in the consumption of nutrients and/or enrichment of food, and in the use of vitamin and food supplements. Some methodological factors, such as the day and time of collecting samples or the time elapsed since the last breastfeeding and the last meal, could contribute to this variability. Additionally, differences in methods of analysis also represent an important factor of variation. Finally, the methods employed for hydrolysis and extraction of an organic matrix of vitamins can affect the concentration of the same in breast milk [62].

Nourishing an infant with milk from his or her own mother results in better growth and nutritional status (including the level of vitamins A and E) than that observed in infants fed formula. Moreover, breast milk composition may be affected by obstetric characteristics, such as a premature delivery. In the present study, the composition of retinol and α-tocopherol in breast milk was negatively affected by premature birth and pregestational overweight and obesity. Furthermore, the concentration of these vitamin precursors was lower in the breast milk of women that had undergone a high-risk pregnancy compared to those having had a normal pregnancy.

Studies that explore the association between neonatal/maternal characteristics and the concentration of retinol and α-tocopherol in breast milk are important for determining the subgroups of newborns at risk for a vitamin A and E deficiency. This information should lead to strategies (e.g., vitamin supplementation) to target the subgroups at risk. Moreover, this approach can broaden the understanding of the influence of maternal factors such as gestational age on the adaptation capacity of mechanisms for transferring retinol and α-tocopherol to the mammary gland.

Certain elements of this study could be considered as limitations, including the lack of an evaluation of the nutritional state and diet of the participants. Another limitation is that a determination of fat in breast milk samples was not made. However, in other populations a high negative correlation has been shown between the concentration of serum cholesterol, the BMI, and the level of tocopherol and retinol. In addition, it must be kept in mind that all of the women participating in this study were of a low socioeconomic level, meaning that the results obtained cannot be generalized to all Mexican women during the period of breastfeeding.

7. Conclusions

Since the nutritional needs of a woman are sharply increased during pregnancy, it can be a challenge to meet these needs if careful attention is not paid to an adequate consumption of nutrients. Any inadequate dietary alteration can affect the health of the mother-fetus binomial. Deficiencies in micronutrients are related to gestational diabetes, preeclampsia, eclampsia, delayed intrauterine growth, low birth weight of the neonate, premature separation of the placenta, premature childbirth, spontaneous abortion, and congenital anomalies. Moreover, maternal nutrition determines the quality of breast milk. The concentration of vitamins A and E in breast milk depend on the concentration of the same in the mother. Hence, a maternal deficiency translates into the same problem for the neonate.

Even though the women in the high-risk pregnancy group showed a deficiency of vitamins A and E in their breast milk, the unique biological benefits of this milk justify the promotion of breast feeding as the optimal method of nourishing neonates. In these cases, it should be recommended that the woman increase her consumption of certain nutrients during pregnancy. Additionally, after childbirth, she should consider the use of supplements to produce milk of adequate quality and, thus, meet the needs of the baby and prevent a deficiency of micronutrients.

When the concentration of vitamins A and E are low in the breast milk of mothers after a high-risk pregnancy, we also recommend supplements for a child who receives nutrition exclusively from the mother. This supplementation should begin during the first days of life and continue until the infant initiates a complementary diet. Some studies have demonstrated that a deficiency in vitamins A and E in newborns, above all those with premature birth, increases the frequency of cases of bronchopulmonary dysplasia, intraventricular hemorrhage, periventricular leukomalacia, retinopathy, and necrotizing enterocolitis. Currently, there is not enough information to evaluate the possible benefits or adverse effects of supplementation during pregnancy.

In the current study, maternal overweight and obesity, as well as preterm birth, were associated with a low concentration of vitamins A and E in breast milk. It is necessary to determine whether the level of physical activity and the individual metabolism influence the quantity of food that each woman needs to achieve an optimal nutritional state and an adequate production of milk. The length and intensity of lactation also significantly affects the nutritional needs of the mother, although this is rarely considered.

Finally, during the period of breast feeding both the mother and child are at risk for a deficiency of vitamins A and E, especially in developing countries like Mexico and, thus, represent a public health problem. Moreover, if the concentration of vitamins A and E are low in the mother, the child is susceptible to suffering a like deficiency.

This study improves the knowledge about the content of vitamins A and E in breast milk from mothers after a high-risk pregnancy. Future research could include other nutrients that are also important for the development of the breast-fed child, as well as evaluate the nutritional intake of women during a high-risk pregnancy.

Acknowledgments: We are grateful to all of the mothers that participated in this study, as well as to all of the nursing personnel of the Neonatal Intensive Care Unit for the help provided in carrying out the present research.

Author Contributions: RS and HMR conceived and designed the experiments; RS, HMR, RMH, JMEP, and MEFQ performed the experiments; RS, HMR, CR, MEFQ and DV analyzed the data; HMR, RMH, DV, and CR, contributed reagents/materials/analysis tools; RS, HMR wrote the paper, all authors reading and approved this paper.

Conflicts of Interest: The authors declare no conflict of interest.

Abbreviations

HPLC	High-performance liquid chromatography
BMI	Body mass index
WHO	World Health Organization
PAHO	Pan American Health Organization
IQR	Interquartile range

1. Simmons, H.A.; Goldberg, L.S. 'High-risk' pregnancy after perinatal loss: Understanding the label. *Midwifery* **2011**, *27*, 452–457. [CrossRef] [PubMed]
2. Aune, D.; Saugstad, O.D.; Henriksen, T.; Tonstad, S. Maternal body mass index and the risk of fetal death, stillbirth, and infant death: A systematic review and meta-analysis. *JAMA* **2014**, *311*, 1536–1546. [CrossRef] [PubMed]
3. Secretaría de Salud. *Encuesta Nacional de Salud y Nutrición 2012, Resultados Nacionales*; Instituto Nacional de Salud Pública: Cuernavaca, Mexico, 2012.
4. Institute of Medicine Report Brief. *Weight Gain during Pregnancy: Reexamining the Guidelines*; National Academies Press: Washington, DC, USA, 2009.
5. Langford, A.; Joshu, C.; Chang, J.J.; Myles, T.; Leet, T. Does gestational weight gain affect the risk of adverse maternal and infant outcomes in overweight women? *Matern. Child Health J.* **2011**, *15*, 860–865. [CrossRef] [PubMed]
6. Surapaneni, K.M. Oxidant–antioxidant status in gestational diabetes patients. *J. Clin. Diagn. Res.* **2007**, *1*, 235–238.
7. Resende, F.B.; Clemente, H.A.; Bezerra, D.F.; Grilo, E.C.; de Melo, L.R.; Bellot, P.E.; Dantas, R.C.; Dimenstein, R. Alpha-tocopherol concentration in serum and colostrum of mothers with gestational diabetes mellitus. *Rev. Paul. Pediatr.* **2014**, *32*, 178–186. [CrossRef] [PubMed]
8. Debier, C.; Larondelle, Y. Vitamins A and E: Metabolism, roles and transfer to offspring. *Br. J. Nutr.* **2005**, *93*, 153–174. [CrossRef] [PubMed]
9. Lira, L.Q.; Dimenstein, R. Vitamin A and gestational diabetes. *Rev. Assoc. Med. Bras.* **2010**, *56*, 355–359. [CrossRef] [PubMed]
10. Krzyzanowska, K.; Zemany, L.; Krugluger, W.; Schernthaner, G.H.; Mittermayer, F.; Schnack, C.; Rahman, R.; Brix, J.; Kahn, B.B.; Schernthaner, G. Serum concentrations of retinol-binding protein 4 in women with and without gestational diabetes. *Diabetologia* **2008**, *51*, 1115–1122. [CrossRef] [PubMed]
11. Resende, F.B.; De Lira, L.Q.; Grilo, E.C.; Lima, M.S. Dimenstein, R. Gestational diabetes: A risk of puerperal hypovitaminosis A? *An. Acad. Bras. Cienc.* **2015**, *87*, 463–470. [CrossRef] [PubMed]
12. Dewey, K.G.; Begum, K. Long-term consequences of stunting in early life. *Matern. Child Nutr.* **2011**, *7* (Suppl. 3), 5–18. [CrossRef] [PubMed]
13. Ibrahim, S.A.; Abd el-Maksoud, A.; Nassar, M.F. Nutritional stunting in Egypt: Which nutrient is responsible? *East. Mediterr. Health J.* **2002**, *8*, 272–280. [PubMed]
14. Fares, S.; Sethom, M.M.; Khouaja-Mokrani, C.; Jabnoun, S.; Feki, M.; Kaabachi, N. Vitamin A, E, and D deficiencies in Tunisian very low birth weight neonates: Prevalence and risk factors. *Pediatr. Neonatol.* **2014**, *55*, 196–201. [CrossRef] [PubMed]
15. Weissgerber, T.L.; Gandley, R.E.; McGee, P.L.; Spong, C.Y.; Myatt, L.; Leveno, K.J.; Thorp, J.M., Jr.; Mercer, B.M.; Peaceman, A.M.; Ramin, S.M.; et al. Haptoglobin phenotype, preeclampsia risk and the efficacy of vitamin C and E supplementation to prevent preeclampsia in a racially diverse population. *PLoS ONE* **2013**, *8*, e60479. [CrossRef] [PubMed]
16. Weissgerber, T.L.; Gandley, R.E.; Roberts, J.M.; Patterson, C.C.; Holmes, V.A.; Young, I.S.; McCance, D.R. Haptoglobin phenotype, pre-eclampsia, and response to supplementation with vitamins C and E in pregnant women with type-1 diabetes. *BJOG* **2013**, *120*, 1192–1199. [CrossRef] [PubMed]
17. Bártfai, L.; Bártfai, Z.; Nedeczky, I.; Puho, E.H.; Bánhidy, F.; Czeizel, A.E. Rate of preterm birth in pregnant women with vitamin E treatment: A population-based study. *J. Matern. Fetal Neonatal Med.* **2012**, *25*, 575–580. [CrossRef] [PubMed]
18. Schmölz, L.; Birringer, M.; Lorkowski, S.; Wallert, M. Complexity of vitamin E metabolism. *World J. Biol. Chem.* **2016**, *7*, 14–43. [CrossRef] [PubMed]
19. Stam, J.; Sauer, P.J.J.; Boelm, G. Can we define an infant's need from the composition of human milk? *Am. J. Clin. Nutr.* **2013**, *98*, 521S–528S. [CrossRef] [PubMed]

20. American College Obstetrician and Gynecologists Committee on Practice bulletin–Obstetrics. ACGO Practice Bulletin. Clinical Management Guidelines for Obstetrician-Gynecologists, No. 30, September 2001 (replaces Technical Bulletin No. 200, December 1994); Gestational diabetes. Available online: http://c.ymcdn.com/sites/chronicdisease.site-ym.com/resource/resmgr/Womens_Health_Council_GDM/pb030_gestational_diabetes_r.pdf (accessed on 1 July 2016).

21. American College Obstetrician and Gynecologists Committee on Practice bulletin–Obstetrics. ACGO Practice Bulletin. Diagnosis and Management of Preeclampsia and Eclampsia, No. 33, January 2002; American College Obstetrician and Gynecologists. Available online: https://www.scribd.com/document/116952914/No-33-Diagnosis-and-Management-of-Preeclampsia-and-Eclampsia (accessed on 1 July 2016).

22. Xue, X.; You, J.; He, P. Simultaneous determination of five fat-soluble vitamins in feed by high-performance liquid chromatography following solid-phase extraction. *J. Chromatogr. Sci.* **2008**, *46*, 345–350. [CrossRef] [PubMed]

23. Rish, L.; Yaqoob, M.; Waseem, A.; Nabi, A. Vitamin A determination in milk sample based on the luminol-periodate chemiluminescence system. *J. Nutr. Sci. Vitaminol.* **2014**, *60*, 9–16. [CrossRef]

24. IOM (Institute of Medicine) and NRC (National Research Council). *Weight Gain During Pregnancy: Reexamining the Guidelines*; The National Academies Press: Washington, DC, USA, 2009.

25. Schweigert, F.J.; Bathe, K.; Chen, F.; Büscher, U.; Dudenhausen, J.W. Effect of the stage of lactation in humans on carotenoid levels in milk, blood plasma and plasma lipoprotein fractions. *Eur. J. Nutr.* **2004**, *43*, 39–44. [CrossRef] [PubMed]

26. Quiles, J.L.; Ochoa, J.J.; Ramirez-Tortosa, M.C.; Linde, J.; Bompadre, S.; Battino, M.; Narbona, E.; Maldonado, J.; Mataix, J. Coenzyme Q concentration and total antioxidant capacity of human milk at different stages of lactation in mothers of preterm and full-term infants. *Free Radic. Res.* **2006**, *40*, 199–206. [CrossRef] [PubMed]

27. Ahmed, L.; Nazrul Islam, S.; Khan, M.N.; Huque, S.; Ahsan, M. Antioxidant micronutrient profile (Vitamin E, C, A, copper, zinc, iron) of colostrum: Association with maternal characteristics. *J. Trop. Pediatr.* **2004**, *50*, 357–358. [CrossRef] [PubMed]

28. Szlagatys-Sidorkiewicz, A.; Zagierski, M.; Jankowska, A.; Łuczak, G.; Macur, K.; Baczek, T.; Korzon, M.; Krzykowski, G.; Martysiak-Żurowska, D.; Kamińska, B. Longitudinal study of vitamins A, E and lipid oxidative damage in human milk throughout lactation. *Early Hum. Dev.* **2012**, *88*, 421–424. [CrossRef] [PubMed]

29. De Lira, L.Q.; Ribeiro, P.P.; Grilo, E.C.; Lima, M.S.; Dimenstein, R. Alpha-tocopherol level in serum and colostrum of breastfeeding women and association with maternal variables. *Rev. Bras. Ginecol. Obstet.* **2012**, *34*, 362–368. (In Portuguese) [PubMed]

30. Shi, Y.D.; Sun, G.Q.; Zhang, Z.G.; Deng, X.; Kang, X.H.; Liu, Z.D.; Ma, Y.; Sheng, Q.H. The chemical composition of human milk from Inner Mongolia of China. *Food Chem.* **2011**, *127*, 1193–1198. [CrossRef] [PubMed]

31. Martysiak-Zurowska, D.; Szlagatys-Sidorkiewicz, A.; Zagierski, C. Concentrations of alpha- and gamma-tocopherols in human breast milk during the first months of lactation and in infant formulas. *Matern. Child Nutr.* **2013**, *9*, 473–482. [CrossRef] [PubMed]

32. Garcia, L.R.; Ribeiro, K.D.; Araújo, K.F.; Azevedo, G.M.; Pires, J.F.; Batista, S.D.; Dimenstein, R. Níveis de alfa-tocoferol no soro e leite maternos de puérperas atendidas em maternidade pública de Natal. *Rio Grande do Norte Rev. Bras. Saude. Matern. Infant.* **2009**, *9*, 423–428. [CrossRef]

33. Sakurai, T.; Furukawa, M.; Asha, M.; Kanno, T.; Kojima, T.; Yonekubo, A. Fat-soluble and water-soluble vitamin contents of breast milk from Japanese women. *J. Nutr. Sci. Vitaminol.* **2005**, *5*, 239–247. [CrossRef]

34. Engle-Stone, R.; Haskell, M.J.; Nankap, M.; Ndjebayi, A.O.; Brown, K.H. Breast milk retinol and plasma retinol-binding protein concentrations provide similar estimates of vitamin A deficiency prevalence and identify similar risk groups among women in Cameroon but breast milk retinol underestimates the prevalence of deficiency among young children. *J. Nutr.* **2014**, *144*, 209–217. [PubMed]

35. Tanumihardjo, S.A.; Russell, R.M.; Stephensen, C.B.; Gannon, B.M.; Craft, N.E.; Haskell, M.J.; Lietz, G.; Schulze, K.; Raiten, D.J. Biomarkers of nutrition for development (BOND)-vitamin A Review. *J. Nutr.* **2016**, *146*, 1816S–1848S. [CrossRef] [PubMed]

36. Kodentsova, V.M.; Vrzhesinskaya, O.A. Evaluation of the vitamin status in nursing women by vitamin content in breast milk. *Bull. Exp. Biol. Med.* **2006**, *141*, 323–327. [CrossRef] [PubMed]

37. Kamao, M.; Tsugawa, N.; Suahra, Y.; Okano, T. Determination of fat-soluble vitamins in human plasma, breast milk, and food samples: Application in nutrition survey for establishment of "Dietary Reference Intakes for Japanese". *J. Health Sci.* **2007**, *53*, 257–262. [CrossRef]

38. Tijerina-Sáenz, A.; Innis, S.M.; Kitts, D.D. Antioxidant capacity of human milk and its association with vitamins A and E and fatty acid composition. *Acta Paediatr.* **2009**, *98*, 1793–1798. [CrossRef] [PubMed]

39. Antonakou, A.; Chiou, A.; Andrikopoulos, N.K.; Bakoula, C.; Matalas, A.L. Breast milk tocopherol content during the first six months in exclusively breastfeeding Greek women. *Eur. J. Nutr.* **2011**, *50*, 195–202. [CrossRef] [PubMed]

40. Szlagatys-Sidorkiewicz, A.; Zagierski, M.; Luczak, G.; Macur, K.; Baczek, T.; Kaminska, B. Maternal smoking does not influence vitamin A and E concentrations in mature breastmilk. *Breastfeed. Med.* **2012**, *7*, 285–289. [CrossRef] [PubMed]

41. Wallingford, J.; Underwood, B. Vitamin A deficiency in pregnancy, lactation and the nursing child. In *Vitamin A deficiency and Its Control*; Bauernfeind, J., Ed.; Academic Press: Orlando, FL, USA, 1986; pp. 101–152.

42. Agne-Djigo, A.; Idohou-Dossou, N.; Kwadjode, K.M.; Tanumihardjo, S.A.; Wade, S. High prevalence of vitamin A deficiency is detected by the modified relative dose-response test in six-month-old Senegalese breast-fed infants. *J. Nutr.* **2012**, *142*, 1991–1996. [CrossRef] [PubMed]

43. Tyndall, J.A.; Okoye, V.; Elumelu, F.; Dahiru, A.; Pariya, H.B. Vitamin A and iron deficiency in pregnant women, lactating mothers and their infants in Adamawa State, Nigeria: A prospective cohort study. *Am. J. Food Nutr.* **2012**, *2*, 14–20. [CrossRef]

44. Azeredo, V.B.; Trugo, N.M. Retinol, carotenoids, and tocopherols in the milk of lactating adolescents and relationships with plasma concentrations. *Nutrition* **2008**, *24*, 133–139. [CrossRef] [PubMed]

45. Tokusoglu, O.; Tansug, N.; Aksit, S.; Dinc, G.; Kasirga, E.; Ozcan, C. Retinol and α-tocopherol concentrations in breast milk of Turkish lactating mothers under different socio-economic status. *Int. J. Food Sci. Nutr.* **2008**, *59*, 166–174. [CrossRef] [PubMed]

46. Debier, C. Vitamin E during pre- and postnatal periods. *Vitam. Horm.* **2007**, *76*, 357–373. [PubMed]

47. Sziklai-László, I.; Majchrzak, D.; Elmadfa, I.; Cser, M.A. Selenium and vitamin E concentrations in human milk and formula milk from Hungary. *J. Radioanalytical Nuclear Chem.* **2009**, *279*, 585–590. [CrossRef]

48. Fujita, M.; Shell-Ducan, B.; Ndemwa, P.; Brindle, E.; Lo, Y.J.; Kombe, Y.; O'Connor, K. Vitamin A Dynamics in breastmilk and liver stores: A life history perspective. *Am. J. Hum. Biol.* **2011**, *23*, 664–673. [CrossRef] [PubMed]

49. De Lira, L.Q.; Lima, M.S.; de Medeiros, J.M.; da Silva, I.F.; Dimenstein, R. Correlation of vitamin A nutritional status on alpha-tocopherol in the colostrum of lactating women. *Matern. Child Nutr.* **2013**, *9*, 31–40. [CrossRef] [PubMed]

50. Pires Medeiros, J.F.; Ribeiro, K.D.; Lima, M.S.; das Neves, R.A.; Lima, A.C.; Dantas, R.C.; da Silva, A.B.; Dimenstein, R. α-tocopherol in breast milk of women with preterm delivery after a single postpartum oral dose of vitamin E. *Br. J. Nutr.* **2016**, *115*, 1424–1430. [CrossRef] [PubMed]

51. Haug, M.; Laubach, C.; Burke, M.; Harzer, G. Vitamin E in human from mothers of preterm and term infants. *J. Pediatr. Gastroenterol. Nutr.* **1987**, *6*, 605–609. [CrossRef] [PubMed]

52. Bishara, R.; Dunn, M.S.; Merko, S.E.; Darling, P. Nutrient composition of hindmilk produced by mothers of very low mothers of very low birth weight infants born at less than 28 weeks gestation. *J. Hum. Lact.* **2008**, *24*, 159–167. [CrossRef] [PubMed]

53. Grilo, E.C.; Lira, L.Q.; Dimenstein, R.; Ribeiro, K.D. Influence of prematurity and birth weight on the concentration of α-tocopherol in colostrum milk. *Rev. Paul. Pediatr.* **2013**, *31*, 473–479. [CrossRef] [PubMed]

54. Souza, G.; Dolinsky, M.; Matos, A.; Chagas, C.; Ramalho, A. Vitamin A concentration in human milk and its relationship with liver reserve formation and compliance with the recommended daily intake of vitamin A in preterm and full term infants in exclusive breastfeeding. *Arch. Gynecol. Obstet.* **2015**, *291*, 319–325. [CrossRef] [PubMed]

55. Ho, M.Y.; Yen, Y.H. Trend of nutritional support in preterm infants. *Pediatr. Neonatol.* **2016**, *57*, 365–370. [CrossRef] [PubMed]

56. Shamim, A.A.; Schulze, K.; Merrill, R.D.; Kabir, A.; Christian, P.; Shaikh, S.; Wu, L.; Ali, H.; Labrique, A.B.; Mehra, S.; et al. First-trimester plasma tocopherols are associated with risk of miscarriage in rural Bangladesh. *Am. J. Clin. Nutr.* **2015**, *101*, 294–301. [CrossRef] [PubMed]

57. Cohen, J.M.; Kramer, M.S.; Platt, R.W.; Basso, O.; Evans, R.W.; Kahn, S.R. The association between maternal antioxidant levels in midpregnancy and preeclampsia. *Am. J. Obstet. Gynecol.* **2015**, *213*, 695.e1–695.e13. [CrossRef] [PubMed]

58. Wei, X.; Peng, R.; Cao, J.; Kang, Y.; Qu, P.; Liu, Y.; Xiao, X.; Li, T. Serum vitamin A status is associated with obesity and the metabolic syndrome among school-age children in Chongqing, China. *Asia Pac. J. Clin. Nutr.* **2016**, *25*, 563–570. [PubMed]

59. Hrolfsdottir, L.; Schalkwijk, C.G.; Birgisdottir, B.E.; Gunnarsdottir, I.; Maslova, E.; Granström, C.; Strøm, M.; Olsen, S.F.; Halldorsson, T.I. Maternal diet, gestational weight gain, and inflammatory markers during pregnancy. *Obesity (Silver Spring)* **2016**, *24*, 2133–2139. [CrossRef] [PubMed]

60. McCurdy, C.E.; Schenk, S.; Hetrick, B.; Houck, J.; Drew, B.G.; Kaye, S.; Lashbrook, M.; Bergman, B.C.; Takahashi, D.L.; Dean, T.A.; et al. Maternal obesity reduces oxidative capacity in fetal skeletal muscle of Japanese macaques. *JCI Insight* **2016**, *1*, e86612. [CrossRef] [PubMed]

61. Lima, M.S.R.; Dimenstein, R.; Ribeiro, K.D.S. Vitamin E concentration in human milk and associated factors: A literature review. *J. Pediatr. (Rio J.)* **2014**, *90*, 440–448. [CrossRef] [PubMed]

62. Fares, S.; Sethom, M.M.; Kacem, S.; Ksibi, I.; Feki, M.; Jebnoun, S.; Kaabachi, N. Retinol and alpha-tocopherol in the colostrum of lactating Tunisian women delivering prematurely: Associations with maternal characteristics. *Pediatr. Neonatol.* **2016**, *57*, 120–126. [CrossRef] [PubMed]

63. Debier, C.; Pottier, J.; Goffe, C.H.; Larondelle, Y. Present knowledge and unexpected behaviors of vitamins A and E in colostrum and milk. *Livest. Prod. Sci.* **2005**, *98*, 135–147. [CrossRef]

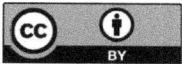

MDPI

Article

Breastmilk Production in the First 4 Weeks after Birth of Term Infants

Jacqueline C. Kent *, Hazel Gardner and Donna T. Geddes

School of Chemistry and Biochemistry, The University of Western Australia, Crawley 6009, Australia; Hazel.Gardner@uwa.edu.au (H.G.); Donna.Geddes@uwa.edu.au (D.T.G.)
* Correspondence: Jacqueline.Kent@uwa.edu.au; Tel.: +61-8-6488-1208

Received: 30 September 2016; Accepted: 21 November 2016; Published: 25 November 2016

Abstract: Breastmilk provides the ideal nutrition for the infant, and exclusive breastfeeding is recommended for the first 6 months. Adequate milk production by the mother is therefore critical, and early milk production has been shown to significantly affect milk production during established lactation. Previous studies indicate that milk production should reach the lower limit of normal for established lactation (440 mL per day) by day 11 after birth. We have used test-weighing of term infants before and after each breastfeed over 24 h to measure milk production in the first 4 weeks of lactation in mothers with and without perceived breastfeeding problems to provide information on how often milk production is inadequate. Between days 11 and 13, two-thirds of the mothers had a milk production of less than 440 mL per day, and between days 14 and 28, nearly one-third of the mothers had a milk production of less than 440 mL per day. The high frequency of inadequate milk production in early lactation and the consequence of suboptimal milk production in later lactation if left untreated suggest that objective measurement of milk production can identify mothers and infants at risk and support early intervention by a lactation specialist.

Keywords: breastfeeding; milk production; insufficient milk

1. Introduction

There is a sound evidence base for the health advantages of breastfeeding for infants and their mothers, and a dose-response relationship has been demonstrated [1]. As such, any breastfeeding should be encouraged and full breastfeeding achieved if possible. Milk production and adequacy at 6 weeks after birth, for mothers of both healthy breastfeeding term infants and non-nursing preterm infants, have been shown to have a significant relationship with milk production 4–6 days after birth [2,3]. Hill et al. therefore suggest that interventions that promote an adequate milk supply by the first week postpartum are critical [2]. These include skin-to-skin contact and milk removal (breastfeeding or expressing) within an hour of birth and frequent milk removal during the first 24 h after birth. Early initiation of lactation, particularly breastfeeding or expressing within an hour of birth, has been shown to lead to a higher rate of breastfeeding beyond 6 weeks for term infants [4]. Skin-to-skin contact between mother and infant for the first hour after birth results in earlier effective breastfeeding [5] and an increased likelihood of breastfeeding 1–4 months after birth than when the infant was swaddled in blankets [6]. There is also a positive effect of the number of breastfeeds in the first 24 h on milk production on days 3 and 5 after birth [7]. It is important, therefore, to know if milk production is adequate during early lactation. The lower limit of normal daily milk production for established lactation has been calculated to be 440 g [8]. During the first week of lactation, on day 5, daily milk transfer during breastfeeding is 415 ± 123 g (combined data from a total of 305 breastfeeding mothers [7,9–14]). For mothers who were exclusively expressing breastmilk, one study of mothers of term infants measured a milk production of 973 ± 176 g per day on day 5 [15]. There is limited data on milk production during the second week after birth, but data from 10 mothers showed a daily milk transfer of 653 ± 154 g with a slightly higher milk yield of 668 ± 163 g due to some mothers occasionally pumping their breastmilk [11]. Hill et al. reported a lower milk production of 556 ± 187 g, but some of those mothers were supplementing [3]. Taken together, published data indicate that 92% of term mothers produce at least 440 g per day by 2 weeks of lactation.

It has been reported that 58% of term mothers experience problems with breastfeeding, including a perception of insufficient milk supply, in the first 2 weeks and this is associated with a lack of confidence in breastfeeding [16]. A perception of insufficient milk supply is given as a reason for the introduction of supplementary infant formula [17,18]. If breastmilk supply is actually inadequate supplementary feeds are necessary. If supplementary feeds are given instead of breastfeeds they could have a negative impact on milk supply. Measurement of milk production using in-home 24-h test-weighing is being used increasingly by lactation consultants and general practitioners as a clinical tool to either reassure mothers that their breastfeeding patterns and milk production are normal, or to guide advice to increase or decrease milk production or breastmilk transfer [19]. We aim to use 24-h milk profiles during the establishment of lactation to try to verify that full milk production is achieved by 2 weeks of lactation in mothers without perceived breastfeeding problems and, in a vulnerable population, how frequently milk supply is not adequate indicating that intervention would be appropriate.

2. Materials and Methods

A convenience sample of mothers within 4 weeks after the birth of a singleton, term infant ($\geq$37 weeks gestational age at delivery, birth weight $\geq$2500 g) who were fully or partially breastfeeding [20] were invited to participate between June 2009 and April 2016. We recruited mothers under the care of general practitioners or lactation consultants for perceived breastfeeding problems, and volunteers for studies undertaken by the research group (e.g., Prime et al. [21]) who were without perceived breastfeeding problems. Demographics were recorded and the participants were loaned accurate digital scales (BabyWeigh™, Medela Inc., McHenry, IL, USA, resolution 2 g, accuracy ± 0.034%) to measure their milk profile. This involved the participants test-weighing their infants in their own homes [22] before and after each breastfeed or supplementary feed and recording amounts of breastmilk expressed. All measurements of breastfeed amounts and milk production are measured in grams but expressed in mL because the density of milk is 1.03 g·mL^{-1}. Data were recorded either on paper or entered on a password-protected website accessed by invitation only. Breastfeeding parameters were calculated: the total amount of milk transferred from the mother to the infant while breastfeeding (total breastfeeding transfer), the amount of breastmilk expressed during the 24-h period (total breastmilk expressed), the total amount of milk produced by both breasts in the 24-h period (total breastmilk production = total breastfeeding transfer + total breastmilk expressed), and the total infant milk intake (total breastfeeding transfer plus expressed breastmilk and/or supplementary formula). The duration of each feed was taken from the time of weighing before to the time of weighing after the feeding.

Analysis used R version 3.2.1 GUI Snow Leopard (The R Foundation for Statistical Computing, Vienna, Austria) [23] with the base package and the library nlme [24] for linear mixed effects models. Summary statistics are presented as mean ± SD where the Shapiro-Wilk test indicated normality, or median (interquartile range) otherwise. Groups were compared on demographic and milk intake variables using two-tailed independent samples Student's *t*-test where the Shapiro-Wilk test indicated normality, and Kruskal-Wallis rank sum test otherwise. Linear mixed effects analyses of the relationship between demographic and milk intake variables and total milk production were carried out with random effects of different intercepts for each mother. Differences were considered to be significant where $p < 0.05$.

All participants supplied written, informed consent to participate in the studies, which were approved by the Human Research Ethics Committee at The University of Western Australia (RA/4/1/4103) and Women and Newborn Health Service (1746/ew).

3. Results

Sixty-two percent of participants who agreed to participate completed 24-h milk profiles between 6 and 28 days after birth. There were 13 participants without perceived breastfeeding problems (6 female infants, all Caucasian, 4 primiparous, 12 vaginal delivery) and 103 participants with perceived breastfeeding problems (50 female infants). Complete demographics were available for 48 participants (43 Caucasian, 32 primiparous, 28 vaginal delivery). Seventy-six of these provided information regarding their breastfeeding problems. The most common was a perception of insufficient milk supply (59 participants), but pain (11 participants) and positioning and attachment (10 participants) were also mentioned. Seventy-five of the participants with perceived breastfeeding problems were supplementing their infants with expressed breastmilk and/or infant formula, 45 using expressed breastmilk alone, 25 using infant formula and expressed breastmilk, and 5 participants used formula but no expressed breastmilk. The characteristics of the participants are presented in Table 1.

Table 1. Characteristics and breastfeeding parameters of participants without and with perceived breastfeeding problems.

| | Perceived Breastfeeding Problems | | *p* Value |
	No	Yes	
n	13	103	
Birth weight (g)	3498 (293)	3450 (3206, 3739)	0.051
Gestational age at delivery (weeks^{+days})	39^{+2} (1^{+3})	39^{+6} (38^{+7}, 40^{+3})	0.025
Feed frequency (breasts)	12 (3)	12 (4)	0.50
Average feed duration (min)	17 (5)	15 (13, 21)	0.052
Average feed amount (mL)	63 (27)	30 (20, 45)	<0.001
Total breastfeeding transfer (mL·day^{-1})	693 (174)	399 (211)	<0.001
Total breastmilk expressed (mL·day^{-1})	160 (*n* = 1)	168 (78, 272) (*n* = 68)	
Supplementary infant formula (mL·day^{-1})	0	135 (80, 272) (*n* = 72)	
Total infant milk intake (mL·day^{-1})	699 (168)	567 (164)	0.007

Data are presented as mean (SD) or median (IQR). Comparisons between measures for participants with and without perceived breastfeeding problems were made using Student's *t*-test where the Shapiro-Wilk test indicated normality, and Kruskal-Wallis rank sum test otherwise.

There were no significant differences between the groups for birth weight, frequency of breastfeeds, duration of breastfeeds, or total breastmilk production, but there were significant differences between the two groups for gestational age at delivery, average feed amount, total breastfeeding transfer, and total infant milk intake. Those with perceived breastfeeding problems who were supplementing with infant formula had a significantly lower average feed amount and total breastfeeding transfer ($p < 0.001$).

There were no significant relationships between infant age, birth weight, gestational age at delivery or average feed duration on total breastfeeding transfer ($p > 0.13$), but there were significant relationships between average feed duration and average feed amount ($R^2 = 0.08$, $p = 0.003$), feed frequency and average feed amount ($R^2 = 0.10$, $p = 0.010$), feed frequency and total breastfeeding transfer ($R^2 = 0.05$, $p = 0.018$), and average feed amount and total breastfeeding transfer ($R^2 = 0.62$, $p < 0.001$).

All measurements of total milk production are shown in Figure 1. Twenty-nine measurements were made between 6 and 13 days of lactation. For those with perceived breastfeeding problems the total breastmilk production of 14 was ≥440 mL and 12 was <440 mL. Of the participants without perceived breastfeeding problems two had a total breastmilk production of 624 and 678 mL, and one who had a total breastmilk production of 338 mL at 1.4 weeks was an experienced breastfeeding mother (parity 4) who subsequently produced 722 mL at 5.1 weeks.

Eighty-seven measurements were made between 14 and 28 days of lactation. For the 77 of those with perceived breastfeeding problems, the total breastmilk production of 53 was ≥440 mL, and for 24 was <440 mL. All 10 participants without perceived breastfeeding problems had a total breastmilk production of ≥ 440 mL.

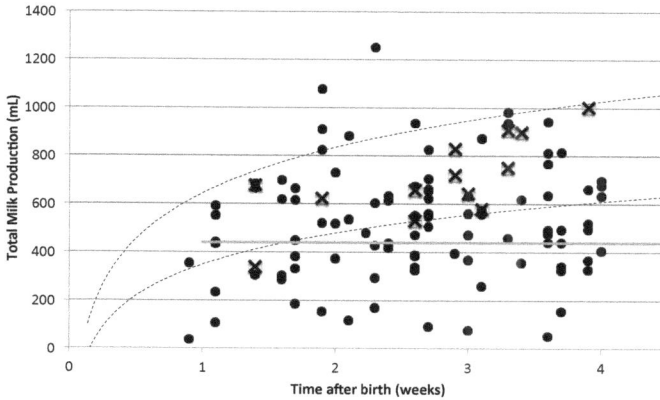

Figure 1. Total milk production of mothers with (circles) and without (crosses) perceived breastfeeding problems. The dotted lines indicate the mean ± SD of milk production derived from the literature [7,9–14,25]. The horizontal grey line indicates the lower limit of normal for established lactation [8].

4. Discussion

The current data from all but one of the participants who did not have any perceived breastfeeding problems support the findings of limited published data suggesting that full milk production is normally reached by the second week of lactation. Even for mothers with perceived breastfeeding problems, over half were producing more than 440 mL per day in the first 13 days after birth.

It is normal for infants to lose weight after birth, and a recent study has demonstrated that the time of the nadir of weight occurs 52.3 h after birth with a loss of 218 g and a weight ratio (weight divided by birth weight) of 0.933 [26]. Compared with infants who were breastfed less than 7 times a day in the first 24 h after birth, infants who were breastfed 7 or more times received significantly more breastmilk, had a maximum weight loss that was 1% lower (5.8% compared with 6.8%), started to regain weight 19 h earlier, and had more than regained their birth weight by 7 days after birth [9]. Although there was no statistically significant difference in the feed frequency between those with and without breastfeeding problems, we observed that 11 of the participants with perceived breastfeeding problems had a feed frequency of <7, a mean total breastfeeding transfer of 195 mL, and a mean total breastmilk production of 344 mL. It is possible that this low production is a result of early infrequent breastfeeding. We suggest that if fully breastfed infants have not regained their birth weight by 7 days after birth the mother's milk profile should be measured during the second week. If it is shown to be low (<440 mL) then early remedial action could be taken, which could include correction of positioning and attachment, increase in feeding frequency, and use of galactogogues. If an ample milk supply is demonstrated the infant should be assessed.

There were small effects of average feed duration and frequency on average feed amount, and a small effect of feed frequency on total breastfeeding transfer. However, the frequency and duration of breastfeeds for this population was very close to the average for mothers of exclusively breastfed infants between 4 and 26 weeks of lactation [17]. The most significant factor affecting total breastfeeding transfer was the average feed amount. This suggests that, while infants should be fed often and feed times should not be unnecessarily restricted, the major contributor to low total breastfeeding transfer is the amount of milk transferred during each breastfeed. About two-thirds of the mothers with perceived breastfeeding problems were already expressing breastmilk, suggesting that milk was possibly available but the infant was unable to remove sufficient milk during breastfeeding. The attention of the lactation specialist on good positioning and attachment and investigation of other possible reasons for poor milk transfer is reinforced by these data. The one participant who had a low measured milk production at 1.4 weeks gave only one extra breastfeed but doubled the amount transferred during each breastfeed and more than doubled her milk production by 5 weeks, illustrating that milk production can be increased during the early weeks as the infant becomes more effective at breastfeeding.

5. Study Limitations

Investigation of breastmilk production of mothers with and without breastfeeding problems in early lactation would benefit from a more detailed history of the initiation of lactation from the time of birth, including time of first breastfeed, skin-to-skin care, assessment of attachment, frequency of breastfeeds, and frequent measurements of the infants' weights in the first week after birth. Measurement of 24-h milk profiles at 7 and 14 days after birth would allow identification of the factors that are most important in optimizing breastfeeding milk transfer. Weighing an infant before and after every feeding for 24 h can be demanding, so while this technique is very useful, it is not appropriate for all lactating mothers.

6. Conclusions

The high frequency of inadequate milk production in early lactation and the consequence of suboptimal milk production in later lactation if left untreated underline the importance of early identification of mothers and infants at risk. Measurement of milk profile during the second week of lactation provides an objective measure of breastfeeding milk transfer and total breastmilk production. These measures, considered with the infant's weight changes, can provide an indication that early intervention by a lactation specialist to improve milk production is warranted.

Acknowledgments: The authors thank the mothers for their participation. Funding was provided by an unrestricted research grant from Medela AG, Baar, Switzerland.

Author Contributions: J.K. and D.G. conceived and designed the experiments; J.K. performed the experiments; J.K. analyzed the data; H.G. retrieved and analysed published data for comparison; J.K. wrote the paper, in consultation with H.G. and D.G.

Conflicts of Interest: The authors declare no conflict of interest. The funding sponsors had no role in the design of the study; in the collection, analyses, or interpretation of data; in the writing of the manuscript, and in the decision to publish the results.

References

1. Allen, J.; Hector, D. Benefits of breastfeeding. *N. S. W. Public Health Bull.* **2005**, *16*, 42–46. [PubMed]
2. Hill, P.D.; Aldag, J.C. Milk volume on day 4 and income predictive of lactation adequacy at 6 weeks of mothers of nonnursing preterm infants. *J. Perinat. Neonatal Nurs.* **2005**, *19*, 273–282. [CrossRef] [PubMed]
3. Hill, P.D.; Aldag, J.C.; Chatterton, R.T.; Zinaman, M. Comparison of milk output between mothers of preterm and term infants: The first 6 weeks after birth. *J. Hum. Lact.* **2005**, *21*, 22–30. [CrossRef] [PubMed]
4. DiGirolamo, A.M.; Grummer-Strawn, L.M.; Fein, S.B. Effect of maternity-care practices on breastfeeding. *Pediatrics* **2008**, *122*, S43–S49. [CrossRef] [PubMed]
5. Moore, E.R.; Anderson, G.C. Randomized controlled trial of very early mother-infant skin-to-skin contact and breastfeeding status. *J. Midwifery Womens Health* **2007**, *52*, 116–125. [CrossRef] [PubMed]

6. Moore, E.R.; Anderson, G.C.; Bergman, N. Early skin-to-skin contact for mothers and their healthy newborn infants. *Cochrane Database Syst. Rev.* **2012**. [CrossRef]

7. Yamauchi, Y.; Yamanouchi, I. Breast-feeding frequency during the first 24 h after birth in full-term neonates. *Pediatrics* **1990**, *86*, 171–175. [PubMed]

8. Kent, J.C.; Mitoulas, L.; Cox, D.B.; Owens, R.A.; Hartmann, P.E. Breast volume and milk production during extended lactation in women. *Exp. Physiol.* **1999**, *84*, 435–447. [CrossRef] [PubMed]

9. Casey, C.E.; Hambidge, K.M.; Neville, M.C. Studies in human lactation: Zinc, copper, manganese and chromium in human milk in the first month of lactation. *Am. J. Clin. Nutr.* **1985**, *41*, 1193–1200. [PubMed]

10. Casey, C.E.; Neifert, M.R.; Seacat, J.M.; Neville, M.C. Nutrient intake by breast-fed infants during the first five days after birth. *Am. J. Dis. Child.* **1986**, *140*, 933–936. [CrossRef] [PubMed]

11. Neville, M.C.; Keller, R.; Seacat, J.; Lutes, V.; Neifert, M.; Casey, C.; Allen, J.; Archer, P. Studies in human lactation: Milk volumes in lactating women during the onset of lactation and full lactation. *Am. J. Clin. Nutr.* **1988**, *48*, 1375–1386. [PubMed]

12. Saint, L.; Smith, M.; Hartmann, P.E. The yield and nutrient content of colostrum and milk of women from giving birth to 1 month post-partum. *Br. J. Nutr.* **1984**, *52*, 87–95. [CrossRef] [PubMed]

13. Evans, K.C.; Evans, R.G.; Royal, R.; Esterman, A.J.; James, S.L. Effect of caesarean section on breast milk transfer to the normal term newborn over the first week of life. *Arch. Dis. Child. Fetal Neonatal Ed.* **2003**, *88*, F380–F382. [CrossRef] [PubMed]

14. Arthur, P.G.; Smith, M.; Hartmann, P.E. Milk lactose, citrate, and glucose as markers of lactogenesis in normal and diabetic women. *J. Pediatr. Gastroenterol. Nutr.* **1989**, *9*, 488–496. [CrossRef] [PubMed]

15. Roderuck, C.; Williams, H.H.; Macy, I.G. Metabolism of women during the reproductive cycle; the utilization of thiamine during lactation. *J. Nutr.* **1946**, *32*, 249–265. [PubMed]

16. Ertem, I.O.; Votto, N.; Leventhal, J.M. The timing and predictors of the early termination of breastfeeding. *Pediatrics* **2001**, *107*, 543–548. [CrossRef] [PubMed]

17. Righard, L. Are breastfeeding problems related to incorrect breastfeeding technique and the use of pacifiers and bottles? *Birth* **1998**, *25*, 40–44. [CrossRef] [PubMed]

18. Segura-Millan, S.; Dewey, K.G.; Perez-Escamilla, R. Factors associated with perceived insufficient milk in a low-income urban population in Mexico. *J. Nutr.* **1994**, *124*, 202–212. [PubMed]

19. Kent, J.C.; Hepworth, A.R.; Langton, D.B.; Hartmann, P.E. Impact of measuring milk production by test weighing on breastfeeding confidence in mothers of term infants. *Breastfeed Med.* **2015**, *10*, 318–325. [CrossRef] [PubMed]

20. Labbok, M.; Krasovec, K. Toward consistency in breastfeeding definitions. *Stud. Fam. Plan.* **1990**, *21*, 226–230. [CrossRef]

21. Prime, D.K.; Garbin, C.P.; Hartmann, P.E.; Kent, J.C. Simultaneous breast expression in breastfeeding women is more efficacious than sequential breast expression. *Breastfeed Med.* **2012**, *7*, 442–447. [CrossRef] [PubMed]

22. Arthur, P.G.; Hartmann, P.E.; Smith, M. Measurement of the milk intake of breast-fed infants. *J. Pediatr. Gastroenterol. Nutr.* **1987**, *6*, 758–763. [CrossRef] [PubMed]

23. R Development Core Team. *R: A Language and Environment for Statistical Computing*; R Foundation for Statistical Computing: Vienna, Austria, 2011.

24. Pinheiro, J.; Bates, C.J.; DebRoy, S.; Sarkar, D.; R Development Core Team. *Nlme: Linear and Nonlinear Mixed Effects Models*, R package version 3.1-102; R Foundation for Statistical Computing: Vienna, Austria, 2011.

25. Dollberg, S.; Lahav, S.; Mimouni, F.B. A comparison of intakes of breast-fed and bottle-fed infants during the first two days of life. *J. Am. Coll. Nutr.* **2001**, *20*, 209–211. [CrossRef] [PubMed]

26. Fonseca, M.J.; Severo, M.; Santos, A.C. A new approach to estimating weight change and its reference intervals during the first 96 h of life. *Acta Paediatr.* **2015**, *104*, 1028–1034. [CrossRef] [PubMed]

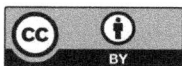

nutrients

MDPI

Article

Effect of Human Milk Appetite Hormones, Macronutrients, and Infant Characteristics on Gastric Emptying and Breastfeeding Patterns of Term Fully Breastfed Infants

Zoya Gridneva [1,*], Sambavi Kugananthan [1,2], Anna R. Hepworth [1], Wan J. Tie [1], Ching T. Lai [1], Leigh C. Ward [3], Peter E. Hartmann [1] and Donna T. Geddes [1]

1 School of Chemistry and Biochemistry, The University of Western Australia, Crawley, Perth, Western Australia 6009, Australia; 21141062@student.uwa.edu.au (S.K.); anna.hepworth@uwa.edu.au (A.R.H.); ash.tie@uwa.edu.au (W.J.T.); ching-tat.lai@uwa.edu.au (C.T.L.); peter.hartmann@uwa.edu.au (P.E.H.); donna.geddes@uwa.edu.au (D.T.G.)
2 School of Anatomy, Physiology and Human Biology, The University of Western Australia, Crawley, Perth, Western Australia 6009, Australia
3 School of Chemistry and Molecular Biosciences, The University of Queensland, St. Lucia, Brisbane, Queensland 4072, Australia; l.ward@uq.edu.au
* Correspondence: zgridneva@gmail.com; Tel.: +61-8-6488-4428

Received: 29 September 2016; Accepted: 22 December 2016; Published: 28 December 2016

Abstract: Human milk (HM) components influence infant feeding patterns and nutrient intake, yet it is unclear how they influence gastric emptying (GE), a key component of appetite regulation. This study analyzed GE of a single breastfeed, HM appetite hormones/macronutrients and demographics/anthropometrics/body composition of term fully breastfed infants ($n = 41$, 2 and/or 5 mo). Stomach volumes (SV) were calculated from pre-/post-feed ultrasound scans, then repeatedly until the next feed. Feed volume (FV) was measured by the test-weigh method. HM samples were analyzed for adiponectin, leptin, fat, lactose, total carbohydrate, lysozyme, and total/whey/casein protein. Linear regression/mixed effect models were used to determine associations between GE/feed variables and HM components/infant anthropometrics/adiposity. Higher FVs were associated with faster (-0.07 [-0.10, -0.03], $p < 0.001$) GE rate, higher post-feed SVs (0.82 [0.53, 1.12], $p < 0.001$), and longer GE times (0.24 [0.03, 0.46], $p = 0.033$). Higher whey protein concentration was associated with higher post-feed SVs (4.99 [0.84, 9.13], $p = 0.023$). Longer GE time was associated with higher adiponectin concentration (2.29 [0.92, 3.66], $p = 0.002$) and dose (0.02 [0.01, 0.03], $p = 0.005$), and lower casein:whey ratio (-65.89 [-107.13, -2.66], $p = 0.003$). FV and HM composition influence GE and breastfeeding patterns in term breastfed infants.

Keywords: human milk; term breastfed infants; gastric emptying; feeding frequency; ultrasound; stomach volumes; appetite hormones; macronutrients; feed volume; anthropometrics; body composition

1. Introduction

Breastfeeding and its longer duration are associated with reduced risks of developing obesity and other chronic non-communicable diseases later in life [1,2]. This unique protection could be the result of many mechanisms associated with both nutritive and non-nutritive components of human milk (HM) [3] as well as breastfeeding patterns and behaviour [4,5]. It has been shown that HM has the pleiotropic role, providing immune and anti-inflammatory protection [6,7] and endocrine, developmental, neural, and psychological benefits [2]. Non-nutritive HM components such as hormones, growth factors, neuropeptides, and anti-inflammatory and immune-modulating agents influence the growth, development, and function of the gastrointestinal (GI) tract during early infancy [8], while some micronutrients act as nutritional antioxidants, improving GI functions [9]; however, there is much to be learned about the spectrum of HM programming agents, how their patterns change throughout lactation period, and their short-term effect on the gastric emptying (GE) rate of the breastfed infants.

GE is a process by which ingested food is mechanically and chemically partially broken down and delivered to the duodenum at a controlled rate for further digestion and absorption [10,11]. While well studied in the preterm population [12–14], in healthy term fully breastfed infants the GE rate and its relationship with breastfeeding patterns are not fully understood.

GE rate and patterns are known to depend on the nature and macronutrient composition of the ingested meal. HM or formula in the infant stomach separates into two phases, a liquid phase consisting of water, whey proteins, lactose, etc., and a semi-solid phase consisting of curd formed by casein and lipids. The semi-solid phase typically empties more slowly than the liquid phase. Different proportions of these phases in part explain the difference between GE patterns of formula-fed and breastfed infants—linear and curvilinear, respectively [12,15].

HM has a unique composition, including nutrients, growth factors, immune factors, and hormones. Despite numerous investigations into the different effects of HM and formula, few components, including major macronutrients, have been studied in connection with the GE of breasted term infants.

Fatty acids profiles are not associated with GE rate in preterm infants [16], while in term infants more rapid GE has been attributed to the fat and protein components of feeds with similar lactose concentration and osmolality [17].

Both osmolality and carbohydrate content are known to influence the rate of GE in adults [18], but in infants results are dependent on the type of carbohydrate [19,20].

Proteins from different HM fractions such as whey and casein are resistant to proteolysis in the infant stomach [21] and the protein content of a food has also been shown to influence appetite and its regulation [22]. Infant formula generally empties more slowly than HM in term infants; further, formulas with different casein:whey protein ratio exhibit different GE rates, with casein-predominant formulas emptying slower than whey-predominant formulas [23]. Thus the casein:whey ratio of HM could play an important role in controlling GE in the breastfed infant.

HM lysozyme, also present in whey in a relatively high concentration, catalyzes the hydrolysis of specific bonds in Gram-negative bacteria cell walls and plays multiple roles in digestive strategy, such as controlling the microbiome in the stomach and speeding up the digestion of microbial protein, which may affect gastric motility and GE rate [24,25].

The satiety hormone leptin and the appetite-stimulating hormone adiponectin are also present in HM. Although not transferred to the infant circulation in direct manner, levels of HM leptin and adiponectin from HM have been found to correlate with levels of these hormones in infant serum [26,27] and are known to affect both appetite control and infant body composition (BC) [28,29], but are yet to be investigated in relation to GE in the term infant. In animal models (rat, mouse), injection of leptin into the fourth ventricle has been shown to delay GE [30] and oral administration reduced food intake [31]. Leptin in HM is by far the most studied appetite hormone, but predominantly in skim milk [32]. Leptin measured in skim HM was not associated with time between feeds [33,34] or GE [34] in term breastfed infants, emphasizing the need for studies including whole milk leptin, where the levels of leptin are shown to be higher [32]. Adiponectin has the highest concentration of any appetite hormone in HM. It is present in a biologically active form that is resistant to digestion [35]. In the animal model adiponectin inhibits tension-sensitive gastric vagal afferent mechanosensitivity, modulating satiety signals in both lean and obese animals, while simultaneously increasing the mechanosensitivity of mucosal gastric vagal afferent in the obesity-induced model [36]. In humans, elevated serum levels of adiponectin are associated with more rapid GE in diabetic patients [37]. It is not known whether adiponectin levels impact GE in the infant and this warrants further investigation.

The volume of milk taken at a single feed varies greatly both within and between infants [38]. This may be affected by HM composition, with greater breastfeeding frequency associated with lower total 24-h protein intakes and higher lactose concentrations [39]. This suggests that the variations in HM components between mothers may potentially influence GE rate and time, and therefore feeding patterns.

This study investigated the effects of HM appetite hormones (whole milk adiponectin and leptin, skim milk leptin) and macronutrients (fat, total carbohydrates, lactose, oligosaccharides, total protein, casein and whey protein, lysozyme) on feeding frequency and GE. Further exploration of infant demographics, anthropometrics, and BC was carried out to determine relationships with infant feeding and GE.

2. Materials and Methods

2.1. Participants

Lactating mothers and their infants (*n* = 27) were recruited predominantly through the Australian Breastfeeding Association. Inclusion criteria were: healthy singletons, gestational age ≥ 37 weeks, fully breastfed on demand at the point of measurement. Exclusion criteria were: infant health issues requiring medication that could potentially influence GE rate (e.g., reflux), indications of low maternal milk production or infant growth issues. All mothers provided written informed consent to participate in the study, which was approved by the University of Western Australia, Human Research Ethics Committee (RA/1/4253) and registered with the Australian New Zealand Clinical Trials Registry (ACTRN12616000368437).

2.2. Study Design

Participants arrived at our laboratory at King Edward Memorial Hospital for Women (Subiaco, Perth, WA, Australia) in the morning (09:30–11:30 a.m.) to avoid circadian influence on the outcomes, and stayed for two consecutive breastfeeding sessions. Before the first feed (F1) infants were weighed and had ultrasound stomach volumes recorded (pre-feed residual, R1). Mothers expressed a pre-feed sample (fore-milk) of milk from the feeding breast/breasts and then breastfed their infants as usual. Immediately after F1, infant stomach volumes images and infant weights were taken, and mothers expressed a post-feed (hind-milk) milk sample. Subsequent scans of the stomach were scheduled at 15–20 min intervals (although attending infants' needs caused some variation) until the infant cued for the next feed (F2), when a final stomach volume immediately before F2 was measured (pre-feed residual, R2).

To assess infant BC bioimpedance spectroscopy measurements were taken pre-feed, unless impractical—then they were taken post-feed [40]. Ultrasound skinfold, length, and head circumference measurements were taken post-feed. This combination of two methods for measuring infant BC was used to ensure safe, non-invasive and accurate assessment and to avoid the inherent limitations of a singular technique [41]. Clothing was removed for the measurements except for a dry diaper and a singlet.

2.3. Feeding Frequency

Mothers were asked how frequently their infant feeds, and the self-reported typical time between the feeds (e.g., every three hours) during the week prior to the study session was taken as a proxy measure of feeding frequency.

2.4. Feed Volume Measurement

The volume of milk transferred from a breast/breasts by the infant was determined by weighing the infant immediately before and after the breastfeed using electronic scales (±2.0 g, Medela Electronic Baby Weigh Scales, Medela Inc., McHenry, IL, USA). Milk intake (g) was calculated by deducting the initial weight from the final weight of the infant [42] and was converted to mL (feed volume; FV) using HM density of 1.03 g/mL [43].

2.5. Stomach Measurements with Ultrasound

The infant's stomach was scanned using the Aplio XG (Toshiba, Tokyo, Japan) machine, with a high-resolution PVT-674BT (6MHz) transducer and Parker ultrasonic gel (Fairfield, NJ, USA). Three to nine (median [IQR]: 5 [5; 6]) serial measurements of infant stomachs were taken 3 to 62 min apart (16 ± 10). Scans were performed with the infant in the semi-supine position according to the method validated in preterm infants [44]. Briefly, the sagittal and transverse planes of the stomach were used to measure the longitudinal (L), anterior-posterior (AP) and transverse (T) diameters directly from images on the ultrasound screen using electronic calipers (Figure 1). One experienced sonographer with good intra- and interrater reliability [44] performed all of the measurements. Gastric volume (mL) was calculated from the above measured diameters using following equation for an ellipsoidal body:

$$\text{Stomach volume (mL)} = \text{L (mm)} \times \text{AP (mm)} \times \text{T (mm)} \times 0.52. \tag{1}$$

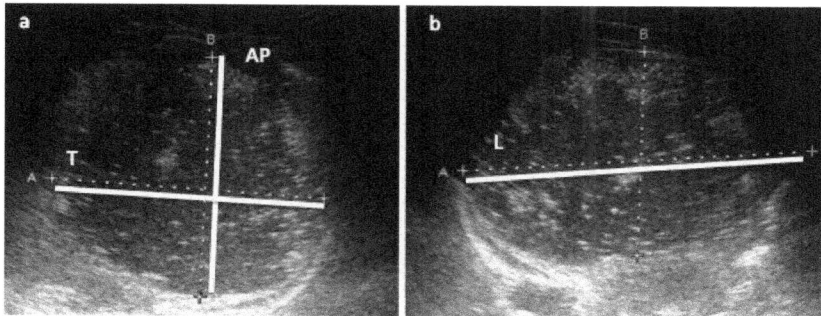

Figure 1. Measurements of infant's stomach with ultrasound. Ultrasound images of infant's stomach: (**a**) transverse view with anterior-posterior (AP) and transverse (T) diameter measurements; (**b**) longitudinal view with longitudinal (L) diameter (maximum length) measurement. Stomach volume (mL) = longitudinal diameter (mm) × anterior-posterior diameter (mm) × transverse diameter (mm) × 0.52.

2.6. Milk Sample Collection

Mothers hand-expressed or pumped small (1–2 mL) pre- and post-feed milk samples into separate 5-mL polypropylene plastic vials (Disposable Products, Adelaide, SA, Australia). Fat concentration was measured (below) and samples were frozen at -20 °C for further biochemical analysis.

2.7. Biochemical Analysis

2.7.1. Fat Content

Percentage fat was measured in pre- and post-feed samples immediately after sample collection with the creamatocrit method [45] using the Creamatocrit Plus device (Medela Inc., McHenry, IL, USA). Fat concentration of the pre- and post-feed milk samples (g/L) was calculated from the cream content of the milk samples, based on the equation [46]:

$$\text{Fat (g/L)} = 3.56 + (5.917 \times \text{cream percentage}). \tag{2}$$

Fat concentration in the volume consumed by the infant was further calculated [47]:

$$Fat\ (g/L) = 0.53 \times Fat_{\text{pre-feed}} + 0.47 \times Fat_{\text{post-feed}}. \tag{3}$$

2.7.2. Sample Preparation

Prior to further analysis, all samples were thawed for two hours at room temperature (RT) and aliquoted into 1.5-mL tubes (Sarstedt, Numbrecht, Germany). Components' concentrations were determined in both pre- and post-feed samples in case of adiponectin, skim and whole milk leptin, fat, and lactose, and in pooled samples in case of total protein, casein, whey protein, total carbohydrates, and lysozyme. Concentrations of pre- and post-feed samples were averaged to arrive at the concentration used for statistical analyses. Whole milk was used for measuring whole milk adiponectin and leptin concentration. Milk samples were defatted (by centrifugation at RT in a Beckman Microfuge 11 (Aberdon Enterprise Inc., Elk Grove Village, IL, USA) at $10,000 \times g$ for 10 min and removing the fat layer by clipping it off with the top of the tube [48]) for analysis of skim milk leptin, total protein, lysozyme, lactose, and total carbohydrates concentrations. The standard assays were adapted for and carried out using a JANUS workstation (PerkinElmer, Inc., Waltham, MA, USA) and measured on EnSpire (PerkinElmer, Inc., Waltham, MA, USA).

2.7.3. Leptin

Leptin concentration in HM was measured using the R & D Systems Human Leptin enzyme linked immunosorbent assay (ELISA) DuoSet kit (Minneapolis, MN, USA) optimized to measure leptin in sonicated skim HM, as previously described by Cannon et al. [33] and further modified to measure leptin in skim and whole HM milk as described by Kuganathan et al. [32]. Recovery of leptin was $97.7\% \pm 9.7\%$ ($n = 10$) with a detection limit of 0.05 ng/mL and an inter-assay CV of <7.2%.

2.7.4. Adiponectin

Adiponectin concentration in whole milk was measured using the Biovendor Human Adiponectin Sandwich ELISA kit (Life Technologies, Asheville, NC, USA). Adiponectin recovery was $96.2\% \pm 3.2\%$ ($n = 10$) with a detection limit of 1 ng/mL and an inter-assay CV of <2.5%.

2.7.5. Protein

Casein and whey proteins were separated by the method fully described by Kunz and Lonnerdal [49], and Khan et al. [50]. Protein concentrations (total protein of skim HM, casein and whey proteins) were measured using the Bradford Protein Assay adapted from Mitoulas et al. [51]. Recovery of protein was $100.6\% \pm 5.2\%$ ($n = 5$) with a detection limit of 0.031 g/L and an inter-assay CV of 7.8% ($n = 18$). Casein:whey ratio was calculated as follows:

$$Casein{:}whey\ ratio = \text{casein concentration/whey protein concentration}. \tag{4}$$

2.7.6. Lysozyme

Lysozyme concentration was determined using a modified turbidimetric assay [52]. Hen egg white lysozyme (EC 3.2.1.17, Sigma, St. Louis, MA, USA) standards (range 0.00075–0.0125 g/L) and skim milk samples were diluted 10-fold with 0.1 M of $Na_2HPO_4/1.1$ mM of citric acid (pH 5.8) buffer. Twenty-five microliters of standards or diluted skim milk samples were placed into the wells of a plate (Greiner Bio-One, Frickenhausen, Germany), 175 µL of *Micrococcus lysodeiltikus* suspension (0.075% *w/v*, ATCC No. 4698, Sigma, St. Louis, MA, USA) was added into each well and plate was incubated at RT for 1 h. The absorbance was measured at 450 nm. Recovery of lysozyme was $97.0\% \pm 5.0\%$ ($n = 8$) with a detection limit of 0.007 g/L and an inter-assay CV of 13.0% ($n = 8$).

2.7.7. Carbohydrates

Defatted milk was deproteinized with trichloroacetic acid [53] before dehydration by sulphuric acid [54]. This technique reliably estimates concentrations and carbon content for monosaccharides, disaccharides, and polysaccharides. Total carbohydrates were analyzed by UV-spectrophotometry. Recovery of total carbohydrates was 101.4% ± 2.1% (*n* = 7) with a detection limit of 0.007 g/L and an inter-assay CV of 3.3% (*n* = 7).

Lactose concentration was measured using the enzymatic spectrophotometric method of Kuhn and Lowenstein [55], adapted from Mitoulas et al. [51], with recovery of 98.2% ± 4.1% (*n* = 10), detection limit of 30 mM and inter-assay CV of 3.5%.

The human milk oligosaccharides (HMO) concentration (g) was calculated by deducting concentration of lactose (g) from concentration of total carbohydrates (g). The glucose and galactose were not measured or accounted for as their concentrations in HM are small and comparable or less than the assays errors [56].

2.8. Hormone and Macronutrient Dose

Doses were defined as the amount of hormone/macronutrient ingested during a breastfeed and calculated as average of the pre- and post-feed HM component concentration, multiplied by the corresponding FV. When an infant fed from both breasts at the breastfeeding session, hormone/macronutrient doses from these individual breastfeeds were calculated separately and added together.

2.9. Infants' Anthropometrics and Body Composition

2.9.1. Anthropometric Measurements

Infants' weight was determined by weighing before breastfeeding using Medela Electronic Baby Weigh Scales (±2.0 g; Medela Inc., McHenry, IL, USA). Clothing was removed except for a dry diaper and a singlet. Infant crown-heel length was measured once to the nearest 0.1 cm using non-stretch tape and headpiece and footpiece, both applied perpendicular to the hard surface. Infant head circumference was measured with non-stretch tape. Infant BMI was calculated according to the following formula:

$$BMI = \text{Body weight (kg)}/(\text{Height (m)})^2. \tag{5}$$

2.9.2. Body Composition with Bioelectrical Impedance Spectroscopy

Infants' whole body bioimpedance were measured using the Impedimed SFB7 bioelectrical impedance analyzer (ImpediMed, Brisbane, Queensland, Australia) applying an adult protocol (wrist to ankle) according to the manufacturer's instructions and analyzed with settings customized for each infant according to Lingwood et al. [57] and Gridneva et al. [41]. Values of resistance (ohm) at frequency of 50 kHz (R_{50}) were determined from the curve of best fit, averaged for analysis purposes and used in the Lingwood et al. age matched (3 and 4.5 mo infants) equations for fat-free mass (FFM) of 2 and 5 mo infants respectively [57]:

$$FFM\ 3\ \text{mo} = 1.458 + 0.498 \times W - 0.197 \times S + 0.067 \times L^2/R_{50} \tag{6}$$

$$FM\ 4.5\ \text{mo} = 2.203 + 0.334 \times W - 0.361 \times S + 0.185 \times L^2/R_{50}, \tag{7}$$

where L is body length (cm), R_{50} is resistance (Ω), S is sex (male = 1, female = 2) and W is infant weight (kg).

%FM was calculated as follows:

$$\%FM = 100(\text{Weight (kg)} - FFM\ \text{(kg)})/\text{Weight (kg)}. \tag{8}$$

2.9.3. Body Composition with Ultrasound Skinfold Measurements

Infant ultrasound skinfold measurements were carried out using the Aplio XG (Toshiba, Tokyo, Japan) ultrasound machine, PLT-1204BX 14-8 MHz transducer and sterile water-based Parker ultrasonic gel (Fairfield, NJ, USA). Single ultrasound scans of four anatomical sites (biceps, subscapular, suprailiac, and triceps) were performed on the left side of the body with minimal compression. Skinfold thickness (skin thickness and the skin–fat interface to fat–muscle interface distance) was measured directly from images on the screen using electronic calipers. One experienced sonographer (DG) with good intra- and interrater reliability [44] performed all of the measurements.

The doubled ultrasound skinfold thickness was used in Brook body density (*d*) age-matched (3–18 mo) equations [58] developed for skinfolds measured with calipers:

$$Male\ d = 1.1690 - 0.0788 \times \log \left(\sum SFT \right) \tag{9}$$

$$Female\ d = 1.2063 - 0.0999 \times \log \left(\sum SFT \right), \tag{10}$$

where *d* is infant body density (kg/L) and $\sum SFT$ is a sum of four skinfolds (mm).

Predicted body density was converted to %FM using the Lohman equation [59]:

$$\%FM = 100 \times (5.28/d - 4.89), \tag{11}$$

where *d* is the infant body density (kg/L).

2.10. Statistical Analysis

Statistical analysis was performed in R 2.9.0 [60] for Mac OSX using additional packages nlme [61]; lattice [62], lattice extra [63], and car [64]; MASS [65], sfsmisc [66] and multcomp [67] for mixed effects modeling, data representation, robust regression, and multiple comparisons of means, respectively. Descriptive statistics are reported as mean ± standard deviation (SD) (range) or median (IQR) unless otherwise stated; model parameters are presented as estimate ± standard error (SE), and, where appropriate, an approximate 95% confidence interval (95% CI).

Measurements missing due to insufficient sample volume: skim milk leptin, whole milk leptin, adiponectin, total protein, whey and casein protein, lactose and total carbohydrate (*n* = 3); lysozyme (*n* = 5). Measurements of fat (*n* = 14) were missing as a result of either insufficient sample volumes or absence of separate feed volumes from breasts where both breast were offered during one feed. Also missing were feeding frequency as reported by mothers (*n* = 6), measurements of length, head circumference, infant BMI, %FM measured with bioelectrical spectroscopy (*n* = 4) and %FM measured with ultrasound skinfolds (*n* = 5).

GE time was determined as the time from the start of F1 to the start of F2 and included the time between two feeds and feed duration. Feed duration was included as up to 80% of HM consumed by term healthy breastfed infants in the first 4–5 min [68]. GE during breastfeeding was defined as the volume of milk to have left the stomach, calculated as the difference between the immediate post-feed stomach volumes and the sum of R1 and FV.

Due to the lack of term infant gastric-emptying studies focusing on stomach volume, no power calculation/sample size determination could be performed for this study. A goal of 20 infants at each two and five months was selected with the expectation that this would be sufficient to show overall patterns. When available, infants were included in both subsets to allow for investigation of longitudinal patterns. Linear mixed effects models allow us to treat the individual feeds as separate, without having to assume independence, when there may be correlations between feeds within infants.

Influences on GE rate were analyzed by first fitting a time curve to the sequential post-feed stomach volumes using linear mixed effects models; as curves differed significantly within and between infants (*p* < 0.001), random time curves were fitted to feeds within infants. Time terms (linear, square root) were selected as per the fractional polynomial method of [69]; this model also considered possible confounding effects of FV (median-centred) and feed duration (median-centred). Interaction terms involving the time curve indicated changes in the GE rate; main effects indicated overall effects on post-feed stomach volumes but not the GE rate. The addition of one term to this base model was used to investigate associations with (a) concentrations/doses of hormones/macronutrients; (b) infant characteristics/anthropometrics/BC; (c) R1. Whether the overall effect of HM component concentrations differs by feed volume was investigated by including interactions between FV and concentration measures. Models using the selected technique did not converge for fat concentration, lysozyme concentration, or lysozyme dose. Omitting the random effect of feed within infant provided converging models, but no evidence of an association with fat or lysozyme was seen. Given the complexity of linear mixed effects models used to analyze GE rate, no further adjustments were performed and $p < 0.05$ was considered to be statistically significant.

Associations between pre-feed residual stomach volumes, FV, immediate post-feed stomach volumes, feed duration, feeding frequency and both hormone and macronutrient concentrations and doses, and infant anthropometrics/BC parameters were tested using robust linear regression. Mixed effects models were considered, but were not significantly better ($p > 0.1$) Robust linear regression (rlm) was chosen so as to address heteroscedasticity in the data and points with high leverage in the majority of the predictors; MM-estimation (M-estimation with Tukey's biweight, initialized by a specific S-estimator) accounting for appropriate covariates was used [65]. Approximate p-values were determined using the Wald test. Multivariate models accounting for FV were used for testing the relationship with FV-dependent predictor (fat dose and concentration).

Possible age differences in HM components, infant characteristics, and GE/breastfeeding parameters were analyzed with either linear mixed effects models or robust linear regression models; model type was determined using likelihood ratio tests. Linear mixed effects models were used to analyze relationships of GE during feed time with HM components and infant characteristics. R1, FV and feed duration were not associated with stomach volume reduction during the feed time, therefore univariate models were run. Multivariate linear mixed effects models accounting for R1, FV and feed duration were used in analysis of relationships of immediate post-feed stomach volumes with HM components and infant characteristics.

Owing to the large number of comparisons, a false discovery rate adjustment [70] was performed on associated subgroupings of results with one or more p-values < 0.05. p-values were considered to be significant at <0.011 for GE time, <0.031 for feeding frequency, <0.038 for R2, and <0.008 for associations between HM components' concentrations.

3. Results

3.1. Participants

Characteristics of the 27 participants (2 months ($n = 20$; longitudinal: 7 females, 7 males; cross-sectional: 2 females, 4 males); 5 months ($n = 21$; longitudinal: 7 females, 7 males; cross-sectional: 6 females); overall $n = 41$ feeds) are described in Table 1. At the study session, infants fed from one ($n = 23$) or both ($n = 18$) breasts.

3.2. Influence of Infant Age

Infant anthropometrics and %FM measured with bioimpedance spectroscopy significantly differed by infant age ($p < 0.001$), while breastfeeding and GE parameters did not change significantly ($p > 0.067$) (Table 1).

Lower whey protein concentration (5.51 ± 0.96 g/L 5 mo vs. 6.41 ± 1.39 g/L 2 mo, $p = 0.034$) and subsequently a higher casein:whey ratio (0.32 ± 0.14 5 mo vs. 0.22 ± 0.07 2 mo, $p = 0.035$) were observed at 5 months. All other measured appetite hormones and macronutrient concentrations did not differ significantly by infant age ($p > 0.053$).

3.3. Analyzed Human Milk Components

Appetite hormones and macronutrient concentrations and doses per feed are presented in Table 2. Higher skim milk leptin concentrations were associated with lower whole milk leptin concentrations (-0.25 [-0.34, -0.16], $p < 0.001$) and higher protein concentrations were associated with higher whey protein concentrations (0.68 [0.41, 0.95], $p < 0.001$). Higher HMO concentrations were associated with higher total carbohydrates concentrations ($p < 0.001$) and lower lactose concentrations ($p < 0.001$).

Table 1. Participant characteristics expressed as mean ± SD and range.

Characteristics	2 mo [a]		5 mo [b]		Total [c]	
	Mean ± SD	Range	Mean ± SD	Range	Mean ± SD	Range
Infant characteristics						
Infant age (weeks)	9 ± 1	6–10	22 ± 1 ***	18–23	16 ± 7	6–23
Infant length (cm)	57 ± 2	53–61	65 ± 2 ***	62–69	61 ± 4	53–69
Infant weight (kg)	5.3 ± 0.8	4.2–6.3	7.2 ± 1.0 ***	5.8–9.5	6.3 ± 1.3	4.2–9.5
Infant BMI	15.9 ± 1.3	13.9–18.1	17.6 ± 1.7 ***	14.9–20.4	16.7 ± 1.7	13.9–20.4
HC (cm)	39 ± 1	37–42	43 ± 2 ***	40–46	41 ± 2	37–46
Fat Mass with BIS (%)	21.4 ± 3.6	11.1–27.1	28.9 ± 3.2 ***	21.7–35.8	25.3 ± 5.0	11.1–35.8
Fat Mass with US (%)	24.2 ± 3.6	17.5–30.5	26.6 ± 3.6	20.8–35.9	25.5 ± 3.8	17.5–35.9
BF/GE characteristics						
Feed volume (mL)	86 ± 34	35–140	85 ± 33	36–180	86 ± 33	35–180
SV after feed 1 (mL)	87 ± 36	32–141	93 ± 41	22–189	90 ± 38	22–189
Feed duration (min)	28 ± 14	11–72	20 ± 8	6–37	24 ± 12	6–72
SV reduction (mL) [d]	5 ± 21	(−42)–33	4 ± 26	(−57)–56	4 ± 24	(−57)–56
GE time (min) [e]	94 ± 29	44–153	88 ± 18	50–140	91 ± 24	44–140
Residual 1 (mL)	6 ± 12	0–50	11 ± 19	0–62	9 ± 16	0–62
Residual 2 (mL)	20 ± 20	0–81	15 ± 15	0–55	18 ± 18	0–81
Feeding frequency (h) [f]	2.3 ± 0.7	1.0–4.0	2.7 ± 0.8	1.5–4.0	2.5 ± 0.7	1.0–4.0

Data are mean ± SD and ranges. [a] $n = 20$; [b] $n = 21$. [c] $n = 41$ feeds. [d] Stomach volume reduction during feed time is calculated as the difference between the sum of residual 1 and feed volume and the immediate stomach volume after Feed 1 . [e] GE time is the time from the start of Feed 1 to the start of Feed 2 (time between feeds plus feed duration). [f] Feeding frequency self-reported by mothers as to how often infant feeds (e.g., every three hours). *** Indicates significant differences ($p < 0.001$) between two- and five-month-old infants. Abbreviations: BF—breastfeeding; BIS—bioimpedance spectroscopy; GE—gastric emptying; HC—head circumference; SV—stomach volume; US—ultrasound.

Table 2. Concentrations and doses of measured HM hormones and macronutrients.

Components	Concentration		Dose Per Feed	
	Mean ± SD	Range	Mean ± SD	Range
Adiponectin (ng/mL, ng)	10.02 ± 4.08	6.18–22.58	868.62 ± 491.32	238.60–2536.91
WM leptin (ng/mL, ng)	0.51 ± 0.18	0.23–1.10	44.80 ± 24.30	10.15–115.03
SM leptin (ng/mL, ng)	0.28 ± 0.12	0.20–0.84	24.8 ± 15.0	6.91–73.00
Total protein (g/L, g)	11.29 ± 2.56	7.60–24.16	0.99 ± 0.39	0.35–2.29
Casein (g/L, g)	1.54 ± 0.53	0.69–3.45	0.14 ± 0.07	0.04–0.29
Whey protein (g/L, g)	5.97 ± 1.26	3.82–9.08	0.52 ± 0.19	0.17–0.95
Casein:whey ratio	0.27 ± 0.11	0.10–0.73	n/a [a]	n/a [a]
Lysozyme (g/L, g)	0.14 ± 0.12	0.05–0.48	0.01 ± 0.01	0.003–0.030
TCH (g/L, g)	82.72 ± 7.89	67.08–97.49	7.28 ± 2.62	3.28–15.18
Lactose (g/L, g)	65.84 ± 5.14	53.49–77.94	5.86 ± 2.22	2.19–12.06
HMO (g/L, g)	16.88 ± 9.89	(−10.86) [b]–35.77	1.42 ± 0.94	(−1.09) [b]–3.78
Fat (g/L, g)	42.74 ± 12.10	17.42–66.79	3.57 ± 1.45	0.64–6.40

Data are mean ± SD and ranges, $n = 41$ feeds. [a] Casein:whey ratios for doses are the same as for concentrations. [b] Negative values are seen for human milk oligosaccharides (HMO) when lactose measurements are higher than total carbohydrates. Abbreviations: SM—skim milk; TCH—total carbohydrates; WM—whole milk.

3.4. Gastric Emptying Rate

The overall decreasing curvilinear pattern of GE (linear: 0.04 [-0.17, 0.24], $p = 0.72$; square root: -10.5 [-12.7, -8.2], $p < 0.001$) is shown in Figure 2. Higher FVs were associated with faster

$(-0.07 \, [-0.10, \, -0.03], \, p < 0.001)$ GE rate (Figure 3) and higher overall post-feed stomach volumes $(0.82 \, [0.53, \, 1.12], \, p < 0.001)$. No association was seen between feed duration and post-feed stomach volume $(-0.25 \, [-0.68, \, 0.18], \, p = 0.23)$.

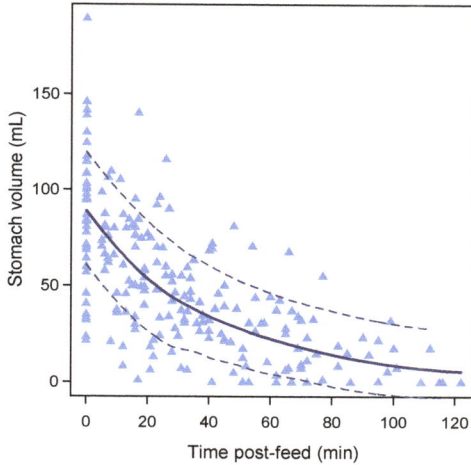

Figure 2. Overall curvilinear pattern of gastric emptying ($n = 41$ feeds). The lines represent the overall pattern of changes in stomach volume as measured by ultrasound imaging. Bold line represents local regression smoother (LOESS, span = 0.9). Dotted lines represent confidence interval.

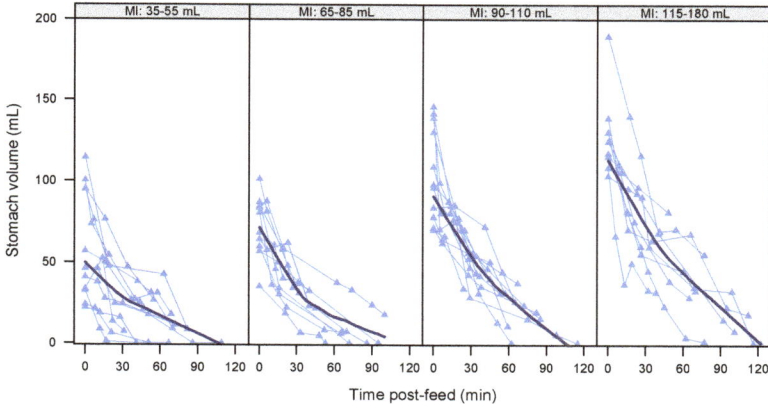

Figure 3. Gastric emptying of individual feeds in term breastfed infants ($n = 41$ feeds). Feeds are grouped by milk intake (MI) to illustrate the effect of the feed volumes; approximately equal numbers are included in each panel. Data points represent stomach volumes calculated from ultrasound images; connecting lines link measurements from the same feed. Bold line represents local regression smoother (LOESS, span = 0.9).

Immediate post-feed stomach volumes were not associated with R1 ($p = 0.91$).

After accounting for time post-feed, FV, and feed duration, as per the above model, larger R1 volumes $(0.55 \, [0.24, \, 0.86], \, p = 0.003)$ and higher whey protein concentrations $(4.99 \, [0.84, \, 9.13], \, p = 0.023)$ were associated with larger post-feed stomach volumes, while the casein:whey ratio $(2.2 \pm 0.88, \, p = 0.030)$ and lactose concentration $(-0.04 \pm 0.02, \, p = 0.037)$ modified the GE curve depending on

FV. Higher casein:whey ratios at lower FVs were associated with faster GE, and at higher FVs with slower GE, while higher lactose concentrations at lower FVs were associated with slower GE, and at higher FVs with faster GE. No other associations with post-feed stomach volumes or changes to the GE curves were found (Table 3).

Table 3. HM components and infant characteristics and their associations with feed variables and gastric emptying.

Predictors	Feed Volume [a]		Gastric Emptying Time [a]		Post-Feed Stomach Volumes [b]	
	Estimate ± SE (95% CI)	*p*-Value	Estimate ± SE (95% CI)	*p*-Value	Estimate ± SE (95% CI)	*p*-Value
Concentrations						
Adiponectin (ng/mL)	1 ± 1.3 (−36.6, 134.5)	0.44	2.3 ± 0.7 (0.9, 3.7)	**0.002** [c]	1.3 ± 0.7 (−0.2, 2.7)	0.081
Whole milk leptin (ng/mL)	9.9 ± 29.9 (−36.6, 134.5)	0.74	6.8 ± 15.8 (−24.2, 37.8)	0.67	−9.5 ± 13.3 (−35.8, 16.9)	0.48
Skim milk leptin (ng/mL)	49 ± 43.6 (−36.6, 134.5)	0.26	6.7 ± 24.3 (−41, 54.4)	0.78	39.8 ± 18.4 (−0.8, 80.3)	0.054
Total protein (g/L)	−2.1 ± 2.1 (−6.2, 1.9)	0.30	−0.9 ± 1.1 (−3.1, 1.3)	0.41	1.1 ± 1 (−1.2, 3.4)	0.30
Whey protein (g/L)	−5.5 ± 4.2 (−13.8, 2.7)	0.19	5.8 ± 2.2 (1.6, 10.1)	0.011	5 ± 1.9 (0.8, 9.1)	**0.023**
Casein (g/L)	2.6 ± 10.2 (−17.4, 22.5)	0.80	−12.4 ± 4.7 (−21.5, −3.2)	0.013	−2 ± 4.4 (−11.6, 7.6)	0.66
Casein:whey ratio	24.5 ± 46.1 (−65.9, 114.9)	0.59	−65.9 ± 21 (−107.1, −24.7)	**0.003**	−17.3 ± 20.1 (−61.4, 26.9)	0.41
Lysozyme (g/L)	−81.4 ± 46.2 (−172, 9.1)	0.079	−19.5 ± 28.3 (−75, 36)	0.49	23.3 ± 15.4 (−7.2, 53.8)	0.13
Total carbohydrates (g/L)	−1.1 ± 0.7 (−2.3, 0.2)	0.12	−0.6 ± 0.4 (−1.3, 0.1)	0.10	−0.5 ± 0.3 (−1.2, 0.1)	0.089
Lactose (g/L)	0.7 ± 1.1 (−1.4, 2.7)	0.51	0.2 ± 0.6 (−0.9, 1.3)	0.76	0.03 ± 0.49 (−1, 1.1)	0.96
HMO (g/L)	−0.8 ± 0.5 (−1.9, 0.2)	0.13	−0.4 ± 0.3 (−1, 0.2)	0.16	−0.4 ± 0.2 (−0.9, 0.1)	0.13
Fat (g/L)	−0.69 ± 0.6 (−1.8, 0.5)	0.26	−0.1 ± 0.3 (−0.6, 0.5)	0.79	−0.1 ± 0.3 (−0.9, 0.6)	0.71
Doses						
Adiponectin (ng)	n/a [d]	n/a [d]	0.02 ± 0.01 (0.01, 0.03)	**0.005**	0.01 ± 0.01 (−0.003, 0.03)	0.094
Whole milk leptin (ng)	n/a	n/a	−0.1 ± 0.2 (−0.4, 0.2)	0.44	−0.2 ± 0.2 (−0.5, 0.2)	0.28
Skim milk leptin (ng)	n/a	n/a	−0.2 ± 0.2 (−0.7, 0.3)	0.38	0.4 ± 0.2 (−0.1, 0.8)	0.086
Total protein (g)	n/a	n/a	−25.9 ± 12.4 (−50.2, −1.7)	0.040	15 ± 13.1 (−13.7, 43.7)	0.27
Whey protein (g)	n/a	n/a	47.6 ± 18.7 (10.8, 84.3)	0.015	50.6 ± 24.3 (−2.8, 104)	0.061
Casein (g)	n/a	n/a	−119 ± 53.3 (−223.4, −14.6)	0.030	0.4 ± 47.6 (−104.2, 105.1)	0.99
Lysozyme (g)	n/a	n/a	−276.2 ± 370.7 (−1002.9, 450.4)	0.46	395.5 ± 258.3 (−114.7, 905.6)	0.13
Total carbohydrates (g)	n/a	n/a	−4.1 ± 1.8 (−7.6, −0.5)	0.030	−4.6 ± 3 (−11.2, 2.1)	0.16
Lactose (g)	n/a	n/a	−5.8 ± 2.7 (−11.1, −0.6)	0.037	−3.1 ± 5.4 (−15.1, 8.9)	0.58
HMO (g)	n/a	n/a	−3.1 ± 3.1 (−9.2, 3)	0.32	−3.2 ± 2.7 (−9.1, 2.8)	0.27
Fat (g)	n/a	n/a	−2.8 ± 2.7 (−8.1, 2.4)	0.30	−4.9 ± 2.8 (−12.7, 2.8)	0.15

Table 3. *Cont.*

Predictors	Feed Volume [a]		Gastric Emptying Time [a]		Post-Feed Stomach Volumes [b]	
	Estimate ± SE (95% CI)	*p*-Value	Estimate ± SE (95% CI)	*p*-Value	Estimate ± SE (95% CI)	*p*-Value
Demographics						
Infant sex (Male)	−2.2 ± 10.7 (−23.1, 18.8)	0.84	−1.5 ± 7.5 (−16.3, 13.2)	0.84	−8.4 ± 4.6 (−17.8, 1.1)	0.081
Infant age (months)	−0.9 ± 3.6 (−7.9, 6)	0.80	−1.8 ± 2.5 (−6.6, 3)	0.47	−1.5 ± 1.4 (−4.5, 1.6)	0.32
Anthropometrics						
Infant length (cm)	−0.03 ± 1.3 (−2.6, 2.6)	0.98	−1.3 ± 0.9 (−3, 0.4)	0.15	−0.5 ± 0.6 (−1.8, 0.8)	0.44
Infant weight (kg)	0.7 ± 4.1 (−7.4, 8.8)	0.87	−2.3 ± 2.9 (−7.9, 3.4)	0.43	−2.3 ± 1.8 (−6.3, 1.7)	0.23
Head circumference (cm)	−2.5 ± 2.6 (−7.5, 2.5)	0.34	−1.4 ± 1.8 (−4.9, 2.1)	0.42	−1.8 ± 1.2 (−4.5, 0.8)	0.15
Infant BMI	−0.2 ± 3.2 (−6.5, 6)	0.94	−1.5 ± 2.2 (−5.8, 2.8)	0.48	−3.2 ± 1.5 (−6.6, 0.2)	0.062
Body composition						
Fat mass with US (%)	0.6 ± 1.4 (−2.2, 3.4)	0.67	−0.3 ± 0.9 (−2.2, 1.5)	0.71	−0.6 ± 0.7 (−2.1, 1.0)	0.42
Fat mass with BIS (%)	0.4 ± 1.1 (−1.8, 2.5)	0.74	−0.4 ± 0.7 (−1.9, 1)	0.56	−0.5 ± 0.5 (−1.5, 0.5)	0.35

Data are parameter estimate ± SE and 95% CI, *n* = 41 feeds. [a] Effects of predictors taken from univariate regression models; [b] Effects of predictors taken from linear mixed effects models that accounted for postprandial time, feed volume and feed duration. [c] After the false discovery rate adjustment the *p*-values were considered to be significant at <0.011 for GE time (bold font); [d] n/a—dosage is dependent on feed volume. Abbreviations: BIS—bioimpedance spectroscopy; HMO—human milk oligosaccharides; US—ultrasound skinfolds.

3.5. Feed Volume, Feed Duration, and Gastric Emptying during Breastfeeding

Higher FVs were associated with higher stomach volumes measured immediately post-feed (0.79 [0.51, 1.07], *p* < 0.001) and longer GE times (0.24 [0.03, 0.46], *p* = 0.033). FV was not associated with either concentrations of measured HM components or infant's characteristics/anthropometrics/BC (Table 3).

Feed duration was not associated with FV (0.06 [−0.03, 0.15], *p* = 0.20) or R1 volume (0.01 [−0.17, 0.19], *p* = 0.91).

After accounting for R1 (1.07 [0.47, 1.7], *p* = 0.002), FV (1.00 [0.71, 1.3], *p* < 0.001) and feed duration (−0.30 [−0.96, 0.36], *p* = 0.34), immediate post-feed stomach volumes were not associated with either measured HM components (*p* > 0.068) or infant's demographics/anthropometrics/BC (*p* > 0.46). Stomach volume reduction during breastfeeding was not associated with either measured HM components (*p* > 0.11); infant's demographics/anthropometrics/BC (*p* > 0.48); R1, FV or feed duration (*p* > 0.34).

3.6. Gastric Emptying Time

The GE time was not associated with feed duration (0.35 [−0.29, 0.98], *p* = 0.28), but was negatively associated with R2 (−0.63 [−1.05, −0.21], *p* = 0.005) after accounting for FV (*p* < 0.001). Longer GE times were associated with higher adiponectin concentration (2.3 [0.9, 3.7], *p* = 0.002) and dose (0.02 [0.01, 0.03], *p* = 0.005), and lower casein:whey ratio (−65.9 [−107.1, −24.7], *p* = 0.003). No associations with infant characteristics were seen (Table 3).

3.7. Pre-Feed Residuals

Infants cued for F1 and F2 with different residual volumes (R1 and R2) present in their stomachs (Table 1). Larger FVs were associated with smaller R1 volumes (*p* = 0.002), with each

−0.92 [−1.47, −0.37] mL of R1 volume resulting in extra mL of FV. Larger R2 volumes were associated with larger FVs ($p = 0.006$), each additional mL of FV resulting in 0.21 [0.07, 0.35] mL greater R2.

There was no association between R2 and R1 in univariate model (0.11 [−0.19, 0.42], $p = 0.46$). After accounting for FV and GE time ($p < 0.001$ for both) larger R2 volumes were associated with larger R1 volumes (0.36 [0.11, 0.60], $p = 0.005$).

After accounting for FV, R2 was not associated with any concentration of HM components ($p \geq 0.038$ after adjusting for multiple comparisons).

3.8. Feeding Frequency

A longer time between the feeds was seen when infants were longer, heavier, and had higher %FM measured with BIS (Table 4) in univariate models. The associations for length and weight were not significant after accounting for the other ($p > 0.38$); the association for %FM measured with BIS was not significant after accounting for infant length ($p = 0.095$).

Table 4. Associations between infant feeding frequency and HM components and infant characteristics.

Predictors	Feeding Frequency (h) [a]	
	Estimate ± SE (95% CI) [b]	*p*-Value
Concentrations		
Adiponectin (ng/mL)	−0.001 ± 0.03 (−0.06, 0.06)	0.96
Whole milk leptin (ng/mL)	−1.1 ± 0.7 (−2.5, 0.3)	0.13
Skim milk leptin (ng/mL)	0.8 ± 1.6 (−2.3, 4)	0.60
Total protein (g/L)	−0.05 ± 0.05 (−0.15, 0.04)	0.28
Whey protein (g/L)	−0.1 ± 0.1 (−0.3, 0.1)	0.42
Casein (g/L)	0.04 ± 0.2 (−0.4, 0.5)	0.86
Casein:whey protein ratio	0.4 ± 1.1 (−1.7, 2.5)	0.68
Lysozyme (g/L)	−0.4 ± 1.1 (−2.5, 1.7)	0.71
Total carbohydrates (g/L)	0.01 ± 0.02 (−0.03, 0.04)	0.73
Lactose (g/L)	−0.05 ± 0.02 (−0.1, −0.01)	0.031
HMO (g/L)	0.01 ± 0.02 (−0.03, 0.04)	0.73
Fat (g/L)	−0.02 ± 0.01 (−0.04, 0.01)	0.19
Doses		
Adiponectin (ng/mL)	0.0002 ± 0.0003 (−0.0004, 0.0008)	0.50
Whole milk leptin (ng/mL)	−0.002 ± 0.01 (−0.01, 0.01)	0.80
Skim milk leptin (ng/mL)	0.01 ± 0.01 (−0.01, 0.03)	0.59
Total protein (g/L)	0.1 ± 0.3 (−0.5, 0.8)	0.67
Whey protein (g/L)	0.1 ± 0.7 (−1.3, 1.5)	0.89
Casein (g/L)	2.1 ± 2 (−1.7, 5.9)	0.27
Lysozyme (g/L)	−5.7 ± 17.2 (−39.4, 27.9)	0.73
Total carbohydrates (g/L)	0.1 ± 0.1 (0, 0.2)	0.22
Lactose (g/L)	0.04 ± 0.06 (−0.08, 0.17)	0.49
HMO (g/L)	0.3 ± 0.1 (0, 0.5)	0.051
Fat (g/L)	−0.2 ± 0.1 (−0.5, 0)	0.085
Demographics		
Infant sex (Male)	−0.2 ± 0.3 (−0.7, 0.4)	0.53
Infant age (months)	0.2 ± 0.1 (0, 0.3)	0.078
Anthropometrics		
Infant length (cm)	0.1 ± 0.03 (0.04, 0.15)	**0.004** [c]
Infant weight (kg)	0.2 ± 0.1 (0.1, 0.4)	**0.010**
Head circumference (cm)	0.1 ± 0.1 (0, 0.2)	0.23
Infant BMI	0.13 ± 0.1 (0, 0.3)	0.10
Body composition		
% fat mass with US	0.07 ± 0.03 (0, 0.13)	0.040
% fat mass with BIS	0.08 ± 0.02 (0.03, 0.12)	**0.002**

Data are parameter estimate ± SE and 95% CI, *n* = 41 feeds. [a] Feeding frequency self-reported by mothers as to how often infant feeds (e.g., every three hours). [b] Effects of predictors are results of univariate regression model. [c] After the false discovery rate adjustment the *p*-values were considered to be significant at <0.031 (highlighted). Abbreviations: BIS—bioimpedance spectroscopy; HMO—human milk oligosaccharides; US—ultrasound skinfolds.

4. Discussion

Our research shows that HM components, such as adiponectin, whey protein, casein: whey ratios, lactose, total carbohydrates, and oligosaccharides are associated with gastric emptying and breastfeeding patterns of breastfed infants. GE is a mechanism involved in satiety, therefore milk components influencing GE have the potential to affect infant milk intake and therefore growth and development in early life and subsequently health later in life.

Given the assumption that HM composition potentially influences GE [14,71], in term infants we expected the appetite hormones to be associated with infant GE rate such that high concentrations and/or doses of leptin would result in slower GE [30], whereas adiponectin might induce faster GE [37] consistent with both animal and human models. However, neither the concentrations nor doses of these hormones were related to GE rate. Previously skim milk leptin was not found to be associated with either GE rate or GE time [33,34], which we have confirmed with this larger study cohort. It was speculated that whole milk leptin, which is known to be of higher concentration, might be the reason for the negative finding [32]. While our measures of whole milk leptin were typically higher, there is an opinion that values of this magnitude are unlikely to contribute considerably to infant serum levels [72] so only the local pathways would be engaged in GE regulation. As such we were unable to find a relationship between whole milk leptin and GE. This is in contrast to animal studies showing reduced GE [30] or food intake [31] after injection or oral administration of leptin, respectively. However, it is possible that the long-term energy expenditure regulatory effect of leptin [73] may mask its short-term satiety effect on GE. Alternatively, if levels of leptin are contributing significantly to serum levels, there is a possibility that the number of receptors in the stomach of the young infant is low. Further, short-term satiety signaling through hypothalamic neurons is not fully mature, both of which would allow the infant to maintain a high physiological drive to feed to ensure adequate growth [28,73]. Gender differences in infant serum leptin levels associated with adiposity [74] have also been speculated to play a role in gastric response to HM leptin, although we did not find any relationships between infant sex/adiposity and both GE rate and GE time.

In contrast to leptin, we found that increased levels and doses of adiponectin were associated with longer GE times. This finding may partially explain the growth-regulating effect of adiponectin in infants in the first six months of life [29], when high HM adiponectin concentration is associated with lower infant weight and adiposity. Further adiponectin is 20-fold higher in concentration compared to leptin and is therefore likely to have greater biological significance [75]. The lack of association between adiponectin and GE rate is in agreement with studies of rats that showed that gastric epithelium and glands are populated with adiponectin receptors, which downregulate gastric motility [36,76]. Conversely, the findings are in contrast to studies of type 2 diabetic adults, in which elevated levels of adiponectin were associated with faster GE [37]. Further, other HM hormones such as ghrelin, cholecystokinin, and insulin may counteract or interact synergistically with leptin [77,78] and/or adiponectin.

Our study examined an extensive array of macronutrients beyond fat, total protein and lactose. Consistent with the findings of Cannon et al. [34] there were no associations with fat and total protein and either GE rate or GE time. Studies in dogs indicate that all three major macronutrients activate the ileal brake, resulting in reduction of GE; limited human studies support the findings for fat and carbohydrates while associations with protein are not so straightforward [79,80]. We were unable to find associations between the HM fat content and GE consistent with findings of Khan et al. [39] and Kent et al. [38] regarding the feeding frequency. This may be because lipids initiate the ileal brake when they reach the ileum via hydrolysis of triacylglycerol into fatty acids, thereby producing a delay in GE in humans [79]. Further analysis of HM fatty acids may shed more light on GE in breastfed infants.

However, we have found that higher whey protein concentrations are associated with larger post-feed stomach volumes, although we did not see any interaction with time, so no effect on GE rate was detected. This contradicts the results of studies of GE conducted on breastfed and formula-fed infants or studies of formula with different casein:whey ratio [15,81] in which a fast or slow GE rate was explained by concentrations of whey protein or casein, respectively. Previous studies, however, could not adequately analyze the effect of the whey protein concentration in conjunction with volume, as they only reported gastric half-emptying time, restricted monitoring time, and/or controlled infants' volume intakes. The whey fraction of HM is highly soluble in the gastric juices and rapidly empties from the stomach compared to other proteins such as casein. Whey isolate, however, was associated with a lower gastric inhibitory polypeptide (GIP) response in adults, consistent with decreased rate of GE [82]. It may very well be that whey protein speeds up the initial stage of GE (probably during the breastfeeding time), but once it activates jejunal or ileal brakes the overall GE is reduced.

While lactose is related to GE rate, it is affected by FV; at the middle range FVs (71–108 mL) lactose has no relationship with GE, whereas at lower FVs higher lactose concentrations are associated with slower GE, and at higher FVs with faster GE. These results are consistent with Khan et al. [39], who reported an association of higher lactose concentration with increased feeding frequency. These findings could be an important addition to the evaluation of the digestive and metabolic effect of lower breastfeeding frequency and larger FVs, common in Western countries, contrary to the lactation practices in traditional societies [83].

In terms of casein:whey ratios the effect is opposite to that of lactose where at lower FVs higher casein:whey ratios are associated with faster GE, and at higher FVs with slower GE, which may explain the contradictory findings for casein associations with GE rate in previous studies [14,23]. Cows' milk casein was found to activate the ileal brake in adults, resulting in reduced food intake, although its effect on GE was not significant [84]. The finding of smaller volumes resulting in more rapid GE rate might be explained by the time casein spends in the acidic environment of the stomach. While soluble whey proteins rapidly enter the small intestine mostly intact, casein transit is delayed due to the curd formation. When it exits the stomach it is mainly in the form of degraded peptides [85]. If the FVs are small some casein may exit intact, thereby speeding up GE, while if the FVs are large, casein curdles and degrades to the opioid peptides that slow down GE [86]. However, this mechanism does not explain why higher casein:whey ratios of HM were associated with shorter GE time, which could be due to the smaller amounts of whey protein reaching the small intestine and having less effect on jejunal or ileal brakes [80]. Our finding that higher whey protein concentrations are associated with larger post-feed stomach volumes further supports this possible explanation.

Further, *k*-casein has been shown to inhibit the binding of *Helicobacter pylori* to human mucosa in vitro [87]. *Helicobacter pylori* are Gram-negative bacteria present in the stomach, and are known to downregulate levels of ghrelin and leptin in the stomach [88], which may significantly affect GE. The protective action of HM *k*-casein is reinforced by lysozyme, one of the major whey proteins. While we have not seen any significant associations between lysozyme and GE, lysozyme contributes to the control of the GI bacterial population [89], and could be upregulated to control the bacterial population in the GI tract [90] and increase digestion of microbial protein [24], all of which could potentially influence GE. In a clinical study of preterm infants, lysozyme added to donor HM or formula was associated with increased body weight, normalization of the stool, and improved feed tolerance [91]. While all of this suggests that lysozyme could potentially have an effect on GE in certain circumstances, given that we have studied a healthy population the magnitude of the effect could be insignificant.

GE during feed administration has been previously documented in preterm infants. In this study, an average of 20% of feed volume is emptied from the stomach during breastfeeding compared with 10% in preterm [92]. This is probably due to a more mature GI tract in term infants and the effect of both larger FVs and present pre-feed residuals, which were associated with faster GE rate, but not to the longer feed duration time in term infants or milk composition as no associations were found.

While we speculated that milk composition might regulate the milk intake of the infant and/or the residual volume in the stomach prior to cueing for the next feed, we were unable to show this. Rather, FV is more strongly associated with GE rate than variations in milk composition.

Gastric mechanosensation is an important factor in the regulation of satiation during food intake. Indeed, gastric distention is an important determinant of GE [93], and volume-related suppression of GE rate has been reported in animal models [94]. The observed volume-related acceleration of GE with larger FVs emptying more quickly in term breastfed infants is consistent with our previous findings [34]. The biggest effect of volume was seen after the feed and as the post-prandial period progressed the magnitude of this effect decreased (Figure 2). This may also explain the variability in the time between each feed for an infant over a 24-h period [33,38]. Feeding frequency decreases between one and three months of lactation, while milk intake during each breastfeeding session increases, with both parameters remaining constant up to six months [95]. This is attributed to the fact that as infants mature they become able to consume larger FVs [38], resulting in a longer time between feeds. Also, larger FVs are generally consumed at night or in the early morning when the frequency of feeding declines [33,38]. This decline in feeding frequency also coincides with higher nocturnal concentrations of leptin and fat, and lower concentrations of lactose in HM [33], although relationships between both feeding frequency and FV and these components' concentrations are yet to be evaluated.

The recommendations for breastfeeding are to feed on demand. Interestingly, we found that the majority of infants cued for a feed when milk was still present in the stomach, albeit in variable volumes (Table 1). This suggests that the reduction of gastric distension, which regulates hunger sensations, plays a greater role in signaling time to feed [96]. Further, it may be beneficial to the developing infant to have the gastric mucosa exposed to HM anti-inflammatory components such as lysozyme or immunomodulatory agents and growth factors, all of which contribute to the maturation of the GI tract [8]. Thus it may be detrimental to prescribe decreasing the frequency of feeding in breastfed infants or expect the infant stomach to be empty in order to feed again [97].

Furthermore, interesting associations were observed between infant milk intake and volumes remaining in the stomach prior to the first and second feed. Smaller residual volumes prior to the first feed were associated with greater milk intakes, and greater milk intakes were associated with larger volumes in the stomach prior to feeding again. This suggests that breastfed infants may appear to be consuming HM volumes in a variable pattern, but due to varying residuals may actually be feeding to a predetermined stomach volume, which is also supported by the positive relationship between both pre-feed residuals (R1, R2). In fasting adults ghrelin was found to increase and spontaneously decrease at the time points of the customary meals [98], supporting the involvement of the brain in GI tract regulation. Further studies monitoring two or more consecutive feeds or even 24-h GE measurements and analyses of ghrelin in HM would clarify this finding.

In healthy adults post-lag GE and colonic transfer is reported to be faster in men than in women [99]. In this study infant sex, age, anthropometrics, and BC were not associated with GE and breastfeeding parameters, with the exception of feeding frequency. Feeding frequency decreases in the first three months of lactation and then remains stable until six months [95,100]. The absence of a significant association between feeding frequency and age, together with associations with anthropometric and body composition parameters, illustrates that feeding frequency is dictated by the growth and development of an infant rather than the infant age. These findings further underline the need for breastfeeding on demand, with the frequency linked to individual infant growth rates rather than scheduled feeding, which could exert a detrimental effect on infant growth.

While the monitoring of a single feed limits the analysis possibilities, examination of multiple feeds requires the study to be carried out in the mother's home for long periods of time. The sample size is not a limitation of the study, as although no associations between milk composition and GE rate were detected, we were able to clearly show a relationship between FV and GE rate as well as associations between milk composition and other GE parameters.

5. Conclusions

Human milk appetite hormones and macronutrients and feed volume affect gastric emptying and feeding patterns in term breastfed infants. Adiponectin, whey protein, and casein:whey ratio are associated with GE, while the effects of casein:whey ratios and lactose concentrations on GE vary with feed volume. Larger feed volumes result in a faster GE rate. Thus, milk composition and feed volume play an important role in appetite regulation via gastric function.

Acknowledgments: All authors read and approved the final manuscript. The authors are grateful to all participants for their time and effort. The authors would like to thank Anna M. Cannon for establishing the methodology of appetite hormones assays (leptin) in human milk. This study was supported by an Australian Postgraduate Award from the University of Western Australia (Australia) and an unrestricted research grant from Medela AG (Switzerland).

Author Contributions: Zoya Gridneva conceived and designed of the study, collected the data, performed biochemical analysis, performed the statistical analyses, and wrote the manuscript; Sambavi Kugananthan adapted the methods for measuring adiponectin and leptin in whole milk, performed the hormone analysis, and critically reviewed the manuscript; Anna R. Hepworth was involved in research design, data analysis, and interpretation, and critically reviewed the manuscript; Wan J. Tie performed biochemical analysis and critically reviewed the manuscript; Ching T. Lai performed biochemical analysis, provided technical support, and critically reviewed the manuscript; Leigh C. Ward provided technical and educational support, contributed to the design of the study, and critically reviewed the manuscript; Peter E. Hartmann substantially contributed to the conception and design of the study, contributed reagents/materials/analysis tools for research, and critically reviewed the manuscript; Donna T. Geddes conceived and designed of the study, carried out the ultrasonography component of the study, provided the ultrasound images, and critically reviewed the manuscript. All authors have read and approved the final manuscript as submitted and agree to be accountable for all aspects of the work.

Conflicts of Interest: The authors declare that Medela AG provided an unrestricted research grant to Donna T. Geddes, from which salaries to Donna T. Geddes, Anna R. Hepworth, Wan J. Tie, Ching T. Lai, and Peter E. Hartmann were paid. Medela AG provided a Top-up Scholarship for Zoya Gridneva, and has provided speaker's fees to Donna T. Geddes for educational lectures. The funding sponsors had no role in the design of the study; in the collection, analyses, or interpretation of data; in the writing of the manuscript, or in the decision to publish the results. Author Leigh C. Ward provides consultancy services to ImpediMed Ltd. ImpediMed Ltd. had no involvement in the inception and conducting of this research or in the writing of the manuscript.

1. Geddes, D.; Prescott, S. Developmental origins of health and disease: The role of human milk in preventing disease in the 21(st) century. *J. Hum. Lact.* **2013**, *29*, 123–127. [CrossRef] [PubMed]

2. Marseglia, L.; Manti, S.; D'Angelo, G.; Cuppari, C.; Salpietro, V.; Filippelli, M.; Trovato, A.; Gitto, E.; Salpietro, C.; Arrigo, T. Obesity and breastfeeding: The strength of association. *Women Birth* **2015**, *28*, 81–86. [CrossRef] [PubMed]

3. Savino, F.; Liguori, S.; Fissore, M.; Oggero, R. Breast milk hormones and their protective effect on obesity. *Int. J. Pediatr. Endocrinol.* **2009**. [CrossRef]

4. Bartok, C. Babies fed breastmilk by breast versus by bottle: A pilot study evaluating early growth patterns. *Breastfeed. Med.* **2011**, *6*, 117–124. [CrossRef] [PubMed]

5. Sievers, E.; Oldigs, H.D.; Santer, R.; Schaub, J. Feeding patterns in breast-fed and formula-fed infants. *Ann. Nutr. Metab.* **2001**, *46*, 243–248. [CrossRef]

6. Le Huërou-Luron, I.; Bouzerzour, K.; Ferret-Bernard, S.; Ménard, O.; Le Normand, L.; Perrier, C.; Le Bourgot, C.; Jardin, J.; Bourlieu, C.; Carton, T.; et al. A mixture of milk and vegetable lipids in infant formula changes gut digestion, mucosal immunity and microbiota composition in neonatal piglets. *Eur. J. Nutr.* **2016**, 1–14. [CrossRef] [PubMed]

7. Manti, S.; Lougaris, V.; Cuppari, C.; Tardino, L.; Dipasquale, V.; Arrigo, T.; Salpietro, C.; Leonardi, S. Breastfeeding and il-10 levels in children affected by cow's milk protein allergy: A restrospective study. *Immunobiology* **2016**. [CrossRef] [PubMed]

8. Goldman, A.S. Modulation of the gastrointestinal tract of infants by human milk. Interfaces and interactions. An evolutionary perspective. *J. Nutr.* **2000**, *130*, S426–S431.

9. Hanson, C.; Lyden, E.; Furtado, J.; Van Ormer, M.; Anderson-Berry, A. A comparison of nutritional antioxidant content in breast milk, donor milk, and infant formulas. *Nutrients* **2016**, *8*, 681. [CrossRef] [PubMed]

10. Hunt, J. A possible relation between the regulation of gastric emptying and food intake. *Am. J. Physiol.* **1980**, *239*, G1–G4. [PubMed]

11. Hellstrom, P.; Gryback, P.; Jacobsson, H. The physiology of gastric emptying. *Best Pract. Res. Clin. Anaesthesiol.* **2006**, *20*, 397–407. [CrossRef] [PubMed]
12. Gomez, H.; Hornoy, P.; Liehn, J. Ultrasonography and gastric emptying in children: Validation of a sonographic method and determination of physiological and pathological patterns. *Pediatr. Radiol.* **2003**, *33*, 522–529. [CrossRef] [PubMed]
13. Carlos, M.; Babyn, P.; Marcon, M.; Moore, A. Changes in gastric emptying in early postnatal life. *J. Pediatr.* **1997**, *130*, 931–937. [CrossRef]
14. Perrella, S.; Hepworth, A.; Simmer, K.; Geddes, D. Influences of breast milk composition on gastric emptying in preterm infants. *J. Paediatr. Gastroenterol. Nutr.* **2015**, *60*, 264–271. [CrossRef] [PubMed]
15. Cavell, B. Gastric emtying in preterm infants. *Acta Paediatr. Scand.* **1979**, *68*, 725–730. [CrossRef] [PubMed]
16. Armand, M.; Hamosh, M.; Mehta, N.; Angelus, P.; Rhilpott, J.; Henderson, T.; Dwyer, N.; Lairon, D.; Hamosh, P. Effect of human milk or formula on gastric function and fat digestion in the premature infant. *Pediatr. Res.* **1996**, *40*, 429–437. [CrossRef] [PubMed]
17. Cavell, B. Gastric emptying in infants fed human milk or infant formula. *Acta Paediatr. Scand.* **1981**, *70*, 639–641. [CrossRef] [PubMed]
18. Vist, G.; Maughan, R. The effect of osmolality and carbohydrate content on the rate of gastric emptying of liquids in man. *J. Physiol.* **1995**, *486*, 523–531. [CrossRef] [PubMed]
19. Hunt, L.; Antonson, D.; Paxson, C.J.; Vanderhoff, J. Osmolality of carbohydrate solutions and gastric emptying in the newborn. *Am. J. Dis. Child.* **1982**, *136*, 448–451. [CrossRef] [PubMed]
20. Husband, J.; Husband, P.; Mallinson, C. Gastric emptying of starch meals in the newborn. *Lancet* **1970**, 290–292. [CrossRef]
21. Lonnerdal, B. Bioactive proteins in human milk: Mechanisms of action. *J. Pediatr.* **2010**, *156*, S26–S30. [CrossRef] [PubMed]
22. Michaelsen, K.; Larnkjaer, A.; Molgaard, C. Amount and quality of dietary proteins during the first two years of life in relation to NCD risk in adulthood. *Nutr. Metab. Cardiovasc. Dis.* **2012**, *22*, 781–786. [CrossRef] [PubMed]
23. Billeaud, C.; Guillet, J.; Sandler, B. Gastric emptying in infants with or without gastro-oesophageal reflux according to type of milk. *Eur. J. Clin. Nutr.* **1990**, *44*, 577–583. [PubMed]
24. Wang, G.; Lo, L.; Forsberg, L.; Maier, R. Helicobacter pylori peptidoglycan modifications confer lysozyme resistance and contribute to survival in the host. *mBio* **2012**, *3*, e00409-12. [CrossRef] [PubMed]
25. Artym, J.; Zimecki, M. Milk-derived proteins and peptides in clinical trials. *Postepy Hig. Med. Dosw.* **2013**, *67*, 800–816. [CrossRef]
26. Savino, F.; Sardo, A.; Rossi, L.; Benetti, S.; Savino, A.; Silvestro, L. Mother and infant body mass index, breast milk leptin and their serum leptin values. *Nutrients* **2016**, *8*, 383. [CrossRef] [PubMed]
27. Wang, Y.Y.; Zhang, Z.J.; Yao, W.; Morrow, A.; Peng, Y.M. Variation of maternal milk adiponectin and its correlation with infant growth. *Zhonghua Er Ke Za Zhi* **2011**, *49*, 338–343. [PubMed]
28. Miralles, O.; Sanchez, J.; Palou, A.; Pico, C. A physiological role of breast milk leptin in body weight control in developing infants. *Obesity* **2006**, *14*, 1371–1377. [CrossRef] [PubMed]
29. Woo, J.; Guerrero, M.; Altaye, M.; Ruiz-Palacios, G.; Martin, L.; Dubert-Ferrandon, A.; Newburg, D.; Morrow, A. Human milk adiponectin is associated with growth in two independent cohorts. *Breastfeed. Med.* **2009**, *4*, 101–109. [CrossRef] [PubMed]
30. Smedh, U.; Hakansson, M.L.; Meister, B.; Uvnas-Moberg, K. Leptin injected into the fourth ventricle inhibits gastric emptying. *Neuroreport* **1998**, *9*, 297–301. [CrossRef] [PubMed]
31. Sanchez, J.; Oliver, P.; Miralles, O.; Ceresi, E.; Pico, C.; Palou, A. Leptin orally supplied to neonate rats is directly uptaken by the immature stomach and may regulate short-term feeding. *Endocrinology* **2005**, *146*, 2575–2582. [CrossRef] [PubMed]
32. Kugananthan, S.; Lai, C.T.; Gridneva, Z.; Mark, P.J.; Geddes, D.T.; Kakulas, F. Leptin levels are higher in whole compared to skim human milk, supporting a cellular contribution. *Nutrients* **2016**, *8*, 711. [CrossRef] [PubMed]
33. Cannon, A.; Kakulas, F.; Hepworth, A.; Lai, C.; Hartmann, P.; Geddes, D. The effects of leptin on breastfeeding behaviour. *Int. J. Environ. Res. Public Helath* **2015**, *12*, 12340–12355. [CrossRef] [PubMed]

34. Cannon, A.M.; Gridneva, Z.; Hepworth, A.; Lai, C.T.; Tie, W.J.; Khan, S.; Hartmann, P.E.; Geddes, D.T. The relationship of human milk leptin and macronutrients with gastric emptying in term breastfed infants. *Pediatr. Res.* **2016**, under review.

35. Newburg, D.; Woo, J.; Morrow, A. Characteristics and potential functions of human milk adiponectin. *J. Pediatr.* **2010**, *156*, S41–S46. [CrossRef] [PubMed]

36. Kentish, S.J.; Ratcliff, K.; Li, H.; Wittert, G.A.; Page, A.J. High fat diet induced changes in gastric vagal afferent response to adiponectin. *Physiol. Behav.* **2015**, *152*, 354–362. [CrossRef] [PubMed]

37. Iwase, M.; Iino, K.; Oku, M.; Nohara, S.; Asano, T.; Doi, Y.; Iida, M. Serum high-molecular weight adiponectin is related to early postprandial glycemic increases and gastric emptying in patients with type 2 diabetes mellitus. *Diabetes Metab. Res. Rev.* **2009**, *25*, 344–350. [CrossRef] [PubMed]

38. Kent, J.C.; Mitoulas, L.R.; Cregan, M.D.; Ramsay, D.T.; Doherty, D.A.; Hartmann, P.E. Volume and frequency of breastfeedings and fat content of breast milk throughout the day. *Pediatrics* **2006**, *117*, e387–e395. [CrossRef] [PubMed]

39. Khan, S.; Hepworth, A.R.; Prime, D.K.; Lai, C.T.; Trengove, N.J.; Hartmann, P.E. Variation in fat, lactose, and protein composition in breast milk over 24 h: Associations with infant feeding patterns. *J. Hum. Lact.* **2013**, *29*, 81–89. [CrossRef] [PubMed]

40. Gridneva, Z.; Hepworth, A.; Ward, L.; Lai, C.T.; Hartmann, P.; Geddes, D.T. Bioimpedance spectroscopy in the infant: Effect of milk intake and extracellular fluid reservoirs on resistance measurements in term breastfed infants. *Eur. J. Clin. Nutr.* **2016**, *70*, 843–851. [CrossRef] [PubMed]

41. Gridneva, Z.; Hepworth, A.R.; Ward, L.C.; Lai, C.T.; Hartmann, P.E.; Geddes, D.T. Determinants of body composition in breastfed infants using bioimpedance spectroscopy and ultrasound skinfolds—Methods comparison. *Pediatr. Res.* **2016**, in press. [CrossRef] [PubMed]

42. Arthur, P.; Hartmann, P.; Smith, M. Measurement of the milk intake of breast-fed infants. *J. Paediatr. Gastroenterol. Nutr.* **1987**, *6*, 758–763. [CrossRef]

43. Neville, M.C.; Keller, R.; Seacat, J.; Lutes, V.; Neifert, M.; Casey, C.; Allen, J.; Archer, P. Studies in human lactation: Milk volumes in lactating women during the onset of lactation and full lactation. *Am. J. Clin. Nutr.* **1988**, *48*, 1375–1386. [PubMed]

44. Perrella, S.; Hepworth, A.; Simmer, K.; Geddes, D. Validation of ultrasound methods to monitor gastric volume changes in preterm infants. *J. Paediatr. Gastroenterol. Nutr.* **2013**, *57*, 741–749. [CrossRef] [PubMed]

45. Fleet, I.; Linzell, J. A rapid method of estimating fat in very small quantities of milk. *J. Physiol.* **1964**, *175*, 15–17.

46. Meier, P.; Engstrom, J.; Zuleger, J.; Motykowski, J.; Vasan, U.; Meier, W.; Hartmann, P.E.; Williams, T.M. Accuracy of a user-friendly centrifuge for measuring creamatocrits on mothers' milk in the clinical setting. *Breastfeed. Med.* **2006**, *1*, 79–87. [CrossRef] [PubMed]

47. Mitoulas, L.R. Short- and Long-Term Variation in the Production, Content and Composition of Human Milk Fat. Ph.D. Thesis, The University of Western Australia, Crawley, WA, Australia, 2000.

48. Keller, R.; Neville, M. Determination of total protein in human milk: Comparison of methods. *Clin. Chem.* **1986**, *32*, 120–123. [PubMed]

49. Kunz, C.; Lonnerdal, B. Human milk proteins: Separation of whey proteins and their analysis by polyacrylamide gel electrophoresis, fast protein liquid chromatography (FPLC) gel filtration, and anion-exchange chromatography. *Am. J. Clin. Nutr.* **1989**, *49*, 464–470. [PubMed]

50. Khan, S.; Casadio, Y.; Lai, C.; Prime, D.; Hepworth, A.; Trengove, N.; Hartmann, P. Investigation of short-term variations in casein and whey proteins in breast milk of term mothers. *Hepatol. Nutr.* **2012**, *55*, 136–141. [CrossRef] [PubMed]

51. Mitoulas, L.R.; Kent, J.C.; Cox, D.B.; Owens, R.A.; Sherriff, J.L.; Hartmann, P.E. Variation in fat, lactose and protein in human milk over 24 h and throughout the first year of lactation. *Br. J. Nutr.* **2002**, *88*, 29–37. [CrossRef] [PubMed]

52. Selsted, M.; Martinez, R. A simple and ultrasensitive enzymatic assay for the quantitative determination of lysozyme in the picogram range. *Anal. Biochem.* **1980**, *109*, 67–70. [CrossRef]

53. Euber, J.; Brunner, J. Determination of lactose in milk products by high-performance liquid chromatography. *J. Dairy Sci.* **1979**, *62*, 685–690. [CrossRef]

54. Albalasmeh, A.; Berhe, A.; Ghezzehei, T. A new method for rapid determination of carbohydrate and total carbon concentrations using UV spectrophotometry. *Carbohydr. Polym.* **2013**, *97*, 253–261. [CrossRef] [PubMed]

55. Kuhn, N.; Lowenstein, J. Lactogenesis in the rat. Changes in metabolic parameters at parturition. *Biochem. J.* **1967**, *105*, 995–1002. [CrossRef] [PubMed]

56. Newburg, D.; Neubauer, S. Carbohydrates in milks: Analysis, quantities, and significance. In *Handbook of Milk Composition*; Jensen, R., Ed.; Academic Press, Inc.: San Diego, CA, USA, 1995; pp. 273–349.

57. Lingwood, B.; Van Leeuwen, A.; Carberry, A.; Fitzgerald, E.; Callaway, L.; Colditz, P.; Ward, L. Prediction of fat-free mass and percentage of body fat in neonates using biolelectrical impedance analysis and anthropometric measures: Validation against pea pod. *Br. J. Nutr.* **2012**, *107*, 1545–1552. [CrossRef] [PubMed]

58. Brook, C. Determination of body composition of children from skinfold measurements. *Arch. Dis. Child.* **1971**, *46*, 182–184. [CrossRef] [PubMed]

59. Lohman, T. Body composition in children and youth. In *Advances in Pediatric Sport Sciences*; Boileau, R.A., Ed.; Human Kinetics Publishers: Champaign, IL, USA, 1984; pp. 29–57.

60. R Core Team. *R: A Language and Environment for Statistical Computing*; R Foundation for Statistical Computing: Vienna, Austria, 2009.

61. Pinheiro, J.; Bates, D.; DebRoy, S.; Sarkar, D.; Team, T.R.C. nlme: Linear and Nonlinear Mixed Effects Models. R Package Version 3.1-128. 2016. Available online: http://CRAN.R-project.org/package=nlme (accessed on 20 May 2016).

62. Sarkar, D. *Lattice: Multivariate Data Visualization with R*; Springer: New York, NY, USA, 2008.

63. Sarkar, D.; Andrews, F. *LatticeExtra: Extra Graphical Utilities Based on Lattice*, R Package Version 0.6-28, 2016. Available online: http://CRAN.R-project.org/package=latticeExtra (accessed on 20 May 2016).

64. Fox, J.; Weisberg, S. *An R Companion to Applied Regression*; Sage: Thousand Oaks, CA, USA, 2011.

65. Venables, W.N.; Ripley, B.D. *Modern Applied Statistics with S*, 4th ed.; Springer: New York, NY, USA, 2002.

66. Maechler, M. Sfsmisc: Utilities from Seminar Fuer Statistik Eth Zurich. R Package Version 1.1-0. 2016. Available online: http://cran.r-project.org/package=sfsmisc (accessed on 20 May 2016).

67. Hothorn, T.; Bretz, F.; Westfall, P. Simultaneous inference in general parametric models. *Biom. J.* **2008**, *50*, 346–363. [CrossRef] [PubMed]

68. Cannon, A.M.; Sakalidis, V.S.; Lai, C.T.; Perrella, S.L.; Geddes, D.T. Vacuum characteristics of the sucking cycle and relationships with milk removal from the breast in term infants. *Early Hum. Dev.* **2016**, *96*, 1–6. [CrossRef] [PubMed]

69. Royston, P.; Altman, D.G. Regression using fractional polynomials of continuous covariates: Parsimonious parametric modelling. *J. R. Stat. Soc. Ser. C Appl. Stat.* **1994**, *43*, 429–467. [CrossRef]

70. Curran-Everett, D. Multiple comparisons: Philosophies and illustrations. *Am. J. Physiol. Regul. Integr. Comp. Physiol.* **2000**, *279*, R1–R8. [PubMed]

71. Meyer, R.; Foong, R.; Thapar, N.; Kritas, S.; Shah, N. Systematic review of the impact of feed protein type and degree of hydrolysis on gastric emptying in children. *BMC Gastroenterol.* **2015**, *15*, 137. [CrossRef] [PubMed]

72. Lonnerdal, B.; Havel, P.J. Serum leptin concentrations in infants: Effects of diet, sex, and adiposity. *Am. J. Clin. Nutr.* **2000**, *72*, 484–489. [PubMed]

73. Bouret, S.G.; Draper, S.J.; Simerly, R.B. Trophic action of leptin on hypothalamic neurons that regulate feeding. *Science* **2004**, *304*, 108–110. [CrossRef] [PubMed]

74. Petridou, E.; Mantzoros, C.S.; Belechri, M.; Skalkidou, A.; Dessypris, N.; Papathoma, E.; Salvanos, H.; Lee, J.H.; Kedikoglou, S.; Chrousos, G.; et al. Neonatal leptin levels are strongly associated with female gender, birth length, IGF-I levels and formula feeding. *Clin. Endocrinol.* **2005**, *62*, 366–371. [CrossRef] [PubMed]

75. Savino, F.; Benetti, S.; Liguori, S.; Sorrenti, M.; Cordero Di Montezemolo, L. Advances of human milk hormones and protection against obesity. *Cell. Mol. Biol.* **2013**, *59*, 89–98. [PubMed]

76. Gonzalez, C.R.; Caminos, J.E.; Gallego, R.; Tovar, S.; Vazquez, M.J.; Garces, M.F.; Lopez, M.; Garcia-Caballero, T.; Tena-Sempere, M.; Nogueiras, R.; et al. Adiponectin receptor 2 is regulated by nutritional status, leptin and pregnancy in a tissue-specific manner. *Physiol. Behav.* **2010**, *99*, 91–99. [CrossRef] [PubMed]

77. Perry, B.; Wang, Y. Appetite regulation and weight control: The role of gut hormones. *Nutr. Diabetes* **2012**, *2*, e26. [CrossRef] [PubMed]

78. Chaudhri, O.; Small, C.; Bloom, S. Gastrointestinal hormones regulating appetite. *Philos. Trans. R. Soc. Lond. B Biol. Sci.* **2006**, *361*, 1187–1209. [CrossRef] [PubMed]

79. Maljaars, P.W.J.; Peters, H.P.F.; Mela, D.J.; NMasclee, A.A.M. Ileal brake: A sensible food target for appetite control. A review. *Physiol. Behav.* **2008**, *95*, 271–281. [CrossRef] [PubMed]

80. Van Citters, G.W.; Lin, H.C. Ileal brake: Neuropeptidergic control of intestinal transit. *Curr. Gastroenterol. Rep.* **2006**, *8*, 367–373. [CrossRef] [PubMed]

81. Khoshoo, V.; Brown, S. Gastric emptying of two whey-based formulas of different energy density and its clinical implication in children with volume intolerance. *Eur. J. Clin. Nutr.* **2002**, *56*, 656–658. [CrossRef] [PubMed]

82. Stanstrup, J.; Schou, S.S.; Holmer-Jensen, J.; Hermansen, K.; Dragsted, L.O. Whey protein delays gastric emptying and suppresses plasma fatty acids and their metabolites compared to casein, gluten, and fish protein. *J. Proteome Res.* **2014**, *13*, 2396–2408. [CrossRef] [PubMed]

83. Hale, T.W.; Hartmann, P.E. *Hale and Hartmann's Textbook of Human Lactation*, 1st ed.; Hale Publishing, L.P.: Amarillo, TX, USA, 2007.

84. Van Avesaat, M.; Troost, F.J.; Ripken, D.; Hendriks, H.F.; Masclee, A.A.M. Ileal brake activation: Macronutrient-specific effects on eating behavior? *Int. J. Obes.* **2015**, *39*, 235–243. [CrossRef] [PubMed]

85. Boirie, Y.; Dangin, M.; Gachon, P.; Vasson, M.P.; Maubois, J.L.; Beaufrere, B. Slow and fast dietary proteins differently modulate postprandial protein accretion. *Proc. Natl. Acad. Sci. USA* **1997**, *94*, 14930–14935. [CrossRef] [PubMed]

86. Daniel, H.; Vohwinkel, M.; Rehner, G. Effect of casein and beta-casomorphins on gastrointestinal motility in rats. *J. Nutr.* **1990**, *120*, 252–257. [PubMed]

87. Stromqvist, M.; Falk, F.; Bergstrom, S.; Hansson, L.; Lonnerdal, B.; Normark, S.; Hernell, O. Human milk kappa-casein and inhibition of helicobacter pylori adhesion to human gastric mucosa. *J. Pediatr. Gastroenterol. Nutr.* **1995**, *21*, 288–296. [CrossRef] [PubMed]

88. Francois, F.; Roper, J.; Joseph, N.; Pei, Z.; Chhada, A.; Shal, J.R.; Olivares De Perez, A.Z.; Perez-Perez, G.I.; Blaser, M.J. The effect of *H. pylori* eradication on meal-associated changes in plasma ghrelin and leptin. *BMC Gastroenterol.* **2011**, *11*, 37. [CrossRef] [PubMed]

89. Montagne, P.; Cuilliere, M.L.; Mole, C.; Bene, M.C.; Faure, G. Changes in lactoferrin and lysozyme levels in human milk during the first twelve weeks of lactation. *Adv. Exp. Med. Biol.* **2001**, *501*, 241–247. [PubMed]

90. Rubio, C.A. The natural antimicrobial enzyme lysozyme is up-regulated in gastrointestinal inflammatory conditions. *Pathogens* **2014**, *3*, 73–92. [CrossRef] [PubMed]

91. Bol'shakova, A.M.; Shcherbakova, E.G.; Ivanova, S.D.; Medvedeva, M.M.; Zhuravleva, T.P. Lysozyme in the feeding of premature infants with mixed pathology. *Antibiotiki* **1984**, *29*, 784–790. [PubMed]

92. Perrella, S.L.; Hepworth, A.R.; Simmer, K.N.; Hartmann, P.E.; Geddes, D.T. Repeatability of gastric volume measurements and intragastric content using ultrasound in preterm infants. *J. Pediatr. Gastroenterol. Nutr.* **2014**, *59*, 254–263. [CrossRef] [PubMed]

93. Hellstrom, P.; Naslund, E. Interactions between gastric emptying and satiety, with special reference to glucagon-like peptide-1. *Physiol. Behav.* **2001**, *74*, 735–741. [CrossRef]

94. Lorenz, D.N. Gastric emptying of milk in rat pups. *Am. J. Physiol.* **1985**, *248*, R732–R738. [PubMed]

95. Kent, J.; Hepworth, A.; Sherriff, J.; Cox, D.; Mitoulas, L.; Hartmann, P. Longitudinal changes in breastfeeding patterns from 1 to 6 months of lactation. *Breastfeed. Med.* **2013**, *8*, 401–407. [CrossRef] [PubMed]

96. Sepple, C.P.; Read, N.W. Gastrointestinal correlates of the development of hunger in man. *Appetite* **1989**, *13*, 183–191. [CrossRef]

97. Lawrence, R.A.; Lawrence, R.M. Practical management of the mother-infant nursing couple. In *Breastfeeding: A Guide for Medical Profession*, 7th ed.; Lawrence, R.A., Lawrence, R.M., Eds.; Mosby/Elsevier: Maryland Heights, MO, USA, 2011; pp. 232–283.

98. Natalucci, G.; Riedl, S.; Zidel, T.; Frisch, H. Spontaneous 24-h ghrelin secretion pattern in fasting subjects: Maintenance of a meal-related pattern. *Eur. J. Endocrinol.* **2005**, *152*, 845–850. [CrossRef] [PubMed]

99. Degen, L.P.; Phillips, S.F. Variability of gastrointestinal transit in healthy women and men. *Gut* **1996**, *39*, 299–305. [CrossRef] [PubMed]

100. Butte, N.; Garza, C.; Smith, E.; Nichols, B. Human milk intake and growth in exclusively breast-fed infants. *J. Pediatr.* **1984**, *104*, 187–195. [CrossRef]

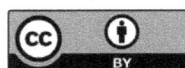

nutrients

MDPI

Article

The Effects of Mild Gestational Hyperglycemia on Exclusive Breastfeeding Cessation

Sergio Verd [1,2,*], **Diego de Sotto** [3], **Consuelo Fernández** [2] and **Antonio Gutiérrez** [4,5]

[1] Department of Primary Care, Balearic Health Authority, Health Sciences Research Institute IUNICS, 10 Alexandre Rosselló Ave, 07002 Palma de Mallorca, Spain

[2] Department of Primary Care, Balearic Health Authority, 07003 Palma de Mallorca, Spain; consuelofernandez@ibsalut.caib.es

[3] Endocrinology Unit, Department of Paediatrics, Hospital Son Espases, Valldemossa Road, 79, 07010 Palma de Mallorca, Spain; diego.desotto@ssib.es

[4] Molecular Biology Unit, Division of Hematology, Son Espases University Hospital, Valldemossa Road, 79, 07010 Palma de Mallorca, Spain; antoniom.gutierrez@ssib.es

[5] Palma de Mallorca Institute of Health Research (IdISPa), Valldemossa Road, 79, 07010 Palma de Mallorca, Spain

* Correspondence: drsverd@gmail.com; Tel.: +34-600505246; Fax: +34-971-799534

Received: 29 September 2016; Accepted: 15 November 2016; Published: 19 November 2016

Abstract: Gestational diabetes increases the risk of a range of adverse perinatal outcomes, including breastfeeding failure, but the best cut-off point for gestational diabetes is unknown. The purpose of this study was to evaluate the association between mild gestational glucose tolerance impairment and the early cessation of exclusive breastfeeding (EBF). This is an observational study of 768 women with full term pregnancies that were screened for gestational diabetes at 24–28 weeks gestation. Subjects were divided into two groups: those with a normal 1-h glucose challenge test and those with an elevated 1-h glucose challenge test but still did not qualify for gestational diabetes. We constructed multivariable logistic regression models using data from 616 women with normal gestational glucose tolerance and 152 women with an isolated positive 1-h glucose challenge test. The risk of early exclusive breastfeeding cessation was found to increase in women with mildly impaired glucose tolerance during pregnancy (adjusted OR, 1.65; 95% CI: 1.11, 2.45). Risks of early EBF cessation were also independently associated with the amount of neonatal weight loss and admission to the neonatal ward. Instead, parity was associated with a decreased risk for shorter EBF duration. Insulin resistance—even in the absence of gestational diabetes mellitus—may be an impeding factor for EBF.

Keywords: breastfeeding; gestational diabetes; neonate; glucose tolerance test; prediabetes; insulin resistance; pregnancy outcomes

---

1. Introduction

The role of maternal metabolic health on early lactation success is only recently gaining recognition. A wide range of entangled factors may contribute to reduced milk supply. We know that gestational diabetes predisposes women to both perinatal depression and undesired weaning [1–3]. Several authors have reported that glucose homeostasis during pregnancy may affect breast development [4] and could correlate with breastfeeding outcomes [5,6]. Insulin resistance may act at the lactocyte level [7]. Pregnant women at risk of metabolic syndrome are prone to delayed onset of lactogenesis stage II (DLII) [8]—a risk factor for early breastfeeding cessation [9]. In recent years, it has been shown that most of the time, variation in onset of lactogenesis stage II (LII) is predicted by 1-h post-glucose challenge (1-hOGTT) at 26 weeks of gestation [8]. This finding is in line with current data suggesting that the correlation between any degree of glucose tolerance impairment and adverse offspring outcome follows a continuous pattern, and that even mild degrees of hyperglycemia may be associated with complications [10].

Taken together, these data suggest that suboptimal maternal glucose tolerance may be a key factor in the establishment of breastfeeding. Despite the rising prevalence of gestational prediabetes, studies on neonatal outcomes of this condition are still scarce. To shed some light on this issue, we conducted a secondary analysis and evaluated the following research question: is there an association between mild gestational hyperglycemia and the early cessation of exclusive breastfeeding (EBF)?

2. Experimental Section

2.1. Enrollment

We enrolled a population-based sample of mother–infant dyads attending a general care pediatric clinic in a middle-class neighborhood in Majorca, Spain. The enrollment phase lasted from January 2007 to December 2012. We invited all mothers who attempted breastfeeding to participate in "a study on infant feeding" upon their first well-child visit. The study was approved by the Institutional Review Boards of the Health Authority of the Balearic Islands, and participants consent was obtained prior to their inclusion in the study.

2.2. Selection Criteria and Data Collection

This analysis was conducted in the context of an ongoing observational study of breastfeeding natural history. The study protocol has previously been described in detail [11,12]. In brief, the study was conducted as a review of medical records from a Pediatric Office where approximately 120 babies are enrolled every year. Prenatal inclusion criteria were: (1) the routinely administered 24 to 28-week gestation 1-hOGTT, and (2) mothers had to be free of gestational diabetes (GDM). Post-birth inclusion criteria were (3) delivery at term (37 weeks of gestation), and (4) the mother initiated breastfeeding as planned. We extracted additional data on patient characteristics and on infant feeding from the prenatal and pediatric medical records. From the pediatric record, information on infant feeding was collected at discharge from the hospital and at the scheduled well-baby visits. Information about the duration of EBF was obtained from pediatric records, information previously collected from mother's report of how the baby was being fed at the time of well-baby visits at 2 weeks, and at 2, 4, 6, and 9 months of age. Duration of EBF was defined as the last notation in the record when the infant was fed only breast milk. According to the WHO, exclusive breastfeeding means that the infant receives only breast milk. No other solids are given, with the exception of vitamins, minerals, or medicines. Of the eligible mother–infant dyads, 768 had information available for all key variables, and were therefore included in the analyses presented here.

2.3. Glucose Challenge Test

According to the recommendations of the American College of Obstetrics and Gynecology (ACOG) [13], standard practice in our setting involves universal screening for GDM in all pregnant women at 24–28 weeks' gestation by a nonfasting 1-h 50 g glucose challenge test. Patients testing positive for the 1-hOGTT (1-h plasma glucose 7.8 mmol/L) were asked to return for a 3-h 100 g oral glucose tolerance test (3-hOGTT).

Categorization. Based on 1-hOGTT and 3-hOGTT, subjects were stratified into the following three glucose tolerance groups:

(i) Normal glucose tolerance (NGT), defined by normal 1-hOGTT results (1-h plasma glucose < 7.8 mmol/L);
(ii) Mild impairment of glucose tolerance (MIGT), defined by a single abnormal value greater than or equal to 7.8 mmol/L, but less than 10.6 mmol/L;

(iii) GDM, requires at least two of the following on the 3-hOGTT: fasting glucose 5.8 mmol/L, 1-h glucose 10.6 mmol/L, 2-h glucose 9.2 mmol/L, or 3-h glucose 8.1 mmol/L.

2.4. Data Analysis

Our outcome measure was discontinuation of EBF. Dichotomization: this variable has been split at the median to form short and normal breastfeeding duration groups. Our primary predictor was MIGT in pregnancy. Patients were allocated to the NGT group or to the MIGT group. Data were analyzed using the IBM-SPSS (V22.0) Package (IBM Corp., Armonk, NY, USA). First, we examined distributions and summary measures for each variable. Table 1 shows, for each study group, continuous variables as median followed by range, while categorical variables are presented as proportions. Univariate differences across the groups were assessed using Mann–Whitney test for continuous variables, and either chi square or Fisher's exact test for categorical variables. Multiple regression analysis was used to identify perinatal factors that independently predicted a short duration of EBF. Covariates considered included parity, glucose tolerance status in pregnancy, delivery type, birth weight, admission to the neonatal ward, and neonatal weight loss at discharge. A series of models were constructed using these covariates. The final models included main effects significant at $p < 0.05$.

Table 1. Patient characteristics.

Variable	NGT: 1-h Plasma Glucose < 7.8 mmol/L (N = 616)	MIGT: 10.6 mmol/L > 1-hOGTT Results ≥ 7.8 mmol/L (N = 152)	p
Gender:			
Male	51%	53%	0.72
Female	49%	47%	
Parity:			
1	64%	65%	1
>1	36%	35%	
Mother's age (years)	33 (20–45)	33 (25–42)	0.064
Gestational weight gain	12 (1–39)	12 (4–27)	0.84
Weeks of gestation	40 (37–42)	40 (37–42)	0.79
Delivery type:			
Eutocic	82%	18%	0.67
Instrumental	80%	20%	
C-section	79%	21%	
Birth weight	3272 (1995–4800)	3395 (2050–4390)	0.018
Birth height	49.5 (33–54)	50 (45.5–53.5)	0.13
Birth head circumference	34.5 (31–37)	34.5 (31–37.5)	0.74
Percent of loss of birth weight to discharge	6 (−0.32–0.21)	7 (−7–13)	0.41

Abbreviations: 1-h post-glucose challenge (1-hOGTT); mild impairment of glucose tolerance (MIGT); normal glucose tolerance (NGT).

3. Results

3.1. Patient Characteristics

Table 1 shows the demographic and perinatal characteristics of the 768 study participants stratified into our two predefined glucose tolerance categories in pregnancy: NGT ($n = 616$) and MIGT ($n = 152$). Around eighty percent (80.2%) of subjects tested in the normal range for glucose tolerance. This was a predominantly middle-class cohort from a general pediatric clinic where most participants had private health insurance. There were no significant differences between the groups with respect to most baseline characteristics, but birth weight was lowest in the NGT group ($p = 0.018$), and birth height was lower in the NGT group than in the MIGT group—though this difference did not reach statistical significance ($p = 0.13$).

3.2. EBF Outcome: Univariate Analysis

Table 2 shows that, upon univariate analysis, the rate of EBF adverse outcomes was significantly higher in the MIGT than in the NGT group (58% vs. 48%; p = 0.03). In fact, in the MIGT cohort, median duration of EBF was 56 days (1–300), while in the NGT cohort, it was significantly longer: 100 days (1–360) (p = 0.045). Other significant findings for decreased EBF duration included parity, gender of the newborn infant, neonatal weight loss at discharge, and admission to the neonatal ward.

Table 2. Results for univariate analysis of exclusive breastfeeding (EBF) duration.

EBF Discontinuation	Before Day 100 (N = 384)	Equal or Later than Day 100 (N = 384)	p
MIGT	58%	42%	0.03 *
NGT	48%	52%	
Gender:			
Male	214 (54%)	169 (43%)	0.001 **
Female	179 (45%)	225 (57%)	
Parity:			
1	271(72%)	214 (57%)	<0.001 ***
>1	107 (28%)	159 (28%)	
Mother's age (years)	33 (18–42)	33 (21–45)	0.92
Gestational weight gain	12 (1–30)	12 (4–39)	0.05
Weeks of gestation	40 (37–42)	40 (37–42)	0.27
Delivery type:			
Eutocic	184 (50%)	207 (57%)	0.38
Instrumental	61 (17%)	55 (15%)	
C-section	119 (33%)	110 (30%)	
Birth weight	3252 (1995–4390)	3330 (2310–4800)	0.02 *
Birth height	49.5 (33–54)	50 (45.5–54)	0.32
Birth head circumference	34.5 (31–37)	34.5 (31–37.5)	0.36
Percent of loss of birth weight to discharge	7 (−7–21)	6 (−32–20)	<0.001 ***

Abbreviations: mild impairment of glucose tolerance (MIGT); normal glucose tolerance (NGT). * p < 0.05; ** p < 0.01; *** p < 0.001.

3.3. EBF Outcome: Multivariate Analysis

We reanalyzed the association between MIGT and EBF outcome after adjustment for significant univariate variables (Table 3). EBF duration—as a dichotomous variable (<100 days)—was independently associated with the MIGT group (OR: 1.65; CI: 1.11–2.45). In addition, neonatal weight loss at discharge and admission to the neonatal ward were identified as significant risk factors for short EBF duration in the multivariable model. Instead, parity was associated with a decreased risk for shorter EBF duration.

Table 3. Multivariate analysis of factors independently associated with reduction in exclusive breastfeeding duration.

	AOR (95% CI)	p
Mildly impaired glucose tolerance	1.65 (1.11–2.45)	0.01
Early neonatal weight loss	1.73 (1.26–2.36)	0.001
Admission to neonatal ward	3.32 (1.04–10.60)	0.04
Parity	0.57 (0.41–0.79)	0.001

Abbreviations: AOR, adjusted odds ratio.

4. Discussion

In this report, we aimed to determine whether an abnormal 1-hOGTT is independently associated with adverse EBF outcomes despite a normal subsequent 3-hOGTT. We have shown that MIGT during pregnancy predicts a shortened breastfeeding duration. To our knowledge, there is only one other study on the lactational implications of mild gestational hyperglycemia. Interestingly, it shows that testing positive in the 1-hOGTT is the main contributing factor to a delay or failure in the onset of LII [9], and specifically, that DLII is a clinical indicator of women at risk of early postpartum breastfeeding cessation. Three groups have evaluated the effect of DLII on breastfeeding outcomes. Chapman et al. showed that among women planning to breastfeed ≥6 months, women without DLII were more likely to continue breastfeeding [14]. In the analyses by Hruschka and colleagues, immediate postpartum supplementation was associated with DLII [15]. Finally, data from over 2400 mothers showed that DLII was associated with the cessation of any and exclusive breastfeeding at 4-weeks postpartum [9].

Since O'Sullivan first described gestational glucose intolerance, progressively lower thresholds have been proposed for the diagnosis and treatment of GDM. New data have demonstrated that the risk of adverse outcomes increases, even among women with sub-threshold results in fasting and post-load glucose screening [16]. Furthermore, it was recently reported that pregnant women with an isolated abnormal glucose value at 1-hOGTT carry a severe metabolic perturbation, characterized by markedly reduced beta-cell function; their metabolic phenotype resembles that of GDM, and may be associated with the same adverse outcomes as GDM [17]. The Hyperglycemia and Adverse Pregnancy Outcome (HAPO) study showed associations between increasing levels of fasting, 1-h, and 2-h plasma glucose obtained on oral glucose-tolerance testing and each of the adverse perinatal outcomes examined: birth weight above the 90th percentile and cordblood serum C-peptide level above the 90th percentile, premature delivery, shoulder dystocia or birth injury, intensive neonatal care, hyperbilirubinemia, and preeclampsia [18]. The effects of GDM on short-term breastfeeding outcomes have been clearly documented, unlike the effects of MIGT. Yet, women with a history of GDM face challenges with EBF in the critical period for setting up breastfeeding success. A recent systematic review of ten original papers from 1989 to 2013 on the effect of GDM on LII onset shows that all studies consistently identified that LII occurred later among gestationally diabetic mothers than in non-diabetic mothers [19]. LII is characterized by changes in breastmilk components—in particular, a decrease in breastmilk sodium. Conversely, the presence of GDM increases the risk of an elevated breastmilk sodium level on day three postpartum [20]. A case–control study revealed that women diagnosed with low milk supply were significantly more likely to have had GDM compared with women with other lactation outcomes [21]. Poorer sucking patterns have been found among newborn infants of mothers with GDM [22]. A cross-sectional analysis including 2038 women found that the adjusted odds of EBF at hospital discharge were lower among women with GDM compared to women without GDM [23].

Overt GDM is associated with significantly increased risks of adverse breastfeeding outcomes. Whereas, until recently, women with an abnormal 1-hOGTT (with normal 3h-OGTT) were regarded as a false positive result, emerging data suggest that current diagnostic criteria for GDM are too restrictive, and that lesser degrees of hyperglycemia also increase offspring risks [10]. Despite the associated adverse pregnancy outcomes, no international consensus exists that identifies a cut-off value for the definition of GDM. Current criteria of the International Association of Diabetes and Pregnancy Study Groups (IADPSG) are lower than the ACOG 2013 thresholds (fasting glucose 5.1 versus 5.8 mmol/L, or 1-h glucose 10.0 versus 10.6 mmol/L). It has been reported that applying the IADPSG criteria to the population would increase the rate of GDM from 7.3% to 10.3% [24]. A 2013 National Institutes of Health (NIH) panel states that there are clear benefits to the standardization of international diagnostic criteria. Nevertheless, the panel is concerned with the adoption of new criteria that would increase the prevalence of GDM (and the corresponding costs and interventions), without clear demonstration of improvements in health outcomes [25]. Therefore, new tools—such as Capula's index—continue to be developed to improve the accuracy and cost-effectiveness of this screening [26].

A brief literature review shows that it is well established that insulin resistance is a strong predictor of short breastfeeding duration, but the underlying causal contributors remained unclear until very recently. Over the last years, insulin-sensitive gene expression has been shown to be upregulated during the lactation cycle, and insulin is now considered to play a direct role in lactation [27].

The established dogma has been that women are never physiologically unable to lactate, but rather that low milk supply is a mistaken belief on their part. Thus, most interventions have focused on improving breastfeeding education. However, emerging clinical research suggests an important association between suboptimal glucose tolerance and lactation difficulty. Our findings add to the evidence that a woman's metabolic complications adversely affect her lactation outcomes. 1-hOGTT may be a useful clinical indicator to identify women at risk of early postpartum breastfeeding cessation. These results have clinical implications, underlining that breastfeeding support of women with abnormal glucose tolerance should be individualized. Given the current insulin resistance epidemic, caregivers face the challenge of meeting the growing need for clinical guidance of women with both metabolic disturbances and low milk supply. Further translational research is needed to successfully implement interventions that will enable more women to avoid undesired breastfeeding cessation.

These analyses have several limitations. First, this is a secondary analysis. Second, the nature of these data did not allow for evaluation of the contribution of interactions between conditions previously reported (e.g., gestational weight gain and maternal obesity, neonatal weight loss and DLII). Third, our significant findings may be inauthentic due to unmeasured confounding. A factor that influences a woman's ability to breastfeed is the presence of personal or professional support. Other mother-centered factors include social barriers, work-related barriers, or a dislike of breastfeeding. We do not have data on all maternal factors that may affect milk production and composition. Finally, our assessment of metabolic dysregulation was done prenatally. We do not know to what extent maternal metabolic status in the early postpartum is affected.

Strengths of this study include the consistency with existing literature and the prospective design to collect breastfeeding duration and exclusivity data. The study does not rely on later recall of breastfeeding outcomes. Although the study populations and availability of pertinent confounders differed, the current study confirms that 1-hOGTT represents an important metabolic perturbation in pregnancy, characterized not only by increased risk for adverse pregnancy outcomes, but also by early breastfeeding dysfunction. It is becoming clear that long glucose challenge tests are not superior to short glucose challenge tests in the assessment of prenatal glucose tolerance.

Finally, we clearly identified several additional independent risk factors for early breastfeeding cessation (e.g., neonatal weight loss, admission to the neonatal ward, and parity).

5. Conclusions

In summary, women who test positive for 1-hOGTT may be less able to sustain EBF at 100 days. These findings suggest that 1-hOGTT may already identify a high-risk population of mothers in need of interventions to increase breast milk production.

Acknowledgments: We want to thank all mothers who participated in this study. We also acknowledge Silvia Celorio, SHO, for her cooperation in participant recruitment. This project would not have been possible without editorial assistance assistance from Berta Verd.

Author Contributions: All authors contributed extensively to the work presented in this paper. S.V. and D.d.S. conceived the study; C.F. and A.G. developed the methdology; D.d.S. and C.F. monitored data collection; A.G. analyzed the data; S.V. wrote the paper.

Conflicts of Interest: All authors declare: no support from any organisation for the submitted work; no financial relationships with any organisations that might have an interest in the submitted work in the previous 3 years; no other relationships or activities that could appear to have influenced the submitted work.

Nutrients **2016**, *8*, 742

Abbreviations

The following abbreviations are used in this manuscript:

1-hOGTT	1-h post-glucose challenge
3-hOGTT	3-h glucose tolerance test
ACOG	American College of Obstetricians and Gynecologists
DLII	delayed onset of lactogenesis stage II
EBF	exclusive breastfeeding
GDM	gestational diabetes
IADPSG	International Association of Diabetes and Pregnancy Study Groups
LII	lactogenesis stage II
MIGT	mild impairment of glucose tolerance
NGT	normal glucose tolerance

References

1. Herring, S.J.; Rich-Edwards, J.W.; Oken, E.; Rifas-Shiman, S.L.; Kleinman, K.P.; Gillman, M.W. Association of postpartum depression with weight retention 1 year after childbirth. *Obesity* **2008**, *16*, 1296–1301. [CrossRef] [PubMed]
2. Dennis, C.L.; McQueen, K. Does maternal postpartum depressive symptomatology influence infant feeding outcomes? *Acta Paediatr.* **2007**, *96*, 590–594. [CrossRef] [PubMed]
3. Matias, S.L.; Dewey, K.G.; Quesenberry, C.P., Jr.; Gunderson, E.P. Maternal prepregnancy obesity and insulin treatment during pregnancy are independently associated with delayed lactogenesis in women with recent gestational diabetes mellitus. *Am. J. Clin. Nutr.* **2014**, *99*, 115–121. [CrossRef] [PubMed]
4. Vanky, E.; Nordskar, J.J.; Leithe, H.; Hjorth-Hansen, A.K.; Martinussen, M.; Carlsen, S.M. Breast size increment during pregnancy and breastfeeding in mothers with polycystic ovary syndrome: A follow-up study of a randomised controlled trial on metformin versus placebo. *BJOG* **2012**, *119*, 1403–1409. [CrossRef] [PubMed]
5. Nommsen-Rivers, L.A.; Chantry, C.J.; Peerson, J.M.; Cohen, R.J.; Dewey, K.G. Delayed onset of lactogenesis among first-time mothers is related to maternal obesity and factors associated with ineffective breastfeeding. *Am. J. Clin. Nutr.* **2010**, *92*, 574–584. [CrossRef] [PubMed]
6. Stuebe, A.M.; Horton, B.J.; Chetwynd, E.; Watkins, S.; Grewen, K.; Meltzer-Brody, S. Prevalence and Risk Factors for Early, Undesired Weaning Attributed to Lactation Dysfunction. *J. Women's Health* **2014**, *23*, 404–412. [CrossRef] [PubMed]
7. Lemay, D.G.; Ballard, O.A.; Hughes, M.A.; Morrow, A.L.; Horseman, N.D.; Nommsen-Rivers, L.A. RNA sequencing of the human milk fat layer transcriptome reveals distinct gene expression profiles at three stages of lactation. *PLoS ONE* **2013**, *8*, e67531. [CrossRef] [PubMed]
8. Nommsen-Rivers, L.A.; Dolan, L.M.; Huang, B. Timing of stage II lactogenesis is predicted by antenatal metabolic health in a cohort of primiparas. *Breastfeed. Med.* **2012**, *7*, 43–49. [CrossRef] [PubMed]
9. Brownell, E.; Howard, C.R.; Lawrence, R.A.; Dozier, A.M. Delayed onset lactogenesis II predicts the cessation of any or exclusive breastfeeding. *J. Pediatr.* **2012**, *161*, 608–614. [CrossRef] [PubMed]
10. Melamed, N.; Hiersch, L.; Hod, M.; Chen, R.; Wiznitzer, A.; Yogev, Y. Is abnormal 50-g glucose-challenge testing an independent predictor of adverse pregnancy outcome? *J. Matern. Fetal Neonatal Med.* **2012**, *25*, 2583–2587. [CrossRef] [PubMed]
11. Verd, S.; Nadal-Amat, J.; Gich, I.; Leshem, M. Salt preference of nursing mothers is associated with earlier cessation of exclusive breastfeeding. *Appetite* **2010**, *54*, 233–236. [CrossRef] [PubMed]
12. Verd, S.; Barriuso, L.; Gich, I.; Gutiérrez, A.; Nadal-Amat, J.; Carreras, E. Risk of early breastfeeding cessation among symmetrical, small for gestational age infants. *Ann. Hum. Biol.* **2013**, *40*, 146–151. [CrossRef] [PubMed]
13. American College of Obstetricians and Gynecologists. Practice Bulletin No. 137: Gestational diabetes mellitus. *Obstet. Gynecol.* **2013**, *122*, 406–416.
14. Chapman, D.J.; Perez-Escamilla, R. Does delayed perception of the onset of lactation shorten breastfeeding duration? *J. Hum. Lact.* **1999**, *5*, 107–111. [CrossRef]

15. Hruschka, D.J.; Sellen, D.W.; Stein, A.D.; Martorell, R. Delayed onset of lactation and risk of ending full breast-feeding early in rural Guatemala. *J. Nutr.* **2003**, *133*, 2592–2599. [PubMed]

16. Stuebe, A.M.; Landon, M.B.; Lai, Y.; Klebanoff, M.; Ramin, S.M.; Wapner, R.J.; Varner, M.W.; Rouse, D.J.; Sciscione, A.; Catalano, P.; et al. Is There a Threshold Oral Glucose Tolerance Test Value for Predicting Adverse Pregnancy Outcome? *Am. J. Perinatol.* **2015**, *32*, 833–838. [PubMed]

17. Retnakaran, R.; Qi, Y.; Sermer, M.; Connelly, P.W.; Zinman, B.; Hanley, A.J. Isolated hyperglycemia at 1 h on oral glucose tolerance test in pregnancy resembles gestational diabetes mellitus in predicting postpartum metabolic dysfunction. *Diabetes Care* **2008**, *31*, 1275–1281. [CrossRef] [PubMed]

18. HAPO Study Cooperative Research Group; Metzger, B.E.; Lowe, L.P.; Dyer, A.R.; Trimble, E.R.; Chaovarindr, U.; Coustan, D.R.; Hadden, D.R.; McCance, D.R.; Hod, M. Hyperlycemia and adverse pregnancy outcomes. *N. Engl. J. Med.* **2008**, *358*, 1991–2002. [PubMed]

19. De Bortoli, J.; Amir, L.H. Is onset of lactation delayed in women with diabetes in pregnancy? A systematic review. *Diabet. Med.* **2016**, *33*, 17–24. [CrossRef] [PubMed]

20. Galipeau, R.; Goulet, C.; Cgagnon, M. Infant and maternal factors influencing breastmilk sodium among primiparous mothers. *Breastfeed. Med.* **2012**, *7*, 290–294. [CrossRef] [PubMed]

21. Riddle, S.W.; Nommsen-Rivers, L.A. A case control study of diabetes during pregnancy and low milk supply. *Breastfeed. Med.* **2016**, *11*, 80–85. [CrossRef] [PubMed]

22. Bromiker, R.; Rachamim, A.; Hammerman, C.; Schimmel, M.; Kaplan, M.; Medoff-Cooper, B. Immature suckling patterns in infants of mothers with diabetes. *J. Pediatr.* **2006**, *49*, 640–643. [CrossRef] [PubMed]

23. Haile, Z.T.; Oza-Frank, R.; Azulay Chertok, I.R.; Passen, N. Association between history of gestational diabetes and exclusive breastfeeding at hospital discharge. *J. Hum. Lact.* **2015**. [CrossRef] [PubMed]

24. Mayo, K.; Melamed, N.; Vandenbergh, H.; Berger, H. The impact of adoption of the international association of diabetes in pregnancy study group criteria for the screening and diagnosis of gestational diabetes. *Am. J. Obstet. Gynecol.* **2015**, *212*, e1–e9. [CrossRef] [PubMed]

25. Vandorten, J.P.; Dodson, W.C.; Espeland, M.A.; Grobman, W.A.; Guise, J.M.; Mercer, B.M.; Minkoff, H.L.; Poindexter, B.; Prosser, L.A.; Sawaya, G.F.; et al. NIH consensus development conference: Diagnosing gestational diabetes mellitus. *NIH Consens. State Sci. Statements* **2013**, *29*, 1–31.

26. Capula, C.; Chiefari, E.; Borelli, M.; Oliverio, R.; Vero, A.; Foti, D.; Puccio, L.; Vero, R.; Brunetti, A. A new predictive tool for the early risk assessment of gestational diabetes mellitus. *Prim Care Diabetes* **2016**, *10*, 315–323. [CrossRef] [PubMed]

27. Nommsen-Rivers, L.A. Does insulin explain the relationship between maternal obesity and poor lactation outcomes? An overview of the literature. *Adv. Nutr.* **2016**, *7*, 407–414. [CrossRef] [PubMed]

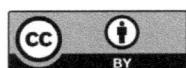

nutrients

MDPI

Article

Increased Calcium Supplementation Postpartum Is Associated with Breastfeeding among Chinese Mothers: Finding from Two Prospective Cohort Studies

Jian Zhao, Yun Zhao *, Colin W. Binns and Andy H. Lee

School of Public Health, Curtin University, Perth 6102, Australia; jian.zhao@postgrad.curtin.edu.au (J.Z.);
c.binns@curtin.edu.au (C.W.B.); andy.lee@curtin.edu.au (A.H.L.)
* Correspondence: y.zhao@curtin.edu.au; Tel.: +61-8-9266-7045

Received: 15 August 2016; Accepted: 26 September 2016; Published: 9 October 2016

Abstract: The calcium supplementation status during the postpartum period among Chinese lactating women is still unclear. The objective of this study is to utilize data from two population-based prospective cohort studies to examine the calcium supplementation status and to identify whether breastfeeding is associated with increased calcium supplementation among Chinese mothers after child birth. Information from 1540 mothers on breastfeeding and calcium supplementation measured at discharge, 1, 3, and 6 months postpartum were extracted to evaluate the association between breastfeeding and calcium supplementation postpartum. A generalized linear mixed model was applied to each study initially to account for the inherent correlation among repeated measurements, adjusting for socio-demographic, obstetric factors and calcium supplementation during pregnancy. In addition, breastfeeding status measured at different follow-up time points was treated as a time dependent variable in the longitudinal analysis. Furthermore, the effect sizes of the two cohort studies were pooled using fixed effect model. Based on the two cohort studies, the pooled likelihood of taking calcium supplementation postpartum among breastfeeding mothers was 4.02 times (95% confidence interval (2.30, 7.03)) higher than that of their non-breastfeeding counterparts. Dietary supplementation intervention programs targeting different subgroups should be promoted in Chinese women, given currently a wide shortage of dietary calcium intake and calcium supplementation postpartum.

Keywords: calcium supplementation; breastfeeding; postpartum; infant; nutrients; generalized linear mixed model; time dependent variable; pooled analysis; China

1. Introduction

The mineral accretion rate of a neonate reaches about 30–40 mg/kg per day, while calcium transfer between mothers and infants is on average 210 mg per day [1–3]. For babies who are breastfed exclusively through the first 6 months, the amount of mineral demand from the mothers is four times greater than that during 9 months of pregnancy [4]. The calcium requirement of mothers during lactation has been the subject of much discussion [5–7]. In 2011, the Institute of Medicine published the calcium dietary reference intakes by life stage, in which Estimated Average Requirement (EAR) of calcium for pregnant and lactating adult women is recommended as 800 mg [8].

Compared to western countries, the lower consumption of dairy products in China results in that most of Chinese residents have calcium intake lower than the adequate intake (AI) [9–11]. In a prospective cohort study of women's health from Shanghai, the median intake of calcium was 485 mg/day, 60% of calcium from plant sources, and only 20% from milk, which was lower than the age group specific AI (800 mg/day for 18–49 years group and 1000 mg/day for over 50 years group) [11,12]. Only 6.25% of perimenopausal women reached the standard of calcium intake in Changsha [13]. The average intake of calcium of Beijing elderly was 505 mg/day, which was about one half of the recommended adequate intake for the elderly [14]. In the National Nutrition and Health Survey of 2002, fewer than 5% reached the adequate intake levels of calcium for all age groups and the prevalence of calcium supplementation during pregnancy was 41.4% [15,16]. Besides cultural preferences, the lower consumption of dairy products in China is attributed to the high rate of lactose intolerance, which is around 80% to 95% [17,18].

The Chinese National Health and Family Planning Commission recommends that pregnant women should have a dietary calcium intake of 1000 mg per day from the second trimester and increase to 1200 mg per day from the third trimester until the end of lactation [19]. However, low dietary calcium intake in lactating women has been reported in different regions of China, as shown in Table 1. This suggests that calcium supplementation for lactating women is an important public health issue to mothers in China based on the current evidence about the benefits of calcium intake during lactation on reducing maternal bone loss [20–23].

Table 1. Dietary calcium intake of lactating women in different regions of China.

Study Location	Study Design	Study Period	Average Daily Dietary Calcium Intake (Postpartum)
Guangzhou [24]	Prospective cohort	2002	786.45 mg (12 weeks)
Hunan [25]	Cross-sectional	2011–2012	426 mg
Beijing, Suzhou & Guangzhou [26]	Cross-sectional	2011–2012	401.4 mg (0–1 month) 585.3 mg (1–2 months) 591.2 mg (2–4 months) 649.0 mg (4–8 months)
Fujian [27]	Prospective cohort	2012	428 mg (2 days) 454 mg (7 days) 595 mg (30 days) 544 mg (90 days)
Shanghai [28]	Prospective cohort	2014–2015	749.3 mg (1–3 days) 781.1 mg (7–9 days) 762.3 mg (14–17 days) 768.4 mg (25–27 days) 678.5 mg (39–41 days)

The calcium supplementation status during postpartum period among Chinese lactating women is still unclear. The objective of the present study is to utilize data from two population-based prospective cohort studies to examine the calcium supplementation status and to identify whether breastfeeding is associated with increased calcium supplementation among Chinese mothers after child birth.

2. Materials and Methods

2.1. Study Participants

Two prospective cohort studies were conducted in an urban area, Chengdu (capital city) and a rural area, Jiangyou (county-level city), Sichuan Province, China between 2010 and 2012. Mothers who gave birth to a healthy singleton infant were invited to participate before discharge. These two studies used the same methodology based on same questionnaires, which had been used in Australia and China [29–31] previously, to interview all consented women face-to-face at discharge, and followed up the participants at one, three and six months postpartum by telephone interviews. The baseline interview collected detailed information on mothers and newborns, including socio-demographic, obstetric characteristics and dietary supplements during pregnancy. The follow-up interviews collected detailed information on lactation patterns and durations and dietary supplements during the postpartum period. The World Health Organization (WHO) standard definition of any breastfeeding was used in these two studies; 'Any breastfeeding' is defined as the infant has received breast milk (direct from the breast or expressed) with or without other drink, formula or other infant food [32].

2.2. Ethical Approval

The two cohort studies were approved by the Human Research Ethics Committee of Curtin University, Perth, Western Australia (approval numbers: HR169/2009 and HR168/2009, respectively). The present study was also approved by the Human Research Ethics Committee of Curtin University (approval number: RDHS-101-15). The data used in this study were de-identified.

2.3. Statistical Analysis

The outcome of the present study is maternal calcium supplementation status (yes or no) measured longitudinally during three different postpartum periods (from discharge to 1 month, from 1 month to 3 months, and from 3 months to 6 months, respectively) at three follow-up time points (namely, 1 month, 3 months and 6 months postpartum). The main variable of interest, any breastfeeding status, was measured longitudinally at three different postpartum time points (discharge, 1 month and 3 months postpartum). Descriptive statistics of mothers' socio-demographic status, obstetric characteristics, calcium supplementation during pregnancy and the three postpartum periods, and any breastfeeding status at the three postpartum time points were obtained and reported. Chi-square test was conducted to compare the calcium supplementation rates between breastfeeding group and non-breastfeeding group at the different follow-up time points. Generalized linear mixed model (GLMM) was used to examine the effect of breastfeeding on calcium supplementation postpartum taking into account inherent correlations among repeated measurements. Furthermore, the breastfeeding status was included as a time-dependent variable in the longitudinal analysis. Random intercept model without covariates (Model I) was run initially to test random intercept effect, and then any breastfeeding status at the different time points and an indicator variable of measurement times were added into the above Model I to be a Model II. Furthermore, subject level socio-demographic covariates such as household annual income, maternal age and maternal education were then added into and adjusted in the Model II to formulate a Model III. Finally, obstetric characteristics such as parity, gravidity, infant gender, infant birth weight and infant gestational week, together with calcium supplementation during pregnancy, were further adjusted in the Model III to become the final Model IV. The above regression analysis was carried out for data set extracted from each cohort study separately, and the results of Model II and final Model IV were reported. In addition, a pooled effect size was calculated using a fixed effect model given that the heterogeneity between the two studies was tested being statistically nonsignificant. All statistical analyses were performed by using SAS 9.4 (SAS Institute Inc., Cary, NC, USA).

3. Results

3.1. Characteristics of Participants

For each cohort, mothers' baseline socio-demographic status, obstetric characteristics and calcium supplementation during pregnancy are presented in Table 2. In the Jiangyou study, 695 mothers were interviewed at baseline, and 648 and 620 mothers remained in the study at 1 month and 3 months postpartum, respectively. Any breastfeeding rate dropped slightly from 93.53% at discharge to 91.05% at 1 month postpartum then continuously to 83.71% at 3 months postpartum. In the other cohort conducted in Chengdu, 845 mothers were interviewed at baseline and 760 mothers were followed up until six months postpartum. Any breastfeeding rate declined from 93.02% at discharge to 87.89% at 1 month postpartum then substantially to 73.42% at 3 months postpartum.

Table 2. Characteristics of participants at baseline by breastfeeding status.

Variable	Cohort in Jiangyou (n = 695)		Cohort in Chengdu (n = 845)	
	BF	Non-BF	BF	Non-BF
Number of participants	650 (93.5)	45 (6.5)	786 (93.0)	59 (7.0)
Household annual income (Chinese yuan)				
<2000	186 (31.0)	9 (23.1)	1 (0.2)	0 (0.0)
2000–5000	309 (51.4)	23 (59.0)	155 (23.5)	12 (24.0)
>5000	106 (17.6)	7 (17.9)	503 (76.3)	38 (76.0)
Maternal age (years)				
<25	373 (57.4)	26 (57.8)	156 (19.9)	5 (8.5)
25–29	163 (25.1)	13 (28.9)	372 (47.3)	28 (47.5)
>29	114 (17.5)	6 (13.3)	258 (32.8)	26 (44.0)
Maternal education				
Secondary school or lower	355 (54.6)	25 (55.6)	90 (11.5)	11 (18.6)
Senior school	215 (33.1)	18 (40.0)	165 (21.0)	11 (18.6)
University or higher	80 (12.3)	2 (4.4)	531 (67.5)	37 (62.8)
Parity				
Primiparous	518 (79.7)	37 (82.2)	700 (89.1)	51 (86.4)
Multiparous	132 (20.3)	8 (17.8)	86 (10.9)	8 (13.6)
Gravidity				
Primigravida	249 (38.3)	18 (40.0)	430 (54.7)	26 (44.1)
Multigravida	401 (61.7)	27 (60.0)	356 (45.3)	33 (55.9)
Infant gender				
Male	328 (50.5)	26 (57.8)	412 (52.4)	34 (57.6)
Female	322 (49.5)	19 (42.2)	374 (47.6)	25 (42.4)
Infant birth weight (g)				
<2500	10 (1.5)	2 (4.4)	13 (1.7)	0 (0.0)
≥2500	640 (98.5)	43 (95.6)	773 (98.3)	59 (100.0)
Infant gestational week				
<37	8 (1.2)	3 (6.8)	9 (1.2)	2 (3.4)
≥37	640 (98.8)	41 (93.2)	777 (98.8)	57 (96.6)
Calcium supplementation during pregnancy				
Yes	410 (63.1)	25 (55.6)	627 (79.8)	47 (79.7)
No	240 (36.9)	20 (44.4)	159 (20.2)	12 (20.3)

Data are presented as *n* (%); BF: any breastfeeding; Non-BF: non-breastfeeding.

3.2. Calcium Supplementation Status during Postpartum Period

Overall, among mothers in the Jiangyou cohort, an inverted U shape of calcium supplementation rates at three different postpartum periods was observed, which corresponded to 13.4%, 19.4% and 17.7%, respectively. While in the Chengdu cohort, a constant decline trend was recorded with 22.5%, 22.2% and 12.0% reported at the three postpartum periods. When considering separately for breastfeeding and non-breastfeeding groups, as shown in Figures 1 and 2, the calcium supplementation rate in the breastfeeding group was statistically significantly higher than that in the non-breastfeeding group for all the different postpartum periods, except between discharge and 1 month in the Jiangyou cohort ($p = 0.36$). In the Jiangyou cohort, calcium supplementation rates ranged from 13.7% to 21.2% for breastfeeding mothers, and ranged from 1.7% to 8.9% for non-breastfeeding mothers. In the Chengdu cohort, calcium supplementation rates reduced from around 23% in the first 3 months postpartum to 14.5% between 3 months and 6 months in breastfeeding mothers, and ranged from 5.0% to 14.1% in non-breastfeeding mothers.

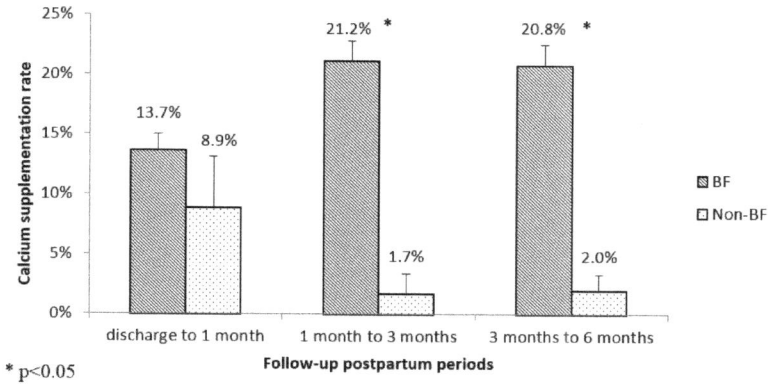

Figure 1. Calcium supplementation postpartum in Jiangyou.

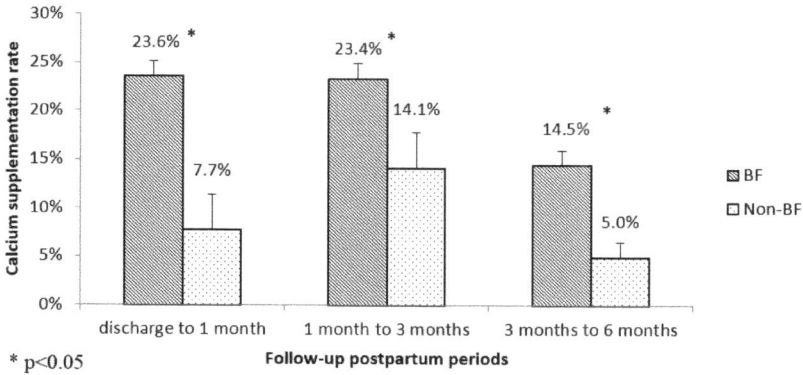

Figure 2. Calcium supplementation postpartum in Chengdu.

3.3. The Association between Breastfeeding and Calcium Supplementation Postpartum

In Model I (without any covariates) for both cohorts, subject random effect was found to be statistically significant. Hence, both the primary variables of interest (i.e., breastfeeding status and the indicator variable of measurement times) were subsequently added into the Model I for examining the association between breastfeeding and calcium supplementation postpartum. As shown in Table 3, the likelihood of calcium supplementation in breastfeeding mothers were 5.85 times (95% confidence interval (CI) (2.50, 13.72)) and 2.88 times (95% CI (1.50, 5.54)) higher of that in non-breastfeeding mothers in Jiangyou and Chengdu, respectively. After adjusting for socio-demographic and obstetric factors as well as calcium supplementation during pregnancy, the odds ratios (ORs) and its 95% CI had changed appreciably to 6.95 and (2.68, 18.04) in the Jiangyou study, and 3.03 and (1.52, 6.02) in the Chengdu study, respectively. The heterogeneity between these two studies was not significant ($I^2 = 0.479$, $p = 0.17$) statistically, therefore a fixed effect model was used to pool the ORs of the two studies. The pooled analysis of these two cohort studies revealed that calcium supplementation postpartum was significantly positively associated with breastfeeding with an adjusted OR = 4.02 with a 95% CI of (2.30, 7.03).

Table 3. Association between breastfeeding status and calcium supplementation postpartum.

Variable	Model II	Model IV
	Crude ORs (95% CI)	Adjusted ORs (95% CI)
Jiangyou Cohort		
Measurement times *		
At discharge (ref)	1	1
1 month	1.72 (1.24, 2.38)	1.90 (1.33, 2.70)
3 months	1.57 (1.12, 2.20)	1.69 (1.18, 2.44)
Breastfeeding status *		
Non-breastfeeding (ref)	1	1
Any breastfeeding	5.85 (2.50, 13.72)	6.95 (2.68, 18.04)
Chengdu Cohort		
Measurement times *		
At discharge (ref)	1	1
1 month	1.02 (0.74, 1.43)	1.02 (0.72, 1.45)
3 months	0.31 (0.21, 0.46)	0.30 (0.20, 0.45)
Breastfeeding status *		
Non-breastfeeding (ref)	1	1
Any breastfeeding	2.88 (1.50, 5.54)	3.03 (1.52, 6.02)
Pooled effect size of two studies		
Non-breastfeeding (ref)	-	1
Any breastfeeding	-	4.02 (2.30, 7.03)

Crude ORs (obtained from Model II): Model included breastfeeding status and the indicator variable of measurement times; Adjusted ORs (obtained from the final Model IV): Model adjusted for socio-demographics variables (household annual income, maternal age and maternal education); obstetric factors (parity, gravidity, infant gender, infant birth weight and infant gestational week); and calcium supplementation during pregnancy; * $p < 0.05$; ref: reference category.

4. Discussion

To our knowledge, the present study is the first population-based study that determines the longitudinal trend of calcium supplementation by Chinese women from discharge to 6 months postpartum and the effect of breastfeeding on calcium supplementation. A relatively low level of calcium supplementation (less than 23%) was observed throughout the postpartum period in either breastfeeding mothers or non-breastfeeding mothers. The pooled effect size after adjusting for socio-demographics variables (household annual income, maternal age and maternal education); obstetric factors (parity, gravidity, infant gender, infant birth weight and infant gestational week); and calcium supplementation during pregnancy reveals that mothers who breastfed their babies were 4.02 times more likely to take calcium supplements compared to their non-breastfeeding counterparts during postpartum. The present result is consistent with previous findings that breastfeeding mothers consumed more calcium than non-breastfeeding counterparts [33–35]. One reason leading to the higher calcium supplementation in breastfeeding mothers may be the general belief that adequate calcium intake is beneficial to breast milk production, and mothers' special attention to infants' calcium intake under the context of wide shortage of calcium intake for Chinese women, in spite of recent evidence demonstrating that calcium supplementation in lactation has no significant effect on increasing calcium content in breast milk [36–38]. The other reason might be mothers' perception of the beneficial effect of calcium supplementation on maternal bone loss during lactating. Some studies found little benefits of calcium supplementation on maternal bone loss during lactating [36,39,40], whereas other studies carried out in the U.S. and Brazil suggested that higher calcium intake during early lactation could minimize the bone loss for the mothers who had daily calcium intake less than 500 mg [20,21]. Further investigation on the factors contributing to difference of calcium supplementation between breastfeeding mothers and non-breastfeeding mothers as well as the effect of calcium supplementation

Nutrients **2016**, *8*, 622

on reducing maternal bone loss during lactation or enhancing maternal skeleton remodeling and remineralization after weaning of breastfeeding is recommended.

Given the habitually lower calcium dietary intake and relatively high lactose intolerance rate in the general Chinese population [12,15,17], calcium supplementation plays an important role on bone health, especially for exclusive breastfeeding women who provide around 300 mg of calcium per day to their babies via breast milk which accompany maternal bone calcium turnover [41].

This study had several strengths. We utilized data from two cohort studies to investigate the longitudinal trends of calcium supplementation at three different postpartum time points (i.e., 1 month, 3 months and 6 months postpartum) and conducted random effect regression modelling accounting for inherent dependency between the repeated measurements. Moreover, since the breastfeeding status was measured longitudinally as well in two cohorts, it was treated as a time-dependent variable in the analysis to account for possible feedback effects between the breastfeeding status and calcium supplementation at different times. In addition, our pooled analysis based on the two individual studies yielded the combined effect size with a larger sample size and higher statistical power. Moreover, calcium supplementation during pregnancy was adjusted in the modelling to control for the consequent effect of calcium intake during pregnancy on calcium supplementation during lactation.

A caveat of this study was that both cohort studies were carried out in Sichuan Province, which may limit the results being able to generalize to other regions of China. Sichuan Basin has special geographic characteristics, where the number of cloudy or rainy days is substantially larger than that in other regions in China, which may lead to a relatively lower level of vitamin D synthesis and calcium deficiency consequently [42]. However, to the best of our knowledge, no data were available currently on calcium supplementation during postpartum in other regions of China for comparison purpose.

5. Conclusions

In conclusion, calcium supplementation during postpartum in Sichuan is variable at different times postpartum with a relatively low level (less than 23%). Although breastfeeding has a substantive effect on calcium supplementation postpartum, dietary supplementation intervention programs and health education targeting different subgroups (e.g., breastfeeding mothers and bottle feeding mothers) should be promoted in Chinese women, given currently a wide shortage of dietary calcium intake and calcium supplementation during postpartum.

Acknowledgments: We would like to thank Li Tang and Chuan Yu from West China Hospital, Sichuan University for providing the two datasets. Jian Zhao would like to acknowledge China Scholarship Council (CSC) for their financial support for his doctoral studies.

Author Contributions: J.Z., Y.Z. and C.W.B. designed the research; J.Z. performed statistical analyses and Y.Z., C.W.B. and A.H.L. provided theoretical and methodological guidance; J.Z., Y.Z. and A.H.L. wrote the manuscript. All authors read and approved the final version of the manuscript.

Conflicts of Interest: The authors declare no conflict of interest.

References

1. Trotter, M.; Hixon, B.B. Sequential changes in weight, density, and percentage ash weight of human skeletons from an early fetal period through old age. *Anat. Rec.* **1974**, *179*, 1–18. [CrossRef] [PubMed]
2. Olausson, H.; Goldberg, G.R.; Laskey, M.A.; Schoenmakers, I.; Jarjou, L.M.; Prentice, A. Calcium economy in human pregnancy and lactation. *Nutr. Res. Rev.* **2012**, *25*, 40–67. [CrossRef] [PubMed]
3. Kalkwarf, H.J.; Specker, B.L.; Ho, M. Effects of calcium supplementation on calcium homeostasis and bone turnover in lactating women. *J. Clin. Endocrinol. Metab.* **1999**, *84*, 464–470. [CrossRef] [PubMed]
4. Kovacs, C.S.; Ralston, S.H. Presentation and management of osteoporosis presenting in association with pregnancy or lactation. *Osteoporos. Int.* **2015**, *26*, 2223–2241. [CrossRef] [PubMed]
5. Thomas, M.; Weisman, S.M. Calcium supplementation during pregnancy and lactation: Effects on the mother and the fetus. *Am. J. Obstet. Gynecol.* **2006**, *194*, 937–945. [CrossRef] [PubMed]

6. Prentice, A. Calcium in pregnancy and lactation. *Annu. Rev. Nutr.* **2000**, *20*, 249–272. [CrossRef] [PubMed]
7. Kovacs, C.S. Calcium and bone metabolism disorders during pregnancy and lactation. *Endocrinol. Metab. Clin. N. Am.* **2011**, *40*, 795–826. [CrossRef] [PubMed]
8. Institute of Medicine. *Dietary Reference Intakes for Calcium and Vitamin D*; National Academies Press: Washington, DC, USA, 2011.
9. Chen, Y.M.; Teucher, B.; Tang, X.Y.; Dainty, J.R.; Lee, K.K.; Woo, J.L.; Ho, S.C. Calcium absorption in postmenopausal Chinese women: A randomized crossover intervention study. *Br. J. Nutr.* **2007**, *97*, 160–166. [CrossRef] [PubMed]
10. Ma, G.; Li, Y.; Jin, Y.; Zhai, F.; Kok, F.J.; Yang, X. Phytate intake and molar ratios of phytate to zinc, iron and calcium in the diets of people in China. *Eur. J. Clin. Nutr.* **2007**, *61*, 368–374. [CrossRef] [PubMed]
11. Wang, Y.; Li, S. Worldwide trends in dairy production and consumption and calcium intake: Is promoting consumption of dairy products a sustainable solution for inadequate calcium intake? *Food Nutr. Bull.* **2008**, *29*, 172–185. [CrossRef] [PubMed]
12. Shin, A.; Li, H.; Shu, X.O.; Yang, G.; Gao, Y.T.; Zheng, W. Dietary intake of calcium, fiber and other micronutrients in relation to colorectal cancer risk: Results from the Shanghai Women's Health Study. *Int. J. Cancer* **2006**, *119*, 2938–2942. [CrossRef] [PubMed]
13. Deng, J.; Huang, Y.M.; Lin, Q. Main sources of dietary calcium in perimenopausal women in Changsha. *Zhong Nan Da Xue Xue Bao Yi Xue Ban* **2008**, *33*, 875–879. [PubMed]
14. Liu, X.; Zhao, X.; Xu, L. Food sources of calcium and iron in the diet of Beijing elderly. *Wei Sheng Yan Jiu* **2004**, *33*, 336–338. [PubMed]
15. He, Y.; Zhai, F.; Wang, Z.; Hu, Y. Status of dietary calcium intake of Chinese residents. *Wei Sheng Yan Jiu* **2007**, *36*, 600–602. [PubMed]
16. Lai, J.; Yin, S.; Ma, G.; Piao, J.; Yang, X. The nutrition and health survery of pregnant women in China. *Acta Nutr. Sin.* **2007**, *29*, 4–8.
17. De Vrese, M.; Stegelmann, A.; Richter, B.; Fenselau, S.; Laue, C.; Schrezenmeir, J. Probiotics—Compensation for lactase insufficiency. *Am. J. Clin. Nutr.* **2001**, *73*, 421S–429S. [PubMed]
18. Wang, Y.G.; Yan, Y.S.; Xu, J.J.; Du, R.F.; Flatz, S.D.; Kuhnau, W.; Flatz, G. Prevalence of primary adult lactose malabsorption in three populations of northern China. *Hum. Genet.* **1984**, *67*, 103–106. [PubMed]
19. National Health and Family Planning Commission of the People's Republic of China. Maternal and Child Health Basic Knowledge and Skills (Trial Version). Available online: http://www.nhfpc.gov.cn/fys/kpxc/201405/0065ee2071204f0c9b52f7cdcbb392f2.shtml (accessed on 5 July 2016).
20. O'Brien, K.O.; Donangelo, C.M.; Ritchie, L.D.; Gildengorin, G.; Abrams, S.; King, J.C. Serum 1,25-dihydroxyvitamin D and calcium intake affect rates of bone calcium deposition during pregnancy and the early postpartum period. *Am. J. Clin. Nutr.* **2012**, *96*, 64–72. [CrossRef] [PubMed]
21. O'Brien, K.O.; Donangelo, C.M.; Zapata, C.L.; Abrams, S.A.; Spencer, E.M.; King, J.C. Bone calcium turnover during pregnancy and lactation in women with low calcium diets is associated with calcium intake and circulating insulin-like growth factor 1 concentrations. *Am. J. Clin. Nutr.* **2006**, *83*, 317–323. [PubMed]
22. Chan, G.M.; McMurry, M.; Westover, K.; Engelbert-Fenton, K.; Thomas, M.R. Effects of increased dietary calcium intake upon the calcium and bone mineral status of lactating adolescent and adult women. *Am. J. Clin. Nutr.* **1987**, *46*, 319–323. [PubMed]
23. Yoneyama, K.; Ikeda, J. The effects of increased dietary calcium intake on bone mineral density in long-term lactating women, and recovery of bone loss caused by long-term lactation with low calcium diet. *Nihon Koshu Eisei Zasshi* **2004**, *51*, 1008–1017. [PubMed]
24. Li, Y.; Liao, D.; Miao, L.; Qian, X. Analysis on dietary investigation of pregnant and lactating women. *Chin. Prim. Health Care* **2004**, *18*, 27–28.
25. Huang, Z. The Dietary Status of 269 Lactating Women and the Content of Minerals in Breast Milk. Master's Thesis, Central South University, Changsha, China, 2014.
26. Yang, T.; Zhang, Y.; Ma, D.; Li, W.; Yang, X.; Wang, P. Survey on the nutrients intake of lactating women in three cities of China. *Acta Nutr. Sin.* **2014**, *36*, 84–86.
27. Chen, H.; Wang, P.; Han, Y.; Ma, J.; Troy, F.A., II; Wang, B. Evaluation of dietary intake of lactating women in China and its potential impact on the health of mothers and infants. *BMC Women's Health* **2012**, *12*, 18. [CrossRef] [PubMed]

28. Kong, X.; Fei, J.; Zhai, Y.; Feng, Y.; Li, J. Dietary survey of lactating mothers during the puerperal state. *China Med. Her.* **2016**, *13*, 49–68.

29. Qiu, L.; Zhao, Y.; Binns, C.W.; Lee, A.H.; Xie, X. A cohort study of infant feeding practices in city, suburban and rural areas in Zhejiang Province, PR China. *Int. Breastfeed. J.* **2008**, *3*, 4. [CrossRef] [PubMed]

30. Xu, F.; Liu, X.; Binns, C.W.; Xiao, C.; Wu, J.; Lee, A.H. A decade of change in breastfeeding in China's far north-west. *Int. Breastfeed. J.* **2006**, *1*, 22. [CrossRef] [PubMed]

31. Scott, J.A.; Landers, M.C.; Hughes, R.M.; Binns, C.W. Factors associated with breastfeeding at discharge and duration of breastfeeding. *J. Paediatr. Child Health* **2001**, *37*, 254–261. [CrossRef] [PubMed]

32. World Health Organization. Indicators for assessing infant and young child feeding practices: Part 1: Definitions. In Proceedings of the Conclusions of a Consensus Meeting, Washington, DC, USA, 6–8 November 2007.

33. Chan, S.M.; Nelson, E.A.; Leung, S.S.; Cheng, J.C. Bone mineral density and calcium metabolism of Hong Kong Chinese postpartum women—A 1-y longitudinal study. *Eur. J. Clin. Nutr.* **2005**, *59*, 868–876. [CrossRef] [PubMed]

34. Laskey, M.A.; Prentice, A.; Hanratty, L.A.; Jarjou, L.M.; Dibba, B.; Beavan, S.R.; Cole, T.J. Bone changes after 3 mo of lactation: Influence of calcium intake, breast-milk output, and vitamin D-receptor genotype. *Am. J. Clin. Nutr.* **1998**, *67*, 685–692. [PubMed]

35. Lopez, J.M.; Gonzalez, G.; Reyes, V.; Campino, C.; Diaz, S. Bone turnover and density in healthy women during breastfeeding and after weaning. *Osteoporos. Int.* **1996**, *6*, 153–159. [CrossRef] [PubMed]

36. Kalkwarf, H.J.; Specker, B.L.; Bianchi, D.C.; Ranz, J.; Ho, M. The effect of calcium supplementation on bone density during lactation and after weaning. *N. Engl. J. Med.* **1997**, *337*, 523–528. [CrossRef] [PubMed]

37. Prentice, A.; Jarjou, L.M.; Cole, T.J.; Stirling, D.M.; Dibba, B.; Fairweather-Tait, S. Calcium requirements of lactating Gambian mothers: Effects of a calcium supplement on breast-milk calcium concentration, maternal bone mineral content, and urinary calcium excretion. *Am. J. Clin. Nutr.* **1995**, *62*, 58–67. [PubMed]

38. Jarjou, L.M.; Prentice, A.; Sawo, Y.; Laskey, M.A.; Bennett, J.; Goldberg, G.R.; Cole, T.J. Randomized, placebo-controlled, calcium supplementation study in pregnant Gambian women: Effects on breast-milk calcium concentrations and infant birth weight, growth, and bone mineral accretion in the first year of life. *Am. J. Clin. Nutr.* **2006**, *83*, 657–666. [PubMed]

39. Zhang, Z.Q.; Chen, Y.M.; Wang, R.Q.; Huang, Z.W.; Yang, X.G.; Su, Y.X. The effects of different levels of calcium supplementation on the bone mineral status of postpartum lactating Chinese women: A 12-month randomised, double-blinded, controlled trial. *Br. J. Nutr.* **2016**, *115*, 24–31. [CrossRef] [PubMed]

40. Cross, N.A.; Hillman, L.S.; Allen, S.H.; Krause, G.F. Changes in bone mineral density and markers of bone remodeling during lactation and postweaning in women consuming high amounts of calcium. *J. Bone Miner. Res.* **1995**, *10*, 1312–1320. [CrossRef] [PubMed]

41. Kovacs, C.S. Maternal mineral and bone metabolism during pregnancy, lactation, and post-weaning recovery. *Physiol. Rev.* **2016**, *96*, 449–547. [PubMed]

42. Wang, J.; Yang, F.; Mao, M.; Liu, D.H.; Yang, H.M.; Yang, S.F. High prevalence of vitamin D and calcium deficiency among pregnant women and their newborns in Chengdu, China. *World J. Pediatr. WJP* **2010**, *6*, 265–267. [CrossRef] [PubMed]

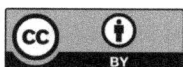

nutrients

MDPI

Article

A Comparison by Milk Feeding Method of the Nutrient Intake of a Cohort of Australian Toddlers

Jane Scott [1,*], Kristina Davey [2], Ellen Ahwong [2], Gemma Devenish [2], Diep Ha [3] and Loc Do [3]

[1] Collaboration for Evidence, Research and Impact in Public Health (CERIPH), School of Public Health, Curtin University, Perth 6102, Australia
[2] School of Public Health, Curtin University, Perth 6102, Australia; kristina.davey@postgrad.curtin.edu.au (K.D.); ellen.pearce@postgrad.curtin.edu.au (E.A.); gemma.Devenish@curtin.edu.au (G.D.)
[3] Australian Research Centre for Population Oral Health, University of Adelaide, Adelaide 5000, Australia; diep.ha@adelaide.edu.au (D.H.); loc.do@adelaide.edu.au (L.D.)
*   Correspondence: jane.scott@curtin.edu.au; Tel.: +61-8-9266-9050

Received: 26 June 2016; Accepted: 12 August 2016; Published: 16 August 2016

Abstract: Breastfeeding is recommended beyond 12 months of age, but little is known about the contribution of breastmilk and infant formula to the nutritional intake of toddlers as they transition to a family diet in the second year of life. This study is a cross-sectional analysis of data collected from a birth cohort study in Adelaide, Australia. Dietary intake data were collected when children were approximately 1 year of age by an interviewer-administered multi-pass 24 h recall and a mother-completed 2 days food diary. Children were categorized according to their milk feeding method, i.e., breastmilk, infant formula, combination or other, and their nutrient intakes compared with recommended nutrient reference values. Complete data were available for 832 children, of which 714 had plausible energy intakes. Breastmilk and formula made a substantial contribution to the nutrient intake of those toddlers, contributing 28% and 34% of total energy, and 16% and 26% of protein intake, respectively when not drunk in combination. In general, Australian toddlers transitioning to the family diet consumed nutritionally adequate diets, although almost one quarter of all children and half of breastfed children with plausible intakes had iron intakes below the estimated average requirement, placing them at risk of iron deficiency.

Keywords: nutritional adequacy; diet; toddler; breastmilk; formula; iron

1. Introduction

Breastfeeding is recommended beyond 12 months of age [1–3], but relatively little is known about the contribution of breastmilk and infant formula to the nutritional intake of toddlers as they transition to a family diet in the second year of life. Similarly, little is known about the nutritional content and adequacy of the diets of Australian children under the age of 2 years. While the Australian National Infant Feeding Survey studied this age group, its focus was on breastfeeding and age of introduction of complementary foods and it did not investigate what and how much children in this age group ate [4]. On the other hand, the 2011–2012 Australian National Nutrition and Physical Activity Survey (NNPAS) [5] and the 2007 Australian National Children's Nutritional and Physical Activity Survey (NCNPAS) [6] only studied the diets of children aged 2 years and older. What data are available on the diets of Australian infants and toddlers aged less than 2 years come from a number of single-center or state-based studies of infants and toddlers of varying ages [7–12]. Relatively little is known about the diets of children as they enter their second year of life [9] and much of what we know about the diets of this age group comes from international studies [13–15].

The objectives of this paper were therefore to (1) estimate the usual intake of a cohort of Australian toddlers and to evaluate their diets relative to the Nutrient Reference Values (NRVs) for Australia and New Zealand [16]; (2) identify the contribution that breastmilk and formula make to the nutrient intake of toddlers; and (3) investigate the relationship between milk feeding method and nutrient adequacy.

2. Materials and Methods

2.1. Design

This study is a cross-sectional analysis of dietary data collected as part of the Study of Mothers' and Infants' Life Events Affecting Health (SMILE), a population-based longitudinal birth cohort study [17]. This study has recruited and is following a cohort of socioeconomically-diverse South Australian newborns from birth and into their third year of life. The primary health outcomes of this study are two related conditions: dental caries and obesity/overweight of young children.

2.2. Setting and Recruitment

In total, 2147 mothers and 2181 newborns, including 34 pairs of twins, were recruited from the three major maternity hospitals in Adelaide, Australia from July 2013 until August 2014. All new mothers who were sufficiently competent in English to be able to understand the description and instructions of the study were invited to participate. Those mothers who indicated their intention to move out of the greater Adelaide area within a year were excluded.

Mothers were recruited, usually within 48 h of giving birth, from the postnatal wards of the participating hospitals. Those agreeing to participate in the study were invited to complete a baseline questionnaire designed to collect mother and family-related information including socio-demographic details such as age, income, education, occupation and postcode. Further details of sample size and recruitment procedures have been reported elsewhere [17].

2.3. Ethical Considerations

The study was approved by the Southern Adelaide Clinical Human Research Ethics Committee (HREC/50.13, approval date: 28 February 2013) and the South Australian Women and Children Health Network (HREC/13/WCHN/69, approval date: 7 August 2013), and received clinical governance clearance from the three participating maternity hospitals. Signed informed consent was obtained from mothers who were advised that their participation was voluntary and that they could withdraw at any time without prejudice.

2.4. Collection and Handling of Dietary Data

Once their child had reached 12 months of age, mothers of the 1919 infants remaining in the study were mailed a food diary and a cover letter explaining that a member of the research team would telephone them to collect a 24 h dietary recall (24 HDR) of their child's intake and explain how to complete the food diary. The 24 HDR was conducted via a telephone interview by a trained dietitian using the five-step multi-pass method [18]. At the end of the 24 HDR interview mothers were allocated two days in the following week to record their child's food intake in the food diary. The days allocated ensured that, together with the 24 HDR, three nonconsecutive days (2 week days and one weekend day) of dietary intake over a 10-day period were recorded. The food diary booklet contained instructions for recording their child's intake and included a detailed example of a one-day food record, as well as photos of food portion sizes and examples of household measures (cups, bowls and spoons), to help mothers estimate amounts consumed when completing both the 24 HDR and the food diary.

The dietary data were entered into FoodWorks® version 8 (Xyris Software) and analyzed using the AUSNUT 2011–2013 food composition database [19]. Foods consumed by children but not included in the AUSNUT database were added utilizing nutrient information gathered from the nutrition information panels of product labels and manufacturer websites. The 24 HDR and the two-day food diary were entered together as a food record by a team of four nutritionists. For quality management purposes, standardization training was conducted and data were entered following a detailed data entry protocol. Cross-checking between the 24 HDR and food diary was conducted for data clarification purposes—for example, where a type of bread (e.g., wholegrain) had been collected as part of the 24 HDR but not recorded by the mother in the food diary.

Breastmilk intake was estimated using the method employed for this age group in the UK 2011 Diet and Nutrition Survey of Infants and Young Children (DNSIYC) [14]. Breastfeeds were recorded in minutes and the amount of milk consumed was calculated as 10 g/min to a maximum of 100 g per feed, as the contribution to nutrient intake after 10 min of breastfeeding is considered minimal in this age group [20]. If within 30 min of the start of the previous feed a second breastfeed was started, it was not considered a new feed, and the breastfeeding time was added to the previous feed to a maximum of 10 min [14]. If the child was breastfed for less than two minutes, this was not considered long enough to contribute to their nutrient intake and was not included [14].

Children were grouped initially into four categories of milk feeding method on the basis of whether or not they had consumed breastmilk and/or formula on one or more days. Formulas included infant formula, defined as suitable for children up to 12 months, and toddler formula. The 'breastmilk group' included toddlers who had received breastmilk but no formula. The 'formula group' included toddlers who had received infant or toddler formula but no breastmilk. The 'combination group' included toddlers who had received both breastmilk and infant or toddler formula. Children in these first three groups may also have consumed (usually in small amounts) animal milk or animal milk substitutes in addition to breastmilk and/or formula. Children in the 'other' group had consumed neither breastmilk nor infant or toddler formula.

2.5. Statistical Analysis

Once entered into FoodWorks® version 8 (Xyris Software, High Gate Hill, Qld, Australia), data were downloaded into an Access database (Microsoft Office, 2013) and imported into SPSS version 22 (IBM SPSS Statistics for Windows, Armonk, NY, USA) for statistical analysis. Descriptive statistics were run to identify outliers and improbable intakes of weight of food, energy and macronutrients, and data were checked and cleaned appropriately. As the child's current weight was unknown, a plausible energy intake was estimated for each child using a sex specific estimated energy requirement (EER) for a reference child of the participant's age [16]. The child's date of birth and the date when the 24 HDR was completed was used to calculate their age. The degree of under and over-reporting was assessed by calculating the ratio of reported energy intake to the EER for each child. Children were deemed to have an implausible intake if they had an average daily energy intake below 0.54 or above 1.46 for their age and sex specific reference EER [7].

Descriptive statistics, including mean values and standard deviations as well as 25th and 75th percentiles, were derived for children with plausible intakes for nutrient intakes averaged across the three days. The data were then transformed to determine the proportion of children with inadequate and excessive intakes compared with the NRVs for children aged 1–3 years [16]. Inadequate intakes were considered to be any value below the Estimated Average Requirement (EAR) and excessive intakes were considered to be any value above the Upper Limit of intake (UL), where relevant.

The mean intake of energy, macronutrients and those micronutrients for which more than 10% of the total sample had inadequate or excessive intakes were reported for each milk feeding group. A one-way ANOVA with a *post hoc* Bonferonni test was used to determine any significant between-group differences in mean intake of each nutrient. The percentage contribution of breastmilk and formula to total intake of energy and nutrients was determined for each group. Due to the small numbers of children with inadequate intakes in some groups, those children who received any formula whether in combination with breastmilk or not were collapsed into a single group for further analysis. The proportion of children with inadequate or excessive intakes in each of these three milk feeding group was then determined. Multivariate binary logistic regression, adjusting for maternal age, education and infant sex, was employed to determine the relationship of milk feeding group and inadequate or excessive intakes of nutrients. A *p*-value of < 0.05 was considered to be statistically significant for all analyses.

3. Results

Of the 1919 children who were mailed a food diary, 1165 had a completed 24 HDR interview (61% response rate) and 844 had returned food diaries (44% response rate). Usable, complete 3 day records were available for 832 children (43%). The participant flow chart is presented in Figure A1.

3.1. Participant Characteristics

Mothers who provided baseline data but did not provide complete dietary data at 12 months were younger (*p* < 0.001), less educated (*p* < 0.001), more socially disadvantaged (*p* < 0.001) and more likely to have been born outside of Australia (*p* < 0.001). However, due to the deliberate over-recruitment of disadvantaged women into the SMILE study [17], women who provided complete dietary data were generally representative of the socioeconomic profile reported by the Pregnancy Outcome Unit for South Australian for births in 2013 with regards to parity and country of birth, but our sample consisted of fewer younger (<25 years) and overweight or obese mothers [21] (Table S1).

The mean age of participant children was 13.1 ± 0.8 months and 54.7% were boys. In total, 118 children had implausible energy intakes (3 under-reporters and 115 over-reporters) and those 714 children with plausible energy intakes represent the analysis population in this study. The characteristics of mother-child dyads with and without plausible dietary data are presented in Table 1. There was no significant association between over-reporting and any of the maternal or child characteristics investigated, with the exception of milk feeding method.

Table 1. Characteristics of mother–child dyads with complete dietary data and of the subsets with plausible and implausible energy intake.

Maternal characteristics	Total (*n* = 832)		Plausible (*n* = 714)		Implausible (*n* = 118)		*p* [a]
	n	%	*n*	%	*n*	%	
Maternal age at birth (years)							
<25	74	8.9	62	8.7	12	10.3	0.583
25–29	259	31.2	227	31.9	32	27.4	
≥30	496	59.8	423	59.4	73	62.4	
Maternal education completed							
School/vocational	358	43.4	310	43.7	48	41.0	0.585
Some university and above	468	56.7	399	56.3	69	59.0	
IRSAD score [b]							
Deciles 1–2	120	14.5	104	14.7	16	13.7	0.941
Deciles 3–4	175	21.2	147	20.7	28	23.9	
Deciles 5–6	172	20.8	147	20.7	25	21.4	
Deciles 7–8	161	19.5	140	19.7	21	17.9	
Deciles 9–10	198	24.0	171	24.1	27	23.1	
Mother's country of birth							
Australia and N. Zealand	613	74.1	519	73.1	94	80.3	0.061
Asia—other	57	6.9	35	4.8	5	1.7	
India	50	6.0	47	6.6	3	2.6	
China	36	4.4	34	3.2	2	6.8	
UK	31	3.7	23	7.3	8	4.3	
Other	40	4.8	35	4.7	5	4.3	
Maternal BMI [c] (kg/m^2)							
<25	476	60.6	413	60.8	63	58.9	0.217
25–29.99	170	21.6	151	22.2	19	17.8	
>30	140	17.8	115	16.9	25	23.4	

Table 1. *Cont.*

	Total		Plausible		Implausible		
	(*n* = 832)		(*n* = 714)		(*n* = 118)		
Parity							
Primiparous	388	48.2	336	48.7	52	45.2	0.489
Multiparous	417	51.8	354	51.3	63	54.8	
Child characteristics							
Child age (mean SD)	13.1	0.8	13.1	0.8	13.0	0.7	0.660 [d]
Infant sex							
Boy	455	54.7	395	55.3	60	50.8	0.366
Girl	377	45.3	319	44.7	58	49.2	
Milk feeding method							
Breastmilk	219	26.3	201	28.3	18	15.3	<0.001
Breastmilk and formula	68	8.2	59	8.3	9	7.6	
Infant formula	314	37.7	275	38.5	39	33.1	
Other	231	27.8	179	25.1	52	44.1	

[a] Chi Square *p* value; [b] Index of Relative Socio-Economic Advantage and Disadvantage (IRSAD) where decile 1 = most disadvantaged and decile 10 = most advantaged; [c] Body Mass Index; [d] Independent *t*-test.

3.2. Nutrient Intake of Children

3.2.1. Comparison of Nutrient Intakes with Nutrient Reference Values

Overall, children had adequate daily intakes of energy, protein and micronutrients, with a few notable exceptions (Table 2). Roughly one in ten children had intakes below the EAR for vitamin C (14.0%), thiamin (14.4%) and calcium (12.6%), while just over two out of ten (22.5%) had intakes below the EAR for iron (Figure 1). Conversely, 18.2% and 14.1% had intakes which exceeded the UL for sodium and zinc (Figure 2), respectively. Dietary fibre intake was generally low in this group.

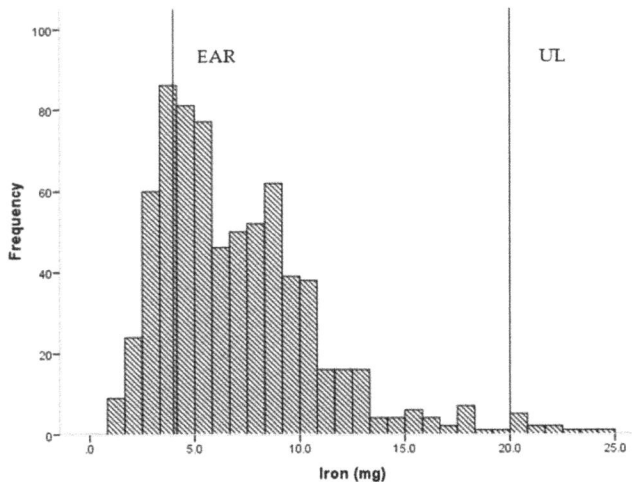

Figure 1. Frequency of intake of iron (*n* = 714) showing estimated average requirement (EAR = 4 mg) and upper limit of intake (UL = 20 mg).

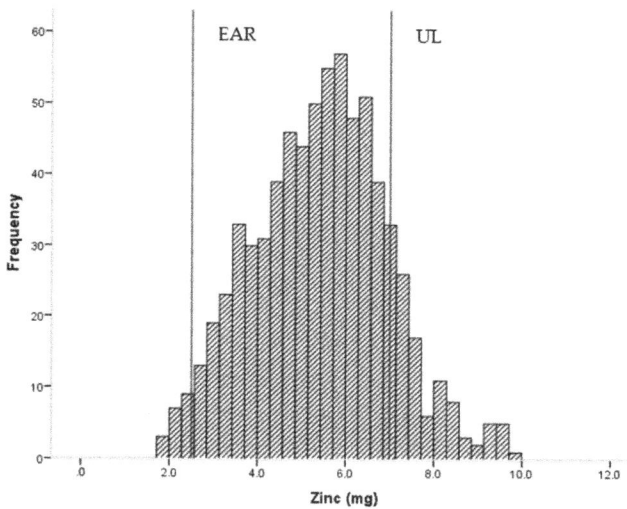

Figure 2. Frequency of intake of zinc ($n = 714$) showing estimated average requirement (EAR = 2.5 mg) and upper limit of intake (UL = 7 mg).

Table 2. Nutrient intakes of children [a] (mean age 13.1 months) and comparison with selected Nutrient Reference Values for children aged 1–3 years.

Average Intake/Day	Mean	SD	25	75	EAR	<EAR%	UL	>UL%
Total mass (kg)	1179	393	993	1322				
Energy (kJ)	3803	714	3297	4378				
Protein (g)	36	11	28	44	12.0	0.0		
Total carbohydrate (g)	107	23	89	123				
Sugar (g)	63	17	51	73				
Total fat (g)	36	9	29	42				
Saturated fat (g)	16.5	5.1	12.8	20.1				
Polyunsaturated fat (g)	4.2	1.6	3.1	5.0				
Monounsaturated fat (g)	12.3	3.4	10.0	14.3				
Dietary fibre (g)	9.6	4.0	6.7	11.8				
Water (g)	1013	386	809	1100				
Sodium (mg)	725	324	487	916			1000	18.2
Potassium (mg)	1467	433	1171	1745				
Calcium (mg)	650	235	481	812	360	12.6	2500	0.0
Phosphorous (mg)	736	229	573	888	380	6.3	3000	0.0
Magnesium (mg)	137	38	110	164	65	2.0		
Iron (mg)	7.1	4.0	4.2	9.0	4	22.5	20	1.5
Zinc (mg)	5.4	1.5	4.4	6.4	2.5	2.2	7	14.1
Vitamin A RE [b] (μg)	726	492	487	851	210	0.4	NA [c]	
Thiamin (mg)	0.8	0.5	0.5	1.0	0.4	14.4		
Riboflavin (mg)	1.4	0.6	1.0	1.8	0.4	2.1		
Niacin equivalents (mg)	16.6	5.5	12.8	19.8	5	0.0	NA [d]	
Folate (μg)	321	130	226	404	120	3.1	NA [d]	
Vitamin C (mg)	61	46	36	80	25	14.0		

NA—not applicable. [a] Children with plausible energy intakes; [b] Retinol equivalents; [c] Upper limit refers to vitamin A from retinol; [d] Upper limit refers to intake from supplements.

3.2.2. Comparison of Nutrient Intakes by Milk Feeding Method

The majority of all 832 children were still receiving breastmilk ($n = 334$, 36%) and/or formula ($n = 374$, 53%); only 26 children (4%) were consuming toddler formula. Of those with plausible energy intakes, 260 children (36%) were consuming breastmilk and 334 children (47%) were consuming formula. Children were categorized according to whether or not they consumed breastmilk and/or formula and the mean intakes of energy, macronutrients and those micronutrient for which more than 10% of children had inadequate or excessive intakes were compared (Table 3). There were a number of significant between-group differences for all nutrients but in general children who did not drink either breastmilk and/or formula had significantly higher intakes of energy, protein, sodium, calcium and a lower intake of vitamin C than the other groups. There was no significant difference in the mean protein and energy intakes of those children in the breastmilk group compared with those in the formula group, although formula made a greater contribution to the total protein (26% vs. 16%) and energy intake (34% vs. 28%) of children than did breastmilk. Those children who drank only breastmilk had significantly lower intakes of zinc than all other groups, while those children who drank only formula had significantly higher intakes of calcium than those children who consumed breastmilk either with or without formula, and significantly higher intakes of zinc and iron than all other groups. Formula contributed 31% and 50% of the total iron intake in those who drank formula with or without breastmilk, respectively.

3.3. Relationship of Milk Feeding Method and Adequacy of Selected Nutrients

Due to the small number of children with inadequate intakes in some groups, those children who received any formula, whether in combination with breastmilk or not, were collapsed into a single group. Those children who were in the breastmilk-only group were significantly more likely than the other milk feeding groups to have intakes of calcium, iron, and thiamin below the EAR (Table 4). Children who drank neither breastmilk nor formula were almost 10 times more likely (AOR 9.64, 95% CI 5.27–17.62) than the breastmilk-only group to have intakes of vitamin C below the EAR, but children who drank formula were less likely (AOR 0.23, 95% CI 0.09–0.59) to have inadequate vitamin C intakes. Almost half (48.8%) of the children in the breastmilk-only group had iron intakes below the EAR while children who consumed formula were less likely (AOR 0.04, 95% CI 0.02–0.07) to have inadequate iron intakes than those who drank breastmilk. Conversely, children in the breastmilk-only group were less likely than all other groups to have intakes of zinc above the UL and less likely than the group that drank neither breastmilk nor formula to have sodium intakes above the UL.

Table 3. Comparison of the mean nutrient intakes of children ‡ by milk feeding group.

| | Milk Feeding Method | | | | | | | | | | | | | | |
| | Breastmilk (n = 201) | | | | Combination—Breastmilk & Formula § (n = 59) | | | | | Formula § (n = 275) | | | | Other (n = 179) | |
	Mean	SD	% CF	% BM	Mean	SD	% CF	% BM	% F	Mean	SD	% CF	% F	Mean	SD
Average intake/day															
Total mass (g)	1102 [a]	263	67	33	1214	1047	58	21	21	1186	264	62	38	1240 [a]	253
Energy (kJ)	3708 [a]	747	72	28	3557 [b]	783	62	20	18	3723 [c]	656	66	34	4111 [a,b,c]	646
Protein (g)	33 [a]	10	84	16	30 [b,c]	10	73	12	15	35 [b,d]	9	74	26	45 [a,c,d]	9
Total carbohydrate (g)	100 [a,b]	25	75	25	102	21	65	16	19	110 [a]	21	66	34	111 [b]	22
Total fat (g)	38 [a]	9	60	40	35	12	49	30	21	33 [a,b]	8	58	42	38 [b]	9
Na (mg)	700 [a,b]	393	89	11	546 [a,c,d]	183	79	8	13	687 [c,e]	279	78	22	872 [b,d,e]	284
Ca (mg)	467 [a,b]	175	72	28	522 [c,d]	191	50	17	33	703 [a,c,e]	177	50	50	815 [b,d,e]	229
Fe (mg)	5.0 [a,b]	3.3	97	3	7.8 [a,c,d]	4.3	68	1	31	9.3 [b,c,e]	3.1	50	50	5.9 [d,e]	4.2
Zinc (mg)	4.2 [a,b,c]	1.2	84	16	5.1 [a,d,e]	2	63	10	27	6.2 [b,d,f]	1.2	56	44	5.6 [c,e,f]	1.2
Thiamin (mg)	0.7 [a,b]	0.5	89	11	0.7 [c]	0.3	72	6	22	0.9 [a,c]	0.4	64	36	0.9 [b]	0.6
Vitamin C (mg)	52 [a,b,c]	21	62	38	69 [a,d]	30	44	20	36	83 [b,e]	58	40	60	36 [c,d,e]	30

‡ Children with plausible intakes; § Infant or toddler formula, CF = Complementary foods and beverages, BM = Breastmilk, F = Infant or toddler formula; Shared superscript letters indicate significant between group differences in the mean intake of that nutrient.

Table 4. Association between milk feeding method and intakes of selected † micronutrients below the estimated average requirement (EAR) or above the upper level (UL) of intake.

	Total (n = 714)		Breastmilk (n = 201)		Formula (n = 334)		Other (n = 179)	
Calcium								
Number (%) below EAR	90	(12.6)	64	(31.8)	19	(5.7)	7	(3.9)
Adjusted # odds ratio (95% CI)			Ref		0.13	(0.07–0.22)	0.09	(0.04–0.19)
Iron								
Number (%) below EAR	161	(22.5)	98	(48.8)	11	(3.3)	52	(29.1)
Adjusted # odds ratio (95% CI)			Ref		0.04	(0.02–0.07)	0.42	(0.27–0.64)
Thiamin								
Number (%) below EAR	103	(14.4)	62	(30.8)	19	(5.7)	22	(12.3)
Adjusted # odds ratio (95% CI)			Ref		0.13	(0.07–0.23)	0.30	(0.17–0.51)
Vitamin C								
Number (%) below EAR	100	(14.0)	15	(7.5)	6	(1.8)	79	(44.1)
Adjusted # odds ratio (95% CI)			Ref		0.23	(0.09–0.59)	9.64	(5.27–17.62)
Zinc								
Number (%) above UL	101	(14.1)	4	(2.0)	75	(22.5)	22	(12.3)
Adjusted # odds ratio (95% CI)			Ref		13.5	(4.85–37.66)	6.35	(2.14–18.85)
Sodium								
Number (%) above UL	130	(18.2)	33	(16.4)	45	(13.5)	52	(29.1)
Adjusted # odds ratio (95% CI)			Ref		0.79	(0.49–1.29)	2.10	(1.28–3.44)

† Nutrients for which 10% or more of children had intakes below the EAR or above the UL; # Adjusted for maternal age, education and infant sex.

4. Discussion

In this study we have described the diets of a cohort of Australian toddlers aged approximately 1 year, an age by which they should have transitioned predominantly to family foods. More than one half and one third of children continued to consume formula or breastmilk, respectively. These 'milks' contributed up to roughly one third of their total energy intake and one quarter of their protein intake when consumed either alone or in combination. A relatively high prevalence of formula feeding (32%) has been reported in another Australian cohort of slightly older toddlers (12–16 months) [9] and 38% of children aged 12–18 months in the UK-based DNSIYC were receiving formula of some kind [14]. The higher prevalence of formula use in our study can be attributed to the younger age of this birth cohort, which had a mean age of 13.1 months at the time that dietary intake was assessed. The Australian Infant Feeding Guidelines (AIFG) encourage the continuation of breastfeeding beyond the first year of life, and while it is recommended that cow's milk not be given as a main drink to infants under the age of 12 months, this restriction is lifted once children enter their second year of life. Furthermore, the AIFG specifically state that "special complementary foods or milks for toddlers are not required for healthy children" [1] (p. 89).

It is unclear why contemporary Australian mothers continue to feed their children formula beyond 12 months of age. However, the advertising of toddler formulas has become increasingly prevalent [22] since Australia became a signatory to the International Code of Marketing of Breastmilk Substitutes (WHA 34.22 1981) which prohibits the advertising of infant formulas. With both products sharing common visual packaging elements such as colour, shape, typeface and logo, toddler milk advertisements appear to function as *de facto* infant formula advertisements with most women not being able distinguish between toddler and infant formulas and referring to both as 'formula' [23,24]. While most toddlers in this study were still consuming 'infant' versions of formula the advertising of toddler formula may have promulgated the perception amongst mothers that formulas of any kind are beneficial to the health of toddlers and are essential to meet the needs of developing toddlers that cannot be met by cow's milk and family foods.

In general, toddlers in this study consumed diets that either met or exceeded their nutritional requirements, with relatively small numbers failing to meet the EAR for any nutrient. A notable exception was our finding that roughly one in five toddlers consumed diets below the EAR of 4 mg/day for iron [16] which placed them at risk of iron deficiency. This is consistent with the findings of a recent Australian study of slightly older toddlers (mean age: 19.6 months) which reported a similar mean iron intake of 6.6 mg/day and that 18.6% of toddlers had inadequate iron intakes [8]. Comparison with international studies is difficult due to differences in the nutrient recommendations between countries and methodological differences in the way in which dietary data are collected. Nevertheless, just over one in 10 (13%) of UK children aged 12–18 months had iron intakes below the Lower Recommended Nutrient Intake (LRNI) of 3.7 mg/day [25]. When this slightly lower cut point was applied to our data, 17.8% of the SMILE cohort had intakes below the UK LRNI for iron. In comparison, less than 1% of toddlers aged 12 to 23 months in the US Feeding Infants and Toddlers Survey (FITS) reportedly consumed diets below the EAR for iron, which for the USA is set lower, at 3 mg/day for this age group [13]. Nevertheless, when the USA cut-off point was used, 8.3% of the SMILE cohort had an average daily iron intake below this level, which remains appreciably higher than that reported in the FITS.

Children in this study who consumed formula, either with or without breastmilk, were unlikely to have inadequate iron intakes. Conn et al. reported a significant difference in the average daily iron intake of breastfed and non-breastfed infants in a younger cohort of children aged 9 months (6.3 mg/day vs. 11.9 mg/day, $p < 0.001$) [7]. Infant formulas are required by law to be fortified with iron, and in our study toddlers consuming formula either in combination with breastmilk or alone received one third to one half of their iron from formula, respectively. On the other hand, while the iron in breastmilk is highly absorbable, the overall levels are low [26] and breastmilk contributed only 3% of the total iron intake in those who were breastfed and not consuming formula. The Euro-Growth study investigated the determinants of iron status in 12-month-old infants and reported that the most important factor positively associated with iron status was the duration of feeding of iron-fortified formula [27].

Foods that children transition to are often poor sources of iron or they may consume low amounts of those foods which are rich in iron [9]. For instance, Byrne et al. reported that the median intake of meat and alternatives amongst a group of Australian toddlers aged 12–16 months was 56 g/day and one quarter had intakes of 28 g/day or less, which is well below the recommended daily intake for this age group of a single 65 g serve of this food group [28]. A low intake of this food group, which is the primary source of iron in the diets of toddlers, is likely to be more of an issue for breastfed toddlers than those who continue to consume appreciable amounts of either infant or toddler formula. Almost one half of children who were breastfed and not consuming formula and one third of children who were not consuming either formula or breastmilk had iron intakes below the EAR, compared with less than 5% of children consuming formula.

While roughly one in ten of all children had calcium and thiamin intakes below the EAR, almost one third of children who were breastfed without receiving formula failed to meet the EAR for both these nutrients. Children from the other milk feeding groups were significantly less likely than those in the breastfed only group to fail to meet the EAR for calcium and thiamin. As with iron, formula contributed a larger proportion of the overall intake of both calcium (50%) and thiamin (36%) in the formula only group than did breastmilk (28% and 11%, respectively) in the breastmilk-only group. This finding is partly explained by the fact that the formula group consumed on average more formula (443 g) than the breastmilk group consumed breastmilk (352 g), and that formula is typically fortified with vitamins and minerals at levels which exceed the highly variable levels of these nutrients found in breastmilk.

The primary limitations of this study are that usual intake of nutrients was estimated by summing and averaging the three days of intake, though this method does not adjust for the day-to-day variability in intake within individuals, which can be achieved with the use of specialist software that was not available to the researchers [29]. Nevertheless, this method is likely to provide more reliable estimates of usual nutrient intake than estimates derived from a single 24 h recall. While less than half of the mothers returned complete dietary data on the intake of their child, the deliberate oversampling of participants from disadvantaged groups means that the sample of women and children in this study are generally representative of the population from which they were drawn.

5. Conclusions

This is one of the first studies to report the contribution of breastmilk and formula to the diets of Australian children as they transition to family foods at the beginning of their second year of life. While the majority of children had intakes which met or exceeded their nutrient requirements, those children who consumed breastmilk only as their milk feed were at greater risk of having intakes below the EAR for iron, calcium and thiamin. This finding should, however, be interpreted with caution and women should continue to be encouraged to breastfeed their children beyond 12 months of age. However, it is possible that breastfeeding mothers may have a misplaced faith in the nutritional superiority of breastmilk over formula and cow's milk as they transition to the family meal. All mothers, regardless of the milk they feed their child, must be educated and encouraged to feed their infant a varied and high-quality diet with adequate serves of the core food groups. In particular, health professionals should advise mothers of the importance of incorporating iron- and calcium-rich complementary foods into their child's diets, both of which are important nutrients required for adequate growth and development of toddlers.

Supplementary Materials: The following is available online at http://www.mdpi.com/2072-6643/8/8/501/s1: Table S1 Comparison of characteristics of participants and non-participants and South Australian pregnancy outcome data for 2013.

Acknowledgments: The SMILE study was supported by a National Health and Medical Research Council Project Grant (APP: 1046219). These funds were not used to cover the costs of this open access publication. We would like to acknowledge Courtney Mizen and Tanya Coelho who assisted with entry of dietary records.

Author Contributions: L.D., J.S. and D.H. conceived and designed the SMILE cohort study; K.D. and E.A. entered and analyzed the data; G.D. wrote the data entry protocol and supervised the data entry; J.S. planned and supervised the analysis of the data and wrote the paper. All authors contributed to the interpretation of results and writing the manuscript, and read and approved the final version.

Conflicts of Interest: The authors declare no conflict of interest. The funding sponsors had no role in the design of the study; in the collection, analyses, or interpretation of data; in the writing of the manuscript, and in the decision to publish the results.

Abbreviations

The following abbreviations are used in this manuscript:

AIFG	Australian Infant Feeding Guidelines
CI	Confidence interval
EAR	Estimated average requirement
IRSAD	Index of Relative Socio-Economic Advantage and Disadvantage
NRV	Nutrient reference value
OR	Odds ratio
RE	Retinol equivalents
UL	Upper level of intake

Appendix A

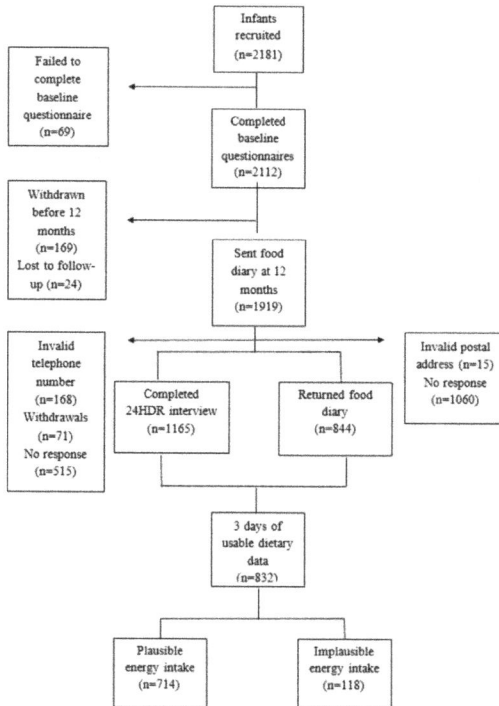

Figure A1. Participant Flow Chart.

1. National Health and Medical Research Council. *Infant Feeding Guidelines*; National Health and Medical Research Council: Canberra, Australia, 2012.
2. WHO/UNICEF. *Global Strategy for Infant and Young Child Feeding*; World Health Organization: Geneva, Switzerland, 2003.
3. Victora, C.G.; Bahl, R.; Barros, A.J.; França, G.V.; Horton, S.; Krasevec, J.; Murch, S.; Sankar, M.J.; Walker, N.; Rollins, N.C.; et al. Breastfeeding in the 21st century: Epidemiology, mechanisms, and lifelong effect. *Lancet* **2016**, *387*, 475–490. [CrossRef]
4. Australian Institute of Health and Welfare. *2010 Australian National Infant Feeding Survey: Indicator Results*; Cat. No. PHE 156; AIHW: Canberra, Australia, 2011.
5. Australian Bureau of Statistics and Food Standards Australia and New Zealand. *4364.0.55.008—Australian Health Survey: Usual Nutrient Intakes, 2011–2012*; Australian Bureau of Statistics: Canberra, Australia, 2015.
6. Commonwealth Scientific Industrial Research Organisation (CSIRO) Preventative Health National Research Flagship and the University of South Australia. *2007 Australian National Children's Nutrition and Physical Activity Survey: Main Findings*; Commonwealth of Australia: Canberra, Australia, 2008.
7. Conn, J.A.; Davies, M.J.; Walker, R.B.; Moore, V.M. Food and nutrient intakes of 9-month-old infants in Adelaide, Australia. *Public Health Nutr.* **2009**, *12*, 2448–2456. [CrossRef] [PubMed]
8. Atkins, L.A.; McNaughton, S.A.; Campbell, K.J.; Szymlek-Gay, E.A. Iron intakes of Australian infants and toddlers: Findings from the Melbourne Infant Feeding, Activity and Nutrition Trial (InFANT) Program. *Br. J. Nutr.* **2016**, *115*, 285–293. [CrossRef] [PubMed]
9. Byrne, R.; Magarey, A.; Daniels, L. Food and beverage intake in Australian children aged 12–16 months participating in the NOURISH and SAIDI studies. *Aust. N. Z. J. Public Health* **2014**, *38*, 326–331. [CrossRef] [PubMed]
10. Lioret, S.; Cameron, A.J.; McNaughton, S.A.; Crawford, D.; Spence, A.C.; Hesketh, K.; Campbell, K.J. Association between maternal education and diet of children at 9 months is partially explained by mothers' diet. *Matern. Child Nutr.* **2015**, *11*, 936–947. [CrossRef] [PubMed]
11. Kavian, F.; Scott, J.; Perry, R.; Byrne, R.; Magarey, A. Assessing dietary intake and growth of infants. *Matern. Paediatr. Nutr. J.* **2015**, *1*, 101.
12. Webb, K.L.; Lahti-Koski, M.; Rutishauser, I.; Hector, D.J.; Knezevic, N.; Gill, T.; Peat, J.K.; Leeder, S.R.; CAPS Team. Consumption of 'extra' foods (energy-dense, nutrient-poor) among children aged 16–24 months from western Sydney, Australia. *Public Health Nutr.* **2007**, *9*, 1035. [CrossRef]
13. Butte, N.F.; Fox, M.K.; Briefel, R.R.; Siega-Riz, A.M.; Dwyer, J.T.; Deming, D.M.; Reidy, K.C. Nutrient intakes of US infants, toddlers, and preschoolers meet or exceed dietary reference intakes. *J. Am. Diet. Assoc.* **2010**, *110*, S27–S37. [CrossRef] [PubMed]
14. Lennox, A.; Sommerville, J.; Ong, K.; Henderson, H.; Allen, R. Diet and Nutrition Survey of Infants and Young Children, 2011, 2013. Available online: http://webarchive.nationalarchives.gov.uk/20130402145952/http://transparency.dh.gov.uk/2013/03/13/dnsiyc-2011/ (accessed on 18 March 2016).
15. Smithers, L.G.; Brazionis, L.; Golley, R.K.; Mittinty, M.N.; Northstone, K.; Emmett, P.; McNaughton, S.A.; Campbell, K.J.; Lynch, J.W. Associations between dietary patterns at 6 and 15 months of age and sociodemographic factors. *Eur. J. Clin. Nutr.* **2012**, *66*, 658–666. [CrossRef] [PubMed]
16. National Health and Medical Research Council and Ministry of Health. *Nutrient Reference Values for Australia and New Zealand*; NHMRC: Canberra, Australia, 2005.
17. Do, L.; Scott, J.; Thomson, W.; Stamm, J.W.; Rugg-Gunn, A.J.; Levy, S.M.; Wong, C.; Devenish, G.; Ha, D.H.; Spencer, A.J. Common risk factor approach to address socioeconomic inequality in the oral health of preschool children—A prospective cohort study. *BMC Public Health* **2014**, *14*, 429. [CrossRef] [PubMed]
18. Australian Bureau of Statistics. 4363.0.55.001—Australian Health Survey: Users' Guide, 2011–2013. 24-h Dietary Recall 2014. Available online: http://www.abs.gov.au/ausstats/abs@.nsf/Lookup/0D6B1FE95EAB8FF3CA257CD2001CA113?opendocument (accessed on 18 March 2016).
19. Food Standards Australia and New Zealand. Ausnut 2011–2013. Australian Food, Supplement and Nutrient Database 2015. Available online: http://www.foodstandards.gov.au/science/monitoringnutrients/ausnut/pages/default.aspx (accessed on 18 November 2015).

20. Kent, J.C.; Mitoulas, L.; Cox, D.B.; Owens, R.A.; Hartmann, P.E. Breast volume and milk production during extended lactation in women. *Exp. Physiol.* **1999**, *84*, 435–447. [CrossRef] [PubMed]

21. Scheil, W.; Jolly, K.; Scott, J.; Catcheside, B.; Sage, L.; Kennare, R. *Pregnancy Outcome in South Australia 2013*; Pregnancy Outcome Unit SA Health, Ed.; Government of South Australia: Adelaide, Australia, 2015.

22. World Health Organization. *International Code of Marketing of Breast-Milk Substitutes*; WHO: Geneva, Switzerland, 1981.

23. Berry, N.J.; Jones, S.C.; Iverson, D. Toddler milk advertising in Australia: Infant formula advertising in disguise? *Australas. Market. J.* **2012**, *20*, 24–27. [CrossRef]

24. Cattaneo, A.; Pani, P.; Carletti, C.; Guidetti, M.; Mutti, V.; Guidetti, C.; Knowles, A. Advertisements of follow-on formula and their perception by pregnant women and mothers in Italy. *Arch. Dis. Child.* **2015**, *100*, 323–328. [CrossRef] [PubMed]

25. Department of Health. *Dietary Reference Values for Food Energy and Nutrients for the United Kingdom*; HMSO: London, UK, 1991.

26. Mcmillan, J.A.; Landaw, S.A.; Oski, F.A. Iron sufficiency in breast-fed infants and the availability of iron from human milk. *Pediatrics* **1976**, *58*, 686–691. [PubMed]

27. Male, C.; Persson, L.A.; Freeman, V.; Guerra, A.; van't Hof, M.A.; Haschke, F.; Euro-Growth Iron Study Group. Prevalence of iron deficiency in 12-mo-old infants from 11 European areas and influence of dietary factors on iron status (Euro-Growth study). *Acta Paediatr.* **2001**, *90*, 492–498. [CrossRef] [PubMed]

28. National Health and Medical Research Council. Eat for Health Educator Guide. National Health and Medical Research Council: Canberra, Australia, 2013. Available online: https://www.nhmrc.gov.au/_files_nhmrc/publications/attachments/n55b_educator_guide_140321.pdf (accessed on 26 June 2016).

29. Piernas, C.; Miles, D.R.; Deming, D.M.; Reidy, K.C.; Popkin, B.M. Estimating usual intakes mainly affects the micronutrient distribution among infants, toddlers and pre-schoolers from the 2012 Mexican National Health and Nutrition Survey. *Public Health Nutr.* **2016**, *19*, 1017–1026. [CrossRef] [PubMed]

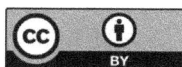

nutrients

MDPI

Article

Compliance with WHO IYCF Indicators and Dietary Intake Adequacy in a Sample of Malaysian Infants Aged 6–23 Months

Geok Lin Khor [1,*], Sue Yee Tan [1], Kok Leong Tan [1], Pauline S. Chan [2] and Maria Sofia V. Amarra [2]

[1] Department of Nutrition and Dietetics, International Medical University, Kuala Lumpur 57000, Malaysia; sueyee_tan@imu.edu.my (S.Y.T.); kokleong_tan@imu.edu.my (K.L.T.)
[2] International Life Sciences Institute South East Asia Region, Singapore 238959, Singapore; paulinechan@ilsisea.org.sg (P.S.C.); sofiaamarra@ilsisea.org.sg (M.S.V.A.)
* Correspondence: khor.geoklin@gmail.com; Tel.: +60-012-383-4830

Received: 3 October 2016; Accepted: 25 November 2016; Published: 1 December 2016

Abstract: Background: The 2010 World Health Organisation (WHO) Infant and Young Child Feeding (IYCF) indicators are useful for monitoring feeding practices. Methods: A total sample of 300 subjects aged 6 to 23 months was recruited from urban suburbs of Kuala Lumpur and Putrajaya. Compliance with each IYCF indicator was computed according to WHO recommendations. Dietary intake based on two-day weighed food records was obtained from a sub-group ($N = 119$) of the total sample. The mean adequacy ratio (MAR) value was computed as an overall measure of dietary intake adequacy. Contributions of core IYCF indicators to MAR were determined by multinomial logistic regression. Results: Generally, the subjects showed high compliance for (i) timely introduction of complementary foods at 6 to 8 months (97.9%); (ii) minimum meal frequency among non-breastfed children aged 6 to 23 months (95.2%); (iii) consumption of iron-rich foods at 6 to 23 months (92.3%); and minimum dietary diversity (78.0%). While relatively high proportions achieved the recommended intake levels for protein (87.4%) and iron (71.4%), lower proportions attained the recommendations for calcium (56.3%) and energy (56.3%). The intake of micronutrients was generally poor. The minimum dietary diversity had the greatest contribution to MAR (95% CI: 3.09, 39.87) ($p = 0.000$) among the core IYCF indicators. Conclusion: Malaysian urban infants and toddlers showed moderate to high compliance with WHO IYCF indicators. The robustness of the analytical approach in this study in quantifying contributions of IYCF indicators to MAR should be further investigated.

Keywords: infant and young child feeding; dietary adequacy; core complementary feeding indicators; micronutrients; dietary diversity

1. Introduction

Culture- and age-appropriate infant and young child feeding (IYCF) practices are well recognized as imperative for child health and survival. In 2008, the World Health Organization (WHO) recommended a set of population-level breastfeeding practices and food-related aspects of child feeding practices appropriate for children aged 6 to 23 months [1]. The questionnaire comprises eight core indicators and seven optional indicators of feeding practices, and offers the advantage of inter-country comparisons of IYCF practices.

In examining indicators of infant and young child feeding practices using data from Demographic and Health Surveys (DHS) of 46 countries between 2002 and 2008, Lutter et al. [2] reported that: (i) few infants and young children benefited from optimal complementary feeding practices; and (ii) less than one-third and only 21% of children aged 6 to 23 months met the minimum criteria for dietary diversity and received a minimum acceptable diet, respectively. Based on India's National Family Health Survey

(2005–2006), involving over 18,000 children aged zero to 23.9 months, Menon et al. [3] reported overall poor status of IYCF practices, especially indicators for complementary feeding, with 16% and 9% complying with minimum dietary diversity and minimum acceptable diet, respectively. A similar finding was reported by Marriot et al. [4], in assessing the WHO IYCF indicators of 14 low-income countries in Africa and Asia. The mean minimum dietary diversity adherence was found low, ranging from 11.3% for ages 6 to 11 months to 25.1% among those aged 18–23 months. The low prevalence of dietary diversity was reflected in poor compliance with minimum acceptable diet which was only 7.7% for infants 6 to 11 months of age and 16.3% for those aged 18–23 months. These recent reviews indicate room for improvement in young child feeding practices in low- to middle-income countries.

The International Life Sciences Institute of Southeast Asia region (ILSI SEA) Expert Panel on Infant and Young Child Nutrition, at its meeting in 2012, highlighted the importance for the region to undertake country-specific assessment of the IYCF indicators in association with measured dietary intakes and nutritional status of infants and young children [5]. In this respect, Cambodia, Indonesia, Philippines and Vietnam have periodic updates on IYCF practices, as reported by Demographic and Health Surveys (DHS) and/or Multiple Indicator Cluster Surveys (MICS) for these countries.

Malaysia is not covered by either the DHS or MICs, and relies instead on its National Health and Morbidity Surveys (NHMS) for IYCF data, such as the Third NHMS undertaken in 2006 [6] and the just-completed 2016 NHMS. There are concerns for inadequate feeding practices in Malaysia in view of recent findings of rather high prevalence of stunting and underweight among young children. Stunting among urban children nationwide was reported at 23.9% in ages 0.5–0.9 years [7], and underweight was reported at 19.6% among children aged 0–4 years [8]. Over-reliance on milk, leading to a lack of dietary diversity, was reported among Malaysian urban children aged one to three years [9]. Hence, this study was undertaken to assess the quality of young child feeding practices and dietary intake adequacy in a sample of infants and toddlers.

2. Methodology

This cross-sectional study was undertaken with the following objectives:

2.1. Objectives

1. To estimate the prevalence of compliance with the WHO IYCF indicators in a total sample of 300 infants and toddlers aged 6.0–23.9 months;
2. To determine dietary intake using a two-day weighed food records of a sub-group of infants and toddlers ($N = 119$), matched for age and sex with the total sample, with dietary intake adequacy computed as the mean adequacy ratio (MAR);
3. To determine the contributions of the WHO core complementary feeding indicators to the MAR values of the sub-group of subjects.

2.2. Subjects

The inclusion criteria for the selection of the study subjects were:

- Infants and children aged 6.0 to 23.9 months
- Malay ethnicity
- Families residing in the urban suburbs of Kuala Lumpur and Putrajaya
- Subjects attending licensed child care centers (registered with the Social Welfare Department of the Ministry of Women, Family and Community Development (Licensed child care centers are obliged to adhere to government regulations including caregiver to child ratio, standards of hygiene and menu guidelines.))
- Consent of the child care center management and parents/caregivers

The exclusion criteria were:

- Mentally or physically disabled infants and children
- Ill at the time of data collection
- Having dietary restrictions

The rationale for including only Malay infants and children of families from urban areas is to minimize the influence of cultural and socio-economic factors on feeding practices of infants and toddlers. Malay is the predominant ethnicity of the Malaysian population.

2.3. Total Sample Size for Determining Compliance with IYCF Indicators

The total sample size was estimated according to the guidelines of the WHO "Indicators for assessing infant and young child feeding practices [1] (Part 2 Measurements). Based on assuming an indicator estimate of 50% and a 95% confidence interval, a minimum number of 225 infants and young children aged 6.0–23.9 months was recommended. It was decided to have a total sample size of 300 subjects in case of dropouts and incomplete questionnaires. Data collection was carried out in 2013–2014.

A list of the licensed child care centers was compiled from various sources including the Association of Registered Care Providers of Selangor and the Ministry of Health Nutrition Division. The child care centers were contacted through emails and phone calls. Out of approximately 100 centers, about one-fifth gave permission for the conduct of this study. Using the snow-ball approach in going from one center to the next, approximately 100 infants and children who met the inclusion criteria were recruited for each of these age groups: 6.0–11.9 months, 12.0–17.9 months and 18.0–23.9 months, with almost an equal proportion of males and females in each age group. As the participants were recruited by convenience sampling, they are not deemed as representative of urban Malay toddlers.

The WHO IYCF indicators questionnaire was translated to the Malay language and pretested before use on five Malay mothers. This is to improve the language, technical contents and length of time used for the interview. Calculation for compliance with each IYCF indicator was in accordance with the formula recommended by WHO [1] (Part 2 Measurements).

2.4. Sub-Group of Toddlers for Two-Day Weighed Food Records and Compliance with Core Complementary Feeding

Only a sub-group of subjects was included for the two-day weighed food records part of the study, given that weighing of food intake was time-consuming. The sub-group of subjects was matched for age and sex to the total sample. In this way, the sub-sample comprised approximately 40 subjects in each of the three age groups of 6.0–11.9 months, 12.0–17.9 months and 18.0–23.9 months, making a total of 120 subjects. This age disaggregation is in accordance with the recommendation for studying the core complementary feeding indicators [1]. Each of the age groups consisted of approximately an equal proportion of male and female subjects. At the end, 119 subjects were included as one questionnaire was found to be incomplete.

Trained research assistants with at least a bachelor-level qualification in nutrition or dietetics carried out the weighing of food intake for two days when the child was in the center from about 7 a.m. until 5 p.m., Monday to Friday. All foods consumed were weighed for two consecutive weekdays but not on a weekend, as the day care centers are closed during the weekends.

For solid or semi-solid foods, the research assistants prepared a duplicate plate of the food items that were given to the child. The individual items were weighed using a kitchen scale that has a weight capacity of 2 kg and a weight graduation of 1 gm (TANITA-KD160WH). The amounts not consumed by the child were deducted from the total amounts weighed. The research assistants checked for ingredients used in preparing the food items by asking the center manager or person who prepared the foods or beverages.

For recording food and beverages consumed by children who were fed individually by the center helpers, the research assistants first identified the ingredients used in preparing the food or beverage, and then estimated the amounts of the food/beverage consumed by the child, based on the serving spoon or cup. As the entire procedure of observation, weighing and calculation for each child was time-consuming, a research assistant could complete the procedure for only three to four subjects a day, on average.

Parents/caregivers were instructed to record foods and beverages, in terms of description and quantity, taken by their child from the time he/she was picked up from the child care center until the following morning when the child was brought back to the center. The research assistants checked the forms and sought clarifications from parents/care givers, particularly for the quantities and types of constituents in the food or beverage consumed at home or outside.

3. Statistical Analyses

Compliance with the IYCF indicators was reported in percentage. Dietary intake was computed in terms of percentage of meeting the Malaysian dietary recommendations (Recommended Nutrient Intakes (RNIs) [10]. The mean adequacy ratio (MAR) was used as an overall measure of dietary adequacy. Several studies have reported MAR values to be positively associated with other indexes of dietary quality [4,11]. In order to compute MAR, one has to calculate first the nutrient adequacy ratio (NAR), which is defined as the ratio of a subject's nutrient intake to the recommended nutrient intake (RNI) of the assessed nutrient, appropriate for the age and sex of the subject.

$$\text{NAR} = \text{Actual nutrient intake (per day)/Recommended nutrient intake (RNI)} \qquad (1)$$

The value for MAR is calculated as the total of all the NARs divided by the total expressed as a percentage. MAR has a range from 0% to 100% with 100% as the ideal [12].

$$\text{MAR} = \sum \text{NARs/Total number of nutrients} \qquad (2)$$

For computing MAR, each of the NARs was truncated as 1, so that a high intake of one nutrient could not compensate for the low intake of another nutrient, as originally conceived by Malden et al. [13] and cited by Vieux et al. [14].

Multinomial logistic regression was used to assess the odds of compliance with the core complementary feeding indicators as the nominal independent variable, and MAR values as the dependent variable. All analyses were performed with SPSS version 22.0 (SPSS Inc., Chicago, IL, USA). A level of <0.05 was set for statistical significance.

Ethics Approval and Consent

The study proposal was approved by the Joint Committee on Research and Ethics of the International Medical University, Kuala Lumpur, Malaysia on 23 September 2013. (Project ID No. IMU R 123/2013). The Study Information Sheet and Written Consent Form in the Malay and English language were also approved by the IMU ethics committee. The Study Information Sheet comprised the following information: What is the purpose of this research? Why you are invited to this research? What is involved in this research? Is there any danger? How does this research help me? Contact persons for further information. After we had explained the information to the parents, one of them signed the Written Consent Form allowing their child to participate in the study.

4. Results

4.1. Total Sample Compliance with IYCF Indicators (N = 300)

The total sample size of 300 children consisted of 105 subjects aged 6.0–11.9 months, 87 aged 12.0–17.9 months, and 98 aged 18.0–23.9 months, with about an equal proportion of male and female subjects in each age group. These children were from young families with mothers having an average age of 30.9 ± 0.3 years, and with 1.4 ± 0.1 of children aged three years or less per family, on average.

Out of the WHO set of 15 IYCF indicators, data was collected for 12 indicators only, as the other three indicators referred to feeding practices for infants aged from zero to under 6 months, whereas these study subjects were aged 6.0–23.9 months. The subjects showed high compliance for several of the assessed indicators, namely (i) Children ever breastfed (99.3%); (ii) Timely introduction of complementary foods at 6–8 months (97.9%); (iii) Minimum meal frequency among non-breastfed children aged 6–23 months (95.2%); and (iv) Consumption of iron-rich foods at 6–23 months (92.3%) (Table 1). In contrast, the other indicators were achieved by relatively lower proportions of the subjects, and these include indicators related to breastfeeding beyond 6 months of age: (i) Continued breastfeeding at 2 years (38.3%); (ii) Continued breastfeeding at 1 year (57.1%); and (iii) Age-appropriate breastfeeding among children aged 6–23 months receiving breast milk as well as solids in the previous day (55.9%).

The minimum acceptable diet indicator was also found to have relatively low compliance among the non-breastfed children (39.5%) and breastfed children (50.6%). The minimum acceptable diet indicator combines compliance with the minimum dietary diversity and minimum meal frequency indicators. Actually, the subjects showed quite high compliance with meeting the latter two indicators separately, which is 78% for minimum dietary diversity, and 95.2% and 69.3% for minimum meal frequency among non-breastfed and breastfed children, respectively. However, in computing the minimum acceptable diet indicator for non-breastfed subjects, the formula includes the criteria of receiving two milk feeds, in addition to meeting the criteria for dietary diversity and meal frequency; moreover, the dairy group is excluded when calculating dietary diversity to avoid "double counting" [1] (WHO Part 2 Measurements). Consequently, the acceptable diet formula becomes more stringent to attain, resulting in a relatively lower prevalence of compliance among the non-breastfed.

Table 1. Compliance (%) with WHO IYCF indicators [1] (WHO, 2010) by total sample (*N* = 300).

Core Indicators	% (*N*) *
1. Early initiation of breastfeeding	
Proportion of children born in the last 24 months who were put to the breast within one hour of birth	76.3 (300)
2. Exclusive breastfeeding under 6 months	-
3. Continued breastfeeding at 1 year	
Proportion of children aged 12–15 months who are fed breast milk during the previous day	57.1 (56)
4. Timely introduction of solid, semi-solid or soft foods	
Proportion of infants aged 6–8 months who receive solid, semi-solid or soft foods during the previous day	97.9 (47)
5. Minimum dietary diversity	
Proportion of children aged 6–23 months who received foods from 4 or more food groups during the previous day	78.0 (300)
6. Minimum meal frequency	
Breastfed children: Proportion of breastfed children aged 6–23 months who received solid, semi-solid, or soft foods the minimum number of times or more during the previous day	69.3 (163)
Non-breastfed children: Proportion of children aged 6–23 months who received solid, semi-solid or soft foods or milk feeds the minimum number of times or more during the previous day	95.2 (125)
Total:	80.6 (288)

Table 1. *Cont.*

7. Minimum acceptable diet	
Breastfed children: Proportion of children aged 6–23 months who had at least a minimum dietary diversity and the minimum meal frequency during the previous day	50.6 (166)
Non-breastfed children: Proportion of children aged 6–23 months who received at least 2 milk feedings and had at least the minimum dietary diversity and the minimum meal frequency during the previous day	39.5 (129)
Total:	45.8 (295)
8. Consumption of iron-rich or iron-fortified foods	
Proportion of children aged 6–23 months who receive an iron-rich food or iron-fortified food that is specially designed for infants and young children, or that is fortified in the home during the previous day	92.3 (298)
Optional Indicators	
9. Children ever breastfed	
Proportion of children born in the last 24 months who were ever breastfed	99.3 (300)
10. Continued breastfeeding at 2 years	
Proportion of children aged 20–23 months who received breast milk during the previous day	38.3 (47)
11. Age-appropriate breastfeeding	-
Proportion of children aged 6–23 months who received breast milk, as well as solid, semi-solid or soft foods during the previous day	55.9 (161)
12. Predominant breastfeeding under 6 months (0–5.9 months)	-
13. Duration of breastfeeding (0–5.9 months)	-
14. Bottle feeding	
Proportion of children aged 0–23 months who are fed with a bottle during the previous day	80.4 (296) **
15. Milk feeding frequency for non-breastfed children	
Proportion of non-breastfed children 6–23 months of age who received at least 2 milk feedings during the previous day	91.3 (127)

* Number of eligible subjects; ** Age studied 6.0–23.9 months.

4.2. Compliance with Core Complementary Feeding Indicators by Sub-Group (N = 119)

Compliance with four of the five core indicators for complementary feeding was investigated among the sub-group of subjects, as only a small number ($N = 13$) of subjects (aged 6 to 8 months) was eligible for computing the indicator on "Timely introduction of solids", which was hence excluded. The sub-group showed generally high compliance with the core complementary feeding indicators (Table 2). There was high compliance with (i) Timely introduction of solid, semi-solid or soft foods (92.3%); (ii) Consumption of iron-rich foods (92.4%); (iii) Minimum meal frequency among both breastfed and non-breastfed children aged 6–23 months (91.7% and 85.5%, respectively); as well as (iv) Minimum dietary diversity (83.2%). A low prevalence for the minimum acceptable diet indicator for non-breastfed (34.6%) and breastfed (68.8%) infants was recorded for the sub-group.

Table 2. Compliance (%) with WHO core complementary feeding indicators by sub-group (*N* = 119).

* Core Complementary Feeding Indicators	Compliance% (*N*)
Minimum dietary diversity	83.2 (119)
Minimum meal frequency	
Breastfed	85.5 (62)
Non-breastfed	91.7 (48)
Minimum acceptable diet	
Breastfed	68.8 (64)
Non-breastfed	34.6 (52)
Consumption of iron-rich or iron-fortified foods	92.4 (119)

* Timely introduction of solid, semi-solid or soft foods indicator was excluded owing to the small number of subjects who were eligible (*N* = 13 aged 6 to 8 months).

4.3. Dietary Intake Adequacy of Sub-Group (N = 119)

Based on the two-day weighed food intake, dietary intake adequacy was computed and described as meeting the Malaysian recommendations for energy and nutrient intake (RNI) [10]. The nutrient adequacy ratio (NAR) value exceeded 1.0 for energy, protein, calcium and iron, indicating that their intakes achieved more than 100% of the recommended levels (RNIs) (Table 3). Mean iron and protein intake were double the RNI recommendation levels, while those for energy and calcium exceeded 100%. The likely dietary sources for these nutrients were animal food including milk, chicken meat, fish and eggs. As for the NAR values for the rest of the nutrients, they ranged from 0.50 for vitamin A to 0.84 for zinc, denoting intake of these nutrients met 50% to 84% of the RNIs, respectively. Relatively high proportions of the subjects achieved the RNI for protein (87.4%) and iron (71.4%), while just over half managed to do so for calcium (56.3%) and energy (56.3%). The proportions of the subjects meeting the rest of the micronutrients were low and these include vitamin A, thiamin, vitamin C niacin, riboflavin and zinc. This finding suggests that the subjects were not consuming sufficient vegetables, fruits, legumes and whole grains.

Table 3. Energy and nutrient intake adequacy (*N* = 119).

Dietary Intake [†]	Percentage of the Recommended Nutrient Intake (RNI) Achieved % ± SD	[a] Nutrient Adequacy Ratio (NAR) Value Mean ± SE
energy	110.7 ± 49.2	1.14 ± 0.05
protein	202.8 ± 101.9	2.07 ± 0.10
calcium	127.5 ± 92.6	1.32 ± 0.10
iron [b]	216.7 ± 181.2	2.44 ± 0.21
zinc	75.7 ± 70.2	0.84 ± 0.10
thiamin	47.6 ± 34.6	0.55 ± 0.06
riboflavin	76.0 ± 51.5	0.82 ± 0.06
niacin	66.5 ± 53.5	0.77 ± 0.07
vitamin C	41.5 ± 39.7	0.57 ± 0.07
vitamin A	42.2 ± 39.6	0.50 ± 0.06
[c] Mean adequacy ratio (MAR)		0.67 ± 0.02

[†] based on two-day weighed food record; [a] NAR for a given nutrient is the ratio of a subject's nutrient intake to the recommended nutrient intake of the assessed nutrient, appropriate for the age and sex of the subject; [b] based on 15% bioavailability; [c] Mean adequacy ratio (MAR) was calculated as the total of all the NARs ($\sum$ NAR for energy and nine nutrients) divided by the total, expressed as a percentage.

For this study, it was arbitrarily decided to compute NAR for energy and nutrients taken by the subjects that met at least 40% of the Malaysian RNIs. Hence, NAR was determined for energy and the following nine nutrients: protein, calcium, iron, zinc, vitamin A, vitamin C, thiamin, riboflavin and niacin. The value for MAR was then calculated as $\sum$ NARs divided by the total (10 in this case) expressed as a percentage.

Overall, the mean adequacy ratio (MAR) value computed was 0.67, indicating that the dietary intake of the subjects met, on average, 67% of the combined RNIs for energy and the nine nutrients under consideration in this study.

4.4. Contributions of Core Complementary Feeding Indicators to Dietary Intake Adequacy (N = 119)

Multinomial logistic regression was used to determine the contributions of the four WHO core complementary feeding indicators as the independent variables to dietary intake adequacy based on MAR values as the dependent variables. Since MAR = 0.67 was generated from the weighed dietary intake in this study, MAR > 0.6 was selected for comparison with MAR $\leq$ 0.5. Among the core complementary feeding indicators, minimum dietary diversity contributed highest to dietary intake adequacy (OR 11.10; 95% CI: 3.09, 39.87) (p = 0.000) (Table 4). The other core complementary feeding indicators showed lower odds of contributing to intake adequacy for the same MAR values. The minimum dietary diversity indicator also showed the highest odds of leading to dietary intake adequacy (OR 5.49; 95% CI: 1.35, 22.22) (p = 0.017) with MAR set at a lower level of (0.5 < MAR $\leq$ 0.6) that is, overall dietary adequacy between 50.1% and 60% (Table 4). Hence, these results suggest that, for this sample of Malaysian urban toddlers, compliance with minimum dietary diversity is of key importance towards attaining dietary intake adequacy.

Table 4. Contributions of WHO core complementary feeding indicators to dietary intake adequacy (N = 119) [†].

Dietary Intake Adequacy Based on Mean Adequacy Ratio (MAR)	Minimum Dietary Diversity	Minimum Meal Frequency	Minimum Acceptable Diet	Consumption of Iron-Rich/Fortified Food
	Odds Ratio (95% CI)			
[b] MAR > 0.6 (more than 60.0%)	11.10 (3.09, 39.87), p = 0.000	6.70 (1.44, 31.16), p = 0.015	4.03 (1.17, 13.87), p = 0.027	2.73 (0.45, 16.48), p = 0.273
0.5 < [a] MAR $\leq$ 0.6 (50.1%–60.0%)	5.49 (1.35, 22.22), p = 0.017	1.60 (0.35, 7.30), p = 0.544	2.96 (0.75, 11.67), p = 0.121	1.33 (0.20, 9.00), p = 0.768

Above results generated using multinomial logistic regression whereby the reference category is MAR $\leq$ 0.5; [†] Dietary adequacy defined as meeting the combined RNIs for energy and nine nutrients (protein, calcium, iron, zinc, vitamin A, vitamin C, thiamin, riboflavin and niacin); NAR = 10 Nutrient adequacy ratio (NAR) for a given nutrient is the ratio of a subject's intake to the current recommended nutrient intake of the assessed nutrient, appropriate for the age and sex of the subject. Mean adequacy ratio (MAR) is the total of all the NARs ($\sum$ NAR for energy and nine nutrients) divided by the 10, expressed as a percentage; 0.5 < [a] MAR $\leq$ 0.6: meeting between 50.1% to 60.0% of the combined RNIs for the 10 NARs; [b] MAR > 0.6: meeting more than 60% of the combined RNIs for the 10 NARs.

5. Discussion

In a sample of urban Malaysian infants and toddlers aged 6 to 23 months, this study highlighted (i) moderate rates of continued breastfeeding beyond 6 months of age; (ii) high proportions of compliance with timely introduction of complementary foods and receiving iron-rich foods; and (iii) moderate to low proportions met the acceptable diet indicator (minimum dietary diversity and minimum meal frequency). Achieving the indicator on acceptable diet is important as it reflects compliance with both the qualitative and quantitative aspects of complementary feeding. Studies have well documented the significant relationships between attaining a minimum acceptable diet and child nutritional status. In assessing the WHO IYCF indicators of 14 low-income countries in Africa and Asia, Marriot et al. [4] found children consuming a minimum acceptable diet had a significantly lower overall probability of being underweight and stunted. Based on India's National Family Health Survey (2005–2006), involving over 18,000 children aged zero to 23.9 months, Menon et al. [3] showed the acceptable diet indicator as a strong predictor of stunting and underweight.

Dietary intake adequacy in terms of MARs was shown to be influenced most by the minimum dietary diversity indicator. This finding is in line with growing global evidence of the usefulness of dietary diversity in predicting dietary quality, including micronutrient intake adequacy among infants and young children [12,15–17]. In evaluating cross-country patterns based on DHS data, Jones et al. [18] reported that achieving minimum dietary diversity reduced the odds of stunting among children in India, Bangladesh and Zambia. Data from the 2007 Bangladesh Demographic and Health Survey of 1508 children aged 6 to 23 months also showed that those who achieved minimum dietary diversity had a significantly higher height for their age [19]. Nguyen et al. [20] reported a strong positive association between maternal and child dietary diversity in Bangladesh, Vietnam and Ethiopia, and hence advocated the measurement of both maternal and child dietary diversity. A low dietary diversity score was significantly associated with poor nutritional status of indigenous children in Malaysia [21]. A lack of dietary diversity is often reported in low-income populations as their diets are predominantly based on starchy staples, as animal food sources are costly and may not be readily available.

Countries are encouraged to conduct periodic surveys using the WHO IYCF indicators to enable comparing trends of breastfeeding and complementary feeding practices within countries and among countries, as well as for identifying populations at risk and evaluating the impacts of interventions [18]. Countries in Southeast Asia generally showed higher compliance with timely introduction of complementary foods than that for dietary diversity, meal frequency and acceptable diet (Table 5). These findings suggest that complementary foods are provided in a timely manner, but the diets tend to lack variety and frequency as recommended. Hence, owing to low achievements of dietary diversity and meal frequency, compliance with a minimum acceptable diet is generally low in the region.

Table 5. Comparison of WHO IYCF practices among countries in Southeast Asia *.

Core Complementary Feeding Indicators	Cambodia 2014 DHS	Indonesia 2012 DHS	Philippines 2008 DHS	Vietnam 2013–2014 MICS5	** Malaysia 2013–2014 Present Study
Timely introduction of complementary foods	82	91.0	89	90.7	97.9
Minimum dietary diversity	48.0	58.2	78.7	76.9	78.0
Minimum meal frequency					
breastfed					
Non-breastfed	74.0	61.4	80.7		69.3
Total	68.0	78.7	48.2	90.5	95.2
Minimum acceptable diet					
breastfed	32.0	34.2	68.2	62.4	50.6
Non-breastfed	26.0	43.0	40.5	54.5	39.5
Consumption of iron-rich/iron-fortified foods	75.8	67.5	78.3		92.3

* Cambodia, Indonesia, Philippines and Vietnam covered by Demographic and Health Surveys (DHS) or Multiple Indicators Cluster Surveys (MICS) [22–25]; ** $N = 300$.

Limitations of Study

The relatively small sample size and the homogeneous subjects preclude generalizing the results to other socio-economic and ethnic population groups of Malaysia. As a cross-section study, interpretation of causality of the data is restricted. The accuracy of the results is also limited by the methods of data collection, particularly relying on weighing of foods and food intake recording by parents/caregivers. There may be bias in the selection of subjects using the convenient snow-ball approach. The dietary results obtained should not be extended to children who do not attend licensed day care centers where the menus are based on the recommendations of the Ministry of Health.

6. Conclusions

Continued efforts remain essential for improving feeding practices to ensure adequate and quality complementary feeding in Malaysia and the region. This study provides an analytic approach at examining the contributions of core complementary feeding indicators to dietary intake adequacy. This approach should be validated with larger subject samples from different socio-economic statuses to verify its usefulness at different population levels.

Acknowledgments: The cooperation of the Nutrition Division, Ministry of Health Malaysia, is much appreciated. Grateful appreciation is also expressed to Chua Ee Yin for data entry and statistical analysis. The authors duly acknowledged the funding of the study by the International Life Sciences, Southeast Asia Region (ILSI SEA Region).

Author Contributions: Khor Geok Lin, Pauline Chan and Sofia Amarra conceptualized the initial proposal. Khor Geok Lin, Tan Sue Yee and Tan Kok Leong designed and supervised the study. Khor Geok Lin was responsible for data analysis, drafting and editing the manuscript. All authors read and approved the final manuscript.

Conflicts of Interest: The authors declare no conflict of interest. The views expressed in the article are solely those of the authors and do not reflect the views of their respective institutions.

1. World Health Organization, Department of Child and Adolescent Health and Development. *Indicators for Assessing Infant and Young Child Feeding Practices. Part II: Measurement*; World Health Organization: Geneva, Switzerland, 2010.

2. Lutter, C.K.; Daelmans, B.M.E.G.; de Onis, M.; Kothari, M.T.; Ruel, M.T.; Arimond, M.; Deitchler, M.; Dewey, K.G.; Blossner, M.; Borghi, E. Undernutrition, poor feeding practices, and low coverage of key nutrition interventions. *Pediatrics* **2011**, *128*, e1418–e1427. [CrossRef] [PubMed]

3. Menon, P.; Bamezai, A.; Subandoro, A.; Ayoya, M.A.; Aguayo, V. Age-appropriate infant and young child feeding practices are associated with child nutrition in India: Insights from nationally representative data. *Matern. Child Nutr.* **2015**, *11*, 73–87. [CrossRef] [PubMed]

4. Marriot, B.P.; White, A.J.; Hadden, L.; Davies, J.C.; Wallingford, J.C. World Health Organization (WHO) infant and young child feeding indicators: Associations with growth measures in 14 low-income countries. *Matern. Child Nutr.* **2012**, *8*, 354–370. [CrossRef] [PubMed]

5. Amarra, M.S.V.; Chan, P.M.S. Proceedings of the 3rd Expert Consultation and Planning Meeting on Infant and Young Child Nutrition-(Part 2). *Malays. J. Nutr.* **2013**, *19*, 139–142. [PubMed]

6. Ministry of Health Malaysia, Institute for Public Health (IPH). *The Third National Health and Morbidity Survey (NHMS III) 2006: Nutritional Status of Adults Aged 18 Years and Above*; Ministry of Health Malaysia: Kuala Lumpur, Malaysia, 2008.

7. Poh, B.K.; Ng, B.K.; Haslinda, M.D.S.; Shanita, S.N.; Wong, J.E.; Budin, S.B.; Ruzita, A.B.; Lai, O.N.; Khouw, I.; Norimah, A.K. Nutritional status and dietary intakes of children aged 6 months to 12 years: Findings of the Nutrition Survey of Malaysian Children (SEANUTS Malaysia). *Br. J. Nutr.* **2013**, *110*, S21–S35. [CrossRef] [PubMed]

8. Ministry of Health Malaysia, Institute for Public Health (IPH). *National Health and Morbidity Survey 2011. Non-Communicable Diseases*; Ministry of Health Malaysia: Kuala Lumpur, Malaysia, 2011.

9. Khor, G.L.; Zalilah, M.S.; Sariman, S.; Huang, S.L.M.; Mohamad, M.; Chan, Y.M.; Chin, Y.S.; Barakatun, N.M.Y. Milk drinking patterns among Malaysian urban children of different household income status. *J. Nutr. Health Sci.* **2015**. [CrossRef]

10. Ministry of Health Malaysia, National Coordinating Committee for Food and Nutrition (NCCFN). *Recommended Nutrient Intakes for Malaysia*; Ministry of Health: Putrajaya, Malaysia, 2005.

11. Torheim, L.E.; Ouattara, F.; Diarra, M.M.; Thiam, F.D.; Barikmo, I.; HatlØy, A.; Oshaug, A. Nutrient adequacy and dietary diversity in rural Mali: Association and determinants. *Eur. J. Clin. Nutr.* **2004**, *58*, 594–604. [CrossRef] [PubMed]

12. Steyn, N.P.; Nel, J.; Labadarios, D.; Maunder, E.M.W.; Salome, H.; Kruger, H.S. Which dietary diversity indicator is best to assess micronutrient adequacy in children 1 to 9 years? *Nutrition* **2014**, *30*, 55–60. [CrossRef] [PubMed]

13. Madden, J.P.; Goodman, S.J.; Guthrie, H.A. Validity of the 24-hr. recall. Analysis of data obtained from elderly subjects. *J. Am. Diet. Assoc.* **1976**, *68*, 143–147. [PubMed]

14. Vieux, F.; Soler, L.G.; Touazi, D.; Darmon, N. High nutritional quality is not associated with low greenhouse gas emissions in self-selected diets of French adults. *Am. J. Clin. Nutr.* **2013**, *97*, 569–583. [CrossRef] [PubMed]

15. Arimond, M.; Ruel, M.T. Dietary diversity is associated with child nutritional status: Evidence from 11 demographic and health surveys. *J. Nutr.* **2004**, *134*, 2579–2585. [PubMed]

16. Kennedy, G.L.; Pedro, M.R.; Seghieri, C.; Nantel, G.; Brouwer, I. Dietary diversity score is a useful indicator of micronutrient intake in non-breastfeeding Filipino children. *J. Nutr.* **2007**, *137*, 472–477. [PubMed]

17. Moursi, M.M.; Arimond, M.; Dewey, K.G.; Tre'che, S.; Ruel, M.T.; Delpeuch, F. Dietary diversity is a good predictor of the micronutrient density of the diet of 6- to 23-month-old children in Madagascar. *J. Nutr.* **2008**, *138*, 2448–2453. [CrossRef] [PubMed]

18. Jones, A.D.; Ickes, S.B.; Smith, L.E.; Mbuya, M.N.N.; Chasekwa, B.; Heidkamp, R.A.; Menon, P.; Zongrone, A.A.; Stoltzfus, R.J. World Health Organization infant and young child feeding indicators and their associations with child anthropometry: A synthesis of recent findings. *Matern. Child Nutr.* **2014**, *10*, 1–17. [CrossRef] [PubMed]

19. Zongrone, A.; Winskell, K.; Menon, P. Infant and young child feeding practices and child undernutrition in Bangladesh: Insights from nationally representative data. *Public Health Nutr.* **2010**, *15*, 1697–1704. [CrossRef] [PubMed]

20. Nguyen, P.H.; Avula, R.; Ruel, M.T.; Saha, K.K.; Ali, D.; Tran, L.M.; Frongillo, E.A.; Menon, P.; Rawat, R. Maternal and child dietary diversity are associated in Bangladesh, Vietnam, and Ethiopia. *J. Nutr.* **2013**, *143*, 1176–1183. [CrossRef] [PubMed]

21. Chua, E.Y.; Zalilah, M.S.; Chin, Y.S.; Norhasmah, S. Dietary Diversity is associated with nutritional status of Orang Asli children in Pahang. *Malays. J. Nutr.* **2012**, *18*, 1–13.

22. National Institute of Statistics, Directorate General for Health, ICF International. *Cambodia Demographic and Health Survey, 2014*; National Institute of Public Health, National Institute of Statistics, Directorate General for Health, ORC Macro: Phnom Penh, Cambodia; ICF International: Rockville, MD, USA, 2015.

23. Statistics Indonesia, National Population and Family Planning Board, Ministry of Health, ICF International. *Indonesia Demographic and Health Survey 2012*; Statistics Indonesia, National Population and Family Planning Board, Ministry of Health: Jakarta, Indonesia; ICF International: Calverton, MD, USA, 2013.

24. Philippine Statistics Authority, ICF International. *Philippines National Demographic and Health Survey 2008*; National Statistics Office (NSO): Quezon City, Philippines; ICF Macro: Calverton, MD, USA, 2009.

25. General Statistics Office, The United Nations Children's Fund. *Viet Nam Multiple Indicator Cluster Survey 2014, Final Report*; General Statistics Office: Hanoi, Vietnam; The United Nations Children's Fund: New York, NY, USA, 2015.

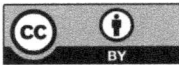

![nutrients logo] *nutrients*

MDPI

Article

Dietary Pattern Trajectories from 6 to 12 Months of Age in a Multi-Ethnic Asian Cohort

Geraldine Huini Lim [1,†], Jia Ying Toh [1,†], Izzuddin M. Aris [1], Ai-Ru Chia [2], Wee Meng Han [3], Seang Mei Saw [4], Keith M. Godfrey [5], Peter D. Gluckman [1,6], Yap-Seng Chong [1,2], Fabian Yap [7,8,9], Yung Seng Lee [1,10,11], Michael S. Kramer [2,12] and Mary Foong-Fong Chong [1,4,13,*]

[1] Singapore Institute for Clinical Sciences (SICS), Agency for Science, Technology and Research (A*STAR), Singapore 117609, Singapore; gerlimhn@gmail.com (G.H.L.); toh_jia_ying@sics.a-star.edu.sg (J.Y.T.); izzuddin_aris@sics.a-star.edu.sg (I.M.A.); pd.gluckman@auckland.ac.nz (P.D.G.); yap_seng_chong@nuhs.edu.sg (Y.-S.C.); yung_seng_lee@nuhs.edu.sg (Y.S.L.)

[2] Department of Obstetrics & Gynaecology, Yong Loo Lin School of Medicine, National University of Singapore, Singapore 119228, Singapore; chiaairu@u.nus.edu (A.-R.C.); michael.kramer@mcgill.ca (M.S.K.)

[3] Department of Nutrition and Dietetics, KK Women's and Children's Hospital, Singapore 229899, Singapore; han.wee.meng@kkh.com.sg

[4] Saw Swee Hock School of Public Health, National University of Singapore, Singapore 117549, Singapore; seang_mei_saw@nuhs.edu.sg

[5] Medical Research Council Lifecourse Epidemiology Unit and National Institute for Health Research Southampton Biomedical Research Centre, University of Southampton and University Hospital Southampton National Health Service Foundation Trust, Southampton SO16 6YD, UK; kmg@mrc.soton.ac.uk

[6] Liggins Institute, University of Auckland, Auckland 1023, New Zealand

[7] Department of Paediatrics, KK Women's and Children's Hospital, Singapore 229899, Singapore; fabian.yap.kp@kkh.com.sg

[8] Department of Paediatrics, Duke-National University of Singapore Graduate Medical School, Singapore 169857, Singapore

[9] Lee Kong Chian School of Medicine, Nanyang Technological University, Singapore 308232, Singapore

[10] Departments of Paediatrics, Yong Loo Lin School of Medicine, National University of Singapore, Singapore 119228, Singapore

[11] Division of Paediatric Endocrinology and Diabetes, Khoo Teck Puat-National University Children's Medical Institute, National University Hospital, National University Health System, Singapore 119074, Singapore

[12] Departments of Pediatrics and of Epidemiology, Biostatistics and Occupational Health, McGill University Faculty of Medicine, Montreal, QC H3A 1A2, Canada

[13] Clinical Nutrition Research Centre, Singapore Institute for Clinical Sciences, Agency for Science, Technology and Research, Singapore 117609, Singapore

* Correspondence: ephmcff@nus.edu.sg; Tel.: +65-6516-4969

† These authors contributed equally to this work.

Received: 28 April 2016; Accepted: 6 June 2016; Published: 15 June 2016

Abstract: Little is known about the dietary patterns of Asian infants in the first year of life, nor of their associations with maternal socio-demographic factors. Based on the Growing Up in Singapore towards healthy Outcomes (GUSTO) mother-offspring cohort, cross-sectional dietary patterns were derived by factor analysis using 24-h recalls and food diaries of infants at 6-, 9- and 12-months of age. Dietary pattern trajectories were modeled by mapping similar dietary patterns across each age using multilevel mixed models. Associations with maternal socio-demographic variables, collected through questionnaires during pregnancy, were assessed using general linear models. In *n* = 486 infants, four dietary pattern trajectories were established from 6- to 12-months. *Predominantly breastmilk:* mainly breastmilk and less formula milk, *Guidelines:* rice porridge, vegetables, fruits and low-fat fish and meat, *Easy-to-prepare foods:* infant cereals, juices, cakes and biscuits and *Noodles (in soup) and seafood:* noodle and common accompaniments. In adjusted models, higher maternal education attainment was correlated with higher start scores on *Predominantly breastmilk,* but lowest education attainment increased its adherence over time. Older mothers had higher start scores on *Easy-to-prepare foods*, but younger mothers had increased adherence over time. Chinese mothers had higher start scores on *Predominantly breastmilk* but greater adherence to *Guidelines* over time, while Indian mothers had higher start scores on *Easy-to-prepare foods* but greater adherence to *Predominantly breastmilk* with time ($p < 0.05$ for all). Changes in trajectories over time were small. Hence, dietary patterns established during weaning are strongly influenced by maternal socio-demographic factors and remain stable over the first year of life.

Keywords: infant dietary patterns; dietary pattern trajectories; first year of life; Asian; factor analysis; multilevel mixed models

---

1. Introduction

Tracking of eating habits through childhood and into adulthood has been observed in different populations [1–4], demonstrating the value of healthful dietary patterns early in life in setting the foundation for life-long eating habits [5]. Thus, besides ensuring an adequate supply of key nutrients and calories to achieve optimal growth, development and health during infancy, the establishment of healthful dietary patterns is also critical.

The importance of healthful dietary patterns during infancy is further supported by recent studies demonstrating associations in infant dietary patterns with growth [6–8] and cognitive outcomes [9,10]. For example, *Health conscious* and *Family foods* dietary patterns, comprising mainly family table foods, at 9-months of age have been related to lower body mass index (BMI) at the same time point [8], while *Discretionary* dietary pattern trajectories, comprising finger foods that are convenient to prepare, from 6 to 24-months appeared have been associated with lower IQ in adolescence [11]. Most of these studies, however, have examined infancy dietary patterns in Caucasian populations and less is known about dietary patterns in Asian infants.

The influence of maternal socio-demographic factors in shaping infancy dietary patterns is widely recognized. Dietary patterns that adhere to infant feeding guidelines are often adopted by mothers with higher educational levels [6,7,12–17], lower BMI [12–14], higher household income [7,14,15] and who are multiparous [8,12,14,17,18]. In contrast, unhealthy infant dietary patterns [19] are associated with younger mothers [6,12,13,15–19] and mothers who smoke [6,14,15,17]. The majority of these have been conducted in Caucasian populations [6,8,12–18,20] with the exception of one study in Japan [18] and another in a multi-ethnic population in America [7]. While it is well established that dietary patterns differ markedly between Asian and Caucasian adults [21,22], the extent to which dietary patterns in Asian infants differ from their Caucasian counterparts and whether maternal predictors of those patterns differ in an Asian infant population remains unexplored.

Weaning represents a transition period during which the diet undergoes rapid changes from milk-based to solid foods, increasing in variety to resemble an adult-like diet. Yet, most studies have limited their scope to a single time-point [7,8,12,17] and may not have adequately accounted for the transitory nature of weaning diets. The concept of modeling dietary patterns longitudinally across time points into dietary trajectories has recently been developed by Smithers *et al.* [11] to address this issue, but no study to date have explored predictors of infant dietary pattern trajectories using this model.

In this study, we aim to better understand the dietary patterns of Asian infants by longitudinally examining the dietary pattern trajectories of infants participating in a multi-ethnic Asian mother-offspring cohort study from 6- to 12-months of age. We also examined potential maternal socio-demographic predictors of these dietary pattern trajectories during this period.

2. Subjects and Methods

Our study is based on the Growing Up in Singapore Towards healthy Outcomes (GUSTO) cohort [23]. Between June 2009 and September 2010, pregnant women 18–50 years of age were recruited from Singapore's two major public maternity units: National University Hospital (NUH) and KK Women's and Children's Hospital (KKH). In brief, the participants were Singapore citizens or permanent residents with the intention to deliver in one of the above-named hospitals, reside in Singapore for the next 5 years, spouses were of the same race, and both parents had a homogenous parental background of Chinese, Malay, or Indian ethnicity. The exclusion criteria included receipt of chemotherapy treatment or psychotropic drugs or the presence of serious medical conditions such as type-1 diabetes mellitus. The study received ethical approval from the institutional review boards of the respective hospitals involved. Written consent was obtained from all participants.

2.1. Maternal and Infant Characteristics

Socio-demographic characteristics such as maternal age, ethnicity, marital and employment status, housing, monthly household income and education level were obtained from the participants during the first clinic visit upon recruitment (<14 weeks gestation). At 26–28 weeks of gestation, self-reported information on pre-pregnancy BMI, tobacco smoking and alcohol consumption were collected. Details on infant gender and birth order were obtained from birth delivery reports.

2.2. Infant Dietary Assessment

Mothers were sent 3-day food diaries to record dietary intakes of their children prior to their postnatal clinic visits at 6-, 9- and 12-months and the diaries were collected at the visits. Instructions and further information on food recording were indicated in the diaries. Mothers who did not complete the food diaries were interviewed by trained personnel at the clinic visits, where a 24-h recall was conducted using the 5-stage, multiple-pass interviewing technique [24]. A set of food pictures and household measurements were provided in the food diaries and during the 24-h recalls to aid in the description of portion size consumed. For the dietary analyses, data from 24-h recalls and 1-day record from the food diaries were used to increase the sample size of the study. Breastmilk consumption via direct breastfeeding was estimated as 780 mL for 6 month-old infants and 600 mL for 9- and 12-month-old infants, based on methods described by Ponza *et al.* [25]. For expressed breastmilk, consumption was quantified according to exact volumes recorded by mothers.

2.3. Identifying Dietary Patterns

Food items from the 24-h recalls (n = 295, 322, 249 at 6, 9 and 12 months, respectively) or 1-day record (chosen by a randomized order) from the food diaries (n = 191, 164, 237 at 6, 9 and 12 months, respectively) were grouped into pre-defined food groups. Food groups with low intakes among the infants ($n < 3$) were further combined based on similarity in culinary usage and nutrient profile [26,27]. A total of 493, 894 and 1137 food items were identified and subsequently grouped into 34, 44 and 61 food groups at 6, 9 and 12 months of age, respectively. Dietary patterns at each time point were extracted by exploratory factor analysis (EFA) using the principal factor method in SPSS version 22.0 (IBM) [28,29] (see Supplementary Materials). EFA solutions were assessed for the magnitude of loadings of food groups, and each pattern was named based on loadings of $\geqslant \pm 0.30$ [9,12,13,15,16]. A dietary pattern score, standardized to a mean of zero and standard deviation of one, was calculated for each subject as a function of the contribution ("loading") that each food made to the pattern. Four dietary patterns were extracted at month-6 and -9 and five dietary patterns at month-12.

2.4. Construction of Dietary Pattern Trajectories

Using multi-level mixed models in Stata version 13.0 (Stata Corporation, College Station, Texas, TX, USA), dietary trajectories were empirically constructed by mapping the dietary patterns extracted by EFA at 6-, 9- and 12-months. This procedure accounts for the repeated measures of dietary pattern scores of each subject. The dietary patterns across the three time-points were examined for their similarity in the types of foods and their loadings to ascertain their suitability to be modeled as trajectories. The mapping of each pattern to a trajectory was based on similar key constituent foods (with high loadings) found in the dietary patterns across the three time-points and this correspondingly determined the name of each trajectory [11]. The model generates estimates of intercepts and slopes. The intercept reflects the trajectory score at the start point of each trajectory (6-months of age), while the slope denotes the rate of change in trajectory scores over time. Details have been previously described by Smithers *et al.* [11].

2.5. Statistical Analysis

Of the 1247 women recruited, 486 singleton subjects with complete birth measurements and dietary records at 6-, 9- and 12-months were included in the final subgroup (illustrated in Supplementary Materials Figure S1). Pearson's chi-square tests and independent sample t-tests were used to compare the characteristics of mothers included in this analysis and those with missing dietary records. Pearson's correlation coefficients were used to assess the correlation between dietary scores derived from 1-day record of the food diaries with the average of the other 2-day records in the subset of mothers who completed the food diaries at the 3 time-points. General linear models were performed to study the associations between dietary trajectory estimates and maternal socio-demographic factors (maternal age, education, ethnicity, employment, BMI at 26-weeks gestation, pre-pregnancy smoking and alcohol status, monthly household income, cohabitation status, parity and infant sex). Socio-demographic factors were stratified into categorical variables and imputations were performed on missing data using the mode. These models were adjusted for potential covariates as described above.

All statistical analyses were performed using the statistical software package SPSS version 22.0 (IBM Corp, New York, NY, USA). A 2-tailed *p*-value of <0.05 was considered to be statistically significant.

3. Results

Maternal and infant characteristics of participants with complete dietary records from 6- to 12-months (n = 486) were similar to those without complete dietary records (n = 438) (Supplementary Materials Table S1). Nonetheless, mothers who provided complete dietary records were more likely to live together with their spouses and had higher monthly household income compared with those who did not provide complete dietary records.

3.1. Dietary Pattern Trajectories

Four dietary pattern trajectories were observed from 6- to 12-months and were labeled *Predominantly breastmilk*, *Guidelines*, *Easy-to-prepare foods* and *Noodles (in soup) and seafood* (Figure 1). The *Predominantly breastmilk* trajectory was characterized by breastmilk feeding that exceeded formula milk, the addition of fresh fruits at 9-months, and bean curd (tofu), high-fat ethnic breads and starchy vegetables at 12-months. The *Guidelines* trajectory followed recommended weaning guidelines [30] and was characterized by rice porridge, low-fat fish and meat, a variety of vegetables and fresh fruits as core foods items throughout the 6–12-month period. This trajectory was also characterized by lower intakes of infant cereal at 9- and 12-months.

The *Easy-to-prepare foods* trajectory consisted of foods that require little preparation (infant cereals, juices, cakes and biscuits, as well as adult table foods such as white rice, green vegetables) at 6-months and progressed to easy-to-prepare foods such as breads, spreads, biscuit and confectionaries at 12-months. The *Noodles (in soup) and seafood* trajectory was pre-dominantly noodle-based and consisted of common accompaniments such as eggs, seafood products, dried preserved fruits and bean curd (tofu) found in noodle soup meals. An additional dietary pattern emerged at 12-months of age but did not fall into any of the dietary trajectories: the *Pulses and grains* pattern. This pattern was distinguished by high intakes of nuts and seeds, grains, legumes and lentils and high energy-dense confectionaries.

A complete list of food items and their loading scores for each dietary pattern and trajectory is provided in the supplementary file (Supplementary Materials Tables S2–S4). Examples of foods consumed in each item are also provided in Supplementary Materials Table S5. Dietary patterns scores derived from 1-day record of the food diaries were found to be significantly correlated with the other 2-days of the same diaries (correlation coefficient ranged from 0.43 to 0.82) for all dietary patterns and all time points except for the *Easy-to-prepare foods* dietary pattern at 9-months (correlation coefficient = 0.123) (Supplementary Materials Tables S6).

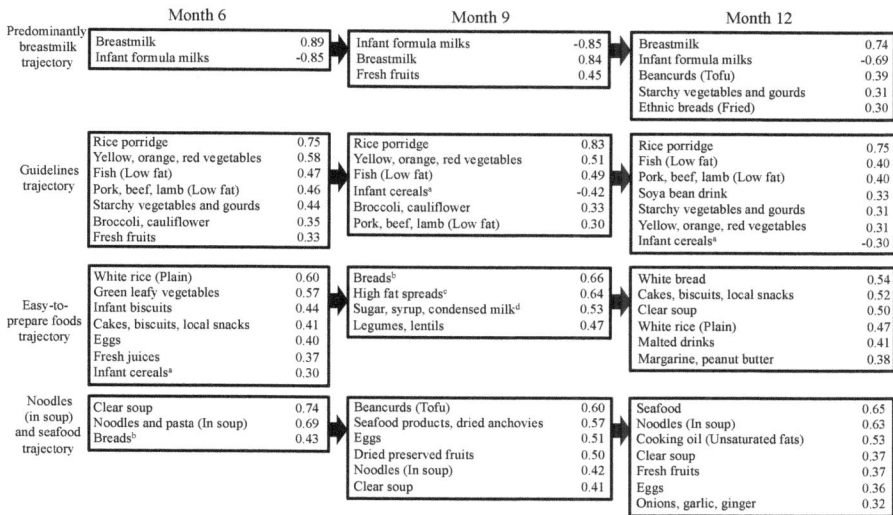

Month 6		Month 9		Month 12	
Predominantly breastmilk trajectory					
Breastmilk	0.89	Infant formula milks	-0.85	Breastmilk	0.74
Infant formula milks	-0.85	Breastmilk	0.84	Infant formula milks	-0.69
		Fresh fruits	0.45	Beancurds (Tofu)	0.39
				Starchy vegetables and gourds	0.31
				Ethnic breads (Fried)	0.30
Guidelines trajectory					
Rice porridge	0.75	Rice porridge	0.83	Rice porridge	0.75
Yellow, orange, red vegetables	0.58	Yellow, orange, red vegetables	0.51	Fish (Low fat)	0.40
Fish (Low fat)	0.47	Fish (Low fat)	0.49	Pork, beef, lamb (Low fat)	0.40
Pork, beef, lamb (Low fat)	0.46	Infant cereals[a]	-0.42	Soya bean drink	0.33
Starchy vegetables and gourds	0.44	Broccoli, cauliflower	0.33	Starchy vegetables and gourds	0.31
Broccoli, cauliflower	0.35	Pork, beef, lamb (Low fat)	0.30	Yellow, orange, red vegetables	0.31
Fresh fruits	0.33			Infant cereals[a]	-0.30
Easy-to-prepare foods trajectory					
White rice (Plain)	0.60	Breads[b]	0.66	White bread	0.54
Green leafy vegetables	0.57	High fat spreads[c]	0.64	Cakes, biscuits, local snacks	0.52
Infant biscuits	0.44	Sugar, syrup, condensed milk[d]	0.53	Clear soup	0.50
Cakes, biscuits, local snacks	0.41	Legumes, lentils	0.47	White rice (Plain)	0.47
Eggs	0.40			Malted drinks	0.41
Fresh juices	0.37			Margarine, peanut butter	0.38
Infant cereals[a]	0.30				
Noodles (in soup) and seafood trajectory					
Clear soup	0.74	Beancurds (Tofu)	0.60	Seafood	0.65
Noodles and pasta (In soup)	0.69	Seafood products, dried anchovies	0.57	Noodles (In soup)	0.63
Breads[b]	0.43	Eggs	0.51	Cooking oil (Unsaturated fats)	0.53
		Dried preserved fruits	0.50	Clear soup	0.37
		Noodles (In soup)	0.42	Fresh fruits	0.37
		Clear soup	0.41	Eggs	0.36
				Onions, garlic, ginger	0.32

Figure 1. Mapping of dietary patterns at age 6, 9 and 12 months to trajectories. Only foods with loadings ⩾±0.30 are shown in the figure. A full list of food items and their loadings are provided in Supplementary Materials. [a] Includes rice, wheat and oat baby cereals; [b] Includes white and whole wheat breads, breads with fillings or toppings, and baked ethnic breads; [c] Includes butter, ghee, peanut butter and margarine; [d] Added to drinks and cereals.

3.2. Characteristics of Study Population with Trajectory Estimates

The dietary pattern trajectory estimates of 486 infants summarized with respect to their maternal and infant characteristics are shown in Supplementary Materials Tables S7 and S8. Ranges of intercepts and slopes are listed in the Supplementary Materials. In general, the slopes were small relative to the intercepts.

3.3. Associations with Trajectory Intercepts

The fully adjusted associations between the intercepts and maternal socio-demographic characteristics are shown in Table 1. Higher *Predominantly breastmilk* trajectory start scores for infants at 6 months were significantly associated with higher maternal education, higher income, Chinese ethnicity, not working outside the home and having more than one child at home. Higher *Guidelines* trajectory intercepts at 6 months were associated with post-secondary education. Male infants had higher *Easy-to-prepare foods* trajectory intercepts at 6 months, while their mothers were more likely to be older (>34 years old) and of Indian ethnicity. No significant maternal factors were associated with the *Noodles (in soup) and seafood* trajectory.

3.4. Associations with Trajectory Slopes

The fully adjusted associations between maternal socio-demographic characteristics and rates of change in dietary trajectory scores (slopes) over the period of 6 to 12-months are shown in Table 2. Mothers of Indian ethnicity, of lower education qualification and primiparous had higher positive slopes for the *Predominantly breastmilk* trajectory. Chinese infants had higher positive slopes for the *Guidelines* trajectory than Malay or Indian infants. Infants with higher slopes for the *Easy-to-prepare foods* trajectory had younger mothers. Chinese infants had higher slopes for the *Noodles (in soup) and seafood* trajectory.

The *Pulses and grain* dietary pattern emerged only at 12-months of age and was associated with Indian ethnicity and mothers with post-secondary education (Supplementary Materials Table S9).

Table 1. Adjusted associations between dietary pattern trajectory intercepts and sociodemographic characteristics ($n = 486$) [a].

Maternal and Child Characteristics	β (95% CI)			
	Predominantly Breastmilk	Guidelines	Easy-to-Prepare Foods	Noodles (in Soup) and Seafood
Maternal characteristics				
Ethnicity				
Indian	−0.245 (−0.463, −0.026) *	0.069 (−0.035, 0.173)	0.123 (0.063, 0.184) ***	0.028 (−0.015, 0.072)
Malay	−0.259 (−0.476, −0.042) *	−0.069 (−0.172, 0.034)	0.031 (−0.029, 0.091)	0.028 (−0.015, 0.071)
Chinese	*Reference*	*Reference*	*Reference*	*Reference*
Maternal Age				
18–29	0.084 (−0.123, 0.292)	−0.026 (−0.125, 0.073)	−0.088 (−0.145, −0.030) **	0.035 (−0.006, 0.076)
30–34	0.040 (−0.161, 0.241)	−0.006 (−0.102, 0.089)	−0.069 (−0.125, −0.014) *	0.034 (−0.005, 0.074)
>34	*Reference*	*Reference*	*Reference*	*Reference*
Maternal Education [b]				
Primary education	−0.781 (−1.021, −0.541) ***	0.081 (−0.033, 0.195)	−0.025 (−0.091, 0.041)	−0.003 (−0.051, 0.044)
Post-secondary	−0.480 (−0.683, −0.277) ***	0.174 (0.077, 0.270) ***	<0.001 (−0.056, 0.056)	−0.007 (−0.047, 0.033)
University and other	*Reference*	*Reference*	*Reference*	*Reference*
Household Income (SGD)				
<1999	−0.441 (−0.746, −0.137) **	−0.065 (−0.21, 0.080)	0.053 (−0.031, 0.137)	−0.013 (−0.073, 0.047)
2000–5999	−0.057 (−0.258, 0.145)	−0.034 (−0.13, 0.061)	0.019 (−0.037, 0.074)	0.029 (−0.010, 0.069)
>6000	*Reference*	*Reference*	*Reference*	*Reference*
Employment				
Unemployed	0.273 (0.096, 0.449) **	0.014 (−0.069, 0.098)	0.009 (−0.040, 0.058)	0.019 (−0.016, 0.054)
Employed	*Reference*	*Reference*	*Reference*	*Reference*
Maternal BMI at 26 weeks [c]				
<18.5–24.9	0.126 (−0.093, 0.344)	0.015 (−0.089, 0.119)	0.010 (−0.050, 0.070)	−0.022 (−0.065, 0.022)
25.0–29.9	0.214 (−0.005, 0.433)	0.059 (−0.045, 0.163)	0.015 (−0.046, 0.075)	−0.009 (−0.052, 0.034)
>30.0	*Reference*	*Reference*	*Reference*	*Reference*
Alcohol [d]				
Yes	0.080 (−0.095, 0.255)	0.030 (−0.053, 0.113)	−0.019 (−0.068, 0.029)	0.013 (−0.021, 0.048)
No	*Reference*	*Reference*	*Reference*	*Reference*
Smoking [d]				
Yes	−0.209 (−0.456, 0.038)	−0.005 (−0.123, 0.112)	0.039 (−0.030, 0.107)	−0.010 (−0.059, 0.039)
No	*Reference*	*Reference*	*Reference*	*Reference*

Table 1. *Cont.*

Maternal and Child Characteristics	β (95% CI)			
	Predominantly Breastmilk	Guidelines	Easy-to-Prepare Foods	Noodles (in Soup) and Seafood
Cohabitation [e]				
Not living together	0.022 (−0.719, 0.762)	0.021 (−0.331, 0.372)	−0.039 (−0.244, 0.165)	0.063 (−0.083, 0.209)
Living together	*Reference*	*Reference*	*Reference*	*Reference*
Infant characteristics				
Gender				
Female	0.027 (−0.122, 0.176)	0.012 (−0.059, 0.082)	−0.042 (−0.083, −0.001) *	−0.016 (−0.045, 0.013)
Male	*Reference*	*Reference*	*Reference*	*Reference*
Parity				
First child	−0.202 (−0.371, −0.033) **	0.014 (−0.066, 0.094)	0.032 (−0.015, 0.079)	0.005 (−0.029, 0.038)
Not first child	*Reference*	*Reference*	*Reference*	*Reference*

Abbreviations: BMI, body mass index. [a] Data shown are multivariable linear model β coefficients and their 95% confidence intervals (95% CIs) obtained from general linear models. Trajectory intercepts are the dependent variable for formed trajectories from age 6 to 12 months and each characteristic was assessed with adjustments for the other characteristics (covariates) [b] Maternal education categorized as primary and secondary education, post-secondary education, as well as university and others; [c] Mother's BMI recorded at 26 weeks of pregnancy (kg/m^2); [d] Status recorded prior to pregnancy; [e] Reflects the marital status; single, separated or divorced mothers as living separately; married mothers as living together. * p-value < 0.05; ** p-value < 0.01; *** p-value < 0.001.

Table 2. Adjusted associations between dietary pattern trajectory slopes and sociodemographic characteristics (n = 486) [a].

Maternal and Child Characteristics	β (95% CI)			
	Predominantly Breastmilk	Guidelines	Easy-to-Prepare Foods	Noodles (in soup) and Seafood
Maternal characteristics				
Ethnicity				
Indian	0.026 (0.013, 0.040) ***	−0.040 (−0.052, −0.028) ***	0.000 (−0.008, 0.008)	−0.013 (−0.020, −0.005) **
Malay	0.013 (−0.001, 0.026)	−0.014 (−0.026, −0.002) *	0.004 (−0.004, 0.012)	−0.013 (−0.021, −0.006) **
Chinese	*Reference*	*Reference*	*Reference*	*Reference*
Maternal Age				
18–29	−8.823×10^{-5} (−0.013, 0.013)	0.005 (−0.007, 0.016)	0.009 (0.001, 0.017) *	−0.005 (−0.012, 0.002)
30–34	0.003 (−0.010, 0.015)	0.007 (−0.004, 0.018)	0.006 (−0.002, 0.013)	−0.003 (−0.010, 0.004)
>34	*Reference*	*Reference*	*Reference*	*Reference*

Nutrients **2016**, *8*, 365

Table 2. *Cont.*

Maternal and Child Characteristics	β (95% CI)			
	Predominantly Breastmilk	Guidelines	Easy-to-Prepare Foods	Noodles (in soup) and Seafood
Maternal Education [b]				
Primary education	0.029 (0.014, 0.044) ***	0.001 (−0.012, 0.015)	0.008 (−0.001, 0.017)	−0.002 (−0.010, 0.007)
Post-secondary	0.013 (0.000, 0.026) *	−0.004 (−0.015, 0.007)	0.003 (−0.004, 0.011)	0.004 (−0.003, 0.011)
University and other	*Reference*	*Reference*	*Reference*	*Reference*
Household Income (SGD)				
<1999	0.002 (−0.017, 0.021)	−0.013 (−0.030, 0.004)	−0.001 (−0.013, 0.010)	−0.001 (−0.011, 0.010)
2000–5999	−0.009 (−0.022, 0.004)	−0.004 (−0.015, 0.007)	−0.001 (−0.009, 0.006)	−0.002 (−0.009, 0.005)
>6000	*Reference*	*Reference*	*Reference*	*Reference*
Employment				
Unemployed	0.007 (−0.004, 0.018)	0.001 (−0.009, 0.011)	0.001 (−0.005, 0.008)	0.002 (−0.004, 0.008)
Employed	*Reference*	*Reference*	*Reference*	*Reference*
Maternal BMI at 26 weeks [c]				
<18.5–24.9	−0.010 (−0.023, 0.004)	0.003 (−0.009, 0.015)	−0.004 (−0.012, 0.004)	0.003 (−0.004, 0.011)
25.0–29.9	−0.008 (−0.022, 0.006)	−0.007 (−0.020, 0.005)	−0.002 (−0.010, 0.006)	0.001 (−0.006, 0.009)
>30.0	*Reference*	*Reference*	*Reference*	*Reference*
Alcohol [d]				
Yes	−0.002 (−0.013, 0.009)	−0.002 (−0.011, 0.008)	0.001 (−0.006, 0.007)	−0.004 (−0.010, 0.002)
No	*Reference*	*Reference*	*Reference*	*Reference*
Smoking [d]				
Yes	0.005 (−0.010, 0.020)	−0.004 (−0.017, 0.010)	−0.002 (−0.012, 0.007)	−0.001 (−0.009, 0.008)
No	*Reference*	*Reference*	*Reference*	*Reference*
Cohabitation [e]				
Not living together	0.011 (−0.035, 0.058)	−0.002 (−0.042, 0.039)	0.018 (−0.010, 0.045)	−0.013 (−0.038, 0.013)
Living together	*Reference*	*Reference*	*Reference*	*Reference*
Infant characteristics				
Gender				
Female	−0.003 (−0.012, 0.006)	−0.005 (−0.014, 0.003)	0.004 (−0.002, 0.009)	−0.001 (−0.006, 0.004)
Male	*Reference*	*Reference*	*Reference*	*Reference*
Parity				
First child	0.014 (0.004, 0.025) **	0.006 (−0.003, 0.016)	−0.006 (−0.012, 0.001)	−0.004 (−0.010, 0.002)
Not first child	*Reference*	*Reference*	*Reference*	*Reference*

Abbreviations: BMI, body mass index. [a] Data shown are multivariable linear model β coefficients and their 95% confidence intervals (95% CIs) obtained from general linear models. Dietary pattern trajectory slopes as the dependent variable for patterns that formed trajectories from age 6 to 12 months and each characteristic was assessed with adjustments for the other characteristics; [b] Maternal education categorized as primary and secondary education, post-secondary education, as well as university and others; [c] Mother's BMI recorded at 26 weeks of pregnancy (kg/m^2); [d] Status recorded prior to pregnancy; [e] Reflects the marital status; single, separated or divorced mothers as living separately; married mothers as living together. * *p*-value < 0.05; ** *p*-value < 0.01; *** *p*-value < 0.001.

4. Discussion

Using multi-level modeling, we integrated food intakes at 6-, 9- and 12-months of age and identified four well-defined dietary patterns and their trajectories over that time period. A key observation was that the rates of change (slopes) of the trajectory scores were much smaller than the differences in the start scores (intercepts) in groups defined by maternal socio-demographic characteristics. This suggests that the maternal characteristics that predict dietary patterns at 6-months of age also largely determine the adherence to the same dietary patterns trajectories for the first year of life. To our knowledge, this is the first study to examine these dietary patterns and associations in an Asian population.

4.1. Dietary Patterns

In our study, the *Predominantly breastmilk* pattern resembles the "breastfeeding" pattern and "longer breastfeeding, late contemporary food introduction and use of home-made foods" reported in the ALSPAC [12] and EDEN studies [8,13], respectively. This pattern was characterized by higher intake of breastmilk and lower intake of formula milk and was accompanied by intakes of fruits and vegetables. The *Guidelines* pattern in our study corresponds to the healthy/prudent eating pattern [7,8,14–17,20] and was characterized by higher intakes of fruits, vegetables, whole grains, poultry and fish. While continued breastfeeding is encouraged during complementary feeding (6–12 months of age), the emphasis in current guidelines for this period is to offer infants a variety of food groups, rather than the type of milk taken [31,32]. The *Easy-to-prepare foods* pattern corresponds to an unhealthy eating pattern characterized by intakes of sugary desserts, high-fat foods and refined grains [6,15,17,18]. Lastly, the *Noodles (in soup) and seafood* pattern, which has not been observed in other studies, appears to reflect Asian adult eating patterns. It resembles the "use of adults' foods" in the EDEN study [8,13].

4.2. Associations between Maternal Factors and Trajectory Intercepts

The trajectory intercept values obtained from the mixed models represents the start point of each dietary pattern trajectory (at 6-months of age). To our knowledge, only three cohort studies to date have reported results for infant dietary patterns at 6-months of age [7,12,17]. Similar to the ALSPAC study [12], higher start scores of our *Predominantly breastmilk* trajectory at 6-months was associated with higher maternal education attainment. The IFPS II study reported that a higher "formula" dietary pattern (reverse of breastmilk) at 6-months of age was negatively associated with maternal education [7]. The relationship we observed with household income is not surprising, as income is closely linked to educational attainment. Its effect on breastfeeding status tends to attenuate when adjusted for education attainment [33,34]. The relationship we observed between higher start scores on the *Predominantly breastmilk* trajectory and unemployment is supported by evidence from studies showing that women working part-time or unemployed are more likely than their counterparts to breastfeed [35–37]. In Singapore, working mothers are entitled to 16 weeks of government-paid maternity leave or 12 weeks of maternity leave depending on citizenship, marriage status and duration of employment, but can choose to consume leave non-consecutively [38]. This may in part explain the lower start scores at 6 months on the *Predominantly breastmilk* trajectory for employed mothers when they return to work. Similarly, we found higher educational attainment to be associated with higher start scores of the *Guidelines* trajectory. Mothers with higher education are probably more aware of recommended practices and guidelines for weaning diets. A similar finding was also observed in the IFPS II study [7].

Maternal ethnicity was strongly associated with the start scores of our diet trajectories. Chinese mothers tended to start their infants on the *Predominantly breastmilk* pattern, while Indian ethnicity was associated with the *Easy-to-prepare foods* pattern. Ethnic differences in dietary patterns has also been observed in the American population, where White and African-American mothers scored higher on "guidelines" and "easy-to-prepare foods" patterns compared to their Hispanic counterparts [7], suggesting the importance of culture on diet and weaning practices.

We observed that higher start scores on the *Easy-to-prepare foods* trajectory were also associated with older mothers. In contrast, previous findings suggest that younger mothers tend to provide their children with more convenient foods, perhaps owing to time constraints [39]. Differences in childcare practices among different populations may explain these contrasting findings. For example, young Singaporean couples tend to live with their parents and leave their infants under the grandparents' supervision. Those infants are more likely to be fed traditional, home-prepared weaning meals than ready-to-eat meals.

No key maternal determinant emerged in the full model analyses for the *Noodles (in soup) and seafood* trajectory, suggesting it may be less influenced by cultural or socioeconomic factors.

4.3. Associations between Maternal Factors and Trajectory Slopes

The trajectory slopes represent the rate of change of each dietary pattern trajectory between 6- and 12-months. The means and standard deviations of the trajectory slopes were small ($<0.05 \pm 0.10$) compared to the intercepts ($<0.51 \pm 1.04$), suggesting that infants tend to maintain their dietary patterns over time. The range of the slopes we observed is similar to that reported by Smithers *et al* [11].

Mothers with lowest educational attainment and primiparous had higher slopes for the *Predominantly breastmilk* trajectory, suggesting a greater adherence to this pattern over time. This may not be ideal as the World Health Organization (WHO) recommends that solid foods be introduced shortly after 6-months of age [31] to ensure that infants obtain adequate micronutrients that breastmilk may not supply in sufficient quantity [30,40]. In addition, the variety of food and food textures provided to infants are believed to facilitate the development of oral motor skills and taste preferences and thereby help build a foundation for healthy eating habits [31,32,41].

Mothers in the youngest age group (18–29) tended to have greater adherence to the *Easy-to-prepare foods* trajectory with time, possibly owing to limited knowledge and experience with infant nutrition [39].

Maternal ethnicity continues to be a prevailing determinant of the slope of the dietary pattern trajectories. We observed that while Indian mothers have greater adherence to the *Predominantly breastmilk* trajectory over time, Chinese mothers adhere more to the *Guidelines* and *Noodles (in soup) and seafood* trajectories over time, reflecting a transition to an increasing pattern of table and adult foods. We also observed a *Pulses and grain* dietary pattern emerging at 12-months, particularly in Indian mothers of higher education status.

4.4. Strengths and Limitations

Our study captures the important time points of an infant's weaning diet and fills an important data gap on early feeding patterns. The modeling of dietary pattern trajectories has enabled us to take a longitudinal approach to assessing the overall diet. Compared to conventional cross-sectional analyses, this technique allows us to observe the introduction of new foods through time and the dietary transition during the weaning period. Furthermore, the representation of dietary pattern scores as intercepts and slopes has enabled us to explore the extent to which changes in diet over time are influenced by socio-demographic variables. While the trajectory intercepts signify the cross-sectional dietary pattern scores at 6-months of age, the slopes illuminate the dynamic changes in dietary patterns over time, which cannot be observed in the cross-sectional studies.

Limitations of our study also merit comment. First, single 24-h recalls or 1-day dietary records may not be a good representative of an infant's usual diet due to day-to-day variation in intakes. However, we have demonstrated high correlation of dietary pattern scores across the 3-days of the food diaries, reflecting good reproducibility of the single day dietary records. Second, GUSTO participants were not randomly sampled from the general population, with deliberate over-sampling of Malay and Indian mothers, and were recruited from two maternity hospitals in Singapore. However, these recruitment sites are the two largest maternity hospitals in Singapore and consist of both private and subsidized patients.

Nutrients **2016**, *8*, 365

5. Conclusions

We examined trajectories of four distinct dietary patterns across three time points between 6- and 12-months. The trajectories were largely determined at the start points (intercepts), and changes over time (slopes) were small. This suggests the importance of establishing the "right" diet at the start of complementary feeding, as dietary changes are more difficult once habits are established. By understanding the key maternal socio-demographic factors that influence dietary patterns during complementary feeding, health professionals and policy-makers can provide more targeted and culturally-appropriate support and advice for mothers and their infants.

Supplementary Materials: The following are available online at http://www.mdpi.com/2072-6643/8/6/365/s1, Figure S1: Flowchart of selection process. Only subjects with complete dietary records from 6 to 12 months were included in the analysis (n = 486), Table S1: Comparisons of characteristics between study group and those excluded due to incomplete dietary records from 6 to 12 months, Table S2: Varimax-rotated component matrix loadings of food items on four dietary patterns extracted by EFA at 6 months of age (n = 486), Table S3: Varimax-rotated component matrix loadings of food items on four dietary patterns extracted by EFA at 9 months of age (n = 486), Table S4: Varimax-rotated component matrix loadings of food items on four dietary patterns extracted by EFA at 12 months of age (n = 486), Table S5: Examples of foods consumed under each food item at 6, 9 and 12 months of age, Table S6: Correlation coefficients for dietary pattern scores derived from 1-day record and average of 2-day record of the food diaries, Table S7: Dietary pattern trajectory intercepts and slopes of infants according to characteristics of study sample (n = 486), Table S8: Dietary pattern trajectory intercepts and slopes of infants according to characteristics of study sample (n = 486), Table S9: Associations between "Pulses and grains" dietary pattern scores at 12 months and sociodemographic characteristics (n = 486).

Acknowledgments: This study acknowledges the contribution of the rest of the GUSTO study group, which includes the following: Allan Sheppard, Amutha Chinnadurai, Anne Eng Neo Goh, Anne Rifkin-Graboi, Anqi Qiu, Arijit Biswas, Bee Wah Lee, Birit F.P. Broekman, Boon Long Quah, Borys Shuter, Chai Kiat Chng, Cheryl Ngo, Choon Looi Bong, Christiani Jeyakumar Henry, Cornelia Yin Ing Chee, Yam Thiam Daniel Goh, Doris Fok, Fabian Yap, George Seow Heong Yeo, Helen Chen, Hugo P S van Bever, Iliana Magiati, Inez Bik Yun Wong, Ivy Yee-Man Lau, Jeevesh Kapur, Jenny L. Richmond, Jerry Kok Yen Chan, Joanna D. Holbrook, Joshua J. Gooley, Keith M. Godfrey, Kenneth Kwek, Kok Hian Tan, Krishnamoorthy Niduvaje, Leher Singh, Lin Lin Su, Lourdes Mary Daniel, Lynette Pei-Chi Shek, Marielle V. Fortier, Mark Hanson, Mary Foong-Fong Chong, Mary Rauff, Mei Chien Chua, Michael Meaney, Mya Thway Tint, Neerja Karnani, Ngee Lek, Oon Hoe Teoh, P. C. Wong, Peter D. Gluckman, Pratibha Agarwal, Rob M. van Dam, Salome A. Rebello, Seang-Mei Saw, Shang Chee Chong, Shirong Cai, Shu-E Soh, Sok Bee Lim, Chin-Ying Stephen Hsu, Victor Samuel Rajadurai, Walter Stunkel, Wee Meng Han, Wei Wei Pang, Yap-Seng Chong, Yin Bun Cheung, Yiong Huak Chan and Yung Seng Lee. This study is supported by the Singapore National Research Foundation under its Translational and Clinical Research (TCR) Flagship Programme and administered by the Singapore Ministry of Health's National Medical Research Council (NMRC), Singapore- NMRC/TCR/004-NUS/2008; NMRC/TCR/012-NUHS/2014. Additional funding is provided by the Singapore Institute for Clinical Sciences, Agency for Science Technology and Research(A*STAR), Singapore. Keith M. Godfrey is supported by the National Institute for Health Research through the NIHR Southampton Biomedical Research Centre.

Author Contributions: Geraldine Huini Lim: designed the study, contributed to data collection, performed the statistical analyses, wrote the manuscript, and had primary responsibility for final content. Jia Ying Toh: designed the study, contributed to data collection, wrote the manuscript, and had primary responsibility for final content. Izzuddin M. Aris: contributed to statistical analyses of dietary patterns data. Ai-Ru Chia: contributed to statistical analyses of dietary patterns data. Wee Meng Han: contributed to the conception and design of the study and the acquisition of data. Seang Mei Saw: designed and led the GUSTO study. Keith M. Godfrey: designed and led the GUSTO study, and revised the manuscript for important intellectual content. Peter D. Gluckman: designed and led the GUSTO study; Yap-Seng Chong: designed and led the GUSTO study. Fabian Yap: designed and led the GUSTO study. Yung Seng Lee: designed and led the GUSTO study, and revised the manuscript for important intellectual content. Michael S. Kramer: contributed to statistical analyses of dietary patterns data and revised the manuscript for important intellectual content. Mary Foong-Fong Chong: designed the study, revised the manuscript for important intellectual content, and had primary responsibility for final content. All authors have read and approved the final manuscript.

Conflicts of Interest: Peter D. Gluckman, Keith M. Godfrey and Yap-Seng Chong have received reimbursement for speaking at conferences sponsored by companies selling nutritional products. These authors are part of an academic consortium that has received research funding from Abbot Nutrition, Nestec, and Danone. None of the other authors report any potential conflict of interest.

References

1. Oellingrath, I.M.; Svendsen, M.V.; Brantsaeter, A.L. Tracking of eating patterns and overweight—A follow-up study of Norwegian schoolchildren from middle childhood to early adolescence. *Nutr. J.* **2011**, *10*, 106. [CrossRef] [PubMed]

2. Mikkila, V.; Räsänen, L.; Raitakari, O.T.; Pietinen, P.; Viikari, J. Consistent dietary patterns identified from childhood to adulthood: The cardiovascular risk in Young Finns Study. *Br. J. Nutr.* **2005**, *93*, 923–931. [CrossRef] [PubMed]

3. Bjelland, M.; Brantsæter, A.L.; Haugen, M.; Meltzer, H.M.; Nystad, W.; Andersen, L.F. Changes and tracking of fruit, vegetables and sugar-sweetened beverages intake from 18 months to 7 years in the Norwegian Mother and Child. Cohort Study. *BMC Public Health* **2013**, *13*, 793. [CrossRef] [PubMed]

4. Grieger, J.A.; Scott, J.; Cobiac, L. Dietary patterns and breast-feeding in Australian children. *Public Health Nutr.* **2011**, *14*, 1939–1947. [CrossRef] [PubMed]

5. Birch, L.; Savage, J.S.; Ventura, A. Influences on the Development of Children's Eating Behaviours: From Infancy to Adolescence. *Can. J. Diet. Pract. Res.* **2007**, *68*, s1–s56. [PubMed]

6. Bell, L.K.; Golley, R.K.; Daniels, L.; Magarey, A.M. Dietary patterns of Australian children aged 14 and 24 months, and associations with socio-demographic factors and adiposity. *Eur. J. Clin. Nutr.* **2013**, *67*, 638–645. [CrossRef] [PubMed]

7. Wen, X.; Kong, K.L.; Eiden, R.D.; Sharma, N.N.; Xie, C. Sociodemographic differences and infant dietary patterns. *Pediatrics* **2014**, *134*, e1387–e1398. [CrossRef] [PubMed]

8. Andersen, L.B.; Mølgaard, C.; Michaelsen, K.F.; Carlsen, E.M.; Bro, R.; Pipper, C.B. Indicators of dietary patterns in Danish infants at 9 months of age. *Food Nutr. Res.* **2015**, *59*, 27665. [PubMed]

9. Smithers, L.G.; Golley, R.K.; Mittinty, M.N.; Brazionis, L.; Northstone, K.; Emmett, P.; Lynch, J.W. Dietary patterns at 6, 15 and 24 months of age are associated with IQ at 8 years of age. *Eur. J. Epidemiol.* **2012**, *27*, 525–535. [CrossRef] [PubMed]

10. Gale, C.R.; Martyn, C.N.; Marriott, L.D.; Limond, J.; Crozier, S.; Inskip, H.M.; Godfrey, K.M.; Law, C.M.; Cooper, C.; Robinson, S.M.; *et al.* Dietary patterns in infancy and cognitive and neuropsychological function in childhood. *J. Child. Psychol. Psychiatr.* **2009**, *50*, 816–823. [CrossRef] [PubMed]

11. Smithers, L.G.; Golley, R.K.; Mittinty, M.N.; Brazionis, L.; Northstone, K.; Emmett, P.; Lynch, J.W. Do dietary trajectories between infancy and toddlerhood influence IQ in childhood and adolescence? Results from a prospective birth cohort study. *PLoS ONE* **2013**, *8*, e58904.

12. Smithers, L.G.; Brazionis, L.; Golley, R.K.; Mittinty, M.N.; Northstone, K.; Emmett, P.; McNaughton, S.A.; Campbell, K.J.; Lynch, J.W. Associations between dietary patterns at 6 and 15 months of age and sociodemographic factors. *Eur. J. Clin. Nutr.* **2012**, *66*, 658–666. [CrossRef] [PubMed]

13. Betoko, A.; Charles, M.A.; Hankard, R.; Forhan, A.; Bonet, M.; Saurel-Cubizolles, M.J.; Heude, B.; de Lauzon-Guillain, B. EDEN mother-child cohort study group. Infant feeding patterns over the first year of life: Influence of family characteristics. *Eur. J. Clin. Nutr.* **2013**, *67*, 631–637. [CrossRef] [PubMed]

14. Kiefte-de Jong, J.C.; de Vries, J.H.; Bleeker, S.E.; Jaddoe, V.W.; Hofman, A.; Raat, H.; Moll, H.A. Socio-demographic and lifestyle determinants of "Western-like" and "Health conscious" dietary patterns in toddlers. *Br. J. Nutr.* **2013**, *109*, 137–147. [CrossRef] [PubMed]

15. Ystrom, E.; Niegel, S.; Vollrath, M.E. The impact of maternal negative affectivity on dietary patterns of 18-month-old children in the Norwegian Mother and Child. Cohort Study. *Matern. Child. Nutr.* **2009**, *5*, 234–242. [CrossRef] [PubMed]

16. Lioret, S.; Betoko, A.; Forhan, A.; Charles, M.A.; Heude, B.; de Lauzon-Guillain, B. EDEN Mother–Child Cohort Study Group. Dietary patterns track from infancy to preschool age: Cross-sectional and longitudinal perspectives. *J. Nutr.* **2015**, *145*, 775–782. [CrossRef] [PubMed]

17. Robinson, S.; Marriott, L.; Poole, J.; Crozier, S.; Borland, S.; Lawrence, W.; Law, C.; Godfrey, K.; Cooper, C.; Inskip, H.; *et al.* Dietary patterns in infancy: The importance of maternal and family influences on feeding practice. *Br. J. Nutr.* **2007**, *98*, 1029–1037. [CrossRef] [PubMed]

18. Okubo, H.; Miyake, Y.; Sasaki, S.; Tanaka, K.; Murakami, K.; Hirota, Y. Osaka Maternal and Child Health Study Group. Dietary patterns in infancy and their associations with maternal socio-economic and lifestyle factors among 758 Japanese mother-child pairs: The Osaka Maternal and Child. *Health Study Matern. Child. Nutr.* **2014**, *10*, 213–225. [CrossRef] [PubMed]

19. Oddy, W.H.; Herbison, C.E.; Jacoby, P.; Ambrosini, G.L.; O'Sullivan, T.A.; Ayonrinde, O.T.; Olynyk, J.K.; Black, L.J.; Beilin, L.J.; Mori, T.A.; *et al.* The Western dietary pattern is prospectively associated with nonalcoholic fatty liver disease in adolescence. *Am. J. Gastroenterol.* **2013**, *108*, 778–785. [CrossRef] [PubMed]

20. Brazionis, L.; Golley, R.K.; Mittinty, M.N.; Smithers, L.G.; Emmett, P.; Northstone, K.; Lynch, J.W. Characterization of transition diets spanning infancy and toddlerhood: A novel, multiple-time-point application of principal components analysis. *Am. J. Clin. Nutr.* **2012**, *95*, 1200–1208. [CrossRef] [PubMed]

21. Smith, Z.; Knight, T.; Sahota, P.; Kernohan, E.; Baker, M. Dietary patterns in Asian and Caucasian men in Bradford: Differences and implications for nutrition education. *J. Hum. Nutr. Diet.* **1993**, *6*, 323–333. [CrossRef]

22. Vergne, S.; Sauvant, P.; Lamothe, V.; Chantre, P.; Asselineau, J.; Perez, P.; Durand, M.; Moore, N.; Bennetau-Pelissero, C. Influence of ethnic origin (Asian v. Caucasian) and background diet on the bioavailability of dietary isoflavones. *Br. J. Nutr.* **2009**, *102*, 1642–1653. [PubMed]

23. Soh, S.E.; Tint, M.T.; Gluckman, P.D.; Godfrey, K.M.; Rifkin-Graboi, A.; Chan, Y.H.; Stünkel, W.; Holbrook, J.D.; Kwek, K.; Chong, Y.S.; *et al.* Cohort profile: Growing Up in Singapore Towards healthy Outcomes (GUSTO) birth cohort study. *Int. J. Epidemiol.* **2014**, *43*, 1401–1409. [CrossRef] [PubMed]

24. Conway, J.M.; Ingwersen, L.A.; Vinyard, B.T.; Moshfegh, A.J. Effectiveness of the US Department of Agriculture 5-step multiple-pass method in assessing food intake in obese and nonobese women. *Am. J. Clin. Nutr.* **2003**, *77*, 1171–1178. [PubMed]

25. Ponza, M.; Devaney, B.; Ziegler, P.; Reidy, K.; Squatrito, C. Nutrient intakes and food choices of infants and toddlers participating in WIC. *J. Am. Diet. Assoc.* **2004**, *104*, s71–s79. [CrossRef] [PubMed]

26. Gao, X.; Chen, H.; Fung, T.T.; Logroscino, G.; Schwarzschild, M.A.; Hu, F.B.; Ascherio, A. Prospective study of dietary pattern and risk of Parkinson disease. *Am. J. Clin. Nutr.* **2007**, *86*, 1486–1494. [PubMed]

27. Crozier, S.R.; Robinson, S.M.; Borland, S.E.; Inskip, H.M.; SWS Study Group. Dietary patterns in the Southampton Women's Survey. *Eur. J. Clin. Nutr.* **2006**, *60*, 1391–1399. [CrossRef] [PubMed]

28. Joliffe, I.T.; Morgan, B.J. Principal component analysis and exploratory factor analysis. *Stat. Methods Med. Res.* **1992**, *1*, 69–95. [CrossRef] [PubMed]

29. Michels, K.B.; Schulze, M.B. Can dietary patterns help us detect diet-disease associations? *Nutr. Res. Rev.* **2005**, *18*, 241–248. [CrossRef] [PubMed]

30. Foote, K.D.; Marriott, L.D. Weaning of infants. *Arch. Dis. Child.* **2003**, *88*, 488–492. [CrossRef] [PubMed]

31. World Health Organization. WHO Guidelines Approved by the Guidelines Review Committee. In *Infant and Young Child. Feeding: Model. Chapter for Textbooks for Medical Students and Allied Health Professionals*; World Health Organization: Geneva, Switzerland, 2009.

32. Health Promotion Board. *Healthy Start for Your Baby*; Health Promotion Board: Singapore, Singapore, 2012.

33. Heck, K.E.; Braveman, P.; Cubbin, C.; Chávez, G.F.; Kiely, J.L. Socioeconomic status and breastfeeding initiation among California mothers. *Public Health Rep.* **2006**, *121*, 51–59. [PubMed]

34. Celi, A.C.; Rich-Edwards, J.W.; Richardson, M.K.; Kleinman, K.P.; Gillman, M.W. Immigration, race/ethnicity, and social and economic factors as predictors of breastfeeding initiation. *Arch. Pediatr. Adolesc. Med.* **2005**, *159*, 255–260. [CrossRef] [PubMed]

35. Hawkins, S.S.; Griffiths, L.J.; Dezateux, C.; Law, C. Millennium Cohort Study Child Health Group. Maternal employment and breast-feeding initiation: Findings from the Millennium Cohort Study. *Paediatr. Perinat. Epidemiol.* **2007**, *21*, 242–247. [CrossRef] [PubMed]

36. Khoury, A.J.; Moazzem, S.W.; Jarjoura, C.M.; Carothers, C.; Hinton, A. Breast-feeding initiation in low-income women: Role of attitudes, support, and perceived control. *Womens Health Issues* **2005**, *15*, 64–72. [CrossRef] [PubMed]

37. Barton, S.J. Infant feeding practices of low-income rural mothers. *MCN Am. J. Matern Child. Nurs.* **2001**, *26*, 93–97. [CrossRef] [PubMed]

38. Ministry of Manpower. Maternity Leave Eligibility and Entitlement, 2016. Available online: http://www.mom. gov.sg/employment-practices/leave/maternity-leave/eligibility-and-entitlement (accessed on 1 June 2016).

39. Bava, C.M.; Jaeger, S.R.; Park, J. Constraints upon food provisioning practices in "busy" women's lives: trade-offs which demand convenience. *Appetite* **2008**, *50*, 486–498. [CrossRef] [PubMed]
40. Dewey, K.G. Nutrition, growth, and complementary feeding of the breastfed infant. *Pediatr. Clin. N. Am.* **2001**, *48*, 87–104. [CrossRef]
41. WHO. Report by the Secretariat. In *Infant and Young Children Nutrition; Global Strategy for Infant and Young Child Feeding*; WHA55.25 Geneva: Fifty-fifth World Health Assembly; WHO: Geneva, Switerzland, 2002.

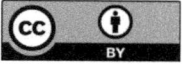

![nutrients logo]

![MDPI logo]

Article

Food and Nutrient Intake among 12-Month-Old Norwegian-Somali and Norwegian-Iraqi Infants

Navnit Kaur Grewal [1,*], Lene Frost Andersen [2], Cathrine Solheim Kolve [1], Ingrid Kverndalen [1] and Liv Elin Torheim [1]

[1] Department of Nursing and Health Promotion, Faculty of Health Sciences, Oslo and Akershus University College of Applied Sciences, P.O. Box 4 St. Olavs Plass, 0130 Oslo, Norway; cathrinekolve@gmail.com (C.S.K.); ingrid.kverndalen@hotmail.com (I.K.); liv.elin.torheim@hioa.no (L.E.T.)

[2] Department of Nutrition, Institute of Basic Medical Sciences, University of Oslo, P.O. Box 1046 Blindern, 0317 Oslo, Norway; l.f.andersen@medisin.uio.no

* Correspondence: navnit-kaur.grewal@hioa.no; Tel.: +47-6723-6665

Received: 12 August 2016; Accepted: 19 September 2016; Published: 28 September 2016

Abstract: The aim of the present paper was to describe food and nutrient intake among 12-month-old Norwegian-Somali and Norwegian-Iraqi infants, with a focus on iron and vitamin D intake. A cross-sectional survey was conducted from August 2013 through September 2014. Eighty-nine mothers/infants of Somali origin and 77 mothers/infants of Iraqi origin residing in Eastern Norway participated in the study. Data were collected using two 24-h multiple-pass recalls. Forty percent of the Norwegian-Somali infants and 47% of the Norwegian-Iraqi infants were breastfed at 12 months of age ($p = 0.414$). Median energy percentages (E%) from protein, fat and carbohydrates were within the recommended intake ranges, except the level of saturated fats (12–13 E%). Median intakes of almost all micronutrients were above the recommended daily intakes. Most of the infants consumed iron-enriched products (81%) and received vitamin D supplements (84%). The median intakes of iron and vitamin D were significantly higher among infants receiving iron-enriched products and vitamin D supplements compared to infants not receiving such products ($p < 0.001$). The findings indicate that the food and nutrient intake of this group of infants in general seems to be in accordance with Norwegian dietary recommendations. Foods rich in iron and vitamin D supplements were important sources of the infants' intake of iron and vitamin D and should continue to be promoted.

Keywords: food; nutrient intake; infants; immigrants; Norway

1. Introduction

The first two years of a child's life are particularly important as this is a period of rapid growth when nutritional needs are high [1,2]. Knowledge about infants' and toddlers' food and nutrient intake is therefore important to evaluate their diet and identify potential challenges. In Norway, national dietary surveys of infants and toddlers have been performed at the ages of 6, 12 and 24 months [3–5]. Due to methodological issues, infants and toddlers of immigrant mothers were excluded from these surveys, and separate surveys for these children have been called for by the Norwegian Directorate of Health [6].

Consequently, compared to infants of Norwegian-born parents, less is known about the food and nutrient intake of infants of immigrant parents in Norway. However, some previous smaller studies of Norwegian immigrant children have shown some potential nutrition challenges, such as high prevalence of iron and vitamin D deficiencies and a relatively high added sugar intake [7–9]. It has further been suggested that immigrant children may be introduced to cow's milk at a younger age than ethnic Norwegian children, although inconsistent trends have been observed [9]. As cow's milk contains very little iron, consumption >500 mL/day has been associated with reduced iron stores in young children [10,11]. However, intake of fortified foods seems to improve iron status in late infancy [12].

To address the paucity of data on food and nutrient intake and infant feeding practices among Norwegian children with immigrant backgrounds, the InnBaKost study was initiated in 2012. Information on breastfeeding and complementary feeding practices among 6-month-old Norwegian-Somali and Norwegian-Iraqi infants was recently published [13]. The present paper aimed to describe and compare food and nutrient intake among 12-month-old Norwegian-Somali and Norwegian-Iraqi infants, with a focus on iron and vitamin D intake.

2. Materials and Methods

2.1. Subjects and Design

A cross-sectional survey was carried out from August 2013–September 2014. Mothers born in Somalia or Iraq and living in Oslo, Akershus or Buskerud were eligible for inclusion. These two immigrant groups were chosen, as they are the two non-Western immigrant groups in Norway with the highest number of births per year [14]. Children on a special diet due to serious illness were excluded. If the mother had twins or triplets, only one child was included by random selection.

Mothers who participated in the InnBaKost survey of 6-month-old infants [13] were contacted again when their children turned 12 months old. These mothers had not received any information about the results in the 6-months survey or dietary counselling which could influence dietary habits at the infants' 12 months of age. In the 6-month survey, 107 Norwegian-Somali mothers and infants and 80 Norwegian-Iraqi mothers and infants participated [13]. Of these, 70 Norwegian-Somali infants and 61 Norwegian-Iraqi infants participated in the 12-month follow-up survey. Seven of the Somali-born mothers and eight of the Iraqi-born mothers declined to participate further, while 30 Somali-born mothers and 11 Iraqi-born mothers could not be reached. Along with the mothers/infants participating in the 6-month survey, 19 additional Somali-born mothers and 16 additional Iraqi-born mothers were recruited. The additional mothers were recruited through lists obtained from the National Population Register. Mothers who were not reached from these lists in the 6-month survey were approached again when the infants were 12 months. A total sample of 89 Norwegian-Somali infants and 77 Norwegian-Iraqi infants were included for the present analysis.

To collect data on the food intake of the 12-month-old infants, two 24-h multiple-pass recalls were conducted face-to-face as closely as possible to the child's 12-month birthday. Eight trained female fieldworkers speaking the relevant language performed the interviews in Somali, Arabic, Kurdish or Norwegian. A total of 8% ($n = 13$) only completed one single 24-h recall. For mothers who were unable to meet in person, the interview was conducted over the telephone. Of all the participants, 3% ($n = 5$) had both interviews conducted over the telephone, while 4% ($n = 7$) had one of the two interviews conducted over the telephone. The interviews were conducted at a time and place chosen by individual mothers. The average time between the two 24-h recalls was 2 weeks. For 7% of the participants, there were more than 4 weeks between the two interviews. Approximately 78% of all the dietary recalls were collected for intakes on weekdays and 22% were collected for intakes on weekends among Norwegian-Somali infants, and the numbers were 83% and 17%, respectively, for Norwegian-Iraqi infants. In both groups, over 85% of the recall days were reported as representative of the usual daily dietary intake of the child. Each mother who completed the two 24-h recalls received a voucher for a baby shop worth approximately US $25.

The Regional Committees for Medical and Health Research Ethics (2012/957) approved the study, and informed consent was obtained from all the participating mothers.

2.2. 24-h Multiple-Pass Recall Method

The 24-h multiple-pass recall method was used to collect data on the 12-month-old Norwegian-Somali and Norwegian-Iraqi infants. The method was first developed and pilot tested on 12 Somali-born and Iraqi-born mothers from January to June 2013 [15].

Briefly, in this dietary recall method, the mothers were to be interviewed twice about the exact food and beverage intake of their children during the preceding 24 h. A 24-h period was defined as from the time the child woke up the previous day until the time the child woke up the day of the interview.

The dietary recall was divided into three passes. In the first pass, the mothers were asked to report everything that their children had consumed the previous day, including during the night. Each breastfeeding occurrence was also to be reported. In the second pass, mothers were asked to provide additional detailed information about each item of food and drink consumed by the children. This included type of product, brand names, cooking methods, amounts and leftovers. For homemade dishes, the mothers were asked for the recipes, and the list of ingredients was recorded. The third pass was a review of the recall, and the mothers were given the opportunity to provide any additional information regarding the children's food and drink consumption. During the last pass, the field workers were also instructed to prompt for information about foods and drinks not mentioned that were considered to be easy to forget, such as snacks, fruits, water, juices and supplements, which the field workers read from a list.

Two photographic booklets previously used in Norwegian national dietary surveys, were utilized during the interviews as an aid to estimate portion sizes. The *Spedkost* booklet [4] containing 17 colour photograph series of infant portion sizes of selected foods and drinks was mostly employed. The *Norkost* booklet [16] containing a series of adult portion sizes was mainly used to estimate portion sizes of different kinds of bread.

A picture library containing 405 pictures divided into 19 folders on an iPad was used to help identify the types of foods/drinks/products given to the children. The development of the picture library has been described in more detail elsewhere [15].

2.3. Questionnaire and Background Characteristics

A questionnaire with 19 questions on five topics was used to collect additional information about the infants. The questions related to breastfeeding (whether the infant was breastfed, and if so, the frequency of breastfeeding), the age of introduction to various foods and drinks, whether the infant had any allergies/intolerances, the use of dietary supplements and arenas for receiving infant nutrition information.

In Norway, healthcare personnel routinely measure the length and weight of children during regular check-ups at children's health clinics, including at 12 months of age. Participating mothers were asked to bring their infant's health cards to the interview in order to record these data. Other background characteristics, such as infants' gender, mothers' age, mothers' age when they immigrated to Norway, number of children, parental education levels and fathers' origins, were already provided from the 6-month survey. The same questions were asked of newly recruited mothers. All mothers were also asked to provide information on current work status and person/place in charge of day-care for the infants. When possible, other persons in charge of the day-care of the infant during the recall days were consulted on the infants' dietary intake during those hours.

2.4. Food Intake and Nutrient Calculations

Information from the 24-h recalls was manually coded by nutritionists. All foods and beverages consumed by each child were converted into grams of edible portions. For recipes, a modified version of the summing method was applied to calculate the intake of each ingredient [17]. A breast milk intake of 124 mL per feed or an intake of 497 mL for children whose mothers reported to have breastfed their children four times or more was used, as described by Grewal et al. [15]. The daily nutrient intakes (averaged over the two days) were computed using a food database and a dietary calculation system (KBS, version 7.2, database AE-10) developed at the Department of Nutrition, University of Oslo, Oslo, Norway. The food database used is mainly based on the official Norwegian food composition table but is also continuously supplemented with data on new food items and nutrient content. Relevant food products missing from KBS were added, and the nutrient content was based on the nutrient content listed on the products' nutritional label. Nutrients from dietary supplements and from fortified foods consumed during the recall days were included in the calculated nutrient intake. The calculated average daily nutrient intake from the two recalls was compared to the recommended intake ranges for macronutrients and recommended daily intakes (RI) for micronutrients [18].

2.5. Statistical Analysis

Data from the questionnaire and background characteristics were manually entered into the statistical software package IBM SPSS Statistics version 22.0. Data about the food and nutrient intakes estimated from KBS were transferred to SPSS. All data were further processed and analysed in SPSS. Energy intake information acquired during the telephone interviews ($n = 12$) did not differ from those who completed two face-to-face 24-h recalls and were therefore included in the analyses. Mothers who only completed one 24-h recall were also included.

The weight and length of the children were converted into Z-scores for weight-for-age, height-for-age and weight-for-height according to 2006 WHO child growth standards [19] using WHO Anthro (version 3.2.2, January 2011, Geneva, Switzerland) and macros. Cow's milk and yoghurt were categorized as 'dairy products' in the analysis. Infant formula and infant cereals were categorized as 'iron-enriched products'.

Iron intake was compared between infants receiving and not receiving dairy products and between infants receiving and not receiving iron-enriched products. The intake of dairy products and the intake of iron-enriched products were tested by different background characteristics. The intake of vitamin D was compared between infants receiving and not receiving vitamin D supplements. The intake of vitamin D supplements was tested by different background characteristics. The data did not adhere to a normal distribution, and continuous variables are presented as median and 25th and 75th percentiles (P_{25}–P_{75}) and were tested using a Mann-Whitney U test. Categorical variables were tested using a Chi-square test.

3. Results

Selected characteristics of the infants and their parents are presented in Table 1. The Norwegian-Somali infants had significantly higher Z-scores for height-for-age (1.4 vs. 0.6, $p = 0.001$) but not for weight-for-height (0.7 vs. 0.2, $p = 0.087$) compared to the Norwegian-Iraqi infants. The Somali-born mothers were younger (29 years vs. 32 years, $p = 0.026$), had lived in Norway for a longer period of time (10 years vs. 7 years, $p = 0.012$) and a higher percentage were working at the time of interviewing (27% vs. 13%, $p = 0.026$) compared to the Iraqi-born mothers. A higher proportion of the Iraqi-born mothers had higher education compared to the Somali-born mothers (64% vs. 38%, $p = 0.001$).

3.1. Breastfeeding

At 12 months of age, 40% of the Norwegian-Somali infants and 47% of the Norwegian-Iraqi infants were breastfed ($p = 0.414$). The median breastfeeding frequency among those breastfeeding was 4.5 times a day in both groups.

Table 1. Characteristics of the infants and parents sampled (n = 166).

Characteristics	Total (n = 166) [†]		Somali Origin (n = 89) [†]		Iraqi Origin (n = 77) [†]		p-Value *
Infants							
Boys/girls [‡]	55/45		60/40		49/51		0.154
Weight at 12 months (g) [‡]	10,000	(9286–11,100)	10,270	(9779–11,811)	9708	(9093–10,575)	0.001
Boys	10,120	(9470–11,293)	10,350	(9824–11,800)	9940	(8600–10,885)	0.034
Girls	9815	(9175–10,960)	10,185	(9481–12,104)	9460	(9100–10,500)	0.012
Length at 12 months (cm) [‡]	77.5	(75.0–79.9)	78.9	(77.0–81.5)	76.5	(74.4–78.3)	<0.001
Boys	78.0	(75.6–80.5)	78.3	(76.8–81.0)	77.8	(74.4–79.3)	0.110
Girls	77.0	(75.0–79.0)	79.5	(76.5–82.8)	76.0	(74.1–77.4)	<0.001
Z-score							
Weight-for-age	0.5	(0.0–1.5)	0.9	(0.2–1.9)	0.4	(0.0–1.1)	0.020
Height-for-age	0.8	(0.8–1.7)	1.4	(0.4–2.4)	0.6	(0.0–1.1)	0.001
Weight-for-height	0.3	(−0.4–1.2)	0.7	(−0.4–1.5)	0.2	(−0.4–0.9)	0.087
Mothers							
Age (years) [‡]	30.0	(27.0–34.0)	29.0	(27.0–33.0)	32.0	(27.0–36.5)	0.026
Age when immigrated to Norway [‡]	22.0	(15.0–26.3)	20.0	(12.0–24.0)	23.0	(19.0–29.0)	0.001
Number of years lived in Norway [‡]	10.0	(5.0–14.0)	10.0	(5.0–15.0)	7.0	(3.0–13.0)	0.012
Education [‡]							0.001
No/basic education	50		62		36		
High school/higher education	50		38		64		
Current employment status [‡]							0.026
Not working	79		73		87		
Working (full-time/part-time)	21		27		13		
Primiparous [‡]	28		28		27		0.891
Fathers							
Origin [‡]							0.001
Somalia./Iraq	92		95		88		
Other	8		5		12		
Education [‡]							0.102
No/basic education	28		29		27		0.285
High school/higher education	63		59		68		
Do not know	9		12		5		
Responsible for child during daytime [‡]							0.021
Mother	58		48		68		
Others (e.g., partner, day-care, etc.)	19		21		17		
Mother and others	23		31		15		

* Comparison of parents and infants of Somali and Iraqi origin. [†] Percentages for categorical variables, and medians (25th and 75th percentiles) for continuous variables; [‡] Data on gender are missing for three infants from Somalia. The lengths of 44 infants are missing (37 from Somalia and 7 from Iraq). The weights of 42 infants are missing (33 from Somalia and 9 from Iraq). Among male infants, data on length are missing for 26 infants and data on weight are missing for 26 infants. Among female infants, data on length are missing for 16 infants and data on weight are missing for 15 infants. The ages of four Somali-born mothers are missing. The ages when immigrated to Norway are missing for six Somali-born mothers and two Iraqi-born mothers. Mothers' and fathers' highest completed education is missing for four mothers and five fathers from Somalia. Current work status is missing for one Somali-born mother and one Iraqi-born mother. Primiparous data and father's origin is missing for four Somali-born mothers. Who is responsible for the child during daytime is missing for one Norwegian-Iraqi infant. These are not included in the analysis.

3.2. Food Intake

Data from the 24-h recalls on daily intakes of various types of foods and drinks among all infants are presented in Table 2. Percentages of and intake among consumers are presented in Table 3. Norwegian-Somali infants had significantly higher median daily intakes of commercial infant cereals, commercial fruit purees, fish/fish products, yoghurt and cow's milk compared to the Norwegian-Iraqi infants (Table 2). Norwegian-Iraqi infants, on the other hand, had significantly higher daily intakes of refined flour bread, cake, meat and meat products, eggs, fruits and berries, added sugar, tea and water than Norwegian-Somali infants (Table 2).

Commercial infant cereals and fruit purees, potatoes and fish/fish products were consumed by a significantly higher proportion of Norwegian-Somali infants compared to Norwegian-Iraqi infants, while bread, grain products, cake, meat, eggs, fruit/berries and tea were more commonly consumed by Norwegian-Iraqi infants (Table 3).

3.3. Energy and Nutrient Intake

The average energy and nutrient intake from the 24-h recalls are shown in Table 4. The median energy intake among Norwegian-Somali infants was 3791 kJ compared to 4122 kJ among Norwegian-Iraqi infants ($p = 0.059$). The median energy percentages (E%) from protein, fat and carbohydrates were within the recommended intake ranges in both groups; however, the intake of saturated fats was above the recommended upper level of 10 E%. The intake of added sugar, on the other hand, was below 5 E% in both groups.

The main sources of saturated fat intake in the total diet of the Norwegian-Somali infants were cow's milk (which contributed with 22%), breast milk (22%), commercial infant cereals (9%) and cheese (8%) (data not shown). The main sources of saturated fats among the Norwegian-Iraqi infants were breast milk (23%), meat and meat products (11%), cow's milk (9%) and cheese (9%). Yoghurt was the main source of the added sugar intake among both the Norwegian-Somali and Norwegian-Iraqi infants (38% vs. 23%).

The median intake of all micronutrients, except iron and niacin in both groups and zinc among Norwegian-Somali infants were above the RI.

3.4. Factors Associated with Iron Intake

The main sources of dietary iron were commercial infant cereals (which contributed with 51% among Norwegian-Somali vs. 34% among Norwegian-Iraqi infants), iron supplements (13% vs. 9%), infant formula (10% vs. 19%) and bread and other grain products (10% vs. 8%). During the recall days, 6% of the Norwegian-Somali infants and 8% of the Norwegian-Iraqi infants received supplements containing iron ($p = 0.574$, data not shown). Table 5 shows the percentage of the infants receiving dairy products and iron-enriched products and also median intakes of iron among infants receiving dairy products and iron-enriched products. There were no significant differences between the two groups regarding the proportion who had received dairy products, whether it concerned any dairy products or more than 500 g dairy products per day. A higher proportion of Norwegian-Somali infants had received iron-enriched products compared to Norwegian-Iraqi infants (88% vs. 73%, respectively; $p = 0.015$). Intakes of iron did not differ significantly between infants receiving dairy products compared to infants not receiving dairy products. However, the median intake of iron was significantly higher among infants receiving iron-enriched products (8.1 mg/day) compared to infants not receiving iron-enriched products (3.7 mg/day; $p < 0.001$). Neither intake of dairy products nor intake of iron-enriched products differed significantly between genders, according to mothers' ages, number of years lived in Norway, education level, current work status or number of children.

Table 2. Median intake of foods and drinks (g/day) among all infants at 12 months of age.

	Total (n = 166)		Somali Origin (n = 89)		Iraqi Origin (n = 77)		p-Value *
	Median	(P$_{25}$, P$_{75}$)	Median	(P$_{25}$, P$_{75}$)	Median	(P$_{25}$, P$_{75}$)	
Infant foods							
Breastmilk	0	(0, 372)	0	(0, 310)	0	(0, 454)	0.139
Infant formula	0	(0, 190)	0	(0, 103)	0	(0, 275)	0.092
Commercial infant cereal [†]	125	(0, 275)	200	(102, 300)	58	(0, 150)	<0.001
Commercial infant dinners	0	(0, 0)	0	(0, 0)	0	(0, 0)	0.762
Commercial fruit puree	0	(0, 3)	0	(0, 45)	0	(0, 0)	0.004
Commercial baby drinks	0	(0, 0)	0	(0, 0)	0	(0, 0)	0.884
Bread	17	(4, 31)	18	(0, 31)	16	(6, 31)	0.281
100% sifted flour	0	(0, 0)	0	(0, 0)	0	(0, 4)	0.001
<50% wholemeal flour	0	(0, 0)	0	(0, 0)	0	(0, 8)	<0.001
>50% wholemeal flour	4	(0, 21)	9	(0, 30)	0	(0, 16)	0.055
Grain products	13	(4, 30)	11	(2, 30)	14	(6, 29)	0.268
Cake	0	(0, 7)	0	(0, 0)	6	(0, 15)	<0.001
Potatoes	13	(0, 26)	16	(6, 26)	10	(0, 27)	0.090
Vegetables	37	(22, 66)	41	(26, 67)	33	(16, 64)	0.239
Meat/meat products	17	(0, 35)	5	(0, 23)	24	(11, 49)	<0.001
Fish/fish products	0	(0, 17)	9	(0, 21)	0	(0, 0)	<0.001
Eggs	0	(0, 0)	0	(0, 0)	0	(0, 22)	<0.001
Fruit and berries	43	(7, 90)	36	(0, 58)	58	(22, 121)	<0.001
Yoghurt	41	(0, 94)	57	(0, 110)	25	(0, 63)	0.009
Cheese	2	(0, 12)	1	(0, 11)	3	(0, 13)	0.512
Margarine, butter and oils	4	(2, 8)	4	(2, 8)	4	(2, 8)	0.602
Added sugar	0	(0, 0)	0	(0, 0)	0	(0, 2)	0.045
Drinks							
Cow's milk	60	(0, 320)	188	(0, 344)	26	(0, 245)	0.025
Whole milk	0	(0, 0)	0	(0, 0)	0	(0, 0)	0.623
Partly skimmed milk	31	(0, 250)	110	(0, 313)	3	(0, 185)	0.013
Skimmed milk	0	(0, 0)	0	(0, 0)	0	(0, 0)	0.127
Nido	0	(0, 0)	0	(0, 0)	0	(0, 0)	0.127
Juice	0	(0, 30)	0	(0, 30)	0	(0, 30)	0.187
Soda/squash with sugar	0	(0, 0)	0	(0, 0)	0	(0, 0)	0.872
Soda/squash, light	0	(0, 0)	0	(0, 0)	0	(0, 0)	0.397
Tea	0	(0, 0)	0	(0, 0)	0	(0, 0)	0.028
Water	180	(120, 270)	160	(98, 248)	187	(126, 299)	0.041

* Comparison of the intake of foods and drinks among infants of Somali and Iraqi origin, Mann–Whitney U test; [†] Prepared with water, infant formula, Nido and/or cow's milk.

Table 3. Percentage of consumers and median intake of foods and drinks (g/day) among consumers at 12 months of age.

	Total (n = 166)			Somali Origin (n = 89)			Iraqi Origin (n = 77)			p-Value *
	% Consumers	Median	(P$_{25}$-P$_{75}$)	% Consumers	Median	(P$_{25}$-P$_{75}$)	% Consumers	Median	(P$_{25}$-P$_{75}$)	
Infant foods										
Breastmilk	43	434	(310–497)	40	372	(248–455)	47	474	(326–497)	0.414
Infant formula	31	330	(217–540)	26	291	(192–492)	36	385	(240–649)	0.143
Commercial infant cereal †	74	200	(109–300)	88	214	(125–305)	57	140	(75–298)	<0.001
Commercial infant dinners	13	95	(44–148)	14	95	(42–134)	12	98	(45–173)	0.729
Commercial fruit puree	25	50	(45–98)	34	50	(45–100)	14	45	(45–90)	0.004
Commercial baby drinks	2	40	(26–88)	2	40	(-)	3	63	(-)	0.883
Bread	79	23	(11–35)	70	25	(16–36)	90	17	(8–33)	0.002
100% sifted flour	18	12	(5–17)	8	25	(13–38)	30	10	(4–15)	<0.001
<50% wholemeal flour	24	16	(6–23)	12	19	(8–23)	36	13	(5–25)	<0.001
>50% wholemeal flour	52	21	(11–33)	57	25	(15–33)	46	17	(8–33)	0.128
Grain products	84	18	(9–32)	75	18	(9–39)	91	17	(8–31)	0.020
Cake	37	17	(6–19)	16	11	(5–14)	62	14	(6–19)	<0.001
Potatoes	71	20	(12–34)	82	18	(11–28)	58	22	(13–37)	0.001
Vegetables	95	38	(25–68)	94	43	(27–69)	96	34	(18–67)	0.605
Meat/meat products	72	24	(13–46)	60	21	(8–31)	86	32	(16–51)	<0.001
Fish/fish products	46	18	(11–37)	65	16	(10–31)	23	29	(16–43)	<0.001
Eggs	21	28	(13–45)	11	10	(4–34)	33	28	(22–45)	0.001
Fruit and berries	80	55	(31–101)	64	54	(38–88)	99	59	(25–123)	<0.001
Yoghurt	70	63	(36–107)	70	95	(50–112)	70	46	(20–75)	0.948
Cheese	53	10	(4–20)	52	10	(4–18)	55	11	(4–21)	0.713
Margarine, butter and oils	95	4	(2–8)	94	4	(2–8)	96	5	(2–8)	0.605
Added sugar	22	4	(1–8)	17	2	(1–9)	29	4	(2–7)	0.070
Drinks										
Cow's milk	68	248	(60–420)	71	286	(152–440)	64	121	(29–404)	0.327
Whole milk	17	173	(23–250)	15	245	(179–392)	20	28	(15–170)	0.403
Partly skimmed milk	58	215	(60–368)	65	239	(117–365)	51	180	(32–375)	0.058
Skimmed milk	1	11	(-)	0	-	(-)	3	11	(-)	0.126
Nido	3	156	(68–537)	1	156	(-)	5	169	(49–689)	0.126
Juice	45	31	(19–93)	38	53	(29–105)	52	30	(13–91)	0.076
Soda/squash with sugar	16	31	(15–100)	16	45	(16–100)	17	31	(14–105)	0.841
Soda/squash, light	2	43	(31–58)	3	35	(-)	1	60	(-)	0.385
Tea	8	15	(5–30)	3	63	(-)	13	13	(4–23)	0.021
Water	100	180	(120–270)	100	160	(98–248)	100	187	(126–299)	-

* Comparison of the percentage of consumers among infants of Somali and Iraqi origin, Chi-square test; † Prepared with water, infant formula, Nido and/or cow's milk.

Table 4. Average energy and nutrient intake among infants of Somali and Iraqi origin at 12 months of age.

	RI† (1–2 Years)	Total (n = 166)		Somali Origin (n = 89)		Iraqi Origin (n = 77)		p-Value *
		Median	(P25–P75)	Median	(P25–P75)	Median	(P25–P75)	
Energy intake (kJ)		3945	(3235–4562)	3791	(2989–4544)	4122	(3454–4751)	0.059
Protein (E%)	10–15	14.5	(12.3–17.0)	14.8	(12.8–17.6)	13.8	(11.7–16.2)	0.074
Total fat (E%)	30–40	35.0	(30.0–39.3)	33.8	(29.9–37.6)	36.5	(32.5–40.9)	0.004
Saturated fat	<10	12.1	(10.1–14.7)	11.7	(9.7–13.7)	12.7	(11.1–15.6)	0.001
Monounsaturated fatty acids		12.6	(10.3–14.5)	11.8	(9.4–13.9)	13.4	(11.3–15.0)	0.002
Polyunsaturated fatty acids		5.7	(4.8–6.8)	5.3	(4.4–6.5)	6.1	(5.3–7.3)	0.003
Total carbohydrates (E%)	45–60	48.5	(44.8–51.9)	49.5	(46.8–51.9)	47.2	(42.9–52.1)	0.048
Added sugars	<10	3.2	(1.3–5.9)	4.0	(1.5–6.1)	2.5	(1.3–5.0)	0.063
Fibre (g)		7.4	(5.4–10.3)	7.4	(5.3–10.2)	7.4	(5.5–10.9)	0.753
Vitamin A (µg)	300 (RAE)	666	(483–878)	717	(574–933)	561	(400–874)	0.011
Vitamin D (µg)	10	12.6	(8.6–17.4)	13.9	(10.2–17.7)	11.7	(7.2–17.0)	0.029
Vitamin E (mg)	4 (µ-TE) ‡	10.5	(5.3–14.6)	12.1	(8.5–15.4)	7.3	(4.6–12.3)	<0.001
Thiamine (mg)	0.5	0.61	(0.42–0.80)	0.62	(0.42–0.80)	0.60	(0.41–0.80)	0.864
Riboflavin (mg)	0.6	0.72	(0.44–1.00)	0.77	(0.48–1.08)	0.66	(0.44–0.86)	0.039
Niacin (mg)	7 (NE) ‡	6.3	(4.4–8.6)	6.1	(4.5–8.3)	6.5	(4.4–8.7)	0.593
B6 (mg)	0.5	0.56	(0.39–0.75)	0.50	(0.37–0.73)	0.60	(0.44–0.82)	0.033
Folate (µg)	60	95	(72–135)	85	(66–121)	108	(80–151)	0.002
B12 (µg)	0.6	1.8	(0.8–2.9)	2.1	(1.1–3.0)	1.3	(0.6–2.6)	0.022
Vitamin C (mg)	25	72	(46–113)	74	(45–110)	69	(48–121)	0.755
Calcium (mg)	600	727	(519–954)	777	(587–984)	633	(480–938)	0.017
Iron (mg)	8	7.1	(4.6–10.3)	7.3	(4.9–10.3)	6.7	(4.5–11.4)	0.523
Zinc (mg)	5	5.1	(3.9–6.4)	4.8	(3.9–6.0)	5.3	(4.0–6.9)	0.117

* Comparison of infants of Somali and Iraqi origin, Mann–Whitney U test; † RI = Recommended intake ranges for macronutrients and recommended daily intakes for micronutrients. ‡ TE = tocopherol equivalent, NE = niacin equivalent.

Table 5. Percentage of Norwegian-Somali and Norwegian-Iraqi infants receiving dairy products and iron-enriched products and median iron intake (mg/day) among infants receiving dairy products and iron-enriched products.

	Total	Somali Origin	Iraqi Origin	p-Value [†]	Iron mg/Day		p-Value [‡]
	(n = 166)	(n = 89)	(n= 77)		Median	(P$_{25}$-P$_{75}$)	
Dairy products							
No (n = 21)	13	9	16	0.199	9.4	(5.2–11.1)	0.327
Yes (n = 145)	87	91	84		7.0	(4.5–10.2)	
Dairy products							
≤500 g/day (n = 140)	84	80	90	0.082	7.2	(4.8–10.7)	0.170
>500 g/day (n = 26)	16	20	10		6.4	(4.2–8.9)	
Iron-enriched products *							
No (n = 32)	19	12	27	0.015	3.7	(2.6–5.5)	<0.001
Yes (n = 145)	81	88	73		8.1	(5.7–11.2)	

* Include infant formula and infant cereals; [†] Tested by Chi-square test; [‡] Tested by Mann–Whitney U test.

3.5. Factors Associated with Vitamin D Intake

Vitamin D supplements comprised more than half of the vitamin D intake in both groups (61% among Norwegian-Somali infants vs. 52% among Norwegian-Iraqi infants). Other sources of vitamin D were commercial infant cereals (19% in both groups), infant formula (7% vs. 17%) and fish and fish products (6% vs. 3%) among Norwegian-Somali and Norwegian-Iraqi infants, respectively. During the recall days, a total of 84% of the infants had received vitamin D supplements. Significantly more among the Norwegian-Somali infants compared to the Norwegian-Iraqi infants had received vitamin D supplements during the recall days (94% vs. 71%, respectively; $p < 0.001$) The median (P_{25}–P_{75}) intake of vitamin D among those receiving vitamin D supplements was 14.5 (10.8–18.1) µg/day compared to 4.1 (1.5–7.6) µg/day among those not receiving vitamin D supplements ($p < 0.001$). The intake of vitamin D supplements did not differ significantly between genders, according to mothers' ages, number of years lived in Norway, education level, current work status or number of children.

4. Discussion

The present paper describes the food and nutrient intake in a group of 12-month-old Norwegian infants of mothers who immigrated to Norway from Somalia and Iraq. The findings indicate that the nutrient intake in this group of infants in general seems to be in accordance with Norwegian dietary recommendations, with the possible exception of certain micronutrients. The intake of added sugar was low, whereas the median intake of saturated fats exceeded the recommendations.

4.1. Breastfeeding

In this group of infants with immigrant backgrounds, 40% of the Norwegian-Somali infants and 47% of the Norwegian-Iraqi infants were breastfed at 12 months of age, with a median frequency of 4.5 times a day. This is quite similar to the 46% found to be breastfed in the Norwegian national dietary survey of infants at 12 months of age who had an average breastfeeding frequency of 3.5 times a day [4]. Breastfeeding patterns have been shown to vary between ethnic subgroups in a society, but also to depend on country of residence [20–22]. Data from a nationally representative population based cohort study from Ireland [21] and the National Survey of Children's Health in the US [22] reported higher breastfeeding initiation and longer duration among immigrant mothers compared to the native mothers. However, the breastfeeding prevalence in Ireland and the US were in general lower than what is common in Norway and other Scandinavian countries [23]. This may explain the opposite findings and the greater differences between immigrant and native mothers compared to our findings.

4.2. Food Intake

Commercial infant cereals, bread, potatoes and vegetables, fruit and berries, meat/meat products and fish/fish products were the most commonly consumed foods among the Norwegian-Somali and Norwegian-Iraqi infants. These foods were also consumed by a high proportion of infants in the Norwegian national dietary survey [4]. Commercial infant dinners were consumed by a higher proportion of infants in the national dietary survey compared to infants in the present survey [4]. Homemade dinners were also more common than commercial infant dinners at 6 months of age among Norwegian-Somali and Norwegian-Iraqi infants [13]. The lower use of commercial infant dinners among the children with immigrant background may be due, as reported in a study of Somali mothers in the US, to concerns about the lack of freshness of commercially produced baby foods and also the practice of feeding children the same foods as adults [24].

One important consideration when comparing these results is that the Norwegian national dietary survey used a semi-quantitative food frequency questionnaire (FFQ) to assess the infants' dietary intake at 12 months of age [4], while the present study used repeated 24-h recalls due to limited knowledge about Norwegian-Somali and Norwegian-Iraqi infants' diets. Thus, any comparison between the two studies should be undertaken with caution because the results from the national dietary survey represent the infants' intake over a longer period of time.

4.3. Energy and Nutrient Intake

The energy intake among both Norwegian-Somali and Norwegian-Iraqi infants was lower than the mean intake of 5100 kJ reported in the national dietary survey, which only reported the energy and nutrient intake of non-breastfed infants [4]. The average daily energy requirement for boys and girls at 12 months of age is 337 kJ/kg and 333 kJ/kg, respectively, according to Nordic nutrition recommendations [25]. Based on the median weights of the infants in the sample, Norwegian-Somali infants would have an average daily energy requirement of 3440 kJ and Norwegian-Iraqi infants would have an average daily energy requirement of 3252 kJ, which is lower than the average energy intake found in this study. However, the quality of the data on weight and height may have some limitations as each child health clinic may differ in terms of accuracy in reporting the measurements and the measurements may have been taken a few weeks before or after the 24-h recalls were performed. In addition, the weights of several infants were not registered, which may also have affected the median weights reported in this study. Furthermore, breast milk amounts were only estimated and this, along with possible misreporting of dietary intakes, may give inaccurate energy intake data.

The median E% of protein, total fat and carbohydrates were all within the recommended intake ranges [18]. Saturated fat was above the recommended 10 E%. However, one of the major sources of saturated fats in the diet was breast milk, which is recommended to give to infants until 12 months of age and beyond [18]. Other main sources of saturated fats was cow's milk and meat and meat products. Parents could reduce the infants' intake of saturated fats by changing high-fat dairy products with low-fat products as well as using lean cuts of meat. The intake of added sugar was appreciably lower than the recommended upper level of 10 E%, which is a positive finding. These results are quite similar to those reported in the national dietary survey, where saturated fats accounted for 12 E% and added sugar only accounted for 4 E%. Previous studies of young children with immigrant backgrounds in Norway and other countries have suggested that high sugar and sweetened beverage intake could be prevalent in this group [9,26–28]. However, the studies from Norway were conducted several years ago, and it could be that the trend of reducing the intake of added sugar, which has been reflected in the national dietary surveys, is also the case for this group of children. In the national dietary surveys, the intake of added sugar decreased from 10 E% in 1999 to 4 E% in 2007 due to the reduced intake of sugary drinks among Norwegian infants and the reduced levels of added sugar in commercial infant products [4,29]. In addition, a qualitative survey among Somali-born mothers in Norway revealed that most mothers thought that their infants at 12 months were too young to be given sugar [30]. However, the older siblings were usually eating candy and the majority of mothers had sweets available at home at all times, which may indicate that sweets and sugary drinks may be introduced at a later stage in the child's life.

4.4. Factors Associated with Iron Intake

Iron deficiency has been reported to be prevalent among both immigrant and non-immigrant children in Europe [7,31,32], however, some studies have suggested a higher prevalence among immigrant children [7,32]. The consumption of milk with low iron content and the excessive consumption of cow's milk have been reported in the literature to be factors that may cause iron deficiency [32,33]. On the other hand, iron-enriched products may be a protective factor against inadequate iron intake [32].

In the present study, we found no significant differences in iron intake among infants who consumed dairy products compared to those who did not consume dairy products. There were no significant differences among those who consumed more than 500 g/day of dairy products compared to those who consumed less. Still, high consumption of cow's milk is not recommended as it may inhibit the iron absorption [34]. Higher iron intakes were observed among infants who received iron-enriched products compared to those who did not receive these products. This has also been found among one-year-old children in other studies [12,35]. The majority of infants in the present study received iron-enriched products; however, the median intake of iron was lower than the RI [18] and the intake reported in the national dietary survey (12.8 mg/day) [4] for both Norwegian-Somali and Norwegian-Iraqi infants. The higher intakes of iron among the infants in the national dietary survey may be explained by a lower consumption of cow's milk (92 g/day), with only 51% consumers, and a higher consumption of commercial infant cereals (293 g/day) and infant formula (144 g/day), with 82% and 40% consumers, respectively [4]. Commercial infant cereals and infant formula were the two major sources of iron in the diet of the infants in the national dietary survey, followed by bread and meat/meat products [4].

4.5. Factors Associated with Vitamin D Intake

The intake of vitamin D exceeded the recommended levels for both Norwegian-Somali and Norwegian-Iraqi infants. Severe vitamin D deficiency has been reported to be prevalent among 6-week-old infants of immigrant backgrounds in Norway who did not receive vitamin D supplements [8]. In the present study, vitamin D supplements were given to the majority of Norwegian-Somali and Norwegian-Iraqi infants, as was seen in the 6-month survey [13]. The proportion was lower among the Norwegian-Iraqi infants. Vitamin D supplements were more commonly given in this sample compared to the 67% reported in the national dietary survey; those infants also had lower average intake of vitamin D (6.8 µg/day) [4]. Those not receiving vitamin D supplements in the present survey were more likely to have much lower intakes of vitamin D than those receiving vitamin D supplements and also lower intakes than the RI of 10 µg/day [18]. Vitamin D supplementation has recently been reported by Moffat et al. [36] to be almost similar and high among both immigrants and Canadian-born mothers, although less so for refugee mothers. According to their findings, current public education on vitamin D supplementation delivered by nurses and other health educators seems to be similarly effective for Canadian and immigrant parents [36]. A study by Madar et al. showed significant improvement in vitamin D status among infants with immigrant backgrounds in Norway after receiving free vitamin D supply together with tailor-made information handouts [37]. Vitamin D supplements are provided for free to of non-Western immigrant backgrounds at child health centres in Norway due to concerns about inadequate vitamin D intakes in this group. [38]. The findings of this study suggest that this information may have reached the majority of the participating mothers.

4.6. Strengths and Limitations of the Study

Two very specific subgroups of the Norwegian population were chosen for the study, which is an important strength of the survey. According to lists from the National Population Register, the participating Norwegian-Somali and Norwegian-Iraqi infants accounted for approximately 19% and 27%, respectively, of all Norwegian-Somali and Norwegian-Iraqi infants who turned 12 months old during the recruitment period in the three Norwegian counties included. Recruitment challenges are widely reported in studies among immigrant populations [39], and was also observed in the present study. The advantage was the use of bilingual field workers, which enabled the recruitment of mothers with limited Norwegian language skills. A possible limitation is the relatively large number of mothers lost to follow-up at 12 months, although new mothers were recruited. However, a comparison of background characteristics from the 6-month survey [13] and a description of the two immigrant groups by Statistics Norway [40] suggest that the mothers are to some extent representative of Somali-born and Iraqi-born mothers in these three counties in Norway.

In general, the dietary assessment of infants can be complicated by the fact that dietary habits change rapidly in infancy. A review by Burrows et al. has indicated that weighed food records may provide the best dietary estimates for younger children from 0.5 to 4 years old [41]. However, the 24-h multiple-pass recall is less time consuming and is reportedly used more frequently among immigrant populations, along with FFQs [39,42]. The recalls were mainly performed face-to-face, which may be a benefit as potential misunderstandings can be easily clarified in a personal interview. On the other hand, the presence of a field worker may cause a perception of authority on the part of the mothers, which could lead to social desirability response bias [43].

Although the macronutrient composition may reflect the true dietary practices of the two immigrant groups, reporting errors such as underreporting or overreporting may contribute to apparently low or high intakes of certain foods [41]. For infants in particular, not all foods served are necessarily consumed as some is wasted. Furthermore, the mothers may share the responsibility for their children with other adults (e.g., partners, grandparents and day-care), and it may be more difficult for the mothers to assess children's intake during the hours they were not present [44].

In addition, biochemical indicators of iron and vitamin D status were not measured in the present study, which is necessary in order to assess the infants' iron and vitamin D status.

5. Conclusions

The findings of this study indicate that the food and nutrient intake of Norwegian-Somali and Norwegian-Iraqi infants in general seems to be in accordance with the Norwegian dietary recommendations. The intake of dairy products was generally higher among Norwegian-Somali infants compared to Norwegian-Iraqi infants, but dairy product intake did not seem to affect iron intake. Iron-enriched products and vitamin D supplements were important sources of the infants' iron and vitamin D intake. Vitamin D supplements and foods rich in iron should continue to be promoted. Infants with immigrant backgrounds are excluded from the Norwegian national dietary surveys, and the present study contributes with information about food and nutrient intake among two of these groups living in Norway. More research to investigate infant feeding practices among immigrant groups in Norway is needed.

Acknowledgments: The present study was financed and supported by the Norwegian Research Council (grant number 213460/H10). We would like to thank the field workers who assisted with the data collection and also the mothers/infants who participated in the study.

Author Contributions: N.K.G. designed the study and participated in the data collection, carried out the data analysis and wrote the manuscript. L.F.A. and L.E.T. designed the study, assisted in the data analysis and provided advice during all stages of the work. C.S.K. and I.K. coded the information from the 24-h recalls. All authors contributed to the development of the manuscript, including the drafting and editing of the manuscript. All authors read and approved the final manuscript.

Conflicts of Interest: The authors declare no conflict of interest.

References

1. Chomtho, S.; Wells, J.C.; Williams, J.E.; Davies, P.S.; Lucas, A.; Fewtrell, M.S. Infant growth and later body composition: Evidence from the 4-component model. *Am. J. Clin. Nutr.* **2008**, *87*, 1776–1784. [PubMed]
2. Victora, C.G. Nutrition in early life: A global priority. *Lancet* **2009**, *374*, 1123–1125. [CrossRef]
3. Øverby, N.C.; Kristiansen, A.L.; Andersen, L.F.; Lande, B. *Spedkost—6 Måneder. Landsomfattende Kostholdsundersøkelse Blant 6 Måneder Gamle Barn (Norwegian National Dietary Survey among 6-Month Old Infants)*; Norwegian Directorate of Health: Oslo, Norway, 2008.
4. Øverby, N.C.; Kristiansen, A.L.; Andersen, L.F.; Lande, B. *Spedkost—12 Måneder. Landsomfattende Kostholdsundersøkelse Blant 12 Måneder Gamle Barn (Norwegian National Dietary Survey among 12-Month Old Infants)*; Norwegian Directorate of Health: Oslo, Norway, 2009.
5. Kristiansen, A.L.; Andersen, L.F.; Lande, B. *Småbarnskost—2 år. Landsomfattende Kostholdesundersøkelse Blant 2 år Gamle Barn (Norwegian National Dietary Survey among 2-Year Old Children)*; Norwegian Directorate of Health: Oslo, Norway, 2009.
6. Lande, B.; Andersen, L.F.; Bærug, A.; Trygg, K.; Lund-Larsen, K.; Bjørneboe, G.E.A. Development of a method for use in a national representative dietary survey among norwegian infants and children—Spedkost/småbarnskost. *Nor. J. Epidemiol.* **2000**, *10*, 43–50.
7. Wandel, M.; Fagerli, R.A.; Olsen, P.T.; BorchIohnsen, B.; Ek, J. Iron status and weaning practices among norwegian and immigrant infants. *Nutr. Res.* **1996**, *16*, 251–265. [CrossRef]

8. Madar, A.A.; Stene, L.C.; Meyer, H.E. Vitamin d status among immigrant mothers from pakistan, turkey and somalia and their infants attending child health clinics in Norway. *Br. J. Nutr.* **2009**, *101*, 1052–1058. [CrossRef] [PubMed]

9. Kumar, B.; Wandel, M. Nutritional challenges among immigrant children and youth in Norway. In *Global Migration and Education*; Adams, L.D., Kirova, A., Eds.; Lawrence Erlbaum Associates: Mahwah, NJ, USA, 2007; pp. 67–81.

10. Maguire, J.L.; Lebovic, G.; Kandasamy, S.; Khovratovich, M.; Mamdani, M.; Birken, C.S.; Parkin, P.C.; Kids, T.A. The relationship between cow's milk and stores of vitamin d and iron in early childhood. *Pediatrics* **2013**, *131*, e144–e151. [CrossRef] [PubMed]

11. Soh, P.; Ferguson, E.L.; McKenzie, J.E.; Homs, M.Y.; Gibson, R.S. Iron deficiency and risk factors for lower iron stores in 6–24-month-old New Zealanders. *Eur. J. Clin. Nutr.* **2004**, *58*, 71–79. [CrossRef] [PubMed]

12. Thorisdottir, A.V.; Ramel, A.; Palsson, G.I.; Tomassson, H.; Thorsdottir, I. Iron status of one-year-olds and association with breast milk, cow's milk or formula in late infancy. *Eur. J. Clin. Nutr.* **2013**, *52*, 1661–1668. [CrossRef] [PubMed]

13. Grewal, N.K.; Andersen, L.F.; Sellen, D.; Mosdol, A.; Torheim, L.E. Breast-feeding and complementary feeding practices in the first 6 months of life among norwegian-somali and norwegian-iraqi infants: The innbakost survey. *Public Health Nutr.* **2016**, *19*, 703–715. [CrossRef] [PubMed]

14. Statistics Norway. Statbank Norway. Available online: http://www.ssb.no/statistikkbanken/SelectTable/hovedtabellHjem.asp?KortNavnWeb=innvbef&CMSSubjectArea=befolkning&StatVariant=&PLanguage=0&checked=true (accessed on 10 July 2015).

15. Grewal, N.K.; Mosdol, A.; Aunan, M.B.; Monsen, C.; Torheim, L.E. Development and pilot testing of 24-h multiple-pass recall to assess dietary intake of toddlers of somali- and iraqi-born mothers living in Norway. *Nutrients* **2014**, *6*, 2333–2347. [CrossRef] [PubMed]

16. Totland, T.H.; Melnæs, B.K.; Lundberg-Hallén, N.; Helland-Kigen, K.M.; Lund-Blix, N.A.; Myhre, J.B.; Johansen, A.M.W.; Løken, E.B.; Andersen, L.F. *Norkost 3—En Landsomfattende Kostholdsundersøkelse Blant Menn og Kvinner i Norge i Alderen 18–70 år, 2010–2011 (Norwegian National Dietary Survey among Adults 18–70 Years, 2010–2011)*; Norwegian Directorate of Health: Oslo, Norway, 2012.

17. Bergström, L. *Nutrient Losses and Gains in the Preparation of Foods*; National Food Administration: Uppsala, Sweden, 1994.

18. Norwegian Directorate for Health. *Recommendations for Diet, Nutrition and Physical Activity (Anbefalinger om Kosthold, Ernæring og Fysisk Aktivitet)*; Norwegian Directorate of Health: Oslo, Norway, 2014.

19. World Health Organization. The WHO Child Growth Standards. Available online: http://www.who.int/childgrowth/standards/en/ (accessed on 10 April 2015).

20. Van Rossem, L.; Vogel, I.; Steegers, E.A.P.; Moll, H.A.; Jaddoe, V.W.V.; Hofman, A.; Mackenbach, J.P.; Raat, H. Breastfeeding patterns among ethnic minorities: The generation r study. *J. Epidemiol. Community Health* **2010**, *64*, 1080–1085. [CrossRef] [PubMed]

21. Ladewig, E.L.; Hayes, C.; Browne, J.; Layte, R.; Reulbach, U. The influence of ethnicity on breastfeeding rates in Ireland: A cross-sectional study. *J. Epidemiol. Community Health* **2014**, *68*, 356–362. [CrossRef] [PubMed]

22. Singh, G.K.; Kogan, M.D.; Dee, D.L. Nativity/immigrant status, race/ethnicity, and socioeconomic determinants of breastfeeding initiation and duration in the United States, 2003. *Pediatrics* **2007**, *119* (Suppl. S1), S38–S46. [CrossRef] [PubMed]

23. Ibanez, G.; Martin, N.; Denantes, M.; Saurel-Cubizolles, M.J.; Ringa, V.; Magnier, A.M. Prevalence of breastfeeding in industrialized countries. *Rev. Epidemiol. Sante Publique* **2012**, *60*, 305–320. [CrossRef] [PubMed]

24. Steinman, L.; Doescher, M.; Keppel, G.A.; Pak-Gorstein, S.; Graham, E.; Haq, A.; Johnson, D.B.; Spicer, P. Understanding infant feeding beliefs, practices and preferred nutrition education and health provider approaches: An exploratory study with somali mothers in the USA. *Mater. Child Nutr.* **2010**, *6*, 67–88. [CrossRef] [PubMed]

25. Nordic Councel of Ministers. *Nordic Nutrition Recommendations 2012 Part 1: Summary, Principles and Use*; Nordic Council of Ministers: Copenhagen, Denmark, 2013.

26. Schneider, S.; Jerusalem, M.; Mente, J.; De Bock, F. Sweets consumption of preschool children—Extent, context, and consumption patterns. *Clin. Oral Investig.* **2013**, *17*, 1301–1309. [CrossRef] [PubMed]

27. De Hoog, M.L.; Kleinman, K.P.; Gillman, M.W.; Vrijkotte, T.G.; van Eijsden, M.; Taveras, E.M. Racial/ethnic and immigrant differences in early childhood diet quality. *Public Health Nutr.* **2014**, *17*, 1308–1317. [CrossRef] [PubMed]

28. Sahota, P.; Gatenby, L.A.; Greenwood, D.C.; Bryant, M.; Robinson, S.; Wright, J. Ethnic differences in dietary intake at age 12 and 18 months: The born in Bradford 1000 study. *Public Health Nutr.* **2015**, *19*, 1–9. [CrossRef] [PubMed]

29. Lande, B.; Andersen, L.F. *Spedkost 12 Måneder—Landsomfattende Kostholdsundersøkelse Blant Spedbarn i Norge (Norwegian National Dietary Survey among 12-Month Old Infants)*; Norwegian Directorate of Health: Oslo, Norway, 2005.

30. Lyngstad, J. Understanding Infant Feeding Practices, Relations to the Health Clinic and Experiences of Receiving Conflicting Advices: A Qualitative Study with Somali Mothers Living in Oslo. Master's Thesis, Faculty of Health Sciences, Department of Health, Nutrition and Management, Oslo and Akershus University College of Applied Sciences, Oslo, Norway, 2014.

31. Bramhagen, A.C.; Svahn, J.; Hallstrom, I.; Axelsson, I. Factors influencing iron nutrition among one-year-old healthy children in Sweden. *J. Clin. Nurs.* **2011**, *20*, 1887–1894. [CrossRef] [PubMed]

32. Verga, M.E.; Widmeier-Pasche, V.; Beck-Popovic, M.; Pauchard, J.Y.; Gehri, M. Iron deficiency in infancy: Is an immigrant more at risk? *Swiss Med. Wkly.* **2014**, *144*, w14065. [CrossRef] [PubMed]

33. Ziegler, E.E. Consumption of cow's milk as a cause of iron deficiency in infants and toddlers. *Nutr. Rev.* **2011**, *69* (Suppl. S1), S37–S42. [CrossRef] [PubMed]

34. Domellof, M.; Braegger, C.; Campoy, C.; Colomb, V.; Decsi, T.; Fewtrell, M.; Hojsak, I.; Mihatsch, W.; Molgaard, C.; Shamir, R.; et al. Iron requirements of infants and toddlers. *J. Pediatr. Gastroenterol. Nutr.* **2014**, *58*, 119–129. [CrossRef] [PubMed]

35. Virtanen, M.A.; Svahn, C.J.; Viinikka, L.U.; Raiha, N.C.; Siimes, M.A.; Axelsson, I.E. Iron-fortified and unfortified cow's milk: Effects on iron intakes and iron status in young children. *Acta Paediatr.* **2001**, *90*, 724–731. [CrossRef] [PubMed]

36. Moffat, T.; Sellen, D.; Wilson, W.; Anderson, L.; Chadwick, S.; Amarra, S. Comparison of infant vitamin d supplement use among Canadian-born, immigrant, and refugee mothers. *J. Transcult. Nurs.* **2015**, *26*, 261–269. [CrossRef] [PubMed]

37. Madar, A.A.; Klepp, K.I.; Meyer, H.E. Effect of free vitamin D (2) drops on serum 25-hydroxyvitamin d in infants with immigrant origin: A cluster randomized controlled trial. *Eur. J. Clin. Nutr.* **2009**, *63*, 478–484. [CrossRef] [PubMed]

38. Norwegian Directorate of Health. Gratis Vitamin D-tilskudd Til Spedbarn Med IKKE-Vestlig Innvandrerbakgrunn (Free Vitamin D Supplement to Infants with Non-Western Immigrant Backgrounds). Available online: http://www.matportalen.no/kosthold_og_helse/tema/kosttilskudd/gratis_vitamin_d-tilskudd_til_spedbarn_med_ikke-vestlig_innvandrerbakgrunn (accessed on 12 June 2015).

39. Ngo, J.; Gurinovic, M.; Frost-Andersen, L.; Serra-Majem, L. How dietary intake methodology is adapted for use in European immigrant population groups—A review. *Br. J. Nutr.* **2009**, *101* (Suppl. S2), S86–S94. [CrossRef] [PubMed]

40. Henriksen, K. *Levekår og Kjønnsforskjeller Blant Innvandrere Fra ti Land (Living Conditions and Gender Differences among Immigrants from Ten Countries)*; Statistics Norway: Oslo, Norway, 2010.

41. Burrows, T.L.; Martin, R.J.; Collins, C.E. A systematic review of the validity of dietary assessment methods in children when compared with the method of doubly labeled water. *J. Am. Diet. Assoc.* **2010**, *110*, 1501–1510. [CrossRef] [PubMed]

42. Garduno-Diaz, S.D.; Husain, W.; Ashkanani, F.; Khokhar, S. Meeting challenges related to the dietary assessment of ethnic minority populations. *J. Hum. Nutr. Diet.* **2014**, *27*, 358–366. [CrossRef] [PubMed]

43. Hebert, J.R.; Clemow, L.; Pbert, L.; Ockene, I.S.; Ockene, J.K. Social desirability bias in dietary self-report may compromise the validity of dietary intake measures. *Int. J. Epidemiol.* **1995**, *24*, 389–398. [CrossRef] [PubMed]

44. Livingstone, M.B.; Robson, P.J.; Wallace, J.M. Issues in dietary intake assessment of children and adolescents. *Br. J. Nutr.* **2004**, *92* (Suppl. S2), S213–S222. [CrossRef] [PubMed]

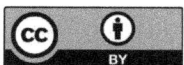

nutrients

MDPI

Article

Food Consumption and Nutrient Intake by Children Aged 10 to 48 Months Attending Day Care in The Netherlands

R. Alexandra Goldbohm [1,*], Carina M. Rubingh [2], Caren I. Lanting [1,*] and Koen F. M. Joosten [3]

[1]   Netherlands Organisation for Applied Scientific Research TNO, Schipholweg 77–89,
      Leiden 2316 ZL, The Netherlands
[2]   Netherlands Organisation for Applied Scientific Research TNO, Utrechtseweg 48,
      Zeist 3700 AJ, The Netherlands; carina.dejong@tno.nl
[3]   Erasmus University Medical Centre, Erasmus MC-Sophia Children's Hospital, Dr. Molewaterplein 60,
      Rotterdam 3015 GJ, The Netherlands; k.joosten@erasmusmc.nl
*   Correspondence: ra.goldbohm@ziggo.nl (R.A.G.); caren.lanting@tno.nl (C.I.L.); Tel.: +31-888-666-226 (C.I.L.)

Received: 2 June 2016; Accepted: 9 July 2016; Published: 14 July 2016

Abstract: The diet of young children is an important determinant of long-term health effects, such as overweight and obesity. We analyzed two-day food consumption records from 1526 young children (10–48 months old) attending 199 daycare centers across The Netherlands. Data were observed and recorded in diaries by caregivers at the day nursery and by parents at home on days that the children attended the daycare center. According to national and European reference values, the children had an adequate nutrient intake with exception of low intakes of total fat, *n*-3 fatty acids from fish and possibly iron. Intakes of energy and protein were substantially higher than recommended and part of the population exceeded the tolerable upper intake levels for sodium, zinc and retinol. Consumption of fruit, fats, fish, and fluids was substantially less than recommended. The children used mostly (semi-)skimmed milk products and non-refined bread and cereals, as recommended. Two thirds of the consumed beverages, however, contained sugar and contributed substantially to energy intake. In young children, low intakes of *n*-3 fatty acids and iron are a potential matter of concern, as are the high intakes of energy, protein, sugared beverages, and milk, since these may increase the risk of becoming overweight.

Keywords: young children; nutrition; dietary habits; childcare

---

1. Introduction

Proper nutrition of young children promotes optimal growth and development. The right amount of energy and nutrients also reduces the risk for developing overweight and obesity, dental caries, and gastrointestinal problems like constipation and diarrhea. In addition, there is some evidence that diet quality and especially breakfast consumption is related to cognitive functioning and academic performance of children [1,2]. Unfavorable dietary habits may have long-term implications, especially since childhood overweight tends to track into adulthood [3] and overweight and obesity are major risk factors for cardiovascular disease, type 2 diabetes mellitus, and cancer [4]. Early childhood is a critical period for prevention of diet-related disease later in life; dietary habits tend to be established at an early age and are maintained throughout later life [5].

In The Netherlands, about 40% of children until four years of age attend childcare [6]. Childcare providers are in a unique position to educate parents about healthy eating, to encourage children to eat healthy, and to provide a healthy environment for children to eat, grow and develop. In the current study, food consumption was registered in a large population of young children

(10–48 months old) attending day care across The Netherlands. Intakes of energy, macro- and micronutrients and on consumption of a complete set of food groups (e.g., bread, milk products, sweetened beverages) were established and compared with current recommendations. Some of the results have been published previously [7,8]; however, these were based on a smaller sample and only comprised a small selection of macronutrients and a few food groups.

2. Materials and Methods

2.1. Study Population

Details on the recruitment methods were previously published [7]. In brief, 199 childcare centers located across the Netherlands, were recruited between 2011 and 2014 to participate in the study, which was originally offered to all childcare centers in The Netherlands by Nutricia Nederland BV, Zoetermeer, The Netherlands, as a service to support their nutrition policy. Children between the age of 10 and 48 months who were attending the nursery for at least two days per week could participate in the study. The manager of the childcare center invited the children's parents to participate in the study and obtained written and signed informed consent from them. The study has been conducted in accordance with the Declaration of Helsinki and complied with national and EU data protection laws (Directive 95/46/EC). According to Dutch law, approval by a medical-ethical committee is exempted for this type of observational research.

2.2. Dietary Intake Assessment

Details on the assessment methods were previously published [7,8]. In brief, at the childcare center, food and beverage consumption was recorded on a structured poster by the carers for all children participating in the study during two days. Dutch children attending a childcare center usually eat breakfast and the main (hot) meal at home and lunch and a morning and afternoon snack at the childcare center. Few childcare centers serve a hot meal during lunchtime or in the evening. For the food and beverages consumed at home, a parent completed a structured diary at the same two days. Berdien van Wezel Dieticians (The Hague, The Netherlands), were responsible for data collection. Trained dieticians instructed carers and parents, supervised the recording and were responsible for coding and computer entry of the consumption data using the FoodFigures system [9].

2.3. Data Processing

A raw data set containing, for each child, records with food codes and a quantity (g or mL), eating occasion (e.g., breakfast), day and location (home or childcare center) per food code was exported from the FoodFigures system. Data checking and calculation of nutrient intake and food group consumption was performed using a software application in SAS [10,11] specifically developed for processing of dietary data [12]. The Dutch food composition database (NEVO), edition 2013, was used for calculation of nutrient intake [13]. In this edition of the NEVO database, dietary fiber is considered an energy-contributing nutrient (2 kcal/g fiber). A few food codes were derived from the NEVO database of 2011 or from an additional food composition database. Data were checked for inconsistencies and completeness of the records, i.e., two days, both at the childcare center and at home, should be present for each child. Potential outliers at the high and the low end of the quantity of consumed foods were listed and checked in the original diaries and posters. After correction of the database, a final check on potential outliers of the calculated nutrient intake was performed.

2.4. Data Analysis

Mean daily energy and nutrient intake was calculated for all children and for each age group (i.e., 10 and 11 months old and 1, 2 and 3 years old, which included children ⩾12–<24 months, ⩾24–<36 months, and ⩾36–<48 months, respectively). As (energy-adjusted) nutrient intake differed very little between boys and girls, their results are not separately presented. We used the "Statistical Program to

Assess Dietary Exposure" (SPADE) to transform the nutrient intake from the two days into a theoretical "usual" intake distribution of the population [14]. For all nutrients, we used the SPADE model for daily intakes, except for *n*-3 fish fatty acids and folic acid for which the module for episodical intakes was used and docosahexaenoic acid, for which no model was found that fitted the required criteria. We followed the European Food Safety Authority's (EFSA) guidance [15] to compare the usual intake distribution with dietary reference values (specifically, Adequate Intake and Tolerable Upper Intake Levels (TUIL)) as established by the Health Council of The Netherlands (HCN) [16–18] and, if relevant, more recent ones from the EFSA [19]. For this comparison, we assumed that the usual intake based on the two weekdays that the children attended the childcare center is representative for their true usual intake.

Furthermore, individual foods were divided into food groups to calculate the mean daily consumption of each food group. We defined several food group classifications. The first, a classic one, was based on type of food (e.g., meat, meat products, and poultry; bread; fruit). We used a second one, based on the food based dietary guidelines ("Schijf van Vijf") published by The Netherlands Nutrition Centre (NNC) [20], to compare mean daily consumption of the relevant food groups with the recommendations that apply to children from 1 to 3 years old. Finally, we subdivided the foods grouped according to the NNC classification in preferable or neutral foods and foods that should be eaten by exception only [21]. Preferable foods contribute positively to a diet preventive for chronic diseases, whereas "by exception" foods contribute negatively to such a diet. Classification of foods is based on their content of saturated fat, trans fat, sodium, dietary fiber and added sugar. For example, full-fat milk products (as opposed to skimmed milk) are classified as by-exception food, just as milk products and beverages with added sugar. The contribution of these food groups to the intake of selected nutrients was also calculated. Furthermore, we simulated the effect of replacing liquid cow's milk by formula among exclusive cow's milk users on usual iron and protein intake. In this simulation, liquid cow's milk was replaced by young children's formula (with a nutrient composition according to Nutrilon, Zoetermeer, The Netherlands, a brand from the Nutricia company).

3. Results

3.1. Study Population

Table 1 presents the characteristics of the study population (*n* = 1526). Body weight and height are not presented, as they were not considered sufficiently accurate and comprised a high proportion of missing values.

Table 1. Characteristics of the study population.

		n	%
Gender	Boy	759	49.7
	Girl	683	44.8
	Missing	84	5.5
Age	10–11 months old	31	2.0
	1 year old	411	26.9
	2 years old	497	32.6
	3 years old	410	26.9
	Missing	177	11.6
Zip-code based socioeconomic status of childcare centers	Low	381	25.0
	Medium	848	55.6
	High	218	14.3
	Missing	79	5.2
Number of days per week that the child attended childcare center	2 days	939	61.5
	3 days	348	22.8
	4 days	68	4.5
	5 days	16	1.1
	Missing	155	10.2
Hot meal at childcare center	Yes	315	20.6
	No	1189	77.9
	Missing	22	1.4

Between 19 and 67 (mean 41) food records were available per child. A food record comprises the consumption of a given quantity of a given food or beverage at a given occasion (e.g., breakfast). 14 children were breastfed (11 of whom were 12 months or younger).

3.2. Nutrient Intake

Table 2 displays the average daily intake of macronutrients (mean and standard deviation), both in absolute amount as in energy density. Boys had a higher mean energy intake than girls (5483 kJ versus 5271 kJ). All gender differences in intake of macronutrients were attributable to the higher energy intake by boys. However, the intake relative to energy was very similar for boys and girls (see supplementary materials Table S1). The absolute intakes of micronutrients (Table 2) were also somewhat higher for boys than for girls (see supplementary materials Table S1). According to their parents, 92% of the children had received a vitamin D supplement on at least one of the two study days.

Table 2. Mean daily nutrient intake by children attending childcare by age (mean of 2 days).

Nutrient	Unit	Total Group (n = 1526)[1] Mean	SD	10–11 Months (n = 31) Mean	SD	1 Year (n = 411) Mean	SD	2 Years (n = 497) Mean	SD	3 Years (n = 410) Mean	SD
Energy	kJ	5383	958	4241	795	4954	822	5424	872	5841	923
Protein	g	45	9	32	8	43	9	45	8	48	10
	en%	14.1	2.2	12.6	2.2	14.6	2.4	13.9	2.0	13.9	2.1
Carbohydrates	g	174	34	136	27	159	30	177	32	189	33
	en%	54.4	5.1	54.2	5.9	54	5.3	54.8	5.0	54.5	4.8
Mono- and disaccharides	g	100	25	79	18	91	24	102	24	108	26
	en%	31.2	5.7	31.4	5.5	30.7	6.1	31.7	5.3	31.1	5.7
Polysaccharides	g	75	16	58	15	69	14	75	15	81	16
	en%	23.4	3.4	23.1	3.6	23.6	3.6	23.3	3.1	23.4	3.3
Fat	g	42	11	34	10	38	10	42	10	45	11
	en%	29.1	4.6	30.4	5.5	28.7	4.8	28.9	4.5	29.3	4.3
Saturated fatty acids	g	14.8	3.8	12.6	4.7	13.5	3.4	14.8	3.7	16.1	3.8
	en%	10.4	1.8	11.2	2.8	10.3	1.9	10.3	1.8	10.4	1.7
Monounsaturated fatty acids	g	14.4	4.5	11.7	4.3	12.9	4.2	14.4	4.5	15.8	4.4
	en%	10.0	2.3	10.4	3.0	9.8	2.4	9.9	2.3	10.2	2.2
Polyunsaturated fatty acids (PUFA)	g	8.6	3.2	6.7	2.3	8.0	3.1	8.6	3.0	9.4	3.4
	en%	6.0	1.8	5.9	1.5	6.1	1.9	5.9	1.7	6.0	1.7
n-3 PUFA	g	1.0	0.4	0.9	0.3	1.0	0.3	1.0	0.4	1.1	0.4
	en%	0.7	0.2	0.8	0.2	0.7	0.2	0.7	0.2	0.7	0.2
ALA (C18:3 (*n*-3) *cis*)	g	1.0	0.3	0.8	0.3	0.9	0.3	1.0	0.3	1.0	0.4
	en%	0.7	0.2	0.7	0.2	0.7	0.2	0.7	0.2	0.7	0.2
EPA (C20:5 (*n*-3) *cis*)	g	0.01	0.03	0.02	0.03	0.02	0.03	0.01	0.02	0.01	0.03
	en%	0	0	0	0	0	0	0	0	0	0
DHA (C22:6 (*n*-3) *cis*)	g	0.02	0.04	0.02	0.04	0.02	0.05	0.02	0.04	0.02	0.04
	en%	0	0	0	0	0	0	0	0	0	0
n-6 PUFA	g	7.3	2.8	5.4	2.0	6.8	2.7	7.3	2.6	8.0	3.0
	en%	5.1	1.6	4.8	1.4	5.1	1.7	5.0	1.5	5.1	1.5
Linoleic acid (C18:2 (*n*-6) *cis*)	g	7.3	2.8	5.4	2.0	6.7	2.7	7.2	2.6	7.9	3.0
	en%	5.0	1.6	4.8	1.4	5.1	1.7	5.0	1.5	5.1	1.5
Trans-unsaturated fatty acids	g	0.4	0.2	0.3	0.2	0.4	0.2	0.4	0.2	0.5	0.2
	en%	0.3	0.1	0.2	0.1	0.3	0.1	0.3	0.1	0.3	0.1
Cholesterol	mg	76.1	38.0	45.9	45.9	69.2	37.2	77.4	38.6	84.4	38.2

Table 2. *Cont.*

Nutrient	Unit	Total Group (n = 1526)[1]		10–11 Months (n = 31)		1 Year (n = 411)		2 Years (n = 497)		3 Years (n = 410)	
		Mean	SD	Mean	SD	Mean	SD	Mean	SD	Mean	SD
Dietary fiber	g	12.6	2.7	12.4	2.6	12.4	2.7	12.5	2.6	13.1	2.7
	g/MJ	2.4	0.4	3.0	0.5	2.5	0.5	2.3	0.4	2.3	0.4
Water	g	1045	248	885	219	988	240	1047	231	1133	245
Sodium	mg	1273	359	790	266	1117	301	1317	340	1420	341
Potassium	mg	1923	405	1435	420	1864	391	1934	377	2010	402
Phosphorus	mg	943	199	715	190	907	189	941	186	997	206
Magnesium	mg	181	38	134	29	172	36	181	34	194	40
Iron	mg	6.3	2.0	8.4	2.5	6.5	2.4	6.0	1.7	6.1	1.7
Calcium	mg	735	186	684	200	734	177	720	177	745	202
Copper	mg	0.61	0.15	0.59	0.13	0.58	0.14	0.60	0.14	0.66	0.15
Selenium	µg	22	6	21	6	21	6	22	6	24	6
Zinc	mg	6.0	1.4	6.0	1.4	6.0	1.4	5.9	1.4	6.1	1.5
Iodine	µg	120	30	118	22	117	31	119	30	124	31
Vitamin A (RAE)	µg	846	568	753	448	746	483	834	568	902	626
Retinol	µg	731	560	648	434	636	479	712	558	787	618
Thiamin (Vitamin B$_1$)	mg	0.58	0.17	0.60	0.20	0.58	0.17	0.57	0.17	0.57	0.17
Riboflavin (Vitamin B$_2$)	mg	1.13	0.29	0.97	0.24	1.09	0.27	1.12	0.29	1.17	0.31
Niacin	mg	7.7	2.5	6.4	2.6	7.4	2.4	7.7	2.5	8.1	2.6
Vitamin B6	mg	0.80	0.27	0.69	0.28	0.79	0.25	0.81	0.28	0.82	0.28
Folate (DFE)	µg	156	47	177	49	162	47	154	50	154	46
Vitamin B$_{12}$	µg	2.95	1.06	1.95	0.79	2.73	0.90	2.94	1.00	3.18	1.19
Vitamin C	mg	93	35	105	29	94	35	92	35	92	35
Vitamin D	µg	3.7	2.8	8.4	3.7	4.7	3.5	3.2	2.1	2.8	1.8
Vitamin E	mg	6.8	2.8	8.0	2.9	6.8	3.0	6.6	2.7	7.0	2.7

[1] The total number of children does not equal the sum of those in the age groups, due to missing data on age. en%: energy percent, i.e., the energy that the nutrient contributes to the total energy intake of a person, expressed as percentage; ALA: alpha-linolenic acid; EPA: eicosapentaenoic acid; DHA: docosahexaenoic acid; RAE: retinol activity equivalents; DFE: dietary folate equivalents; SD: standard deviation

Comparing the transformed usual intake distribution with dietary reference values the following results were found. The intake of most of the assessed macro- and micronutrients was found to be adequate (see supplementary materials Table S2). Exceptions were encountered for:

- Energy: Mean daily intake, both for boys (5.5 MJ) and girls (5.3 MJ), was higher than the requirement established by the HCN (5 MJ for boys, 4.5 MJ for girls between 1 and 3 years old [16] and much higher than the intake considered adequate according to EFSA (3.3–4.9 MJ for boys, 3.0–4.6 MJ for girls [19]).
- Protein: Median usual intake (45 g, 14 energy percent) was approximately three times higher than the Adequate Intake of 5 energy percent [16] or the Population Reference Intake of 11–13 g [19]. Among the children below 1 year, 26% exceeded the TUIL of 15 energy percent for this age. If, among the children that used exclusively cow's milk, liquid cow's milk would be substituted by formula, median usual protein intake would decrease from 14.2 to 12.3 energy percent.
- Fat: Intake was relatively low (29 energy percent). The mean usual intake was within the recommended range (25–40 energy percent) according the HCN recommendation [16], although 11% of the population had an intake below 25 energy percent. The mean intake was lower than the more recent EFSA recommendation (35–40 energy percent for children under 4 years [19]). Less than 5% of the children achieved a usual fat intake of 35 energy percent. No children below the age of 1 year achieved a usual fat intake of 40 energy percent, as recommended by the HCN and EFSA.
- Dietary fiber: With a mean of 12.7 g or 2.3 g/MJ, the usual intake of the children of 1 year and older was below the intake considered as adequate by the HCN (2.8 g/MJ [17]) and not achieved by 92% of them. However, new reference intakes for young children established by EFSA are lower (10 g [19]). These were achieved by the large majority of the children.

- *n*-3 fatty acids from fish, i.e., eicosapentaenoic acid (EPA) and docosahexaenoic acid (DHA): the mean daily intake of DHA by children below 2 years and of EPA + DHA by children above 2 years was far below the intake considered adequate by the HCN or EFSA.

- Iron: The median usual iron intake of 6.0 mg was lower than the Adequate Intake of 8 mg/day [18] and also lower than the Population Reference Intake of 7 mg/day established by EFSA [22]. This implies that iron intake was possibly inadequate. Children receiving formula, most of them in combination with cow's milk, had a median usual intake of 6.8 mg iron, whereas exclusive cow's milk users had a median usual intake of 5.6 mg. If, in the latter group, liquid cow's milk products would be replaced by formula, median usual iron intake would increase to 8.5 mg.

- Sodium: The percentage of children with a usual sodium intake of more than 1200 mg, i.e., the upper limit established by the NNC for young children above 1 year, increased with age from 47% to 81%, whereas the usual intake of all children below 1 year exceeded the upper limit of 400 mg [23].

- Zinc: The median usual intake of 5.9 mg was adequate. However, 17% of the children exceeded the TUIL of 7 mg/day.

- Retinol: 30% of the children exceeded the TUIL of 800 mg retinol. The percentage increased from 27% in the youngest age group to 33% in the oldest age group. Liverwurst spread, popular among young children, appeared to be responsible for the excess intake.

3.3. Food Consumption

Almost all children (98%) had eaten a breakfast on both days, contributing to 20% of the daily energy intake. Only 12 out of 1526 (<1%) children did not have breakfast on any of the days.

Table 3 shows the mean daily consumption of food groups, classified according to type of food, across all age groups. Consumption of potatoes, vegetables, fruits, cereals, and cheese was similar across all age groups. In contrast, consumption of bread and, in accordance, fat spreads doubled over age, just as cakes and biscuits, and meat. Consumption of milk products increased slightly over age, with exception of the much lower consumption (176 g) by children under 1 year. However, this was compensated by the high consumption (411 mL) of follow-on formulae among the youngest age group, 87% of which used formula. Mean consumption of formulae (follow-on or young-child formulae) decreased from 111 mL among the 1-years old (41% users) to 15 mL among the 3-years old (7% users). Consumption of mixed dishes, including baby and young-child meals in jars, also substantially decreased over age. Mean fish consumption was rather low, and did not change with age. We calculated from the food records that the children ate fish once per 10 days on average.

Table 3. Mean daily consumption of food groups (g) by children attending childcare by age (mean of 2 days).

Food Group	Total Group (n = 1526) [1]		10–11 Months (n = 31)		1 Year (n = 411)		2 Years (n = 497)		3 Years (n = 410)	
	Mean	SD	Mean	SD	Mean	SD	Mean	SD	Mean	SD
Potatoes	29	27	25	25	31	28	28	27	28	26
Vegetables	58	39	48	45	60	41	58	39	61	38
Fruit	128	59	129	66	127	58	129	59	130	61
Legumes	1	7	1	4	2	9	1	6	1	6
Bread	100	35	57	29	86	33	103	33	114	33
Cereals (including rice and pasta)	29	29	21	26	30	30	28	28	30	28
Cakes and biscuits	13	12	6	8	11	10	14	12	16	13
Nuts, seeds, savory snacks	1	5	0	0	1	3	1	5	2	6
Milk and milk products	358	158	176	217	333	162	363	143	383	147
Follow-on and young children's formula	63	135	411	226	111	162	35	87	15	61
Cheese	14	11	14	10	15	11	14	11	15	12
Eggs	3	8	1	4	2	7	3	8	3	8
Fish	5	12	2	7	5	12	5	12	6	13
Meat, meat products, poultry	44	25	24	23	40	24	44	22	49	26
Soy and vegetarian products	8	49	0	2	8	54	8	47	10	55
Savory spreads	4	6	0	0	3	6	4	6	4	7
Mixed dishes	20	45	52	78	28	53	15	39	14	35
Soups	10	33	0	1	6	23	12	37	13	39
Sugar, confectionary, sweet spreads	18	13	6	7	13	10	20	12	23	14
Fat spreads, oils, savory sauces	24	11	11	8	20	10	24	11	27	12
Non-alcoholic beverages (excluding milk products)	427	222	182	145	367	204	446	209	508	220

[1] The total number of children does not equal the sum of those in the age groups, due to missing data on age; SD: standard deviation.

3.4. Consumption According to Food-Based Dietary Guidelines

Figure 1 displays the consumption of food groups by children from 1 year, classified according to the food-based dietary guidelines. Figure 1 shows for each defined food group the percentage of children with a consumption quantity (g or mL) below and above the recommended daily consumption. The majority of children did not comply with the recommendations for fruit and cooking fats. Around 40% of the children did not comply with the recommendations for vegetables, potatoes (including rice and pasta), cheese, meat (including poultry, fish and eggs) and beverages (including liquid milk products). Children who ate a hot meal at the childcare center ate more vegetables: Only 30% of them did not comply with the recommendation. A large majority of children complied with the recommendations for bread (including breakfast cereals), fat spreads and milk products.

The food groups were also subdivided into preferable or neutral foods and foods that should be eaten by exception only. Table 4 shows the mean consumption of each food group. More than half of the foods from the potatoes group were eaten as by-exception type. This was due to the consumption of white rice and refined pasta (instead of brown rice and wholemeal pasta). In contrast, bread and breakfast cereals were almost always eaten as wholemeal or "brown" type. Cheese was mostly eaten as full-fat type and therefore classified as by-exception type. Milk products were mostly (79%) consumed as preferable or neutral type, i.e., (semi-)skimmed, non-sweetened milk. Two thirds of the meat group was eaten as by-exception type, mostly because of the saturated fat content of the meat or the salt content of processed meats. Fats and oils, in contrast, were predominantly of the preferable (less-saturated fat) type. Sixty-two percent of the beverages were drunk as by-exception type, mostly because they contained sugars. This percentage is even higher as part of the water (in the preferable group) was used to mix it with fruit juice concentrate or syrup. Thirty-seven percent of the total foods (in g) consumed by the children were by-exception foods (35% at home and 40% at the childcare center). The higher consumption of by-exception foods at childcare centers was mainly attributable to by-exception beverages (see supplementary materials Figure S1).

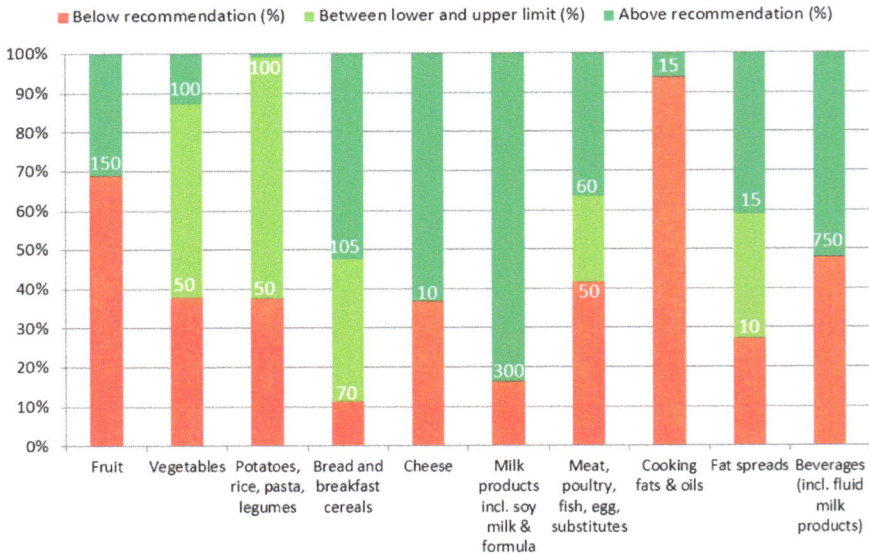

Figure 1. Percentage of children from 1 year old with a daily consumption (g) below, above or in within the range of the recommendation.

Table 4 also lists the contribution of the food groups to mean intake of selected nutrients. Bread, milk products and sweetened beverages were important contributors to energy intake. Milk products contributed most to protein intake, followed by bread and the meat group. Sweetened beverages were by far the largest contributors to intake of sugars, at a distance followed by milk products (contributes mainly lactose), fruit, and sugar and sweet spreads. Bread and potatoes were the main contributors to polysaccharides. Milk products, meats, and fats and oils contributed mostly to intake of fat and saturated fatty acids. However, almost half of the intake of polyunsaturated fatty acids originated from fats and oils. Dietary fiber came mainly from bread and breakfast cereals, followed by vegetables and fruit. Bread was also responsible for one third of the daily sodium intake (which excluded salt added at cooking and at the table), followed by processed meats, cheese and milk products. Fruit, followed at a distance by sweetened beverages (including fruit syrups and juices) and vegetables and milk, contributed most to vitamin C intake.

Table 4. Consumption of food groups [1] and their contribution to intake of selected nutrients among children 1–3 years old.

	Mean	Energy	Protein	MDS	PS	Fat	SFA	PUFA	Water	Dietary Fiber	Sodium	Vitamin C
Basic Foods	g/day	%	%	%	%	%	%	%	%	%	%	%
Fruit	123	6	2	13	3	1	1	2	10	16	0	42
Vegetables	58	1	2	1	1	1	0	1	5	10	1	11
Potatoes, rice, pasta, legumes	23	2	1	0	5	0	0	1	2	4	0	2
Potatoes, rice, pasta, legumes (exception)	30	3	3	0	10	2	1	2	2	3	0	1
Bread and breakfast cereals	98	19	22	3	54	4	3	7	3	42	34	2
Cheese	1	0	0	0	0	0	1	0	0	0	1	0
Cheese (exception)	13	3	5	0	0	8	13	1	1	0	10	0
Milk products including soy milk and formula	333	13	23	16	1	13	21	4	26	4	10	11
Milk products incl. soy milk (exception)	90	6	7	9	2	5	8	2	7	2	4	1
Meat, poultry, fish, egg, substitutes	18	2	9	0	0	2	2	2	1	0	4	0
Meat, poultry, fish, egg, substitutes (exception)	35	8	15	0	2	18	18	12	2	1	13	6
Fats, oils	18	8	0	0	0	26	15	47	1	0	2	0
Fats, oils (exception)	1	0	0	0	0	1	1	1	0	0	0	0
Beverages, excluding milk products	165	0	0	0	0	0	0		16	0	0	1
Beverages, excluding milk products (exception)	267	12	1	39	0	0	0	0	22	3	4	21
Mixed dishes	12	1	1	0	1	1	1	2	1	2	1	0
Mixed dishes (exception)	7	1	1	0	2	1	2	1	0	1	2	0
Non-Basic Foods												
Sugar, sweet spreads	18	5	1	12	1	4	4	2	0	3	0	0
Cakes and biscuits	13	4	2	4	7	3	4	2	0	3	3	0
Confectionary	3	1	0	1	0	1	1	0	0	0	0	0
Nuts, seeds, savory snacks	1	0	0	0	1	1	1	1	0	0	1	0
Sauces	5	1	0	0	0	2	1	4	0	0	1	0
Savory spreads	4	2	2	0	0	5	2	5	0	2	2	0
Soups	9	0	2	0	0	0	0	1	1	0	2	1
Miscellaneous [2]	14	3	2	1	8	1	1	1	1	4	4	0

[1] Division in food groups according to food choice guidelines by the Netherlands Nutrition Center [21]; [2] The sum of all not listed food groups that were consumed in small quantities; MDS: mono- and disaccharides; PS: polysaccharides; SFA: saturated fatty acids; PUFA: polyunsaturated fatty acids.

4. Discussion

This study showed that Dutch children aged 10 to 48 months, at the days they attended childcare, appeared to have an adequate nutrient intake according to national and European reference values with exception of intakes of total fat, *n*-3 fatty acids from fish and possibly iron which were all lower than the reference values. Intakes of energy and protein were substantially higher than recommended and part of the population exceeded the Tolerable Upper Intake Levels for sodium, zinc and retinol. Consumption of fruit and fats was substantially less than recommended according to food-based dietary guidelines. So were, to a lesser extent, components of the hot meal (vegetables, potatoes/rice/pasta, and meat/fish/poultry/eggs) and fluids. The children consumed milk products and bread mostly as recommended with respect to type (i.e., low fat and high fiber types, respectively), but milk consumption was on average higher than recommended. A notably high consumption of sugar-containing beverages contributed substantially to energy intake. Almost all children ate breakfast and received vitamin D supplements at the recorded days.

Results presented here are from a large dataset, which covers a very large variety of childcare centers, located across the country. Some limitations should be mentioned. Firstly, the authors were not involved in the design of the data collection methods, nor in the execution of the data collection. It was therefore difficult to evaluate the quality of the data. However, based on the documentation provided and the performed data checks, we assessed the data to be of sufficient quality to merit publication. Missing data on gender, age, and body weight and height reduced the usefulness of the data. However, comparing our results with those of the Dutch National Food Consumption Survey conducted among young children in 2005/2006 in the age categories of 2- and 3-years old overlapping between the studies, we observed that mean energy intake was very similar between the surveys (5632 kJ/day versus 5645 kJ/day, respectively). The Dutch National Food Consumption Survey concluded, based on comparison of energy intake and energy requirement, that underreporting was not an issue in their survey [24]. We conclude therefore that substantial underreporting is unlikely in our study either. Secondly, there are considerations with respect to the study population and design. During the period of data collection (2011–2014) approximately 40% of Dutch children under the age of 4 attended a childcare center on one or more days per week [6]. Although formal childcare in the Netherlands is partly subsidized depending on family income, parents (in particular mothers) of children attending a childcare center had on average a higher family income, were more educated and worked more hours per week than parents of other children of the same age [25]. The study population was therefore not representative of the total Dutch population of 10 to 48 months old. In addition, response rates were not formally monitored. Furthermore, food consumption was only recorded on days that the children attended the childcare center. Although we assumed—to compare the children's usual nutrient intake distribution with dietary reference values—that the recorded days were representative of a child's diet, this can be questioned, considering the structure of the day, the food provider, and possible peer pressure. Nevertheless, the data are valuable in their own right. They were mostly observed and recorded directly by the food providers, both at home and at the childcare center. The latter is unusual in food consumption surveys.

As concluded from other studies and countries, reviewed by EFSA [19], intake of *n*-3 fatty acids, in particular DHA and EPA, and iron and vitamin D is low among the Dutch young children. The low dietary intake of vitamin D was largely remedied through the high proportion of children (92%) that received a vitamin D supplement. Although some practitioners doubt whether such a high percentage of supplement users is real, communication about the recommendation has improved since 2012. Intake of *n*-3 fatty acids was much lower than recommended. Mean DHA intake by children younger than 2 years is only one fifth of the intake considered as adequate (100 mg/day). Children receiving formula, fortified with DHA, more or less double their DHA intake. If the children of 2 to 4 years old would eat 50 g lean fish and 50 g fatty fish such as salmon per week, as recommended by the NNC, they would easily achieve an adequate intake of DHA and EPA combined. Whether the low *n*-3 fatty acid intake has health consequences is uncertain. As for iron, there is evidence that iron deficit at young age may interfere with cognitive development [26,27]. However, while the usual iron intake of all children in this survey is above the Average Requirement of 3 mg/day for 1–3 years old established by the US Institute of Medicine [28], 25% of the children from 1 year do not achieve the Average Requirement of 5 mg/day recently proposed by EFSA [22]. Recent research in a well-defined, healthy population of 400 young children in The Netherlands has shown that iron deficiency and iron deficiency anemia was detected in 18.8% and 8.5% of the children, respectively, with a lower iron deficiency prevalence among children receiving formula and a higher prevalence among children receiving a large amount (more than 400 mL/day) of cow's milk after adjustment for age [29]. However, iron intake was not assessed in this study.

The high intake of energy and protein among young children is also a universal observation across Europe [19]. They both increase the risk for overweight [30,31]. In particular the 1-year-old are at risk: they use a lot of milk, mostly cow's milk and also formula, and have the highest protein intake. Although no reference value for sugars has been established by the HCN or by EFSA, increasing evidence shows that in particular sugar-sweetened beverages increase the risk of overweight [32]. We also found that usual intake exceeded the Tolerable Upper Intake Level for zinc (17%) and retinol (30%). As the Adequate Intake and TUIL for zinc are very close, such an excess is inevitable and is unlikely to be harmful. The TUIL for retinol intake among young children is based on the relatively low TUIL for pregnant women owing to its teratogenic effects and adjusted to children. Some excess intake is therefore not likely to be harmful for young children. Also, vitamin A intoxication has not been reported in young children in The Netherlands. Excess retinol intake can nevertheless be avoided if childcare centers and parents restrict the consumption of liverwurst (spread) by their young children, in accordance with the NNC guideline. Dietary sodium intake—70% of the children exceeded the TUIL set by the NNC—is difficult to reduce without endangering a balanced diet. Even though the Dutch bread sector made a major effort to reduce the salt content of bread, bread is a main contributor to young children's sodium intake. According to EFSA, however, sodium intake is not a matter of concern [19].

The results of this survey are in particular informative to nutrition policy and education, both for childcare organizations as for parents and youth health care providers. They demonstrate that the young children's food consumption pattern could be substantially improved by a few changes, such as a replacement of sugared beverages by water and some reduction of milk products. For example, milk-based desserts could be replaced by fruit. Childcare centers that serve a hot meal are able to increase the children's daily vegetable consumption. All in all, these changes would result in lower energy and protein intake and higher vegetable and fruit consumption, which may in turn lower the risk of overweight. Reduction of a high milk consumption should be able to enhance iron absorption from the diet, as calcium hampers iron absorption. Stimulating fish consumption, both at home and at day care, is a feasible way to increase intake of *n*-3 fatty acids. Only if, in specific situations, a recommended diet is difficult to achieve, replacement of cow's milk by formula may help to meet some of the dietary recommendations.

5. Conclusions

Dutch 10 to 48-month-old had, at least on the days they attended childcare, mostly an adequate nutrient intake. The intake of *n*-3 fatty acids and of iron however was low, which is in line with European findings. This seems a matter of concern in young children in this survey and most likely in all young children in the Netherlands, although more research is needed on their potential health effects. The high intakes of energy and protein in this population are also a matter of concern as they may increase the risk of becoming overweight.

Almost all children ate breakfast and received vitamin D supplements. They used mostly (semi-) skimmed types of milk products and non-refined bread and cereals, as recommended. However, their relatively high milk consumption and very high consumption of sugared beverages are undesirable and the latter should be replaced mostly by water. The relative low consumption of fruit, vegetables and fish, on the other hand, should be increased.

Supplementary Materials: The following are available online at http://www.mdpi.com/2072-6643/8/7/428/s1, Figure S1: Consumption of foods by 1–3 years old by location, Table S1: Mean daily nutrient intake by children 10–48 months old attending childcare by gender (mean of 2 days), Table S2: Distribution of usual nutrient intake as calculated with SPADE model for daily intakes and comparison of the distribution with dietary reference values.

Acknowledgments: We thank the staff of the participating childcare centers and the parents of the children as well as the dieticians from Berdien van Wezel Dieticians for their roles in data collection. This study, including this publication, was funded by Nutricia Nederland BV.

Author Contributions: R.A.G. and C.M.R. designed the data analysis plan. C.M.R. carried out the data processing and analysis, R.A.G. drafted the manuscript. C.I.L. and K.F.M.J. contributed important intellectual content and expert advice, and critically reviewed the draft manuscript. All authors read and approved the final manuscript.

Conflicts of Interest: R.A.G., C.M.R. and C.I.L. are employees of research institute TNO, which was commissioned by the sponsor to analyze the data from the survey among young children attending childcare and to write an independent report and scientific publication on the results. This publication was contractually agreed with the sponsor before the start of the work. The sponsor was not involved in nor consulted for the data analysis, selection of results to be presented, interpretation of the results, drafting the manuscript, and formulation of the conclusions.

References

1. Hoyland, A.; Dye, L.; Lawton, C.L. A systematic review of the effect of breakfast on the cognitive performance of children and adolescents. *Nutr. Res. Rev.* **2009**, *22*, 220–243. [CrossRef] [PubMed]

2. Florence, M.D.; Asbridge, M.; Veugelers, P.J. Diet quality and academic performance. *J. Sch. Health* **2008**, *78*, 209–215. [CrossRef] [PubMed]

3. Singh, A.S.; Mulder, C.; Twisk, J.W.; van Mechelen, W.; Chinapaw, M.J. Tracking of childhood overweight into adulthood: A systematic review of the literature. *Obes. Rev.* **2008**, *9*, 474–488. [CrossRef] [PubMed]

4. Lanting, C.I.; de Vroome, E.M.; Elias, S.G.; van den Brandt, P.A.; van Leeuwen, F.E.; Kampman, E.; Kiemeney, L.A.; Peeters, P.H.; de Vries, E.; Bausch-Goldbohm, R.A. Contribution of lifestyle factors to cancer: Secondary analysis of Dutch data over 2010 and a projection for 2020. *Ned. Tijdschr. Geneeskd.* **2014**, *159*, A8085. [PubMed]

5. Singer, M.R.; Moore, L.L.; Garrahie, E.J.; Ellison, R.C. The tracking of nutrient intake in young children: The Framingham children's study. *Am. J. Public Health* **1995**, *85*, 1673–1677. [CrossRef] [PubMed]

6. Statistics Netherlands. Minder Kinderen naar Kinderdagverblijven (Less Children in Day Care), 2014. Available online: http://www.cbs.nl/nl-NL/menu/themas/dossiers/jongeren/publicaties/artikelen/archief/2014/2014-4024-wm.htm (accessed on 20 May 2015).

7. Gubbels, J.S.; Raaijmakers, L.G.M.; Gerards, S.M.P.L.; Kremers, S.P.J. Dietary intake by Dutch 1- to 3-year-old children at childcare and at home. *Nutrients* **2014**, *6*, 304–318. [CrossRef] [PubMed]

8. Gubbels, J.S.; Gerards, S.M.; Kremers, S.P. Use of food practices by childcare staff and the association with dietary intake of children at childcare. *Nutrients* **2015**, *7*, 2161–2175. [CrossRef] [PubMed]

9. WebArchitecten vof. FoodFigures. Available online: http://www.foodfigures.nl/ (accessed on 2 May 2015).

10. SAS. *Version 8.2*; SAS Institute Inc.: Cary, NC, USA, 1999–2001.

11. SAS. *Version 9.3*; SAS Institute Inc.: Cary, NC, USA, 1999–2001.

12. Kistemaker, C.; Bouman, M. *Voedselconsumptiepeiling Met SAS. de Ontwikkeling van een Geautomatiseerd Systeem voor de Verwerking van Voedingsenquetes. Deel 2: Beschrijving Functioneel en Systeem Ontwerp (Vertrouwelijk). Rapportnummer V98.799*; TNO Voeding: Zeist, The Netherlands, 1999.

13. NEVO-Online Versie 2013/4.0. Available online: http://nevo-online.rivm.nl/ (accessed on 20 May 2015).

14. Dekkers, A.L.M.; Verkaik-Kloosterman, J.; Rossum, C.T.M.; Ocke, M.C. SPADE, a new statistical program to estimate habitual dietary intake from multiple food sources and dietary supplements. *J. Nutr.* **2014**, *144*, 2083–2091. [CrossRef] [PubMed]

15. EFSA Panel on Dietetic Products, Nutrition and Allergies (NDA). Scientific opinion on principles for deriving and applying dietary reference values. *EFSA J.* **2010**, *8*, 1458.

16. Health Council of The Netherlands. *Dietary Reference Intakes: Energy, Proteins, Fats and Digestible Carbohydrates*; Health Council of The Netherlands: The Hague, The Netherlands, 2001.

17. Health Council of The Netherlands. *Guideline for Dietary Fibre Intake*; Health Council of The Netherlands: The Hague, The Netherlands, 2006.

18. Voedingscentrum (Netherlands Nutrition Centre). Aanbevelingen voor Vitamine, Mineralen en Spoorelementen: Factsheet (Recommendations for Vitamins, Minerals, and Trace Elements), 2014. Available online: http://www.voedingscentrum.nl/nl/pers/factsheets.aspx (accessed on 20 May 2015).

19. EFSA NDA Panel (EFSA Panel on Dietetic Products, Nutrition and Allergies). Scientific opinion on nutrient requirements and dietary intakes of infants and young children in the European Union. *EFSA J.* **2013**, *11*, 3408.

20. Gezond eten met de Schijf van Vijf. Available online: http://www.voedingscentrum.nl/nl/schijf-van-vijf/schijf.aspx (accessed on 20 May 2015).

21. Voedingscentrum (Netherlands Nutrition Centre). *Richtlijnen Voedselkeuze, 1 Maart 2011, Update 12 April 2011 (Guidelines for Food Choice, 12 April 2011)*; Voedingscentrum: Den Haag, The Netherlands, 2011.

22. EFSA NDA Panel (EFSA Panel on Dietetic Products, Nutrition and Allergies). Scientific opinion on dietary reference values for iron. *EFSA J.* **2015**, *13*, 4254.

23. Encyclopedie. Available online: http://www.voedingscentrum.nl/encyclopedie/zout.aspx (accessed on 20 May 2015).

24. Ocké, M.C.; van Rossum, C.T.M.; Fransen, H.P.; Buurma, E.M.; de Boer, E.J.; Brants, H.A.M.; Niekerk, E.M.; van der Laan, J.D.; Drijvers, J.J.M.M.; Ghameshlou, Z. *Dutch National Food Consumption Survey—Young Children 2005/2006*; RIVM: Bilthoven, The Netherlands, 2008.

25. Portegijs, W.; Cloïn, M.; Merens, A. *Krimp in de Kinderopvang*; Sociaal en Cultureel Planbureau: The Hague, The Netherlands, 2014.

26. Lozoff, B.; Jimenez, E.; Smith, J.B. Double burden of iron deficiency in infancy and low socioeconomic status: A longitudinal analysis of cognitive test scores to age 19 years. *Arch. Pediatr. Adolesc. Med.* **2006**, *160*, 1108–1113. [CrossRef] [PubMed]

27. Qubty, W.; Renaud, D.L. Cognitive impairment associated with low ferritin responsive to iron supplementation. *Pediatr. Neurol.* **2014**, *51*, 831–833. [CrossRef] [PubMed]

28. Trumbo, P.; Yates, A.A.; Schlicker, S.; Poos, M. Dietary reference intakes: Vitamin A, vitamin K, arsenic, boron, chromium, copper, iodine, iron, manganese, molybdenum, nickel, silicon, vanadium, and zinc. *J. Am. Diet. Assoc.* **2001**, *101*, 294–301. [CrossRef]

29. Uijterschout, L.; Vloemans, J.; Vos, R.; Teunisse, P.P.; Hudig, C.; Bubbers, S.; Verbruggen, S.; Veldhorst, M.; de Leeuw, T.; van Goudoever, J.B.; et al. Prevalence and risk factors of iron deficiency in healthy young children in the southwestern Netherlands. *J. Pediatr. Gastroenterol. Nutr.* **2014**, *58*, 193–198. [CrossRef] [PubMed]

30. Weber, M.; Grote, V.; Closa-Monasterolo, R.; Escribano, J.; Langehendries, J.; Sain, E.; Giovannini, M.; Verduci, E.; Gruzfeld, S.; Socha, P.; et al. Lower protein content in infant formula reduces BMI and obesity risk at school age: Follow-up of a randomized trial. *Am. J. Clin. Nutr.* **2014**, *99*, 1041–1051. [CrossRef] [PubMed]

31. Hebestreit, A.; Börnhorst, C.; Barba, G.; Siani, A.; Huybrechts, I.; Tognon, G.; Eiben, G.; Moreno, L.A.; Fernández Alvira, J.M.; Loit, H.M.; et al. Associations between energy intake, daily food intake and energy density of foods and BMI z-score in 2–9-year-old european children. *Eur. J. Nutr.* **2014**, *53*, 673–681. [CrossRef] [PubMed]

32. De Ruyter, J.C.; Olthof, M.R.; Seidell, J.C.; Katan, M.B. A trial of sugar-free or sugar-sweetened beverages and body weight in children. *N. Engl. J. Med.* **2012**, *367*, 1397–1406. [CrossRef] [PubMed]

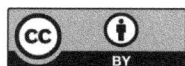

nutrients

MDPI

Article

Introduction of Complementary Foods in a Cohort of Infants in Northeast Italy: Do Parents Comply with WHO Recommendations?

Claudia Carletti, Paola Pani, Lorenzo Monasta, Alessandra Knowles * and Adriano Cattaneo

Clinical Epidemiology and Public Health Research Unit, Institute for Maternal and Child Health IRCCS "Burlo Garofolo", Via dell'Istria 65/1, Trieste 34137, Italy; claudiaveronica.carletti@burlo.trieste.it (C.C.); paola.pani@burlo.trieste.it (P.P.); lorenzo.monasta@burlo.trieste.it (L.M.); adriano.cattaneo@gmail.com (A.C.)
* Correspondence: alessandra.knowles@burlo.trieste.it; Tel.: +39-040-378-5236

Received: 30 September 2016; Accepted: 22 December 2016; Published: 4 January 2017

Abstract: Timing and type of complementary food in infancy affect nutritional status and health later in life. The objective of this paper was to assess complementary feeding practices, looking at timing, type, and compliance with World Health Organization (WHO) recommendations. Data were obtained from a birth cohort of 400 infants, enrolled in Trieste (Italy) between July 2007 and July 2008 and followed up for three years, using a "food introduction timing table". Five WHO recommendations standards were used to assess parental compliance and associated factors. Thirty seven percent of mothers returned the completed "timing table" up until the child was three years of age. Eighty six percent of infants were already receiving complementary foods at six months. The first food type to be introduced was fresh fruit (170 days from birth, median). Overall, infants shared a very similar diet, which was different from the family diet and characterized by delayed introduction of certain food types. Five percent of parents complied with either all five or only one of the WHO recommendations, 34% with three, and 35% with four. The parents' partial compliance with WHO recommendations is probably due to conflicting information received from different sources. This advocates for national evidence-based guidelines, supported and promoted by health professionals.

Keywords: complementary feeding; compliance with WHO recommendation; timing of introduction of complementary food; infant nutrition; Italy

1. Introduction

Complementary feeding is a process that, according to World Health Organization (WHO) [1], should take place between the ages of around six months and two years, this being a crucial period for child growth, development, and health. Studies conducted in low and high-income countries show that inadequate nutrition during this period increases the risk of becoming underweight or overweight, with potentially serious life-long health effects [2–5]. Under- and over-nutrition can coexist in the same country, regardless of the country's economic status, and tend to affect the poorest population groups [6]. The time of introduction of complementary foods, as well as their type, are crucial not only to ensure that nutritional needs are met in the short term, but also to promote good health later in life and to prevent overweight and obesity [7–10].

The WHO recommends, as a public health measure, exclusive breastfeeding up to six months of age, followed by adequate, safe and appropriate complementary foods with breastfeeding continuing up to two years and beyond [1]. This recommendation has been adopted in many countries, including Italy [11]. In conflict with the WHO recommendation, the European Society for Pediatric Gastroenterology Hepatology and Nutrition (ESPGHAN) recommends the introduction of complementary foods no earlier than 17 and no later than 26 weeks of age [12]. This commentary triggered a debate [13], and in 2011 the WHO released a statement reaffirming that exclusive breastfeeding for six months has several advantages over exclusive breastfeeding for three to four months, and should be followed by gradual introduction of solid food alongside breastfeeding [14]. WHO also recommends that, between the ages of 6 and 12 months, the infant's diet should be progressively integrated into a healthy family diet, without restrictions on the types of food that are offered. There is no evidence to support the practice of delaying the introduction of potentially allergenic foods (e.g., tomatoes, fish, eggs), with the exception of the replacement of breast milk or formula with cow milk, which is not recommended before 12 months of age due to its low content in iron [15]. This recommendation is shared by ESPGHAN [12]. Finally, WHO warns against the use of honey in the first 12 months due to the risk of botulism, and recommends that, from six months onwards, infants should make a gradual transition to eating family foods limiting the consumption of commercial complementary foods [1,16] as these may delay the infant's acceptance of the family's normal diet [15].

In spite of these recommendations, data on current feeding practices suggest that the introduction of complementary foods before six months is common in many countries [17,18], including Italy [19,20], where there are no Ministry of Health guidelines on complementary feeding. The national guidelines on the protection, promotion, and support of breastfeeding simply state that "after six months, breast milk, with appropriate complementary feeding, provides an important contribution to the nutrition, health and development of the child" [11]. What "appropriate complementary feeding" means is not clearly explained.

The cohort study aimed at investigating the transition from milk to family foods, and its association with overweight, in a birth cohort of 400 children followed up for 36 months. The prevalence and duration of breastfeeding, the data on nutrient intake at six month of age and on the mothers' socioeconomic status, have already been reported in previous papers [20,21]. The specific objective of the present research was to assess complementary feeding practices, focusing on timing, characteristics, and compliance with the WHO recommendations. Considering that there is very little national data [19,22] describing complementary feeding practices, a better understanding of parents' approach to the introduction of complementary foods could support the development of evidence-based national guidelines on infant feeding.

2. Materials and Methods

Data were obtained from a cohort study conducted at the maternity hospital of Trieste (Institute for Maternal and Child Health Burlo Garofolo), Italy, between July 2007 and July 2011. A cohort of 400 mother-infant pairs was followed up for three years, using telephone interviews and self-reported diaries to investigate feeding practices and attitudes of mothers. The study was approved by the ethics committee of the Institute. The study design, methods, and sampling procedures have already been reported [21]. In brief, mother-infant pairs were enrolled at birth according to the following eligibility criteria: birth weight $\geq$2000 g, no congenital malformation nor severe diseases that required hospital admission, gestational age of 36 completed weeks or more, and residence in the province of Trieste. Upon enrolment, mothers were checked for eligibility and asked to give their informed consent. During the first contact, they were given a feeding diary with instructions on how to record type and quantity of foods over a 24-h period on three separate non-consecutive days at 3, 6, 9, 12, 18, 24, and 36 months of age of the infant [23,24].

At the same time, mothers were also given a "timing of introduction of food timetable" ("food timetable") in which they were asked to record information on the characteristics, preparation and date of introduction of the first food type for each of 17 set food categories. The food timetable was handed back to the researchers when the child was 36 months old, together with the last feeding diary and the data on weight and length/height of the child recorded by the paediatricians at 1, 3, 6, 9, 12, 18, 24 and 36 months, on the occasion of periodic health checks.

The food timetable was divided into food categories: fresh fruit, vegetables (with a separate category for tomatoes because of their potential allergenicity), cereals (with a focus on gluten free pasta and bread), cow milk, milk products, meat, legumes, fish, eggs, cured meats, industrial fruit juice, tubers, honey, sugar (added to drinks or foods), sweets, creamy porridge, and nuts and seeds. For each food category, mothers were asked to record the date of the first tasting and the date from which the food type was fully incorporated in the infant's diet, if different from the date of the first tasting. Mothers were also asked to record the method of preparation (e.g., raw or cooked, homogenized or lyophilized) and the characteristics (e.g., commercial baby food or homemade) of each food item.

WHO recommends appropriate complementary feeding starting from the age of six months, with continued breastfeeding up to two years and beyond. Appropriate complementary feeding is: timely, adequate, safe, and properly fed. On the basis of these indications we derived from the WHO recommendations five standards to assess compliance:

1. introduction at or after 6 months;
2. "minimum dietary diversity";
3. use of homemade vs. commercial baby food;
4. introduction of cow's milk at 12 months or more;
5. introduction of honey at 12 months or more.

Recommendation 1 describes the concept of "timeliness", recommendations 2, 3, and 4 cover "adequateness", meaning that food provides sufficient energy, protein, and micronutrients to meet a growing child's nutritional needs. "Safety" is represented by recommendation 5. With regards to "propriety of feeding" the timing questionnaire did not assess either meal frequency or feeding methods.

The second recommendation is based on a slightly modified version of WHO's "minimum dietary diversity" indicator, by which infants are defined as "compliant" if their diet incorporates four to seven different food categories by the age of 12 months. [25]. The seven food groups used by WHO to codify this indicator are: "grains, roots, and tubers"; "flesh foods (meat and fish)"; "dairy (milk) products"; "legumes and nuts"; "vitamin-A rich fruits and vegetables"; "other fruits and vegetables"; and "eggs". In the present study, "vitamin-A rich fruits and vegetables" were not assessed as an independent group because Italy is considered to be free from vitamin A deficiency [26]. Instead, we chose to allocate to fruits and vegetables two separate categories with the aim of evaluating their independent contribution to the daily diet. Because our timing questionnaire covered a period of three years, we also extracted an index of "maximum dietary diversity" to determine how many children had introduced all seven food categories into their diet by the age of 12 months.

For the third recommendation, we analyzed the consumption of homemade vs. commercial complementary baby food defining the use of the latter as 'high' if it covered at least three out of five food groups (fruit, vegetables, meat, fish, cereals, and milk products) at six months of age. Almost 38% of infants fell into this category.

Differences between groups were examined with Fisher exact two-tailed test for categorical variables and with Mann-Whitney rank-sum test for continuous variables.

In order to perform the logistic regression analyses described below, the sample was divided into two groups based on the timing of the first introduction of complementary food. The cut-off was set at 21 weeks, which was the median of the distribution curve (Figure 1). The 21 weeks value had the additional advantage of falling in the middle of the ESPGHAN recommended window (17 to 26 weeks). This timing distribution was used as dependent variable.

The independent variables reflected the objective of the study to assess compliance with WHO recommendations both as stand-alone variables and as overall compliance with any three out of five. The relation between these independent variables and timing was analyzed using stratified and simultaneous univariate and multivariate logistic regression analyses. The variables included in the simultaneous models are presented in Supplementary Materials Tables S1–S6.

The stratified analysis was carried out considering each of the following variables: mothers' characteristics, including age (≥34 years), body mass index (BMI) before pregnancy (≥25), place of birth (Italy vs. other), level of education (degree or higher vs. lower), occupation, whether she was breastfeeding or had breastfed, if she had allergies or a family history of allergies, if she was or had been a smoker, and type of professional figure (paediatrician or midwife) who provided counselling on complementary feeding.

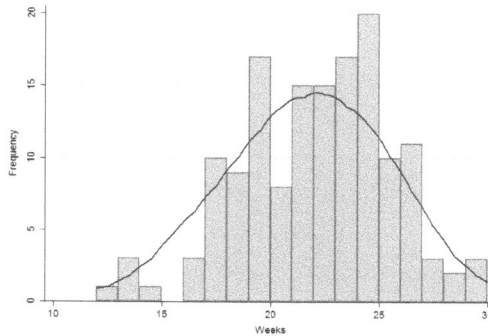

Figure 1. Distribution curve of the timing of first introduction of complementary foods in weeks. The probability density function was estimated with a non-parametric Kernel density estimation (KDE).

The characteristics of the mothers were selected based on literature data. The information on which professional figures were providing counselling on complementary feeding was based on the hypothesis, formulated by the authors but also supported by literature [27,28], that this may influence mothers' behavior.

All the analyses were carried out using Stata IC 14.1 (StataCorp LP, College Station, TX, USA).

3. Results

3.1. Population Characteristics

Four hundred mother-infant pairs were enrolled in the study, but only 148 (37%) completed and returned the food timetable when the child reached 36 months of age. The participation rate declined during the study: after three months 34% (135/400) of mothers had withdrawn from the study. This percentage subsequently followed a fluctuating pattern, rising to 59% (235/400) at 6 months and then dropping to 43% (173/400) and 41% (165/400) at 9 and 12 months, respectively. By the time of the 24-month interview, the study cohort had reduced by 67% (132/400). The characteristics of the mothers and infants of the sub-cohort that completed the timing questionnaire are described in Table 1. No statistically significant differences were observed between the cohort (400) and the sub-cohort (148), as already reported [16,17]. In brief, 89% of mothers (mean age 33.7 years; Standard Deviation 4.4) had a medium-to-high level of education, 95% declared they were employed before birth and 80% were in employment at six months after birth. Most infants (90%) were born between 38 and 42 weeks of gestation and 82% by vaginal delivery. The majority (91%) weighed between 2500 g and 4199 g at birth, and 79% were between 46 and 52 cm long. The infants' mean BMI was calculated at three and six months: 70% and 75% of infants had a BMI that fell within the normal range (between the 15th and the 85th WHO percentile), 15% and 3% were below the 15th percentile, while 15% and 21% were over the 85th percentile, respectively.

Table 1. Characteristics of mothers at enrolment and children at birth.

Mothers	Cohort n (%)	Sub-Cohort n (%)	p *
Age (years)	(n = 399)	(n = 148)	0.713
≤29	90 (23)	29 (20)	
30–34	160 (40)	59 (40)	
≥35	149 (37)	60 (40)	
Born in Italy	(n = 400)	(n = 148)	0.451
Yes	351 (88)	134 (91)	
No	49 (12)	14 (9)	
Education	(n = 348)	(n = 147)	0.158
≤Secondary school	59 (17)	16 (11)	
Completed high school or equivalent	154 (44)	64 (43)	
Bachelor degree or higher	135 (39)	67 (46)	
Employment before birth	(n = 323)	(n = 136)	1.000
Yes	306 (95)	129 (95)	
No	17 (5)	7 (5)	
Employment at 6 months after birth	(n = 218)	(n = 147)	0.790
Yes	176 (81)	117 (80)	
No	42 (19)	30 (20)	
Allergy of mother or of other family member	(n = 263)	(n = 148)	0.812
Yes	64 (24)	38 (26)	
No	199 (76)	110 (74)	
Children	**n (%)**	**n (%)**	**p**
Gestational age (weeks)	(n = 339)	(n = 147)	0.730
36–37	29 (9)	14 (9)	
38–42	310 (91)	133 (91)	
Infant gender	(n = 345)	(n = 148)	0.142
male	173 (50)	85 (57)	
female	172 (50)	63 (43)	
Birth weight (g)	(n = 344)	(n = 148)	0.552
<2500	3 (1)	2 (1)	
2500–4199	324 (94)	136 (92)	
≥4200	17 (5)	10 (7)	
Birth length (cm)	(n = 342)	(n = 148)	0.563
<46	5 (1)	2 (1)	
46–52.9	283 (83)	117 (79)	
≥53	54 (16)	29 (20)	

* *p*-Value is calculated using a two-tailed Fisher Exact test.

3.2. Timing of Complementary Feeding

At six months of age, 73% of infants were still receiving breast milk but, in contrast with WHO recommendations, only 7% were exclusively breastfed; 40% received formula and breast milk, 27% only formula and 26% breast milk and complementary food. One infant was given food other than milk before the age of three months, 7% at three months, 32% at four, 47% at five months. Only 14% of infants were given their first complementary food at six months or more

The median age of introduction of solid foods was 5.2 months (min 2.8; max 7.2). The interval between the first tasting and the complete introduction of the different food categories ranged from 6 to 32 days. The range was narrower for food groups such as dairy products, vegetables, and cereals (6, 6, and 7 days, respectively) and wider for honey, sugar, and cow milk (32, 29, and 22 days, respectively). The timetable of the complete introduction of each food category is reported in Figure 2.

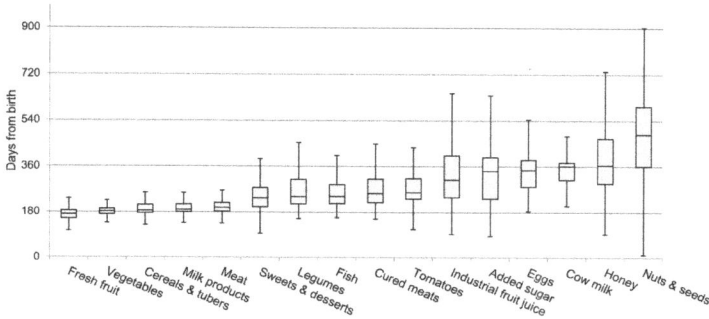

Figure 2. Timing of introduction of the single food groups in days from birth. The ends of the whiskers are set at 1.5*IQR above the third quartile (Q3) and 1.5*IQR below the first quartile (Q1). If the Minimum or Maximum values are outside this range, then they are shown as outliers. IQR = Inter Quartile Range.

In the figure, the cereals/tubers categories and the sweets/desserts categories, which include sweets and creamy porridge, have been merged for representational purposes. The first food group to be introduced was fresh fruit (at a median age of 170 days); followed by vegetables (182 days); cereals, including bread, pasta with gluten, and rice (193 days); milk products (189 days); and meat (197 days). The last food groups to be introduced were cow milk (362 days), honey (365 days), and nuts and seeds (484 days). In 80% of the cases, the first type of food to be offered was the apple, followed by vegetable soup (41%), and baby cereals (41%). The use of gluten-free products (bread, pasta, and desserts) was low (17% of infants) and the timing of their introduction was similar to that of the products with gluten. The introduction of pasta with gluten occurred at a median of 234 days, as opposed to 224 days for gluten-free pasta. The most frequently used commercial baby food types were: milk products (67%), fish (62%), sweets and desserts (61%), cured meat (52%), cereals (52%), meat (49%), fruit (27%), and vegetables (3%).

3.3. Compliance with WHO Recommendations

Table 2 shows the percentage of mothers who complied with the WHO recommendations on complementary feeding. The recommendations to which most mothers adhered were the minimum diversity diet (96%) and the introduction of honey after 12 months of age (80%), while 62% of the mothers complied with the recommendation to limit the use of commercial baby foods. However, the analysis of the "maximum diversity diet" indicated that, by the age 12 months, only 45% of children had introduced all seven food groups and, in particular, eggs and legumes had been introduced by 53% and 74% of infants, respectively.

Table 2. Percentage of mothers who followed the WHO recommendations (*n* = 148).

Items Included in the Score	(*n*)
Introduction of solid foods $\geq$6 months	14% (21)
Reduced use of commercial baby foods	62% (92)
Introduction of cow's milk $\geq$12 months	63% (94)
Introduction of honey $\geq$12 months	80% (118)
Minimum dietary diversity	96% (142)

As shown in Figure 3, eight mothers (5%) complied with all five recommendations and eight (5%) complied with only one, while 34% complied with at least three recommendations. Within this subgroup, the least frequently adhered to recommendation was the introduction of complementary feeding after the age of six months (19%).

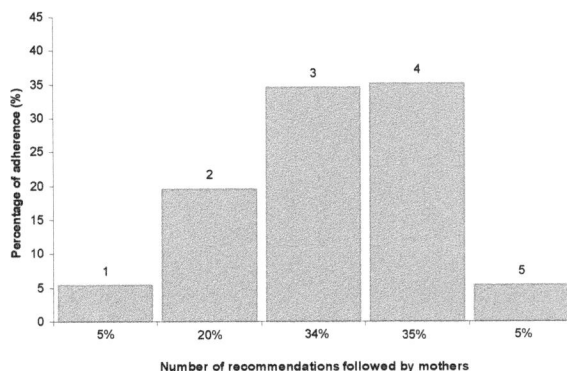

Figure 3. Number of recommendations (0, 1, 2, 3, 4 and 5) followed by mothers and percentage of compliance.

3.4. Regression Analyses

The stratified analyses showed that only few of the outcomes considered were significantly associated with selected mothers' characteristics. The introduction of cow milk after 12 months was significantly associated with the introduction of the first foods at 21 weeks of age or more if mothers were not breastfeeding their infants at six months (66%, $p = 0.03$), did not have a family history of allergy (80%, $p < 0.01$), had a BMI (kg/m^2) of less than 25 (72%, $p = 0.02$), and were younger than 35 years old (76%, $p = 0.02$). The test of homogeneity showed significant differences only between mothers with or without a history of allergy ($p = 0.03$).

Compliance with at least three out of five recommendations was significantly associated with the introduction of the first food at 21 weeks of age or more, if mothers where not breastfeeding their infants at six months (63%, $p = 0.05$), did not have a family history of allergy (74%, $p = 0.01$), had a BMI (kg/m^2) of less than 25 (71%, $p = 0.02$), and if they had received information on infant feeding from a midwife (68%, $p = 0.03$).

The multivariate logistic regression analyses showed no significant associations between the outcomes and maternal characteristics, probably due to the small size of the sample. The results are reported in the Supplementary Materials section (Tables S2–S6).

4. Discussion

As already observed in other studies [20,22,29], the timing of the introduction of complementary foods tends to follow a standard pattern: the infant's diet includes only few categories of food and differs substantially from that of the family, with commercial baby foods taking up a considerable share. Our study shows that the feeding practices of this cohort follow the same pattern and fall short of the WHO recommendations on breast and complementary feeding. Seventy five percent of mothers adhered to three or more out of five WHO recommendations on adequate complementary feeding, but only 5% complied with all five. The lowest rate of compliance related to the recommendation to introduce complementary foods at six months or more, with 86% of infants receiving complementary foods before the age of six months. This percentage is higher than the one reported in a recent study in the Netherlands [14], but close to the data reported in a nutrition survey from the UK [30] and in a WHO multicenter study of comparable sample size conducted in different countries [31]. However, comparisons with other studies are difficult because most of them adopt a cut-off of 17 weeks of age for early introduction, as recommended by ESPGHAN [12].

Despite the evidence that, in terms of prevention of allergies, there is no benefit in delaying the introduction of potentially allergenic foods [15] and that, in fact, early contact with food can induce tolerance and desensitization [32], the mothers in our cohort deferred the introduction of tomatoes, eggs, fish, and nuts and seeds, to between 8 (fish) and 16 months of age (nuts and seeds), as shown in Figure 2. This may have contributed to the lack of "maximum dietary diversity" by 12 months observed in more than half of the infants in our cohort. Indeed, as noted in a recent national survey [33,34], in a developed country such as Italy, without nutritional deficiencies and with high availability of nutrients, the "maximum dietary diversity" index could, and should, be higher.

It has been shown that the process of food learning starts very early and that there is a period in which new foods are relatively easily accepted [35,36]. Because food preferences developed at an early age may have long-lasting influence [37], it would be desirable to expose infants to as many tastes as possible in the first year of life. In her study [38], Cashdan showed that infants introduced to solids unusually late maintain a reduced diet and food range throughout childhood, perhaps as a result of the contraction of the sensitive period.

The partial compliance with WHO recommendations observed in our cohort, has already been reported by others [22,29,39]. Considering that 98% of the mothers in our study declared they received information on complementary feeding from their paediatrician and that in 62% of the cases, this advice was followed, the role of health professionals seems to be crucial, despite the lack of a statistically significant association in our regression analyses.

One of the possible reasons for the lack of correct and consistent information on the timing and type of complementary feeding is that in Italy there are no specific national Ministry of Health guidelines incorporating the WHO recommendations. These are therefore unevenly acquired by health professionals and poorly transferred to parents.

To our knowledge, this is the first study to explore in detail timing of complementary feeding and compliance with WHO recommendations, and associated factors, in Italy. The study does, however, have a number of limitations. The main problem is the loss to follow up of enrolled mother-infant pairs between birth and 36 months of age (37%), which greatly reduced the availability of complete data and thus the power to detect significant associations by multivariate analyses. The second major limitation is the complexity of the food timetable which required regular updating over a long period of time with detailed information regarding newly introduced food types. Although this tool is designed to provide high quality data, in our case this was at the expense of the sample size, making it difficult to compare our results with those of other national surveys.

5. Conclusions

Our paper describes the partial compliance with WHO recommendations on complementary feeding, in northeast Italy. Most of the infants in our cohort were started on complementary foods before the age of six months. They shared a very similar diet, which was very different from the family diet and characterized by the delayed introduction of certain food types. Further research will be needed to clarify the association between compliance with recommendations and socio-economic variables, in order to identify vulnerable groups in the population, including migrant families.

Taken together, our results suggest that Italy would greatly benefit from national evidence-based guidelines on infant feeding to support the development of solid public health strategies. These guidelines should be free from commercial interests, consistently adhered to, and promoted by all health professionals, especially in the light of the considerable influence their advice seems to have on parental practices.

Supplementary Materials: The following are available online at http://www.mdpi.com/2072-6643/9/1/34/s1. Table S1: Association between introduction of first foods after 21 weeks and compliance with WHO recommendations both as stand-alone variables and as overall compliance with any three out of five and selected variables by bivariate logistic regression analysis (n = 148), Table S2: Association between introduction of first foods after 21 weeks and introduction of honey after 12 months adjusted by selected variables by multivariate logistic regression analysis (n = 130), Table S3: Association between introduction of first foods after 21 weeks and introduction of cow milk after 12 months adjusted by selected variables by multivariate logistic regression analysis (n = 130), Table S4: Association between introduction of first foods after 21 weeks and less consumption of baby food adjusted by selected variables by multivariate logistic regression analysis (n = 130), Table S5: Association between introduction of first foods after 21 weeks and minimum dietary diversity recommendation adjusted by selected variables by multivariate logistic regression analysis (n = 130), Table S6: Association between introduction of first foods after 21 weeks and compliance with three out of five WHO recommendations adjusted by selected variables by multivariate logistic regression analysis (n = 130).

Acknowledgments: The authors wish to thank the mothers who participated in the study. The study was funded by the Institute for Maternal and Child Health IRCCS Burlo Garofolo, Trieste, Italy, and was approved by its Ethics Committee (RC 32/06).

Author Contributions: A.C. designed and supervised the study, helped analyze and interpret the results, and revised the manuscript. P.P., C.C. and A.K. conducted the study, collected the data, constructed the database, helped analyze and interpret the results, and wrote the manuscript. L.M. was in charge of the statistical analysis and revised the manuscript. All authors read and approved the final manuscript.

Conflicts of Interest: The authors declare no conflict of interest.

References

1. World Health Organization. *Complementay Feeding: Report of the Global Consultation, and Summary of Guiding Principles for Complementary Feeding of the Breastfed Child*; WHO: Geneva, Switzerland, 2002.
2. Monteiro, P.O.A.; Victora, C.G. Rapid growth in infancy and childhood and obesity in later life—A systematic review. *Obes. Rev.* **2005**, *6*, 143–154. [CrossRef] [PubMed]
3. Reynolds, C.M.; Gray, C.; Li, M.; Segovia, S.A.; Vickers, M.H. Early Life Nutrition and Energy Balance Disorders in Offspring in Later Life. *Nutrients* **2015**, *7*, 8090–8111. [CrossRef] [PubMed]
4. Ersino, G.; Henry, C.J.; Zello, G.A. Suboptimal Feeding Practices and High Levels of Undernutrition Among Infants and Young Children in the Rural Communities of Halaba and Zeway, Ethiopia. *Food Nutr. Bull.* **2016**, *37*, 409–424. [CrossRef] [PubMed]
5. Saaka, M.; Wemakor, A.; Abizari, A.R.; Aryee, P. How well do WHO complementary feeding indicators relate to nutritional status of children aged 6–23 months in rural Northern Ghana? *BMC Public Health* **2015**, *15*, 1157. [CrossRef] [PubMed]
6. World Health Organization; The United Nations Children's Fund. *Global Strategy for Infant and Young Child Feeding*; WHO: Geneva, Switzerland, 2002.
7. Arenz, S.; Ruckerl, R.; Koletzko, B.; von Kries, R. Breast-feeding and childhood obesity—A systematic review. *Int. J. Obes. Relat. Metab. Disord.* **2004**, *28*, 1247–1256. [CrossRef] [PubMed]
8. Huh, S.Y.; Rifas-Shiman, S.L.; Taveras, E.M.; Oken, E.; Gillman, M.W. Timing of solid food introduction and risk of obesity in preschool-aged children. *Pediatrics* **2011**, *127*, 544–551. [CrossRef] [PubMed]
9. Pearce, J.; Taylor, M.A.; Langley-Evans, S.C. Timing of the introduction of complementary feeding and risk of childhood obesity: A systematic review. *Int. J. Obes. (Lond.)* **2013**, *37*, 1295–1306. [CrossRef] [PubMed]
10. De Beer, M.; Vrijkotte, T.G.; Fall, C.H.; van Eijsden, M.; Osmond, C.; Gemke, R.J. Associations of infant feeding and timing of linear growth and relative weight gain during early life with childhood body composition. *Int. J. Obes. (Lond.)* **2015**, *39*, 586–592. [CrossRef] [PubMed]
11. Della Salute, M. *Linee di Indirizzo Nazionali Sulla Protezione, la Promozione ed il Sostegno Dell'allattamento al Seno*; Gazzetta Ufficiale: Roma, Italy, 2008.
12. Agostoni, C.; Decsi, T.; Fewtrell, M.; Goulet, O.; Kolacek, S.; Koletzko, B.; Michaelsen, K.F.; Moreno, L.; Puntis, J.; Rigo, J.; et al. Complementary feeding: A commentary by the ESPGHAN Committee on Nutrition. *J. Pediatr. Gastroenterol. Nutr.* **2008**, *46*, 99–110. [CrossRef] [PubMed]
13. Cattaneo, A.; Williams, C.; Pallas-Alonso, C.R.; Hernandez-Aguilar, M.T.; Lasarte-Velillas, J.J.; Landa-Rivera, L.; Rouw, E.; Pina, M.; Volta, A.; Oudesluys-Murphy, A.M. ESPGHAN's 2008 recommendation for early introduction of complementary foods: How good is the evidence? *Matern. Child Nutr.* **2011**, *7*, 335–343. [CrossRef] [PubMed]
14. World Health Organization. *Exclusive Breastfeeding for Six Months Best for Babies Everywhere*; WHO: Geneva, Switzerland, 2011.

15. Michaelsen, K.F.; Weaver, L.; Branca, F.; Robertson, A. *Feeding and Nutrition of Infants and Young Children*, 87th ed.; WHO Regional Publications, European Series; WHO Regional Office for Europe: Copenhagen, Denmark, 2000.

16. World Health Organization. *Complementary Feeding: Family Foods for Breasfed Infants*; WHO: Geneva, Switzerland, 2000.

17. Scott, J.A.; Binns, C.W.; Graham, K.I.; Oddy, W.H. Predictors of the early introduction of solid foods in infants: Results of a cohort study. *BMC Pediatr.* **2009**, *9*, 60. [CrossRef] [PubMed]

18. Tromp, I.I.M.; Briede, S.; Kiefte-de Jong, J.C.; Renders, C.M.; Jaddoe, V.W.; Franco, O.H.; Hofman, A.; Raat, H.; Moll, H.A. Factors associated with the timing of introduction of complementary feeding: The Generation R Study. *Eur. J. Clin. Nutr.* **2013**, *67*, 625–630. [CrossRef] [PubMed]

19. Giovannini, M.; Riva, E.; Banderali, G.; Scaglioni, S.; Veehof, S.H.; Sala, M.; Radaelli, G.; Agostoni, C. Feeding practices of infants through the first year of life in Italy. *Acta Paediatr.* **2004**, *93*, 492–497. [PubMed]

20. Pani, P.; Carletti, C.; Knowles, A.; Parpinel, M.; Concina, F.; Montico, M.; Cattaneo, A. Patterns of nutrients' intake at six months in the northeast of Italy: A cohort study. *BMC Pediatr.* **2014**, *14*, 127. [CrossRef] [PubMed]

21. Carletti, C.; Pani, P.; Knowles, A.; Monasta, L.; Montico, M.; Cattaneo, A. Breastfeeding to 24 months of age in the northeast of Italy: A cohort study. *Breastfeed. Med.* **2011**, *6*, 177–182. [CrossRef] [PubMed]

22. Schiess, S.; Grote, V.; Scaglioni, S.; Luque, V.; Martin, F.; Stolarczyk, A.; Vecchi, F.; Koletzko, B.; European Childhood Obesity Project. Introduction of complementary feeding in 5 European countries. *J. Pediatr. Gastroenterol. Nutr.* **2010**, *50*, 92–98. [CrossRef] [PubMed]

23. Biro, G.; Hulshof, K.F.; Ovesen, L.; Amorim Cruz, J.A.; EFCOSUM Group. Selection of methodology to assess food intake. *Eur. J. Clin. Nutr.* **2002**, *56*, S25–S32. [CrossRef] [PubMed]

24. Buzzard, M. 24-Hour dietary recall and food record methods. In *Nutritional Epidemiology*, 2nd ed.; Willett, W., Ed.; Oxford University Press: Oxford, UK, 1998; pp. 50–73.

25. World Health Organization; The United Nations Children's Fund. Indicators for assessing infant and young child feeding practices. In Proceedings of the Conclusions of a Consensus Meeting, Washington, DC, USA, 6–8 November 2007; WHO: Geneva, Switzerland, 2008.

26. World Health Organization. *Guideline: Vitamin A Supplementation in Infants and Children 6–59 Months of Age*; WHO: Geneva, Switzerland, 2011.

27. Clayton, H.B.; Li, R.; Perrine, C.G.; Scanlon, K.S. Prevalence and reasons for introducing infants early to solid foods: Variations by milk feeding type. *Pediatrics* **2013**, *131*, 1108–1114. [CrossRef] [PubMed]

28. Baker, J.L.; Michaelsen, K.F.; Rasmussen, K.M.; Sørensen, T.I. Maternal prepregnant body mass index, duration of breastfeeding, and timing of complementary food introduction are associated with infant weight gain. *Am. J. Clin. Nutr.* **2004**, *80*, 1579–1588. [PubMed]

29. Dratva, J.; Merten, S.; Ackermann-Liebrich, U. The timing of complementary feeding of infants in Switzerland: Compliance with the Swiss and the WHO guidelines. *Acta Paediatr.* **2006**, *95*, 818–825. [CrossRef] [PubMed]

30. Lennox, A.; Sommerville, J.; Ong, K.; Henderson, H.; Allen, R. *Diet and Nutrition Survey of Infants and Young Children, 2011*; Department of Health and Food Standards Agency: London, UK, 2013.

31. WHO Multicenter Growth Reference Study Group. Complementary feeding in the WHO Multicenter Growth Reference Study. *Acta Paediatr.* **2006**, *450*, 27–37.

32. Longo, G.; Berti, I.; Burks, A.W.; Krauss, B.; Barbi, E. IgE-mediated food allergy in children. *Lancet* **2013**, *382*, 1656–1664. [CrossRef]

33. Leclercq, C.; Arcella, D.; Piccinelli, R.; Sette, S.; Le Donne, C.; Turrini, A.; INRAN-SCAI 2005-06 Study Group. The Italian National Food Consumption Survey INRAN-SCAI 2005-06: Main results in terms of food consumption. *Public Health Nutr.* **2009**, *12*, 2504–2532. [CrossRef] [PubMed]

34. Sette, S.; Le Donne, C.; Piccinelli, R.; Arcella, D.; Turrini, A.; Leclercq, C.; INRAN-SCAI 2005-6 Study Group. The third Italian National Food Consumption Survey, INRAN-SCAI 2005-06—Part 1: Nutrient intakes in Italy. *Nutr. Metab. Cardiovasc. Dis.* **2011**, *21*, 922–932. [CrossRef] [PubMed]

35. Lange, C.; Visalli, M.; Jacob, S.; Chabanet, C.; Schlich, P.; Nicklaus, S. Maternal feeding practices during the first year and their impact on infants' acceptance of complementary food. *Food Qual. Prefer.* **2013**, *29*, 89–98. [CrossRef]

36. Schwartz, C.; Scholtens, P.A.; Lalanne, A.; Weenen, H.; Nicklaus, S. Development of healthy eating habits early in life. Review of recent evidence and selected guidelines. *Appetite* **2011**, *57*, 796–807. [PubMed]

37. Nicklaus, S.; Remy, E. Early origins of overeating: Tracking between early food habits and later eating patterns. *Curr. Obes. Rep.* **2013**, *2*, 179–184. [CrossRef]

38. Cashdan, E. A sensitive period for learning about food. *Hum. Nat.* **1994**, *5*, 279–291. [CrossRef] [PubMed]

39. O'Donovan, S.M.; Murray, D.M.; Hourihane, J.O.; Kenny, L.C.; Irvine, A.D.; Kiely, M. Adherence with early infant feeding and complementary feeding guidelines in the Cork BASELINE Birth Cohort Study. *Public Health Nutr.* **2015**, *18*, 2864–2873. [CrossRef] [PubMed]

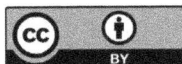

nutrients

MDPI

Article

On the Importance of Processing Conditions for the Nutritional Characteristics of Homogenized Composite Meals Intended for Infants

Elin Östman *, Anna Forslund, Eden Tareke and Inger Björck

Food for Health Science Centre, Lund University, P.O. Box 124, 221 00 Lund, Sweden;
anna.k.forslund@gmail.com (A.F.); eden.tareke@food-health-science.lu.se (E.T.);
inger.bjorck@food-health-science.lu.se (I.B.)
* Correspondence: elin.ostman@food-health-science.lu.se; Tel.: +46-46-222-8318

Received: 25 April 2016; Accepted: 27 May 2016; Published: 3 June 2016

Abstract: The nutritional quality of infant food is an important consideration in the effort to prevent a further increase in the rate of childhood obesity. We hypothesized that the canning of composite infant meals would lead to elevated contents of carboxymethyl-lysine (CML) and favor high glycemic and insulinemic responses compared with milder heat treatment conditions. We have compared composite infant pasta Bolognese meals that were either conventionally canned (CANPBol), or prepared by microwave cooking (MWPBol). A meal where the pasta and Bolognese sauce were separate during microwave cooking (MWP_CANBol) was also included. The infant meals were tested at breakfast in healthy adults using white wheat bread (WWB) as reference. A standardized lunch meal was served at 240 min and blood was collected from fasting to 360 min after breakfast. The 2-h glucose response (iAUC) was lower following the test meals than with WWB. The insulin response was lower after the MWP_CANBol (-47%, $p = 0.0000$) but markedly higher after CANPBol ($+40\%$, $p = 0.0019$), compared with WWB. A combined measure of the glucose and insulin responses ($ISI_{composite}$) revealed that MWP_CANBol resulted in 94% better insulin sensitivity than CANPBol. Additionally, the separate processing of the meal components in MWP_CANBol resulted in 39% lower CML levels than the CANPBol. It was therefore concluded that intake of commercially canned composite infant meals leads to reduced postprandial insulin sensitivity and increased exposure to oxidative stress promoting agents.

Keywords: infant food; glycemia; insulinemia; human; advanced glycation end products; carboxymethyl-lysine; early protein hypothesis; protein quality; carbohydrate digestibility; glycemic index

1. Introduction

In the development of infant formulas, weaning food, and composite infant meals, the main aim has traditionally been to ensure the provision of adequate amounts of essential nutrients. Great interest has therefore been devoted to the availability of certain nutrients, such as protein and selected minerals. Two nutritional quality characteristics that are emphasized in food for adults are the availability of carbohydrates affecting the glycemic response, and the presence of process-induced advanced glycation end products (AGEs), which affect the biological value of the protein. Carbohydrate-rich foods with low glycemic impact were recently classified as relevant for the prevention and treatment of type 2 diabetes, coronary heart disease, and probably obesity [1]. High-glycemic meals have been associated with the increased activation of inflammatory markers in the postprandial phase [2]. Elevated intakes of AGEs are of interest due to their association with cardiometabolic risk markers and pathological conditions such as diabetes [3–5]. In the case of powder-based weaning foods, considerable and varying amounts of AGEs were recently reported in milk powder, infant formulas, and gruel [6,7]. Furthermore, high intakes of ultra-processed food products were recently positively and independently associated with increased prevalence of excess weight gain and obesity in different age groups in Brazil [8]. It is interesting to note that composite canned meals intended for small children are subjected to high-temperature treatment. Excessive heat treatment is known to affect the availability of the carbohydrate component [9], and the homogenization of composite infant meals prior to canning is likely to further increase the availability of the carbohydrate components for digestion and absorption [10]. Additionally, homogenization of the meal components could be expected to boost AGE formation by enhancing the accessibility of the necessary precursors.

Based on the above, we hypothesized that the canning of homogenized composite infant meals may render carbohydrates and protein rapidly available for digestion and absorption, leading to high blood glucose and insulin responses. Furthermore, it was hypothesized that the increased availability of carbohydrates and proteins would result in the formation of higher levels of AGEs than in less harshly processed composite meals. The objectives of the present work were to establish some of the nutritional quality characteristics of canned homogenized composite meals intended for infants, and to compare them with more gently processed alternatives.

2. Methods

Two studies were performed, the first of which involved a commercially canned pasta Bolognese meal and a canned composite meal with beef and white beans (Study 1). In the second study, a commercially canned pasta Bolognese meal (purée with some intact soft pieces) was again used and compared with a similar but microwave heat-treated meal (cracked spaghetti with minced meat and vegetables). Separately boiled cracked spaghetti served with a commercially canned meat sauce was also included. White wheat bread (WWB) was used as a reference [11] in both studies to allow the determination of the glycemic index (GI) and the insulinemic index (II). The GI is defined as the incremental area under the blood glucose curve (iAUC) following the intake of a test meal, expressed as a percentage of an equi-carbohydrate reference meal, eaten by the same subject. The II is calculated similarly, based on the corresponding insulin responses. WWB is a starch-rich product considered to be a more physiologically relevant reference product than pure glucose, due to its more complex food matrix. The meal studies were performed in healthy adults to investigate the postprandial effects on glucose and insulin. In Study 2, non-esterified fatty acids (NEFAs) and triglycerides (TGs) were also analyzed. *N*-carboxymethyl-lysine (CML) was used as a marker of AGEs. The CML contents in some commercially canned composite infant meals and relevant composite frozen meals intended for adults were included for comparison. All test products were heated to eating temperature prior to the analysis of CML, determination of rate of *in vitro* starch hydrolysis, or being served as a test meal.

2.1. General Study Design

Healthy adult volunteers were recruited for the studies. All test subjects gave their informed consent, and were aware that they could withdraw from the study at any time. The studies were approved by the Regional Ethical Review Board in Lund (LU 558-01 and 2012/615). The test meals and the reference meal were served as breakfast in a random order, after overnight fasting. The tests were performed approximately one week apart and commenced at the same time in the morning. Subjects were instructed to maintain their regular lifestyle throughout the period of the study. The day prior to a test they were told to avoid alcohol, excessive physical activity, and food rich in dietary fiber. On the evening (21.00–22.00) before each test, the subjects were instructed to eat a standardized meal consisting of white wheat bread with spread and drink of their own choice. However, the subjects were instructed to have the same evening meal before each test.

2.2. Study 1

Five men and four women aged 24–41 years, with normal body mass indices (23.1 $\pm$ 2.7 kg/m^2; mean $\pm$ SD), normal fasting blood glucose (4.4 $\pm$ 0.05 mmol/L; mean $\pm$ SEM), and who were not taking any medication, participated in the study. The test subjects were recruited and the study performed between October 1999 and February 2000. Test subjects were recruited by advertising on notice boards around the Lund University (LU) campus, and by contacting former volunteers. Two commercially available canned composite meals, "canned Meat&Pasta" and "canned Meat&Beans", intended for infants aged 12 months, were studied. The meals were microwave heated according to the manufacturer's instructions before serving. Both test meals and the reference WWB meal contained 30 g of potentially available carbohydrates [12]. Both the test meals and the reference meal were served with 250 mL water and followed by 150 mL coffee or tea. Finger-prick capillary blood samples were taken repeatedly up to 120 min after ingesting the meal for the analysis of blood glucose concentrations (glucose oxidase-peroxidase reagent) and serum insulin (Insulin ELISA, Mercodia AB, Uppsala, Sweden).

Product Characterization

Levels of CML were determined in freeze-dried samples of selected canned composite infant meals and corresponding frozen ready-to-eat meals intended for adults using gas chromatography mass spectrometry (GC-MS) according to Birlouez-Aragon [3]. The results are presented in Table 1. The *in vitro* rate of starch hydrolysis (hydrolysis index, HI) was analyzed for the meals using the method described by Granfeldt *et al.* [13]. Before HI-analysis, samples of the composite meals were rinsed in a strainer using tap water to obtain the intact pieces of the carbohydrate sources (beans and pasta).

2.3. Study 2

2.3.1. Recipes and Processing Conditions

Canned pasta Bolognese (CANPBol) for infants aged 12 months was bought in the local supermarket, and two other test meals were prepared in the laboratory. In order to investigate the possible advantages of minimal processing of a composite meal, an in-pack pasteurization method was used (MicVac AB, Mölndal, Sweden). The microwave cooked test meal (MWPBol) was based on a recipe resembling that of the CANPBol meal, and contained: 60 g water, 50 g crushed tomatoes (ICA, Solna, Sweden), 17 g carrots, 17 g yellow onions, 16 g minced beef, 13 g manually cracked spaghetti (ICA Italia, Solna, Sweden), 10 g tomato purée (ICA), 10 g celery root, 2 g corn starch (Maizena, Unilever, Solna, Sweden), 2 g rapeseed oil (ICA), 0.15 g iodized salt (Falksalt, Ab Hanson & Möhring, Halmstad, Sweden), 0.2 g dry oregano (Santa Maria, Mölndal, Sweden), 0.1 g dry basil (Santa Maria), and 0.07 g white pepper (Santa Maria). A test meal consisting of separately microwave-cooked pieces of spaghetti (ICA Italia) and canned Bolognese sauce (Felix Köttfärsås Original, Orkla Foods, Eslöv, Sweden) was used to study the effect of preparing the meal components separately (MWP_CANBol). All pasta and canned Bolognese sauce were bought from one batch. In the case of the MWPBol meal, all dried/canned ingredients and minced beef was bought from one batch, but vegetables were bought fresh every week. The minced beef was frozen in portions and thawed prior to the preparation of each serving. Each MWPBol portion was prepared the evening before the test by combining the minced meat with small pieces of the vegetables, crushed tomatoes, spices, and cracked spaghetti. After sealing the tray with plastic film, the portion was cooked in a microwave oven for 8 min, chilled on ice and then stored overnight in a refrigerator. Just before serving, MWPBol meal was reheated in microwave oven for 1.5 min. In the case of the MWP_CANBol meal, cracked spaghetti was boiled in water for 7.5 min using a similar tray sealed with plastic film in microwave oven and stored in the refrigerator overnight. In the morning, the pasta was heated separately for 2 min, and the canned Bolognese sauce was heated separately for 2.5 min, in the microwave oven. The pasta and Bolognese sauce were then mixed on the plate before serving. Each CANPBol portion was weighed on a plate just before serving, and microwave heated for 2.5 min, with breaks for stirring after 1 and 2 min.

2.3.2. Product Characterization

All test and reference meals in Study 2 were standardized so as to contain 35 g available starch, according to Holm *et al.* [12]. The CANPBol meal and the canned Bolognese sauce were analyzed as bought, without preparation. The microwave-cooked spaghetti was re-heated before analysis, and the starch content converted to dry matter basis. The protein contents in the test meals were determined using an elemental analyzer (FlashEA 1112, Thermo Fischer Scientific Inc., Waltham, MA, USA). The fat contents in the commercial products were estimated from the manufacturers' declarations. In the case of WWB, estimates of the protein and fat contents were based on a previous analysis of a similar product [14]. CML was determined using high-pressure liquid chromatography mass spectrometry (HPLC-MS/MS), with an Accela UHPLC pump with an autoinjector coupled to an LTQ VelosPro Orbitrap mass spectrometer (Thermo Scientific, Waltham, MA, USA). The MS/MS was run in positive electrospray ionization ion trap mode, detecting two selected reaction monitoring (SRM) transitions for CML and two for the internal standard. Xcalibur software (ver. 2.2, Thermo Scientific) was used for both data acquisition and evaluation. Samples were prepared by hydrolyzing 0.3 g sample for 12 h at 110 °C, using 6 M HCl, together with isotope-labelled d4-CML (Larodan Fine Chemicals AB, Malmö, Sweden) as internal standard. CML was extracted after hydrolysis using solid phase extraction (Telos*neo*PCX, Teknolab Sorbent AB, Västra Frölunda, Sweden). All the dried samples were reconstituted in 0.01% (v/v) nonafluoropentanoic acid (Sigma-Aldrich, Steinheim, Germany) and centrifuged before analysis. Solid phase extraction, chromatographic parameters, ion source parameters, and the SRM transitions were the same as described by Tareke *et al.* [6,7]. CML analyses were performed on three different days. To check any instrumental inconsistency, duplicates of each sample were analyzed on one occasion. The portion sizes, macronutrient and energy compositions, and the CML contents are presented in Table 2.

2.3.3. Subjects

The inclusion criteria were being a healthy, non-smoker with normal weight (body mass index, BMI, 19–25 kg/m^2), aged 18–40 years, with a stable body weight over the previous two months. Exclusion criteria were being a vegetarian/vegan and/or having food allergies, lactose intolerance, having any disease or taking any medication that might affect the study, as well as being pregnant or lactating.

2.3.4. Sample Collection and Protocol

The subjects arrived at the laboratory at 7:45 a.m. after overnight fasting. A peripheral venous catheter (BD Venflon Dickinson, Helsingborg, Sweden) was inserted into an antecubital vein. Capillary plasma glucose and venous blood samples were collected, after which the individually assigned test meal was served, together with 250 g of tap water (time 0). All meals were tolerated and finished within 10–15 min, except for one test person who needed 20 min to finish eating the CANPBol meal. Blood samples were taken at 15, 30, 45, 60, 90, 120, 240, 270, 300, 330, and 360 min after the beginning of the meal. One hundred and thirty-five minutes after the meal, each subject was given 200 g water to be drunk within 15 min. Two hundred and forty-five minutes after the start of the meal, a standardized lunch, consisting of a ready-to-eat dish of 400 g (2320 kJ) pasta with tomatoes, basil, and mozzarella cheese (Pasta al Pomodoro, Gooh, Lantmännen, Sweden) was served. The lunch meal was served with 250 g tap water, and was to be consumed within 20 min.

2.3.5. Blood Analysis

Blood glucose was analyzed in capillary blood (HemoCue®B-glucose, HemoCue AB, Ängelholm, Sweden). Serum was obtained from venous blood collected in CAT tubes (BD Vacutainer, ref. 368492) and left to clot for 60 min before being centrifuged at 3500 rpm for 10 min at 4 °C. Plasma was obtained in EDTA tubes (BD Vacutainer, ref 368274) and put on ice for a maximum of 30 min until centrifuged at 3500 rpm for 10 min at 4 °C. Samples were then aliquoted in Eppendorf tubes and stored immediately at −20 °C until analysis. Serum insulin and serum TGs were analyzed by a lab at Skåne University Hospital (Clinical Chemistry, Region Skåne, Sweden), whereas NEFAs were analyzed at the department using a colorimetric assay (NEFA C, ACS-ACOD method, WAKO Chemicals GmbH, Neuss, Germany).

3. Statistical Calculations

The least number of subjects required to detect a difference in the GI with a power of 80% at a level of $p < 0.05$, is ten [15]. The sample size in Study 1 was nine, and in order to improve the power of Study 2, twenty-one subjects were included. The iAUCs for glucose and insulin were calculated using GraphPad Prism (GraphPad Software, San Diego, CA, USA) and the trapezoid model. All areas below the baseline were excluded from the calculations. The results are expressed as means ± SEM. Differences resulting in $p < 0.05$ were considered statistically significant.

3.1. Study 1

The 120 min blood glucose and insulin iAUCs were used to determine GI and II, respectively. The statistical differences were evaluated using the general linear model (ANOVA) followed by Tukey's multiple comparisons test using Minitab software (ver. 13, Minitab Inc., State College, PA, USA).

3.2. Study 2

Differences in CML content between the test meals and the reference meal were evaluated with one-way ANOVA using GraphPad Prism (as described above). The composite insulin sensitivity index ($ISI_{composite}$), also called the Matsuda index, was calculated for both the test meals and the reference meal in order to assess the insulin sensitivity.

$ISI_{composite}$ = 10,000/$\sqrt{}$[fasting glucose (mmol/L) × fasting insulin (nmol/L) × glucose iAUC 0–120 min (mmol· min/L) × insulin iAUC 0–120 min (nmol· min/L)] [16,17].

The effects of the test meals and reference meal on glucose and insulin responses, as well as on the NEFA and TG levels, were evaluated using the PROC MIXED SAS procedure. The subject was treated as a random effect and the test meal as a fixed effect. The fixed effect of corresponding baseline (fasting) values was included as a covariate, and time × meal interactions were tested. All models were tested for the normality of residuals. To adjust for multiple comparisons of significant effects, the Tukey–Kramer *post hoc* significance test was performed. Statistical analyses of metabolic outcomes were performed using SAS 9.2 (SAS Institute Inc., Cary, NC, USA) and Minitab software (ver. 16). The data are presented as iAUC values or least-square means (LSMs) ± SEM. The data were also tested for outliers. The fasting level of insulin was found to be an outlier for one subject, and the result was therefore not included in the insulin analyses. In addition, insulin data were lacking for one subject 30 min after the CANPBol meal and for another 240 min after the MWP_CANBol meal. Due to the missing values, those two test meals were excluded from the calculations for insulin. Another subject missed the CANPBol meal, resulting in $n = 20$ for the CANPBol meal for all blood tests except insulin, where $n = 18$.

4. Results

4.1. Study 1

The canned meals intended for infants contained three to four times higher levels of CML (expressed as mg CML/g protein) than frozen meals with similar ingredients but intended for adults (Table 1). The HI for canned beans was 44, which was significantly lower ($p < 0.05$) than the HI of both the canned pasta (109) and WWB reference (100).

The glycemic response to canned Meat&Beans (GI = 48 ± 11) was significantly lower ($p < 0.05$) than that after the reference WWB meal (GI = 100). The GI of canned Meat&Pasta (79 ± 12) did not differ from either of the other two meals. No significant differences were found in the insulin responses, and the II values were 100, 91 ± 13, and 140 ± 30 for WWB, canned Meat&Beans, and canned Meat&Pasta, respectively.

Table 1. *N*-carboxymethyl-lysine (CML) content in canned and homogenized meals intended for infants and in frozen ready-to-eat meals intended for adults.

Meal	CML (mg/g Protein)
Beef stew "Kalops"	
Canned, homogenized	0.33
Frozen	0.08
Hash "Pytt i panna"	
Canned, homogenized	0.45
Frozen	0.14

Results are presented as the mean of two duplicates.

4.2. Study 2

Twenty-one healthy volunteers (14 men and 7 women) participated in Study 2. All female subjects were taking birth control medication. The mean BMI was 21.8 ± 0.3 kg/m^2 and mean age 24.3 ± 0.9 years (±SEM). All subjects had normal fasting blood glucose levels (5.4 ± 0.06 mmol/L). The recruitment of test subjects and the study were performed from November 2012 to March 2013. Recruitment was performed by advertising on notice boards at and around the LU campus as well as by contacting former volunteers. The macronutrient composition and CML content of the various foods are presented in Table 2. All test and reference meals were similar in content of available carbohydrates and the protein and fat levels as well as energy contents were within the same range for all composite test meals. CANPBol and MWPBol contained significantly higher levels of CML compared with MWP_CANBol. The CML-content of WWB was significantly lower than in all test meals.

Table 2. Portion sizes and contents of macronutrients, energy, and CML in the test meals and reference meal in Study 2.

Meal	Portion g	Starch g/Port	Protein g/Port	Fat [1] g/Port	Energy kJ/Port	CML [2,3] mg/Port
WWB	83	35	4.9	0.7	704	0.41 ± 0.04 [a]
CANPBol	467	34	13	11.7	1232	9.75 ± 0.89 [b]
MWPBol	479	36	15	11.5	1292	8.98 ± 0.13 [b]
MWP_CANBol of which:	309	35	12	9.3	1143	5.94 ± 0.64 [c]
Canned Bolognese sauce	130	3.3	7.3	8.9	-	5.94 ± 0.64 [c]
Pasta, uncooked	42	30	4.4	0.4	-	n.a.
Maize starch (Maizena)	2	1.7	-	-	-	n.a.

[1] Estimated from a previous study (WWB) and manufacturers' declarations (commercial products/ingredients). WWB, white wheat bread; CANPBol, canned mixed meal; MWP_CANBol, canned Bolognese sauce served with microwave-cooked spaghetti; MWPBol, microwave-cooked mixed meal; n.a., not analyzed; [2] Values are presented as mean ± SEM, $n = 4$; [3] Values within the row not sharing a superscript letter are significantly different, $p < 0.05$.

4.2.1. Blood Glucose Responses

No differences were observed in fasting glucose levels. There was a significant time × meal interaction ($p < 0.0001$) over the 360 min follow-up (Figure 1). Incremental glucose responses (0–120 min) were significantly lower (31%–63%) following all the test meals than after the WWB meal (Table 3). Furthermore, the glucose response (iAUC and GI) after the MWP_CANBol meal was significantly lower than those after the two other test meals, during the same time period. After the standardized lunch meal (iAUC 240–360) the glucose response following the MWP_CANBol breakfast was significantly lower compared to WWB and CANPBol. The cumulative glucose response over the entire test period (iAUC 0–360 min) showed that overall glycemia following the MWPBol and MWP_CANBol meals was lower than following the CANPBol meal and WWB reference meal.

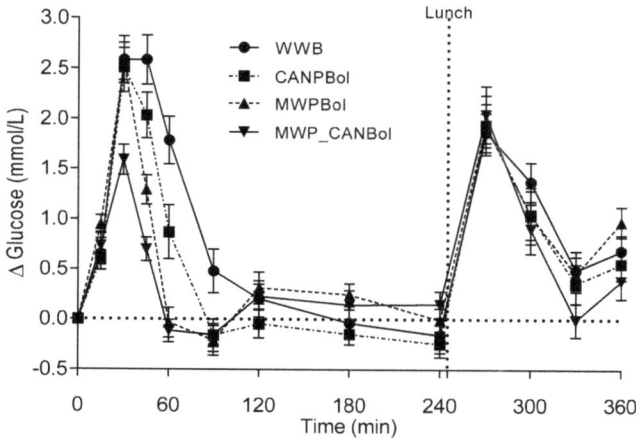

Figure 1. Mean (±SEM) changes in glucose response after the test meals and reference meal and the subsequent standardized lunch (Study 2).

Table 3. Glucose and insulin responses [1], together with a measure of insulin sensitivity after the test meals and the reference meal (Study 2).

	WWB [2]	CANPBol [2]	Δ %	MWPBol [2]	Δ %	MWP_CANBol [2]	Δ %
Glucose							
GI 0–120 min	100 [a]	79 ± 13 [b]	−21	61 ± 5.4 [b]	−39	38 ± 3.6 [c]	−62
iAUC 0–45 min	68.4 ± 6.13 [a]	61.8 ± 5.30 [a]	−10	62.0 ± 3.40 [a]	−9	40.6 ± 4.31 [b]	−41
iAUC 0–120	153 ± 16.0 [a]	104 ± 13.7 [b]	−31	84.6 ± 10.3 [b]	−45	57.4 ± 7.7 [c]	−63
iAUC 240–360	148 ± 18.5 [a]	136 ± 16.3 [a]	−8	120 ± 12.4 [a,b]	−19	92.2 ± 13.1 [b]	−38
iAUC 0–360	312 ± 30.8 [a]	240 ± 31.9 [a,b]	−23	245 ± 37.9 [b]	−22	206 ± 33.3 [b]	−34
Insulin							
II 0–120 min	100 [a]	161 ± 19 [b]	61	129 ± 15 [a,b]	29	57 ± 5.5 [c]	−43
iAUC 0–45 min	5.11 ± 0.79 [a]	8.10 ± 1.02 [b]	59	7.15 ± 0.88 [b]	40	4.01 ± 0.63 [a]	−22
iAUC 0–120	11.3 ± 1.79 [a]	15.8 ± 2.45 [b]	40	12.4 ± 1.90 [a,b]	10	5.95 ± 0.97 [c]	−47
iAUC 0–360	26.4 ± 3.74 [a]	32.2 ± 4.86 [a]	22	26.5 ± 3.81 [a]	0.2	20.2 ± 2.75 [b]	−24
ISI$_{composite}$	703 ± 82 [a]	733 ± 98 [a]	4	865 ± 72 [a]	23	1421 ± 135 [b]	102

[1] Values are presented as mean ± SEM; [2] Values within the same row not sharing superscript letters are significantly different, $p < 0.05$. GI, glycemic index; iAUC, incremental area under the curve; II, insulin index; ISI$_{composite}$, insulin sensitivity index; WWB, white wheat bread; CANPBol, canned mixed meal; MWP_CANBol, canned Bolognese sauce served with microwave-cooked spaghetti; MWPBol, microwave-cooked mixed meal.

4.2.2. Insulin Response

No differences were observed in fasting insulin levels. There was no significant time × meal interaction over the 360 min study period (Figure 2). During the first 45 min, the insulin level was significantly higher following the CANPBol meal (59%) and the MWPBol meal (40%) than the MWP_CANBol meal and the WWB meal. The incremental insulin responses during the periods 0–120 and 0–360 min were significantly lower after the MWP_CANBol meal than after all other meals. In addition, the insulin response during 0–120 min was significantly higher following the CANPBol meal than the WWB reference meal.

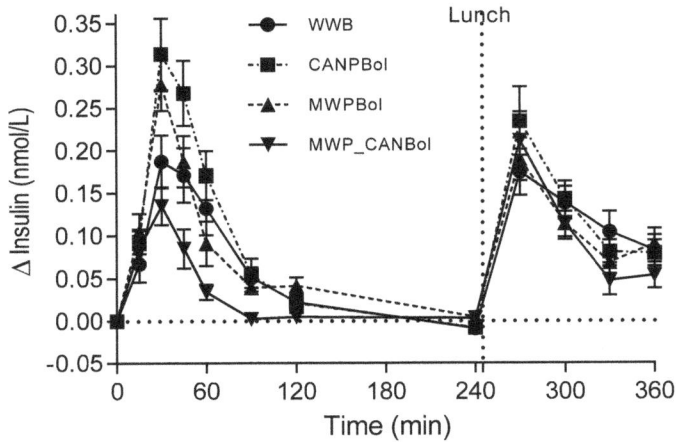

Figure 2. Mean (±SEM) changes in insulin response after the intake of the test meals and reference meal, and subsequent standardized lunch (Study 2).

4.2.3. Blood Lipids

No differences were observed in fasting levels of NEFAs or TGs and no significant time × meal interactions were observed for either of the lipid variables ($p < 0.0001$). Pairwise comparisons of NEFA levels at 240 min showed that they were significantly lower after the MWPBol and MWP_CANBol meals than after the WWB meal ($p = 0.0392$ and 0.0001, respectively, Figure S1). The overall TG response was significantly higher after the CANPBol ($p = 0.0216$) and MWPBol ($p = 0.0008$) meals than after the WWB meal (Figure 3). Furthermore, the level of TGs was significantly higher following the MWPBol meal than after the MWP_CANBol meal ($p = 0.0041$) over the 360 min.

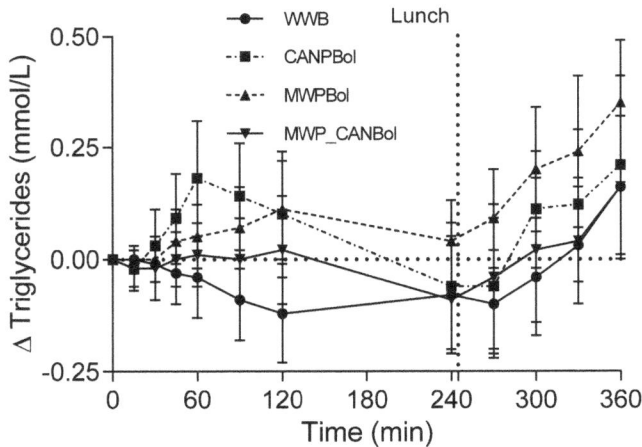

Figure 3. Mean (±SEM) changes in triglyceride response after the intake of the test meals and reference meal, and a subsequent standardized lunch (Study 2).

5. Discussion

The major finding of this study is that canned composite pasta Bolognese meals, processed according to a common procedure for infant meals, elicited substantially higher postprandial metabolic responses in healthy adults than meals intended for adults prepared with conventional cooking conditions. In fact, the infant CANPBol meal elicited an almost two-fold higher postprandial glucose and a 2.6 times higher insulin level during the first 2 h, compared with a meal of canned meat sauce served with gently and separately cooked pasta (MWP_CANBol). When combining the glucose and insulin data in a composite index, $ISI_{composite}$, the insulin sensitivity was improved by 94% after the MWP_CANBol meal, compared with the CANPBol meal. The significantly higher insulin response (+59%) during the first 45 min after the CANPBol meal, compared to the WWB meal, cannot be explained by the corresponding increase in glucose, since this was reduced by 10% (not statistically significant). Instead, we suggest that a fraction of the proteins was rendered highly soluble by the canning process, and may thus exert insulinotrophic effects. Surprisingly, the microwave-cooked composite meal (MWPBol) also led to a significant increase in early insulin response, but no significant differences were found in insulin, compared with WWB, over 120 min. The separately processed meal, MWP_CANBol, resulted in substantially lower glucose (−63%) and insulin (−47%) responses, compared with WWB. Apparently, the canning of Bolognese sauce *per se* did not result in an elevated insulin response, and the reduction in both glucose and insulin is in line with previous findings regarding pasta meals, where a low glucose peak and a late net increment with an accompanying lowering of insulin responses have been reported [18]. Holm *et al.* have previously reported a higher postprandial glycemic response in healthy adults to canned pasta, compared to cooked pasta [9]. They observed glucose responses that were twice as high after canned then after boiled spaghetti, and the insulin response was also significantly increased by canning. A suggested mechanism for the rapid uptake of carbohydrates following the intake of canned pasta was the excessive swelling of the starch, resulting in a very soft and easily digestible texture. The significantly reduced glucose response following the canned Meat&Beans in Study 1 is probably the result of some remaining intact cell structures following homogenization and canning of the composite bean meal [19]. This was also illustrated by the lower *in vitro* rate of starch hydrolysis for the bean component in the canned Meat&Beans meal (HI = 44), than in the canned Meat&Pasta meal (HI = 109) and the WWB reference meal (HI = 100). It should be noted though, that only the intact beans were included in HI-analysis, since they stayed in the strainer after washing. The high HI found for canned pasta is in line with the findings of a previous study indicating that homogenized spaghetti (cooked spaghetti treated for 35 s in a food processor) had a higher GI (73) than intact spaghetti (60), but was still lower than that for bread baked using spaghetti ingredients (100) [18]. Taken together, these findings indicate that canning of pasta disrupts the texture.

The substantial reduction in postprandial glycemic response after the MWP_CANBol meal, compared to the other meals, is further reflected by the improved glucose tolerance following a standardized lunch, manifested by a 38% lower glucose response, than after the WWB breakfast. Another indication of improved insulin sensitivity at the time of lunch (240 min) following the MWP_CANBol breakfast was the reduced NEFA levels. This is in agreement with other reports showing that suppressed NEFA levels between meals improves glucose tolerance following a second meal [20]. The increase in TG levels tended to be higher after the intake of CANPBol than after the other meals over the first postprandial hour. This may be related to a higher availability of lipids from this particular canned composite meal.

It has been suggested that the mechanism behind the increased risk of obesity associated with high protein intakes during infancy may be the protein-associated stimulation of insulin and IGF-1 release [21]. The results of the present study show that insulin stimulation by infant food may be related not only to the quantity of protein, but possibly also to process-induced changes in protein availability. In line with this, hydrolyzed protein appears to stimulate insulin release to a higher extent than intact protein [22].

The CML content in the MWP_CANBol meal was significantly lower than in the MWPBol meal (−34%) and the CANPBol meal (−39%). Gentle processing of the composite meal, as in the case of the MWPBol meal, was, thus, not as effective as expected in terms of reducing CML contents and no significant difference was found between the CML levels in the MWPBol and CANPBol meals. These results indicate that it may be more important to separate the protein- and carbohydrate-rich meal components during processing, than to use gentle heat treatment of a composite meal. The CML comparison in Study 1 indicates that freezing may be an interesting way forward to allow for both gentle and separate heat treatment of the different meal components. It is important to note that the formation of CML renders lysine less available. The fact that lysine is an essential amino acid is one reason to counteract CML formation during processing of all foods, and especially in products intended for infants. Additionally, dietary exposure to CML has repeatedly been linked to impaired metabolism. Consequently, a cross-over study in healthy subjects has shown that exposure to CML-levels of 5.4 mg CML/day (GC-MS analysis) for one month resulted in lower insulin sensitivity, lower plasma levels of omega-3 fatty acids, and higher concentrations of blood lipids than after a low-AGE diet (2.2 mg CML/day) [3]. Similarly, the consumption of a high-AGE diet (24.6 mg CML/day, LC-MS analysis) for one month led to increased fasting insulin and insulin resistance (HOMA-IR), compared to a diet low in AGEs (10.7 mg CML/day), in overweight women [23]. The CML content in one portion of CANPBol was 9.7 mg (LC-MS analysis), and a single meal of canned infant food would thus provide 0.75 mg CML/kg body weight in 12-month-old infants (assuming a body weight of 13 kg). This is more than twice the amount of CML ingested in the case of the high-CML diet previously mentioned where the intake in adults corresponded to 0.35 mg/kg body weight per day [23]. A recent review of randomized controlled trials has shown that high AGE intakes are associated with increased levels of TNF-alpha, which is an established biomarker of inflammation in healthy humans [24]. Furthermore, high postprandial glycemia *per se*, as seen in the current study in the case of CANPBol, has been associated with low-grade inflammation [2,25]. In summary, the intake of canned infant meals appears to result in reduced postprandial insulin sensitivity and high intakes of AGE (measured as CML). The latter is due to favorable conditions for the Maillard reaction, which may result in lower lysine availability and pro-inflammatory responses.

It should be noted that the sample size in Study 1 was lower than that recommended for GI determinations, which may partly explain the larger variation in insulin response after the canned Meat&Pasta meal than after the CANPBol meal. It cannot be excluded that the inclusion of coffee/tea at both test and reference breakfasts in Study 1 may have influenced the postprandial insulin sensitivity and it was therefore removed from the study design in Study 2. Although the metabolic responses to the infant meals were measured in healthy adults, it is reasonable to assume that the differences seen, depending on the type of processing, would be similar in infants.

6. Conclusions

The findings of this study indicate an urgent need for more research on the metabolic effects of food products intended for infants and young children. The importance of considering both the quantity and quality of macronutrients when designing diets for infants was also recently pointed out by Alvisi *et al.* [26]. Gentle and separate processing of meal components seems to have a beneficial impact on human metabolism compared to canning or microwave heated mixed composite meals. With respect to CML contents, conventional cooking and freezing of meal components appears to be more beneficial in comparison with canning.

Supplementary Materials: The following are available online at http://www.mdpi.com/2072-6643/8/6/340/s1, Figure S1: Mean (±SEM) changes in NEFA response after the intake of the test meals and the reference meal (Study 2).

Acknowledgments: The work in Study 1 was funded by The Swedish Research Council Formas, while the work in Study 2 was funded by the Lund University Antidiabetic Food Centre, a VINNOVA VINN Excellence Centre.

Author Contributions: Elin Östman and Inger Björck conceived and designed the experiments; Inger Björck performed the experiments in Study 1; Elin Östman analyzed the data from Study 1; Anna Forslund performed the experiments and analyzed the data in Study 2; Anna Forslund and Eden Tareke performed the experiments and analyzed the data regarding CML; all authors contributed to writing the manuscript; Elin Östman was primarily responsible for the final content.

Conflicts of Interest: The authors declare no conflict of interest.

References

1. Augustin, L.S.A.; Kendall, C.W.C.; Jenkins, D.J.A.; Willett, W.C.; Astrup, A.; Barclay, A.W.; Björck, I.; Brand-Miller, J.C.; Brighenti, F.; Buyken, A.E.; *et al.* Glycemic index, glycemic load and glycemic response: An international scientific consensus summit from the international carbohydrate quality consortium (ICQC). *Nutr. Metab. Cardiovasc. Dis.* **2015**, *25*, 795–815. [CrossRef] [PubMed]
2. Dickinson, S.; Hancock, D.P.; Petocz, P.; Ceriello, A.; Brand-Miller, J. High-glycemic index carbohydrate increases nuclear factor-kappab activation in mononuclear cells of young, lean healthy subjects. *Am. J. Clin. Nutr.* **2008**, *87*, 1188–1193. [PubMed]
3. Birlouez-Aragon, I.; Saavedra, G.; Tessier, F.J.; Galinier, A.; Ait-Ameur, L.; Lacoste, F.; Niamba, C.N.; Alt, N.; Somoza, V.; Lecerf, J.M. A diet based on high-heat-treated foods promotes risk factors for diabetes mellitus and cardiovascular diseases. *Am. J. Clin. Nutr.* **2010**, *91*, 1220–1226. [CrossRef] [PubMed]
4. Stirban, A.; Tschope, D. Vascular effects of dietary advanced glycation end products. *Int. J. Endocrinol.* **2015**, *2015*, 836498. [CrossRef] [PubMed]
5. Vlassara, H.; Cai, W.; Crandall, J.; Goldberg, T.; Oberstein, R.; Dardaine, V.; Peppa, M.; Rayfield, E.J. Inflammatory mediators are induced by dietary glycotoxins, a major risk factor for diabetic angiopathy. *Proc. Natl. Acad. Sci. USA* **2002**, *99*, 15596–15601. [CrossRef] [PubMed]
6. Tareke, E.; Forslund, A.; Lindh, C.; Fahlgren, C.; Östman, E. Isotope dilution esi-lc-ms/ms for quantification of free and total nε-(1-carboxymethyl)-l-lysine and free nε-(1-carboxyethyl)-l-lysine: Comparison of total nε-(1-carboxymethyl)-l-lysine levels measured with new method to elisa assay in gruel samples. *Food Chem.* **2013**, *141*, 4253–4259. [CrossRef] [PubMed]
7. Plaza, M.; Östman, E.; Tareke, E. Maillard reaction products in powder based food for infants and toddlers. *Eur. J. Food Saf. Nutr.* **2016**, *6*, 65–74. [CrossRef]
8. Canella, D.S.; Levy, R.B.; Martins, A.P.B.; Claro, R.M.; Moubarac, J.C.; Baraldi, L.G.; Cannon, G.; Monteiro, C.A. Ultra-processed food products and obesity in brazilian households (2008–2009). *PLoS ONE* **2014**, *9*. [CrossRef] [PubMed]
9. Holm, J.; Koellreutter, B.; Wursch, P. Influence of sterilization, drying and oat bran enrichment of pasta on glucose and insulin responses in healthy subjects and on the rate and extent of *in vitro* starch digestion. *Eur. J. Clin. Nutr.* **1992**, *46*, 629–640. [PubMed]
10. Järvi, A.E.; Karlström, B.E.; Granfeldt, Y.E.; Björck, I.M.E.; Vessby, B.O.H.; Asp, N.-G.L. The influence of food structure on postprandial metabolism in patients with non-insulin-dependent diabetes mellitus. *Am. J. Clin. Nutr.* **1995**, *61*, 837–842. [PubMed]
11. Liljeberg, H.G.M.; Björck, I.M.E. Bioavailability of starch in bread products. Postprandial glucose and insulin responses in healthy subjects and *in vitro* resistant starch content. *Eur. J. Clin. Nutr.* **1994**, *48*, 151–163. [PubMed]
12. Holm, J.; Bjorck, I.; Drews, A.; Asp, N.G. A rapid method for the analysis of starch. *Starch-Starke* **1986**, *38*, 224–226. [CrossRef]
13. Granfeldt, Y.E.; Björck, I.M.E.; Drews, A.; Tovar, J. An *in vitro* procedure based on chewing to predict metabolic response to starch in cereal and legume product. *Eur. J. Clin. Nutr.* **1992**, *46*, 649–660. [PubMed]
14. Rosen, L.A.; Östman, E.M.; Björck, I.M. Effects of cereal breakfasts on postprandial glucose, appetite regulation and voluntary energy intake at a subsequent standardized lunch; focusing on rye products. *Nutr. J.* **2011**, *10*. [CrossRef] [PubMed]
15. Brouns, F.; Bjorck, I.; Frayn, K.N.; Gibbs, A.L.; Lang, V.; Slama, G.; Wolever, T.M.S. Glycaemic index methodology. *Nutr. Res. Rev.* **2005**, *18*, 145–171. [CrossRef] [PubMed]
16. DeFronzo, R.A.; Matsuda, M. Reduced time points to calculate the composite index. *Diabetes Care* **2010**, *33*. [CrossRef] [PubMed]

17. Matsuda, M.; DeFronzo, R.A. Insulin sensitivity indices obtained from oral glucose tolerance testing: Comparison with the euglycemic insulin clamp. *Diabetes Care* **1999**, *22*, 1462–1470. [CrossRef] [PubMed]

18. Granfeldt, Y.; Bjorck, I. Glycemic response to starch in pasta: A study of mechanisms of limited enzyme availability. *J. Cereal Sci.* **1991**, *14*, 47–61. [CrossRef]

19. Tovar, J.; Granfeldt, Y.; Bjorck, I.M. Effect of processing on blood glucose and insulin responses to starch in legumes. *J. Agric. Food Chem.* **1992**, *40*, 1846–1851. [CrossRef]

20. Gonzalez, J.T. Paradoxical second-meal phenomenon in the acute postexercise period. *Nutrition* **2014**, *30*, 961–967. [CrossRef] [PubMed]

21. Holland-Cachera, M.F. Prediction of adult body composition from infant and child measurements. In *Body Composition Techniques in Health and Disease*; Davies, P.S.W., Cole, T.J., Eds.; Cambridge University Press: Cambridge, UK, 1995; pp. 100–135.

22. Koopman, R.; Crombach, N.; Gijsen, A.P.; Walrand, S.; Fauquant, J.; Kies, A.K.; Lemosquet, S.; Saris, W.H.; Boirie, Y.; van Loon, L.J. Ingestion of a protein hydrolysate is accompanied by an accelerated *in vivo* digestion and absorption rate when compared with its intact protein. *Am. J. Clin. Nut.* **2009**, *90*, 106–115. [CrossRef] [PubMed]

23. Mark, A.B.; Poulsen, M.W.; Andersen, S.; Andersen, J.M.; Bak, M.J.; Ritz, C.; Holst, J.J.; Nielsen, J.; de Courten, B.; Dragsted, L.O.; *et al.* Consumption of a diet low in advanced glycation end products for 4 weeks improves insulin sensitivity in overweight women. *Diabetes Care* **2014**, *37*, 88–95. [CrossRef] [PubMed]

24. Clarke, R.; Dordevic, A.; Tan, S.; Ryan, L.; Coughlan, M. Dietary advanced glycation end products and risk factors for chronic disease: A systematic review of randomised controlled trials. *Nutrition* **2016**, *8*. [CrossRef] [PubMed]

25. Esposito, K.; Nappo, F.; Marfella, R.; Giugliano, G.; Giugliano, F.; Ciotola, M.; Quagliaro, L.; Ceriello, A.; Giugliano, D. Inflammatory cytokine concentrations are acutely increased by hyperglycemia in humans: Role of oxidative stress. *Circulation* **2002**, *106*, 2067–2072. [CrossRef] [PubMed]

26. Alvisi, P.; Brusa, S.; Alboresi, S.; Amarri, S.; Bottau, P.; Cavagni, G.; Corradini, B.; Landi, L.; Loroni, L.; Marani, M.; *et al.* Recommendations on complementary feeding for healthy, full-term infants. *Ital. J. Pediatr.* **2015**, *41*. [CrossRef] [PubMed]

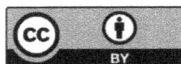

nutrients

MDPI

Article

Sensory Acceptability of Infant Cereals with Whole Grain in Infants and Young Children

Juan Francisco Haro-Vicente [1], Maria Jose Bernal-Cava [1,*], Amparo Lopez-Fernandez [2], Gaspar Ros-Berruezo [2], Stefan Bodenstab [3] and Luis Manuel Sanchez-Siles [3]

[1]   Department of Research and Development, Hero Group, Alcantarilla, Murcia 30820, Spain; jfrancisco.haro@hero.es
[2]   Department of Food Science and Nutrition, University of Murcia, Campus de Espinardo, Espinardo, Murcia 30071, Spain; amparolf@um.es (A.L.-F.); gros@um.es (G.R.-B.)
[3]   Department of Research and Development, Hero Group, Lenzburg 5600, Switzerland; stefan.bodenstab@hero.ch (S.B.); luisma.sanchez@hero.es (L.M.S.-S.)
*   Correspondence: mjose.bernal@hero.es; Tel.: +34-968-898-900

Received: 13 October 2016; Accepted: 6 January 2017; Published: 13 January 2017

Abstract: In many countries, infant cereals are one of the first foods introduced during the complementary feeding stage. These cereals are usually made with refined cereal flours, even though several health benefits have been linked to the intake of whole grain cereals. Prior evidence suggests that food preferences are developed at early stages of life, and may persist in later childhood and adulthood. Our aim was to test whether an infant cereal with 30% of whole grain was similarly accepted both by parents and infants in comparison to a similar cereal made from refined flour. A total of 81 infants between 4 and 24 months old were included in the study. Parent-infant pairs participated in an 8-day experimental study. Acceptance was rated on hedonic scales (4-points for infants and 7-points for parents). Other attributes like color, smell, and taste were evaluated by the parents. Acceptability for infant cereals with whole grain and refined cereals was very similar both for infants (2.30 ± 0.12 and 2.32 ± 0.11, $p = 0.606$) and parents (6.1 ± 0.8 and 6.0 ± 0.9, $p = 0.494$). Therefore, our findings show that there is an opportunity to introduce whole grain cereals to infants, including those who are already used to consuming refined infant cereals, thereby accelerating the exposure of whole grain in early life.

Keywords: acceptability; complementary feeding; infant cereals; whole grain

1. Introduction

Scholars have long established that the complementary feeding stage is very important because of the continued rapid growth and many changes that affect children's health and development [1–3]. These changes have a major influence on nutritional status during infancy and the food preferences during childhood and adulthood [4–6]. For this reason, several authors have strongly recommended the intake of healthy foods from the very beginning of the complementary feeding stage [7–9].

Weaning practices are significantly influenced by cultural beliefs [10,11]. However, in many countries, infant cereals are one of the first foods introduced at the beginning of the complementary period [11–14]. One possible reason stems from their sensorial and digestive properties [15]. For millennia, cereals have been staples for humans and are currently a large part of U.S. Dietary Guidelines [16]. Cereals are a good source of energy and macronutrients, such as carbohydrates, proteins and fats, that are needed for growth. Cereals are also an important source of vitamins, minerals and other essential bioactive compounds necessary for health [17].

Cereals can be consumed as whole grain or refined. Although the definition of whole grain is currently under discussion, the International American Association of Cereal Chemistry (AACC)

defined whole grains as "intact, ground, cracked or flaked caryopsis, whose principal anatomical components—the starchy endosperm, germ, and bran—are present in the same relative proportions as they exist in the intact caryopsis" [18]. In 2010, the Healthgrain Consortium broadened the AACC definition of whole grain to include small losses of components—that is, less than 2% of the grain/10% of the bran. Such losses may occur through processing methods required to ensure the safety and quality of whole grain and are allowed under the above definition [19].

It should be taken into account that until the 19th century, cereals were consumed as whole grain; it was only during the Industrial Revolution with the advent of new milling techniques that the bran and germ were removed from the grain kernel, obtaining refined cereal flours with improved texture and taste and ultimately leading to longer shelf life [20].

Several organizations and scholars have acknowledged the benefits associated with the intake of whole grain cereals for adults and children above two years [21–23]. Moreover, the USDA (US Department of Agriculture) recommends that, during the second semester of life, infants should be gradually introduced to fiber-containing foods, such as whole grain cereals, vegetables, and legumes [10]. Although there is no general agreement regarding daily dietary intake recommendations for whole grain (even for adults) [23,24], these recommendations are important and should be further studied in infants and young children. As eating habits can be molded during complementary feeding time, the early introduction and consumption of infant cereals elaborated with whole grain flour could be desirable [22].

In most countries, commercial infant cereals are made with refined cereal flours (www.innovadatabase.com). One of the main problems found when whole grain is introduced into the diet of an adult is the low sensorial acceptability compared to refined cereal-based foods [23,25]. However, prior research reveals that infants and young children have a higher acceptance of new foods in the complementary feeding period until the age of 18–24 months [26–28]. In this vein, several authors recommend gradually introducing whole grain products by substituting refined cereals as an effective way of incorporating whole grain into consumers' diets [23]. This can be reinforced by the development of technological processes to improve sensorial properties of whole grain products [29,30].

The present study was designed to determine if the intake of an infant cereal-based product with 30% whole grain was similarly accepted both by parents and their children, compared to the same infant cereal without whole grain (refined cereals).

2. Materials and Methods

2.1. Infant Cereal Samples

All infant cereals used in this experiment were commercially available products from HERO ESPAÑA S.A (Murcia, Spain). We selected this brand of multicereals to conduct this study because it is one of the most widely consumed infant cereals on the Spanish market. One of two infant cereals contained 30% of whole grain flour, WGC (new recipe), and the other one 100% refined cereal flours, RC (old recipe). The ingredients for WGC were: hydrolyzed cereal flour (wheat, wheat whole grain, corn, rice, oat, barley, rye, sorghum and millet), minerals, natural flavor and vitamins where the content of wheat whole grain flour was 30% of total cereals. The ingredients of RC were: hydrolyzed cereal flours (wheat, corn, rice, oat, barley, rye, sorghum and millet), minerals, natural flavor and vitamins. The nutritional composition of the two infant cereals used in this study is described in Table 1.

Table 1. Nutritional composition of the two infant cereals used in the study.

Mean Value (100 g)	WGC	RC
Energy (kcal)	380	372
Protein (g)	9.1	8.5
Carbohydrates (g)	78	81.6
Sugars (g)	21	22
Fat (g)	2.3	1.3
Fiber (g)	5.2	3

WGC: Whole Grain Cereal and RC: Refined Cereal.

2.2. Participant Characteristics

There were 81 parents with infants between the ages of 4–24 months recruited through advertisement on the website of the University of Murcia (Spain), as well as in kindergartens and parents' circles. Eligible healthy infants had a gestational age of 37–42 weeks and a birth weight greater than 2500 g and had been fed with gluten-containing cereals prior to enrolment in the experiment. Infants that had food allergies, swallowing or digestion problems, or other medical issues that could influence the ability to eat were excluded. There were an additional 20 pairs excluded because the parents did not complete the study or did not return the questionnaire (See Supplementary Materials). Once all parent-infant pairs were recruited, they were assigned to only one group where they received two packages of infant cereals (WGC and RC). The distribution of samples was counterbalanced to avoid any possible bias. The study protocol was approved by the Research Ethical Committee of the University of Murcia. Written informed consent was obtained from both parents of all participating infants before the inclusion.

2.3. Data Collection

Testing was carried out at home during a period of eight days. For the home-use test, the parents were responsible for conducting the experiment and collecting the data requested in the questionnaire (See Supplementary Materials). Prior to testing, the parents received both detailed written and oral instructions.

2.3.1. Testing

Parents received two coded packs of cereals. During days 1 and 2, infants were accustomed to the first of the two cereals. On the third day, parents evaluated the acceptance. Over days 4 and 5, infants continued eating the cereal which they used to eat before enrollment in the present study. On day 6, the same process started with the second infant cereal—familiarization on days 6 and 7 and, on day 8, evaluation of acceptance. No additional foods or beverages were introduced into the infants' diet during the study. All samples used in this study were packaged into identical foil bags. Each bag was marked with a three-digit randomization code. At the moment of feeding, the samples were counterbalanced and randomized; consequently, a child was fed with one sample on one day and the other sample on the other day. Each parent fed his/her infant in the habitual place, at a normal pace until the infant refused the spoon or bottle three consecutive times. Rejection behaviors are typically turning the head away, closing the mouth firmly, pushing the spoon away, spitting the food out or becoming upset [14,31]. Before each feeding, it was necessary to ensure that the infant was sufficiently hungry. In particular, parents were asked not to feed their infants with infant milk, other beverages, or solid foods for 1 h before the cereal intake [14,32]. Furthermore, testing occurred at approximately the same time of the day and 30 to 60 min before the infants' next scheduled feeding, so that variation of intake was not affected by different levels of hunger or satiation, but rather reflected hedonic response to the food. Regarding mode of preparation, this depended on the parents' habits (using bottle or spoon). Parents performed the sensory evaluation of the same products only after feeding their infants to ensure no interference with their infant's reactions due to non-habitual parent behavior (product testing) during the feeding (days 3 and 8) [14,32].

2.3.2. Measure of Food Acceptance

Parents were first asked to answer questions about their infants, feeding practices as well as socio-demographic information, such as gender, age and education (See Supplementary Materials). Then, parents were asked to score their degree of liking using a 7-point hedonic scale ranging from 1 "dislikes very much" to 7 "likes very much." This test allowed us to evaluate the acceptability of each parent for the sample of cereal. Parents' liking represents one important step to deciding if this type of cereal would be suitable for their infants. For the assessment of the acceptance by children, we used a 4-point hedonic scale [14,31]. This scale uses the following scores: "— " (very negative) if the infant spit out the food, frowned, pushed the spoon away or stopped eating; "−" (negative) if the infant ate a couple of spoonful, grimaced and stopped eating; "+" (positive) if the infant ate some of the food without a specific reaction; "++" (very positive) if the infant accepted the first spoonful immediately and displayed signs of content, such as a relaxed face or a smile [14,31].

2.4. Statistical Analyses

Data are expressed as means $\pm$ standard error of mean (SEM) for the following variables: age of introduction of infant cereals and parent's perception of child's degree of liking. For variables related to sensory analysis, data were expressed as mean $\pm$ standard deviation (SD). The categorical variables were expressed as percentage (%).

Descriptive analysis was employed to describe parents' and infants' characteristics as well as all variables related to consumption, mode of preparation, frequency of intake of infant cereals and sensory analysis. The evaluation of infants' acceptance, assessed by parents, was converted into scores of −3, −1, 1 and 3 so that there were equal intervals between adjacent scores throughout the scale. Taking into account that all variables are not distributed normally (Kolmogorov–Smirnov test), non-parametric analyses were performed: the Wilcoxon test for paired samples was used to detect differences in sensorial variables between the two samples of infant cereals; in the case of cereal feeding practices, variables expressed as percentages as per the Mann–Whitney test were applied in order to detect difference between both age ranges.

All results with a significance level of $p < 0.05$ were considered statistically significant. Statistical analyses of data were performed using the Statistical Package for the Social Sciences (SPSS version 19.0; Inc., Chicago, IL, USA).

3. Results

3.1. Subject Characteristics and Cereal Feeding Practices

The characteristics of the 81parent-infant pairs are presented in Table 2. The mean age of introduction of infant cereals was 5.2 ($\pm$1.3) months. The type of milk used by parents to prepare the cereals was in 55.6% of cases as follows: 21.0% "growing-up" milk; 13.5% cow's milk; 7.4% infant formula; and 2.5% breast milk (Table 3).

Parents were asked about the cereal feeding mode (bottle and/or spoon) and the number of times infants were fed per day (Table 3). The cereal feeding mode was distributed as follows: most infants (70.4%) were taking cereals from a bottle, 16.0% took cereals with a spoon and 13.6% used both bottle and spoon. There were significant differences in the mode of preparation of infant cereals depending on the age group ($p < 0.05$). Cereal bottle feeding was higher in the group of infants between 13 and 24 months of age (80%) as compared to the group of infants below one year. In general, more than 50% of infants took two servings a day, almost 40% took one serving a day, and the rest between three or more servings (7.4%) without significant differences between the two age ranges studied (below and above one year of age) (Table 3).

Table 2. Characteristics of infants and parents who participated in this study.

Characteristics	Group (*n* = 81)
Infants	
Age (by ranges)	
4–6 months	8.6
7–9 months	13.6
10–11 months	16
12–24 months	61.8
Girls	60
Parents	
Men	12
Women	88
Age	
25–30 years	5.3
31–35 years	46
36–40 years	43.4
>41 years	5.3
Number of children	
One child	48
Two children	48
Three children	4

Values expressed as percentage.

Table 3. Cereal feeding practices used for parents to prepare the infant cereals.

	Age Range		
	4–11 Months	12–24 Months	Total
Type of Milk Used			
Breast milk	6.5 (2)	-	2.5 (2)
Infant formula	9.7 (3)	6.0 (3)	7.4 (6)
Follow on formula	77.4 (24)	42 (21)	55.6 (45)
Growing up milk	3.2 (1)	32 (16)	27 (17)
Cow's milk	3.2 (1)	20 (10)	13.6 (11)
Mode of Cereal Feeding [a]			
Bottle	54.8 (17)	80 (40)	70.4 (57)
Spoon	25.8 (8)	10 (5)	16 (13)
Both	19.4 (4)	10 (5)	13.6 (11)
Frequency of Intake			
One serving	48.4 (11)	34 (17)	39.5 (32)
Two serving	41.9 (13)	60 (30)	53.1 (43)
Three or more serving	9.7 (3)	6 (3)	7.4 (6)

Values are expressed as percentage of total infant (number of infants); [a] Superscript indicates that there is significant differences between both groups of age and mode of feeding cereals ($z = -2.281$; $p < 0.05$).

The average amount of WGC and RC cereals consumed by age group is shown in Figure 1. In both cases, over 75% of infants consumed the entire serving of the cereals prepared, with no significant differences between the infant cereals evaluated.

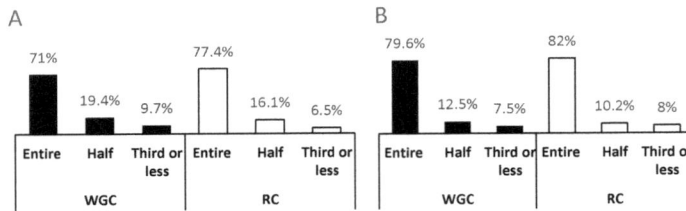

Figure 1. Infants' consumption of the serving of infant cereals prepared by parents. WGC: Whole Grain Cereal; RC: Refined Cereal. Values are expressed as percentage of total infants. (**A**) represents the consumption of cereals by infants 4–11 months of age; (**B**) consumption of cereals by infants 12–24 months of age.

3.2. Parents' Perception of Infants' Liking

As shown in Table 4, parents' rating of their infants' degree of liking was not statistically significant between the two infant cereals evaluated (WGC and RC)—neither within the two age groups ($p = 0.317$, $p = 0.666$ for group 4–11 months and group 12–24 months, respectively) nor in the total sample ($n = 81$, $p = 0.606$). Both infant cereals were highly accepted with average scores higher than 2.

Table 4. Parent's perception of child's degree of liking (mean ± SEM).

Age	WGC ($n = 81$)	RC ($n = 81$)	p-Value
4–11 months	2.35 ± 0.19	2.16 ± 0.18	0.317
12–24 months	2.29 ± 0.16	2.40 ± 0.15	0.666
Total ($n = 81$)	2.3 ± 0.12	2.32 ± 0.11	0.606

WGC: Whole Grain Cereal; RC: Refined Cereal.

3.3. Parents' Acceptability of Infant Cereals

There were no significant differences between WGC and RC in any of the attributes, as shown in Table 5. Parental rating of liking for each attribute did not differ for any infant cereal, indicating that parents reported the same liking for each sample. In general, the score for each attribute was very similar between both samples and overall acceptability was rated very high for both cereal products (6.1 for WGC and 6.0 for RC). In addition, we asked parents why they liked the infant cereals and which attributes influenced their choices. In both cases, the criteria for their choices were similar; for example, about 50% of the parents chose the taste as first choice, followed by aroma (20%), and texture (17%).

Table 5. Sensory evaluation of infant cereals by parents (mean ± SD).

Attributes	WGC	RC	p-Value
Color	6.1 ± 0.9	5.8 ± 1.1	0.090
Aroma	6.3 ± 0.9	6.3 ± 0.8	0.850
Taste	6.2 ± 0.9	6.1 ± 0.9	0.799
Texture	5.9 ± 1.1	6.2 ± 1.1	0.235
Overall acceptability	6.1 ± 0.8	6.0 ± 0.9	0.494

* Values in rows with different superscripts are significantly different ($p < 0.05$).

4. Discussion

The present study reveals that the addition of whole grain in infant cereals was similarly well accepted from the sensorial point of view by both parents and their infants as compared to refined cereals. Importantly, previous studies have observed that early exposure to foods affects infants' later taste acceptance patterns and that infants are able to communicate their acceptance by both quantity of intake and facial expression [32]. In our study, we did not observe any differences in the facial expression or in the intake, and more than 75% of the infants ate the entire cereal serving prepared by their parents. Several factors are likely to explain the high acceptability found in whole grain infant cereals such as the percentage of whole grain used in this study (30%), the milk used for the reconstitution of the cereal (already accepted by the infants) or technology advances in cereal processing which improve the sensorial characteristics of whole grain cereals.

The selected amount of whole grain tested in our study was based on the minimal amount of whole grain with possible beneficial effects. Although there is no defined adequate intake of whole grain for adults or infants, Ferruzi et al. [15] have suggested that a whole grain food should provide 8 g of whole grain per 30 g serving (27 g/100 g) in order to be defined as a whole grain food which is nutritionally meaningful.

Interestingly, it has been reported that the main factor of consumer rejection in whole grain-based products is its bitter taste and rough texture [25,33]. In our study, we did not observe any of these issues. In fact, parents were reporting similar sensory liking scores in taste and texture and high scores in both infant cereals. Our results are similar to those found in students by Magalis et al. (2016), who did not find statistical differences in bitter taste between refined and whole grain products, although sensorial preferences tended toward some refined cereal products [25]. Other sensorial studies in school children have also reported a similar degree of acceptability of whole grain versus refined cereal products, i.e., whole grain products were well accepted [34,35].

Whole grain cereals, as well as vegetables, can be bitter due to their content of polyphenolic compounds [36]. Similar to findings in our study, Lange et al. (2013) and Mennella et al. (2015) reported that when the new foods are introduced (vegetables) with other foods already accepted, the acceptability of new foods was better [14,37]. This effect was related to the reduction of the unpleasant, bitter or sour notes of the vegetables not only by dilution, but also by the sweetness of the milk. The sweetness of breast milk has been estimated as equivalent to a 2.12% solution of sucrose [38]. The sweetness of standard formula milks is similar [39]. Salty and sweet tastes have the characteristic of blocking or masking unpleasant tastes present in many foods, such as a bitter taste in vegetables [38,39]. A clinical study of school-aged children has shown that the presence of diluted solutions of a sweetener (aspartame) along with vegetables increased the liking of vegetables and decreased the perception of bitter taste [40]. For that reason, we could hypothesize that like in vegetables, our infant cereals with whole grain were highly accepted due to the fact that they were reconstituted with infant milk formulas or breast milk previously accepted by the infant. In our study, whole grain cereals were mainly prepared with milk formula and to a lesser extent with breast milk. The presence of sweet taste and its acceptance by infants could mask the bitter notes present in the whole grain cereals, leading the products to be accepted in the same way as the refined product [41,42].

Regarding infant cereal practices, our study shows that the mean age of introduction of cereals was 5.2 months. In Spain, infant cereals are usually the first food introduced at the beginning of weaning and therefore the age of introduction in our study was in line with current recommendations of first introducing products between 4 and 6 months of age [3,43].

The complementary feeding period is a "critical time window" in human development during which eating behaviors are developed [44]. For this reason, timing, type and ways the foods are introduced are important feeding practices in the development of acceptance of healthy food as part of a healthy diet. Cereals play a main role at the beginning of and during the complementary feeding period. The type of cereals consumed (whole grain or refined) may influence both health and nutritional status of infants. In adults, it has been shown that significant consumption of whole grain products is associated with a lower risk of cardiovascular diseases, diabetes, obesity, colon cancer and gastrointestinal health [36]. A previous meta-analysis concluded that there is a negative correlation between intake of whole grain and mortality, with a reduction of 7% in risk associated with each single serving/day increase in whole grain intake [45]. Due to increasing evidence of health benefits associated with whole grains, several authors have strongly recommended implementing strategies for educating consumers to gradually incorporate whole grains into their diets through the substitution of refined cereals [23]. Although the beneficial effects of whole grains have not been demonstrated in infants or young children due to the lack of clinical trials in this age range, the development of healthy dietary habits during early stages of infancy including a diet with whole grain products could be desirable [22].

Two potential risks of the use of whole grain in infant cereals should be taken in account. Firstly, as compared to refined rice, whole grain rice has a higher content of inorganic arsenic, which is concentrated in the bran layers [46,47]. Secondly, in unbalanced diets, excessive fiber content is likely to have negative effects on mineral bioavailability [48]. In order to avoid these issues, we have used whole grain wheat in compliance with European infant legislation (Directive 2006/125/CE) [48]. Also, the fiber content of the cereals used in our study was within commercial standard values.

5. Conclusions

This research was conducted as a preliminary study toward a clinical trial designed to evaluate whole grain effects in infants with ages ranging from 5 to 9 months. Interestingly, we found that infant cereals with 30% whole grain were very well accepted from a sensory point of view by infants between 4 to 24 months as well as by their parents. Moreover, there is a lack of studies showing that refined cereal flours in infants and young children are better from a nutritional point of view than whole grain infant cereals. Throughout most of human development, whole grain cereals—not refined cereals—were naturally consumed. Therefore, there might be an opportunity to (re)introduce whole grain cereals to infants who are accustomed to consuming refined infant cereals, thereby accelerating the exposure of whole grain in early life. This research represents a first step in our understanding of sensory acceptability of whole grain infant cereals in infants aged 4 to 24 months. We encourage future studies to analyze both the acceptability of higher percentages of whole grain in infant cereal-based products as well as possible imprinting of health effects on infants during the complementary feeding period.

Supplementary Materials: The following are available online at http://www.mdpi.com/2072-6643/9/1/65/s1. Data Collection Questionnaire used in study.

Acknowledgments: The present study was funded by Hero Group. We are grateful to all parents who participated in this preliminary study and especially to the kindergartens as well as the university community.

Author Contributions: All authors participated in the conception, design and writing of the manuscript. All authors read and approved the final manuscript.

Conflicts of Interest: All authors declare conflict of interest because the present study was funded by Hero Group. J.F.H.V., M.J.B.C., S.B. and L.M.S.S. are members of the Research and Development Department of Hero Group.

1. World Health Organization. *Guiding Principles for Complementary Feeding of the Breastfed Child*; Pan American Health Organization: Washington, DC, USA, 2003.
2. Butte, N.; Cobb, K.; Dwyer, J.; Graney, L.; Heird, W.; Rickard, K. The Start Healthy Feeding Guidelines for infants and toddlers. *J. Am. Diet. Assoc.* **2004**, *104*, 442–454. [CrossRef] [PubMed]
3. Agostoni, C.; Decsi, T.; Fewtrell, M.; Goulet, O.; Kolacek, S.; Koletzko, B.; Michaelsen, K.F.; Moreno, L.; Puntis, J.; Rigo, J.; et al. ESPGHAN Committee on Nutrition. Complementary Feeding: A Commentary by the ESPGHAN Committee on Nutrition. *J. Pediatr. Gastroenterol. Nutr.* **2008**, *46*, 99–110. [CrossRef] [PubMed]
4. Mennella, J.A.; Trabulsi, J.C. Complementary foods and flavor experiences: Setting the foundation. *Ann. Nutr. Metab.* **2012**, *60*, 40–50. [CrossRef] [PubMed]
5. Schwartz, C.; Scholtens, P.; Lalanne, A.; Weenen, H.; Nicklaus, S. Development of healthy eating habits early in life: Review of recent evidence and selected guidelines. *Appetite* **2011**, *57*, 796–807. [CrossRef] [PubMed]

6. Nicklaus, S. The role of food experiences during early childhood in food pleasure learning. *Appetite* **2016**, *104*, 3–9. [CrossRef] [PubMed]

7. Nicklaus, S.; Boggio, V.; Chabanet, C.; Issanchou, S. A prospective study of food variety seeking in childhood, adolescence and early adult life. *Appetite* **2005**, *44*, 289–297. [CrossRef] [PubMed]

8. Ventura, A.K.; Worobey, J. Early influences on the development of food preferences. *Curr. Biol.* **2003**, *23*, R401–R408. [CrossRef] [PubMed]

9. Nicklaus, S.; Boggio, V.; Chabanet, C.; Issanchou, S. A prospective study of food preferences in childhood. *Food Qual. Prefer.* **2004**, *15*, 805–818. [CrossRef]

10. United States Department of Agriculture. *Infant Nutrition and Feeding. A Guide for Use in the WIC and CSF Programs*; United States Department of Agriculture: Washington, DC, USA, 2009; pp. 101–129.

11. Caroli, M.; Mele, R.M.; Tomaselli, M.A.; Cammisa, M.; Longo, F.; Attolini, E. Complementary feeding patterns in Europe with a special focus on Italy. *Nutr. Metab. Cardiovasc.* **2012**, *22*, 813–818. [CrossRef] [PubMed]

12. Siega-Riz, A.M.; Deming, D.M.; Reidy, K.C.; Fox, M.K.; Condon, E.; Briefel, R.R. Food consumption patterns of infants and toddlers: where are we now? *J. Am. Diet. Assoc.* **2010**, *110*, S38–S51. [CrossRef] [PubMed]

13. Butte, N.F.; Fox, M.K.; Briefel, R.R.; Siega-Riz, A.M.; Dwyer, J.T.; Deming, D.M.; Reidy, K.C. Nutrient intakes of US infants, toddlers, and preschoolers meet or exceed dietary reference intakes. *J. Am. Diet. Assoc.* **2010**, *110*, S27–S37. [CrossRef] [PubMed]

14. Lange, C.; Visalli, M.; Jacob, S.; Chabanet, C.; Schlich, P.; Nicklaus, S. Maternal feeding practices during the first year and their impact on infants' acceptance of complementary food. *Food Qual. Prefer.* **2013**, *29*, 89–98. [CrossRef]

15. Bernal, M.J.; Periago, M.J.; Martínez, R.; Ortuño, I.; Sánchez-Solís, M.; Ros, G.; Romero, F.; Abellán, P. Effects of infant cereals with different carbohydrate profiles on colonic function-randomized and double-blind clinical trial in infants aged between 6 and 12 months—Pilot study. *Eur. J. Pediatr.* **2013**, *172*, 1535–1542. [CrossRef] [PubMed]

16. U.S. Department of Health and Human Services and U.S. Department of Agriculture. Dietary Guidelines for Americans 2015–2020. Available online: http://health.gov/dietaryguidelines/2015/guidelines/ (accessed on 28 November 2016).

17. Topping, D. Cereal complex carbohydrates and their contribution to human health. *J. Cereal Sci.* **2007**, *46*, 220–229. [CrossRef]

18. American Association of Cereal Chemists. Definition of Whole Grain in 1999. Available online: http://www.aaccnet.org/initiatives/definitions/pages/wholegrain.aspx (accessed on 30 September 2016).

19. Van der Kamp, J.; Poutanen, K.; Seal, C.; Richardson, D. The HEALTHGRAIN definition of 'whole grain'. *Food Nutr. Res.* **2014**, *58*. [CrossRef] [PubMed]

20. Cordain, L.; Eaton, S.B.; Sebastian, A.; Mann, N.; Lindeberg, S.; Watkins, B.A.; O'Keefe, J.H.; Brand-Miller, J. Origins and evolution of the Western diet: Health implications for the 21st century. *Am. J. Clin. Nutr.* **2005**, *81*, 341–354. [PubMed]

21. World Health Organization. *Global Strategy on Diet, Physical Activity and Health Worldwide Strategy about "Feeding Regimen, Physical Activity and Health"*; World Health Organization: Washington, DC, USA, 2004.

22. Alexy, U.; Zorn, C.; Kersting, M. Whole grain in children's diet: Intake, food sources and trends. *Eur. J. Clin. Nutr.* **2010**, *64*, 745–751. [CrossRef] [PubMed]

23. Ferruzzi, M.G.; Jonnalagadda, S.S.; Liu, S.; Marquart, L.; McKeown, N.; Reicks, M.; Riccardi, G.; Seal, C.; Slavin, J.; Thielecke, F.; et al. Developing a standard definition of whole-grain foods for dietary recommendations: Summary report of a multidisciplinary expert roundtable discussion. *Adv. Nutr.* **2014**, *5*, 164–176. [CrossRef] [PubMed]

24. Slavin, J.; Tucker, M.; Harriman, C.; Jonnalagadda, S.S. Whole grains: Definition, dietary recommendations, and health benefits. *Cereal Chem.* **2016**, *93*, 209–216. [CrossRef]

25. Magalis, R.M.; Giovanni, M.; Silliman, K. Whole grain foods: is sensory liking related to knowledge, attitude, or intake? *Nut. Food Sci.* **2016**, *46*, 488–503. [CrossRef]

26. Wright, P. Development of food choice during infancy. *Proc. Nutr. Soc.* **1991**, *50*, 107–113. [CrossRef] [PubMed]

27. Cashdan, E. A sensitive period for learning about food. *Hum. Nat.* **1994**, *5*, 279–291. [CrossRef] [PubMed]

28. Olsen, A.; Møller, P.; Hausner, H. Early origins of overeating: Early habit formation and implications for obesity in later life. *Curr. Obes. Rep.* **2013**, *2*, 157–164. [CrossRef]

29. Poutanen, K. Past and future of cereal grains as food for health. *Trends Food Sci. Technol.* **2012**, *25*, 58–62. [CrossRef]

30. Poutanen, K.; Sozer, N.; Della Valle, G. How can technology help to deliver more of grain in cereal foods for a healthy diet? *J. Cereal Sci.* **2014**, *59*, 327–336. [CrossRef]

31. Schwartz, C.; Chabanet, C.; Lange, C.; Issanchou, S.; Nicklaus, S. The role of taste in food acceptance at the beginning of complementary feeding. *Physiol. Behav.* **2013**, *2011*, 646–652. [CrossRef] [PubMed]

32. Forestell, C.A.; Mennella, J.A. Early determinants of fruit and vegetable acceptance. *Pediatrics* **2007**, *120*, 1247–1254. [CrossRef] [PubMed]

33. Bakke, A.; Vickers, Z. Consumer liking of refined and whole wheat breads. *J. Food Sci.* **2007**, *72*, S473–S480. [CrossRef] [PubMed]

34. Burgess-Champoux, T.; Marquart, L.; Vickers, Z.; Reicks, M. Perceptions of Children, Parents, and Teachers Regarding Whole-Grain Foods, and Implications for a School-Based Intervention. *J. Nutr. Educ. Behav.* **2006**, *38*, 230–237. [CrossRef] [PubMed]

35. Chan, H.W.; Burgess-Champoux, T.; Reicks, M.; Vickers, Z.; Marquart, L. White whole-wheat flour can be partially substituted for refined-wheat flour in pizza crust in school meals without affecting consumption. *J. Child Nutr. Manag.* **2008**, *32*.

36. Fardet, A. New hypotheses for the health-protective mechanisms of whole-grain cereals: What is beyond fibre? *Nutr. Res. Rev.* **2010**, *23*, 65–134. [CrossRef] [PubMed]

37. Hetherington, M.M.; Schwartz, C.; Madrelle, J.; Crode, F.; Nekitsing, C.; Vereijken, C.M.J.L.; Weenen, H. A step-by-step introduction to vegetables at the beginning of complementary feeding. The effects of early and repeated exposure. *Appetite* **2015**, *84*, 280–290. [CrossRef] [PubMed]

38. McDaniel, M.R.; Barker, E.; Lederer, C.L. Sensory characterization of human milk. *J. Dairy Sci.* **1989**, *72*, 1149–1158. [CrossRef]

39. Schwartz, C.; Chabanet, C.; Boggio, V.; Lange, C.; Issanchou, S.; Nicklaus, S. À quelles saveurs les nourrissons sont-ils exposés dans la premiére année de vie? To which tastes are infants exposed during the first year of life? *Arch. Pediatr.* **2010**, *17*, 1026–1034. (In French) [CrossRef] [PubMed]

40. Mennella, J.A.; Reed, D.R.; Roberts, K.M.; Mathew, P.S.; Mansfield, C.J. Age-related differences in bitter taste and efficacy of bitter blockers. *PLoS ONE* **2014**, *9*, e103107. [CrossRef] [PubMed]

41. Mennella, J.A.; Reed, D.R.; Mathew, P.S.; Roberts, K.M.; Mansfield, C.J. "A spoonful of sugar helps the medicine go down": Bitter masking by sucrose among children and adults. *Chem. Senses* **2015**, *40*, 17–25. [CrossRef] [PubMed]

42. Capaldi, E.D.; Privitera, G.J. Decreasing dislike for sour and bitter in children and adults. *Appetite* **2008**, *50*, 139–145. [CrossRef] [PubMed]

43. EFSA Panel on Dietetic Products. Nutrition and Allergies. Scientific Opinion on the appropriate age for introduction of complementary feeding of infant. *EFSA J.* **2009**, *7*, 1423–1461.

44. Birch, L.L.; Doub, L.E. Learning to eat: Birth to age 2 years. *Am. J. Clin. Nutr.* **2014**, *99*, 723S–728S. [CrossRef] [PubMed]

45. Ma, X.; Tang, W.G.; Yang, Y.; Zhang, Q.L.; Zheng, J.L.; Xiang, Y.B. Association between whole grain intake and all-cause mortality: a meta-analysis of cohort studies. *Oncotarget* **2016**, *7*, 61996–62005. [CrossRef] [PubMed]

46. Sun, G.X.; Williams, P.N.; Carey, A.M.; Zhu, Y.G.; Deacon, C.; Raab, A.; Feldmann, J.; Islam, R.M.; Meharg, A.A. Inorganic arsenic in rice bran and its products are an order of magnitude higher than in bulk grain. *Environ. Sci. Technol.* **2008**, *42*, 7542–7546. [CrossRef] [PubMed]

47. Signes-Pastor, A.; Carey, M.; Meharg, A.A. Inorganic arsenic in rice-based products for infants and young children. *Food Chem.* **2016**, *191*, 128–134. [CrossRef] [PubMed]

48. Directive 2006/125/CE. Commission Directive 2006/125/EC of 5 December 2006 on Processed Cereal-Based Foods and Baby Foods for Infants and Young Children. Available online: http://eur-lex.europa.eu/legal-content/EN/TXT/PDF/?uri=CELEX:32006L0125&from=EN (accessed on 30 September 2016).

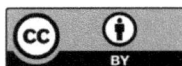

nutrients

MDPI

Article

Usual Intake of Key Minerals among Children in the Second Year of Life, NHANES 2003–2012

Heather C. Hamner *, Cria G. Perrine and Kelley S. Scanlon

National Center for Chronic Disease Prevention and Health Promotion, Centers for Disease Control and Prevention (CDC), Atlanta, GA 30341, USA; hgk3@cdc.gov (C.G.P.); kelley.scanlon@fns.usda.gov (K.S.S.)
* Correspondence: hfc2@cdc.gov; Tel.: +1-770-488-7672

Received: 8 June 2016; Accepted: 26 July 2016; Published: 30 July 2016

Abstract: Iron, calcium, and zinc are important nutrients for the young, developing child. This study describes the usual intake of iron, calcium, and zinc among US children in the second year of life using two days of dietary intake data from the National Health and Nutrition Examination Survey 2003–2012. Estimates were calculated using PC-SIDE to account for within and between person variation. Mean usual iron, calcium, and zinc intakes were 9.5 mg/day, 1046 mg/day, and 7.1 mg/day, respectively. Over a quarter of children had usual iron intakes less than the Recommended Dietary Allowance (RDA) (26.1%). Eleven percent of children had usual calcium intakes below the RDA and over half of children had usual intakes of zinc that exceeded the tolerable upper intake level (UL). Two percent or less had usual intakes below the Estimated Average Requirement (EAR) for iron, calcium, and zinc. Our findings suggest that during 2003–2012, one in four children and one in ten children had usual intakes below the RDA for iron and calcium, respectively. Children who are not meeting their nutrient requirements could be at increased risk for developing deficiencies such as iron deficiency or could lead to a shortage in adequate nutrients required for growth and development. One in every two children is exceeding the UL for zinc, but the interpretation of these estimates should be done with caution given the limited data on adverse health outcomes. Continued monitoring of zinc intake and further assessment for the potential of adverse health outcomes associated with high zinc intakes may be needed.

Keywords: iron; calcium; zinc; young children; usual nutrient intake; NHANES

1. Introduction

Iron, calcium, and zinc are key minerals needed to ensure optimal cognitive development [1,2], bone health [3], and growth [1]. For young children, the American Academy of Pediatrics (AAP) has identified iron and zinc as critical nutrients—especially for children who are exclusively breastfed and are transitioning to the introduction of complementary foods [4]. Although the majority of children 12–23 months of age have transitioned to solid foods, this time period is still an important period of physical and cognitive development and adequate nutrient intakes are needed [5]. Iron, calcium, and zinc are needed throughout early childhood. Iron is important for optimal cognitive development [1]; calcium is critical in the development of bones and teeth and can be especially important during growth spurts [3], and zinc is important in growth [1]. Ensuring adequate intake of iron, calcium, and zinc can help reduce the risk of developing severe deficiencies such as iron deficiency anemia [1,2] or impaired growth, such as rickets [1,3]. Conversely, nutrient intakes exceeding cut points such as the tolerable upper intake level (UL) could lead to adverse consequences; however, limited data are available on functional outcomes for young children with regard to higher intake values [1,3].

Nationally representative data on the nutrient intake for this age group as well as the proportions who are meeting Dietary Reference Intakes, such as the Estimated Average Requirement (EAR), the Recommended Dietary Allowance (RDA), and those exceeding the UL, are lacking. Nutrition intake estimates among this age group can inform clinicians about key nutrient intakes during a critical growth period, as well as provide a basis for population level estimates that can support efforts, such as the United States Department of Agriculture (USDA)/Health and Human Services (HHS) Dietary Guidance Development Project for Birth to 24 Months and Pregnancy (B24/P) [6]. We focus this analysis on three key minerals needed for growth and development (iron, calcium, and zinc) for children 12–23 months of age and present the proportion meeting the EAR, RDA, and those exceeding the UL.

2. Materials and Methods

2.1. National Health and Nutrition Examination Survey

NHANES is an ongoing nationally representative survey of the noninstitutionalized civilian US population [7]. The survey is conducted using a stratified multistage probability design. Data from NHANES are released in 2-year cycles. This analysis includes data from 2003 to 2012. Survey respondents participate in a household interview in which participants are asked a variety of questions including information on demographics and health-related questions and a physical examination in which participants undergo a medical exam and participate in a dietary interview. Analyses reported by race/ethnicity were restricted to non-Hispanic white, non-Hispanic black, and Mexican American respondents because of the small number of individuals of other racial and ethnic groups; however, all race/ethnicities are included in analyses not stratified by race/ethnicity. We limited our analyses to children who were aged 12–23 months at the time of the physical examination. All participants in NHANES provide written informed consent or by proxy for those who are under 7 years of age. The National Center for Health Statistics Research Ethics Review Board provided the following protocol approval numbers for the presented survey years: Protocol #98-12 (NHANES 1999–2004), Protocol #2005-06 (NHANES 2005–2006), Continuation of Protocol #2005-06 (NHANES 2007–2010), and Protocol #2011-17 (NHANES 2011–2012).

2.2. Nutrient Intake

Usual nutrient intake (calories, iron, calcium, and zinc) was estimated using two 24 h dietary recall questionnaires. The first dietary recall was conducted in-person and the second dietary recall was conducted 3–10 days later via telephone. Dietary interviews for children less than 6 years of age were conducted using a proxy (i.e., a parent) who was most familiar with the child's dietary intake [8]. The USDA Food and Nutrient Database for Dietary Studies was used to determine the nutrient amount for foods that are reported in NHANES 2003–2012 [9–13]. Total nutrient intake for day one and day two of the 24 h dietary recall were used in analyses.

2.3. Analytic Sample

There were a total of 1534 children aged 12–23 months at the time of the physical examination from 2003 to 2012 and were eligible to complete a dietary recall. Children were excluded if they reported consuming any breast milk on either day one or day two of the dietary interview ($n = 94$) because nutrient intakes from breast milk were not available and therefore, total nutrient intake could not be calculated. Additionally, children who did not have a dietary intake record for day one and day two, or who had a dietary record that was coded as not reliable, were excluded ($n = 318$), leaving a final sample size of 1122 (78% of the eligible sample who did not consume any breast milk).

2.4. Covariates

Information on age, race/ethnicity, and income to poverty ratio were obtained through the household interview questionnaire. Race/ethnicity was based on respondents'/parental answers to questions on race and Hispanic origin. The income to poverty ratio, a ratio of family income to poverty guidelines, was based on the family's reported household income. The income to poverty ratio was split into three categories: (1) income to poverty ratios <1.85; (2) income to poverty ratios between 1.85 and less than 3.5; and (3) income to poverty ratios ⩾3.5. These income to poverty ratios correspond to income eligibility cut-offs used in the United States Department of Agriculture Women, Infants, and Children Program.

2.5. Statistical Analyses

Using data from the two 24-h dietary recalls, the usual intakes of total caloric intake (for reference), iron, calcium, and zinc for children 12–23 months of age were estimated using software developed by Iowa State University, PC-SIDE version 1.02 (Iowa State University, Ames, IA, USA) and within-person variation of nutrient intake were accounted for across days. In addition, the proportion of children below two specific cut-points, i.e., estimated average requirement (EAR) and recommended dietary allowance (RDA), and the proportion above the cut-points for tolerable upper intake level (UL) for each mineral were assessed. The EAR is the average daily nutrient intake estimated to meet the needs of half the healthy children of this age; whereas, the RDA is the average daily nutrient intake estimated to meet the needs of nearly all healthy children of this age [14]. The UL is the highest average daily intake likely to pose no adverse health effects [14]. Usual intakes were adjusted for the intake day of the week and interview method (in person vs. telephone). Estimates of usual intake and proportions were calculated by sex, race/ethnicity, and income to poverty ratio. Since usual intakes cannot be negative, any estimates that were negative (i.e., lower bound for 95% Confidence Interval (CIs)) were truncated at zero. Additionally, if a cut-point fell on the distribution of intakes such that no individual was included, these values did not have a standard error; thus, a zero value was given and no 95% CIs were provided.

SPSS Complex Samples Design version 23.0 (SPSS Inc., Chicago, IL, USA) was used to account for the survey design and calculate frequencies and Chi-square tests. All analyses were conducted using 10-year dietary weights calculated from day two dietary weights for the period 2003–2012, as recommended by the National Center for Health Statistics, Centers for Disease Control and Prevention [15,16]. For analyses conducted with PC-SIDE, standard errors were calculated using a set of 150 Jackknife replicate weights calculated using the 10-year dietary weights. T-tests were calculated to assess differences in mean usual intakes; statistical significance defined as $p < 0.05$.

3. Results

A total of 1122 children aged 12–23 months of age were included in the analysis. Approximately half of children were male (52%) (weighted percent). Over half (53.6%) of children were non-Hispanic white, 14.4% were non-Hispanic black, and 17.8% were Mexican American (weighted percent). Among the analytic sample, 49.3% reported an income to poverty ratio <1.85 (weighted percent).

Among children 12–23 months of age, the mean usual caloric intake was 1264 kcal/day (95% CI: 1225, 1302). Caloric intake did not differ by sex or income to poverty ratio, but non-Hispanic black children had significantly higher usual caloric intake than either non-Hispanic white children or Mexican American children (1350 kcal/day, 1267 kcal/day, and 1218 kcal/day, respectively) ($p < 0.05$). Mean usual iron intake was 9.5 mg/day (Table 1). Compared to non-Hispanic white and non-Hispanic black children, Mexican-American children had significantly lower reported mean usual iron intake (9.6 mg, 10.2 mg, and 8.5 mg, respectively) ($p < 0.05$). Mean usual calcium intake was 1046 mg/day; no differences were observed by sex, race/ethnicity, or poverty status. Mean usual zinc intake was 7.1 mg/day; girls had significantly lower zinc intake compared to boys (6.9 mg vs. 7.3 mg, respectively) ($p < 0.05$).

Less than 1% of children had usual iron intakes below the EAR (3 mg/day) [1]; however, 26.1% had usual intakes below the RDA (7 mg/day) [1]. Mexican American children had significantly higher proportions below the RDA for iron compared to non-Hispanic white and non-Hispanic black children

(36.4%, 24.3%, and 18.7%, respectively) ($p < 0.05$). No children had usual iron intakes exceeding the UL (40 mg/day) [1].

Table 1. Mean usual iron, calcium, and zinc intake for children age 12 to 23 months [1,2] by select demographic characteristics, NHANES 2003–2012.

	Mean (95% Confidence Interval)		
	Iron (mg)	Calcium (mg)	Zinc (mg)
Total (*n* = 1122)	9.5 (9.0, 10.0)	1046 (1002, 1090)	7.1 (6.9, 7.4)
Sex			
Male (*n* = 574)	9.8 (9.1, 10.5)	1050 (992, 1108)	7.3 (7.0, 7.7) [a]
Female (*n* = 548)	9.1 (8.5, 9.7)	1041 (985, 1097)	6.9 (6.7, 7.2) [b]
Race/ethnicity [3]			
Non-Hispanic white (*n* = 332)	9.6 (8.9, 10.4) [a]	1055 (981, 1128)	7.2 (6.8, 7.6)
Non-Hispanic black (*n* = 261)	10.2 (9.4, 11.1) [a]	983 (909, 1056)	7.2 (6.6, 7.7)
Mexican American (*n* = 357)	8.5 (8.0, 9.1) [b]	1047 (993, 1100)	7.2 (6.8, 7.5)
Poverty status			
Income to poverty ratio <1.85 (*n* = 684)	9.4 (8.8, 9.9)	1020 (973, 1068)	7.2 (6.9, 7.5)
Income to poverty ratio 1.85 to <3.5 (*n* = 204)	9.2 (8.3, 10.1)	1056 (962, 1149)	7.0 (6.5, 7.5)
Income to poverty ratio ≥3.5 (*n* = 174)	9.8 (8.7, 10.9)	1095 (1011, 1180)	7.1 (6.6, 7.6)

[1] Does not include any children who reported consuming breast milk on either day one or day two of the 24-h dietary recall; [2] age in months at time of exam in Medical Examination Center; [3] race/ethnicity subanalyses are limited to those individuals who report being either non-Hispanic white, non-Hispanic black, and Mexican American; values with superscript letters that differ are significantly different, *p*-value < 0.05; abbreviations: National Health and Nutrition Examination Survey (NHANES).

Two percent of children 12–23 months had usual calcium intake below the EAR (500 mg/day) [3] and 11.2% had usual calcium intakes below the RDA (700 mg/day) [3] (Table 2). Non-Hispanic black children and children with an income to poverty ratio <1.85 had significantly higher proportions below the RDA for calcium ($p < 0.05$). There were no children 12–23 months with usual calcium intakes that exceeded the UL (2500 mg/day) [3].

Less than 1% of children had usual zinc intakes below either the EAR (2.5 mg/day) [1] or the RDA (3 mg/day) [1]. Over 50% of children had usual zinc intakes that exceeded the UL (7 mg/day) [1]; no differences by sex, race/ethnicity, or income to poverty ratio were observed.

4. Discussion

Our analyses presented nationally representative usual mean intake for children 12–23 months of age on key minerals needed for healthy growth and development [1,3]. Our findings indicate that one in four children and one in ten children 12–23 months of age are not consuming enough iron and calcium to meet current RDA recommendations, respectively. However, one in two children 12–23 months of age are exceeding the UL for zinc.

Our findings, presented here, are similar to what was reported in the 2008 Feeding Infants and Toddler Study (FITS) [17], a cross-sectional consumer panel survey weighted to be nationally representative. For example, FITS reported usual intake of zinc 7.2 mg/day and our analysis indicated a usual intake of 7.1 mg/day. However, FITS data had slightly lower usual intakes of calories and calcium and higher usual intakes of iron as compared to our results using NHANES (FITS: 1141 kcal/day; 892 mg/day calcium; 10.3 mg/day iron; NHANES: 1264 kcal/day; 1046 mg/day calcium; 9.5 mg/day iron) [17]. The FITS 2008 findings assessed both the proportion below the EAR and the proportion exceeding the UL and found similar results as those presented here. Although FITS is considered nationally representative, it may not be truly representative if the consumer panel used as the sampling frame is not representative of the US population. Although the surveys had slightly different estimates, both came to similar conclusions in regard to nutrient intake of key minerals for children in the second year of life (12–23 months of age).

Table 2. Percent of children aged 12 to 23 months [1,2] not meeting recommendations for iron, calcium and zinc by select demographic characteristics, NHANES 2003–2012 [3].

	% (95% Confidence Interval)								
	Iron			Calcium			Zinc		
	% below EAR (3 mg/Day)	% below RDA (7 mg/Day)	% above UL (40 mg/Day)	% below EAR (500 mg/Day)	% below RDA (700 mg/Day)	% above UL (2500 mg/Day)	% below EAR (2.5 mg/Day)	% below RDA (3 mg/Day)	% above UL (7 mg/Day)
Total (n = 1122)	0.4 (0.2, 0.6)	26.1 (21.7, 30.4)	0	2.0 (1.3, 2.7)	11.2 (8.7, 13.7)	0	0	0.1 (0, 0.2)	50.8 (45.4, 56.1)
Sex									
Male (n = 574)	0.5 (0.1, 0.8)	25.0 (18.9, 31.1)	0	2.8 (1.4, 4.2) [a]	13.1 (8.7, 17.6)	0	0	0.2 (0, 0.3)	46.8 (39.0, 54.6)
Female (n = 548)	0.4 (0, 0.7)	26.9 (20.5, 33.3)	0	1.2 (0.6, 1.8) [b]	9.4 (6.5, 12.4)	0	0	0.1 (0, 0.2)	55.3 (48.2, 62.5)
Race/ethnicity [4]									
Non-Hispanic white (n = 332)	0.3 (0, 0.7) [a,b]	24.3 (18.1, 30.4) [a]	0	2.1 (1.0, 3.1) [a,b]	11.5 (7.0, 16.1) [a,b]	0	0	0 [a]	48.2 (37.6, 58.9)
Non-Hispanic black (n = 261)	0 (0, 0.2) [a]	18.7 (12.7, 24.8) [a]	0	3.6 (1.1, 6.1) [b]	17.4 (10.4, 24.4) [b]	0	0 (0, 0)	0.3 (0.1, 0.4) [b]	51.7 (40.7, 62.6)
Mexican American (n = 357)	0.8 (0.2, 1.4) [b]	36.4 (29.6, 43.1) [b]	0	1.3 (0.5, 2.2) [a]	9.6 (6.4, 12.8) [a]	0	0	0 (0, 0.2) [a]	50.6 (42.4, 58.9)
Poverty status									
Income to poverty ratio <1.85 (n = 684)	0.2 (0.1, 0.4)	23.1 (16.7, 29.4)	0	2.3 (1.3, 3.2)	13.8 (10.2, 17.4) [a]	0	0	0.1 (0, 0.2) [a,b]	50.0 (43.2, 56.7)
Income to poverty ratio 1.85 to <3.5 (n = 204)	0.7 (0.1, 1.4)	32.8 (22.8, 42.8)	0	2.5 (0.8, 4.1)	12.0 (6.9, 17.1) [a,b]	0 (0, 0)	0	0.2 (0, 0.4) [a]	53.3 (42.7, 63.8)
Income to poverty ratio ≥3.5 (n = 174)	0.5 (0, 1.1)	27.8 (19.5, 36.1)	0	1.8 (0.2, 3.4)	9.0 (4.5, 13.4) [b]	0 (0, 0)	0	0 [b]	50.4 (38.0, 62.7)

[1] Does not include any children who reported consuming breast milk on either day one or day two of the 24 h dietary recall; [2] age in months at time of exam in Medical Examination Center; [3] since usual intakes cannot be negative, any estimates that were negative (i.e., lower bound for 95% Confidence Interval (CIs)) were truncated at zero and 95% CIs are provided. If a cut-point fell on the distribution of intakes such that no individual was included, these values did not have a standard error; thus, a zero value was given and no 95% CIs were provided; [4] race/ethnicity subanalyses are limited to those individuals who report being either non-Hispanic white, non-Hispanic black, and Mexican American; values with superscript letters that differ are significantly different; p-value < 0.05; abbreviations: Estimated Average Requirement (EAR), Recommended Dietary Allowance (RDA), Tolerable Upper Intake Level (UL).

Our analysis expanded on the FITS assessment by looking at the proportion of children 12–23 months of age with usual intakes below the RDA. One in every four children, and one in every three children who was Mexican American, reported having an iron intake below the RDA and the intake value recommended by the AAP [1,2]. A recent study by Grimes et al. reported the top food sources of iron for this age group and found ready-to-eat cereals, baby foods, breads, rolls and tortillas, mixed dishes—grains, and cooked cereals were responsible for half of a child's total daily iron intake [18]. These sources are a combination of multiple foods and could represent fortified sources (i.e., ready-to-eat cereals), as well as heme-rich sources (i.e., baby foods with meat) or non-heme sources (i.e., baby foods with fruit and/or vegetables). Adequate intake of iron can help reduce the likelihood of developing iron deficiency and iron deficiency anemia [2]. According to data from NHANES 2007–2010, 13.5% of children 1–2 years of age were considered iron deficient [19]. Given the importance of iron in optimal cognitive development at this age [1,2], the reported estimates of iron deficiency [19] and iron intake suggest the need to ensure young children are consuming adequate iron and to continue monitoring iron status.

Calcium has also been identified as a key mineral to ensuring adequate growth and development of young children, especially for bone health [3]. With the development of the 2011 Institute of Medicine report on calcium and vitamin D, there are now EARs and RDAs for calcium for children 1–3 years of age; these values were not available in the previous 1997 IOM report for calcium and vitamin D [3,20]. Our data indicate that although very few children 12–23 months of age have a usual calcium intake below the EAR, one in ten, and almost one in five non-Hispanic black children (17.4%), have an intake below the RDA. Milk is the main food group that contributes to calcium intake for this age group with over 50% of daily intake of calcium coming from milk [18]. However, trends in beverage consumption indicate a significant decline in milk consumption among 1 year olds (3.8% decline) and an increase in 100% fruit juice consumption (21.9% increase) from 1988–1994 to 2001–2006 [21]. Continued support for ensuring adequate calcium intake through sources like milk is important.

Ensuring adequate zinc intake for young children, especially during the transition from breast milk to complementary foods, has been one of the cornerstones of AAP recommendations [4]. However, our data indicate that over half of children 12–23 months have usual zinc intakes that exceed the UL, which is similar to what Butte et al. reported using FITS [17]. Milk and ready-to-eat cereals were the top two food sources contributing 39.1% of total zinc intake among children 12–23 months of age [18]. Ready-to-eat cereals may be fortified with zinc and could be one of the reasons for higher zinc intakes in this age group. Data were not available on children 1–3 years of age to set a UL value for zinc for this age group[1]; however, data were available from one study among 68 infants 0–6 months of age receiving infant formula with 5.8 mg zinc/L of formula for six months found no adverse effects [22]. Using this study as a basis, the UL value for zinc among children 1–3 years of age was extrapolated and then adjusted for body weight [1]. Two case reports of children receiving ⩾16 mg of zinc for ⩾6 months developed a copper-induced anemia [23,24]; however, evidence of zinc toxicity in young children is not often reported [25,26] and may not be a concern at the population level. Additionally, the potential that the zinc UL for children is too low has been raised [27,28]. Therefore, interpreting whether the proportion of children above the UL for zinc is of concern should be done with caution since limited data are available supporting population-level indications of adverse health outcomes associated with high intake and the relevance of the current UL value has been questioned. Continued monitoring of zinc intake and the potential for adverse health outcomes could be warranted.

This analysis provides pediatricians, other health care providers, and public health practitioners with evidence on the nutritional intake of young children, specifically for key minerals needed for healthy growth and development. Compared with developing countries, children in the United States may not be considered as at risk for specific nutritional deficiencies; however, this analysis indicates that for specific minerals, such as iron, there may be a need for a renewed focus on ensuring children are consuming adequate nutrients. A further assessment of nationally representative data on the nutritional status of young children using biomarkers could help provide context to national level policies and recommendations for foods and food groups to encourage. Biomarkers, with the exception of iron, on this age group are not routinely collected through surveys, such as NHANES, but specific biomarkers may need to be considered given the assessment of current intake and the development of the B24/P Guidance.

This study is subject to several limitations. First, we combined multiple survey years. Although this provides a larger sample size and smaller standard errors, the data span a period of ten years. Sociodemographic characteristics did not differ by survey year; however, we did find that usual caloric intake was significantly higher in 2003–2004. We did not correct for this because we were not assessing trends over time and recommendations, such as the EAR, RDA and UL are set values and are not dependent on total caloric intake. Second, we did not include any nutrient intake coming from dietary supplements, which could contribute to mineral intake. This decision was based on a change in methodology for reporting supplement intake during the survey years included in our analysis. When we assessed the frequency of supplement use in a subset of the population with similar supplement intake methodology, we concluded that the inclusion of dietary supplements would not change the overall interpretation of our results. Specifically, we found that among children 12–23 months of age surveyed in 2007–2012, 13.3% reported consuming any dietary supplement on day 1 Lastly, we limited our analyses to children not reporting the consumption of breast milk during the second year of life on day one or day two of the dietary intake recall. This was done because nutrient intakes were not reported for children who reported consuming any breast milk. A total of 94 children reported some consumption of breastmilk (6% of the original sample). As a result, these findings may not be generalizable to children consuming breast milk during the second year of life. There were also several strengths of this study. First, NHANES is a nationally representative study. Second, usual dietary intake assessment was possible because two 24-h dietary recalls were collected and nutrients examined were consumed on a daily basis and were not episodic. This allowed for the estimation of the proportions of the population at specific cut-points (i.e., EAR, RDA, and UL). Lastly, because we combined survey years, we were able to have adequate sample size to stratify by different sociodemographic factors.

5. Conclusions

During 2003–2012, one in every four and one in every ten children 12–23 months of age is not meeting the recommended iron and calcium intake, respectively. Efforts to ensure children are consuming optimal amounts of both iron and calcium are important for their growth and development. One in every two children 12–23 months of age is exceeding the UL for zinc, but the interpretation of these estimates should be done with caution given the limited data on adverse health outcomes.

Acknowledgments: No funding was secured for this study.

Author Contributions: H.C.H. conceived the research question and analyzed the data; H.C.H., C.G.P. and K.S.S. reviewed and interpreted the statistical analyses and wrote the paper.

Conflicts of Interest: The authors declare no conflicts of interest.

Disclaimer: The findings and conclusions in this report are those of the authors and do not necessarily represent the official position of the Centers for Disease Control and Prevention.

Abbreviations

AAP	American Academy of Pediatrics
B24/P	Birth to 24 Months and Pregnancy
CI	Confidence Interval
EAR	Estimated Average Requirement
FITS	Feeding Infants and Toddler Study
HHS	Health and Human Services
NHANES	National Health and Nutrition Examination Survey
RDA	Recommended Dietary Allowance
UL	Tolerable Upper Intake Level
USDA	United States Department of Agriculture

References

1. Institute of Medicine. *Dietary Reference Intakes: Vitamin A, Vitamin K, Arsenic, Boron, Chromium, Copper, Iodine, Iron, Manganese, Molybedenum, Nickel, Silicon, Vanadium, and Zinc*; National Academy Press: Washington, DC, USA, 2001.
2. Baker, R.D.; Greer, F.R. American Academy of Pediatrics Committe on Nutrition. Clinical report—Diagnosis and prevention of iron deficiency and iron-deficiency anemia in infants and young children (0–3 years of age). *Pediatrics* **2010**, *126*, 1040–1050. [CrossRef] [PubMed]
3. Institute of Medicine. *Dietary Reference Intakes for Calcium and Vitamin D*; The National Academies Press: Washington, DC, USA, 2011.
4. American Academy of Pediatrics Committe on Nutrition. Chapter 6: Complementary feeding. In *Pediatric Nutrition*, 7th ed.; Kleinman, R.E., Greer, F.R., Eds.; American Academy of Pediatrics: Elk Grove Village, IL, USA, 2014.
5. Dewey, K.G.; Vitta, B.S. *Strategies for Ensuring Adequate Nutrient Intake for Infants and Young Children during the Period of Complementary Feeding*; A & T Technical Brief: Washington, DC, USA, 2013; pp. 1–14.
6. Raiten, D.J.; Raghavan, R.; Porter, A.; Obbagy, J.E.; Spahn, J.M. Executive summary: Evaluating the evidnce base to support the inclusion of infants and children from birth to 24 months of age in the Dietary Guidelines for Americans—"The B-24 Project". *Am. J. Clin. Nutr.* **2014**, *99*, 663S–691S. [CrossRef] [PubMed]
7. National Center for Health Statistics. About the National Health and Nutrition Examination Survey. Available online: http://www.cdc.gov/nchs/nhanes/about_nhanes.htm (accessed on 7 March 2016).
8. National Center for Health Statistics. National Health and Nutrition Examination Survey: Dietary Data. Available online: http://wwwn.cdc.gov/Nchs/Nhanes/Search/DataPage.aspx?Component=Dietary& CycleBeginYear=2011 (accessed on 14 December 2015).
9. US Department of Agriculture. Food and Nutrient Database for Dietary Studies, 2.0. Available online: http://www.ars.usda.gov/SP2UserFiles/Place/80400530/pdf/fndds/fndds2_doc.pdf (accessed on 28 July 2016).
10. US Department of Agriculture. Food and Nutrient Database for Dietary Studies, 3.0. Available online: http://www.ars.usda.gov/SP2UserFiles/Place/80400530/pdf/fndds/fndds3_doc.pdf (accessed on 28 July 2016).
11. US Department of Agriculture. Food and Nutrient Database for Dietary Studies, 4.0. Available online: http://www.ars.usda.gov/SP2UserFiles/Place/80400530/pdf/fndds/fndds4_doc.pdf (accessed on 28 July 2016).
12. US Department of Agriculture. Food and Nutrient Database for Dietary Studies, 5.0. Available online: http://www.ars.usda.gov/SP2UserFiles/Place/80400530/pdf/fndds/fndds5_doc.pdf (accessed on 28 July 2016).
13. US Department of Agriculture. Food and Nutrient Database for Dietary Studies 2011–2012. Available online: http://www.ars.usda.gov/SP2UserFiles/Place/80400530/pdf/fndds/fndds_2011_2012_doc.pdf (accessed on 28 July 2016).
14. Institute of Medicine. *Dietary Reference Intakes: Application in Dietary Assessment*; National Academy Press: Washington DC, USA, 2000.

15. National Center for Health Statistics. *National Health and Nutrition Examination Survey: Analytic Guidelines, 2011–2012*; Centers for Disease Control and Prevention: Hyattsville, MD, USA, 2013.

16. Johnson, C.L.; Paulose-Ram, R.; Ogden, C.L.; Carroll, M.D.; Kruszon-Moran, D.; Dohrmann, S.M.; Curtin, L.R. National health and nutrition examination survey: Analytic guidelines, 1999–2010. *Vital Health Stat.* **2013**, *2*, 1–24.

17. Butte, N.F.; Fox, M.K.; Briefel, R.R.; Siega-Riz, A.M.; Dwyer, J.T.; Deming, D.M.; Reidy, K.C. Nutrient intakes of US infants, toddlers, and preschoolers meet or exceed Dietary Reference Intakes. *J. Am. Diet. Assoc.* **2010**, *110*, S27–S37. [CrossRef] [PubMed]

18. Grimes, C.A.; Szymlek-Gay, E.A.; Campbell, K.J.; Nicklas, T.A. Food sources of total energy and nutrients among US infants and toddlers: National Health and Nutrition Examination Survey 2005–2012. *Nutrients* **2015**, *7*, 6797–6836. [CrossRef] [PubMed]

19. Gupta, P.M.; Perrine, C.G.; Mei, Z.; Scanlon, K.S. Iron, anemia, and iron deficiency anemia among young children in the United States. *Nutrients* **2016**, *8*. [CrossRef] [PubMed]

20. Institute of Medicine. *Dietary Reference Intakes for Calcium, Phosphorus, Magnesium, Vitamin D, and Fluoride*; National Academy Press: Washington, DC, USA, 1997.

21. Fulgoini, V.L.; Quann, E.E. National trends in beverage consumption in children from birth to 5 years: Analysis of NHANES across three decades. *Nutr. J.* **2012**, *11*, 1–11. [CrossRef] [PubMed]

22. Walravens, P.A.; Hambidge, M. Growth of infants fed a zinc supplemented formula. *Am. J. Clin. Nutr.* **1976**, *29*, 1114–1121. [PubMed]

23. Botash, A.S.; Nasca, J.; Dubowy, R.; Weinberger, H.L.; Oliphant, M. Zinc-induced copper deficiency in an infant. *Am. J. Dis. Child.* **1992**, *146*, 709–711. [CrossRef] [PubMed]

24. Sugiura, T.; Goto, K.; Ito, K.; Ueta, A.; Fujimoto, S.; Togari, H. Chronic zinc toxicity in an infant who received zinc theraphy for atopic dermatitis. *Acta Paediatr.* **2005**, *94*, 1333–1335. [CrossRef] [PubMed]

25. Krebs, N.F. Update on zinc deficiency and excess in clinical pediatirc practice. *Ann. Nutr. Metab.* **2013**, *62*, 19–29. [CrossRef] [PubMed]

26. Willoughby, J.L.; Bowen, C.N. Zinc deficiency and toxicity in pediatric practice. *Curr. Opin. Pediatr.* **2014**, *26*, 579–584. [CrossRef] [PubMed]

27. King, J.C.; Brown, K.H.; Gibson, R.S.; KrebS, N.F.; Lowe, N.M.; Siekmann, J.H.; Raiten, D.J. Biomarkers of nutrition for development (BOND)—Zinc review. *J. Nutr.* **2016**. [CrossRef] [PubMed]

28. Bertinato, J.; Simpson, J.R.; Sherrard, L.; Taylor, J.; Plouffe, L.J.; Van Dyke, D.; Geleynse, M.; Dam, Y.Y.; Murphy, P.; Knee, C.; et al. Zinc supplementation does not alter sensitive biomarkers of copper status in healthy boys. *J. Nutr.* **2013**, *143*, 284–289. [CrossRef] [PubMed]

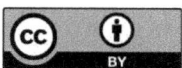

MDPI AG

St. Alban-Anlage 66

4052 Basel, Switzerland

Tel. +41 61 683 77 34

Fax +41 61 302 89 18

http://www.mdpi.com

Nutrients Editorial Office

E-mail: nutrients@mdpi.com

http://www.mdpi.com/journal/nutrients